Surgical Management of the Diabetic Patient

Surgical Management of the Diabetic Patient

Editors

Michael Bergman, M.D.

Clinical Professor of Medicine
New York Medical College
Valhalla, New York
and
Director
Cardiovascular Clinical Research Metabolism
Worldwide Clinical Research
and Development
Bristol-Myers Squibb Pharmaceutical
Research Institute
Princeton, New Jersey

Gregorio A. Sicard, M.D.

Professor
Department of Surgery
Director, Vascular Service
Washington University School of Medicine
St. Louis, Missouri

Raven Press 🦢 New York

Raven Press, Ltd. 1185 Avenue of the Americas, New York, New York 10036

Made in the United States of America.

Library of Congress Cataloging-in-Publication Data

Surgical management of the diabetic patient / editors, Michael
   Bergman, Gregorio A. Sicard.
      p.   cm.
   Includes bibliographical references.
   Includes index.
   ISBN 0-88167-720-5
   1. Diabetics—Surgery.   2. Diabetes—Complications and sequelae.
I. Bergman, Michael.   II. Sicard, Gregorio A.
   [DNLM: 1. Diabetes Mellitus—complications.   2. Intraoperative
Complications—prevention & control.   3. Postoperative
Complications—prevention & control.   WK 835 S961]
RD98.4.S87   1991
616.4′6206—dc20
DNLM/DLC
for Library of Congress   90-9064
                                                                  CIP

9 8 7 6 5 4 3 2 1

To Yetta, Elana, and Danielle Bergman for their love, to Dr. Saim B. Akin whose support will always be appreciated and finally to Mrs. Marilyn Mazza, who has taught me the value of spirit, determination, courage and exemplary commitment to a full life while living with diabetes.

Michael Bergman

To my loving wife Kathy and our children Greg, Jane, Melissa, and Michael who have staunchly supported my work, aspiration, and personal growth, although it often infringes on their lives.

Gregorio A. Sicard

Preface

Diabetes is indeed a unique disease, given its multifarious presentations and propensity for insidiously involving multitudinous organ systems simultaneously. Individuals with diabetes characteristically have significant underlying abnormalities in the absence of overt symptoms. It thus becomes the responsibility of the physician to assiduously investigate the presence of complications. This is particularly critical when diabetic patients undergo surgical procedures. It is not uncommon for certain manifestations (e.g., coronary artery disease, peripheral vascular disease, neuropathy, nephropathy) to become apparent for the first time during the preoperative evaluation. Failure to identify these complications can expose the individuals to greater risk than is already likely, given their diabetic status.

Diabetes care involves participation of a multidisciplinary team to assure a beneficial outcome. Optimally, planning for surgery should start quite early so that last minute decision-making can be averted. As detailed in this book, evaluation of cardiac, renal, ophthalmologic, neurologic, and vascular status needs thorough exploration, preferably performed as an outpatient. Attention and remediation of significant deviation in blood glucose control and correction of other biochemistries, as well as investigation for occult infections (e.g., cystitis) should be entertained preoperatively. The diffuse nature of vasculopathy in diabetic patients continuously tests the skills of the internist and surgeon as they attempt to preserve extremities and, most importantly, provide the patient with a reasonable lifestyle and longevity. Meticulous attention to hemodynamic monitoring, nutrition, wound healing, and metabolic control is continuous throughout the perioperative period. The anesthesiologist and surgeon need to be informed even if subtle clinical findings, such as neuropathy, are present so that positioning, for example, during a lengthy procedure takes this complication into consideration. Similarly, the presence of retinopathy may also require exquisite attention to head positioning.

Pre-discharge planning should be instituted early during hospitalization and, as described in greater detail, requires comprehensive assessment of both the patients' and their families' knowledge and skills related to diabetes management. Counseling and reassurance should be provided to allay anxiety, particularly in a newly diagnosed patient. This may, at times, require referral for individual therapy; participation in a group situation is often invaluable.

This book affords practical information for the detailed assessment of the diabetic patient from the early stages when surgery is considered through the surgical and postsurgical periods as well. Consideration is given to those issues vital to patient well-being at each phase. Specialized surgical interventions are also provided in detail. Scientific information is offered to enhance the understanding of the relationship between the biochemical perturbations of diabetes and its clinical manifestations.

Michael Bergman
Gregorio A. Sicard

Acknowledgments

The editors express their sincere appreciation to all the authors who have shared their expertise to formulate a broadly based resource for practitioners encompassing a variety of specialties. It is the expressed hope and avowed purpose of this book to assist in providing enhanced quality of care to the millions of patients afflicted with diabetes and, in so doing, to improve their lives.

We also express our gratitude to Raven Press for accepting so graciously the ideals and goals that this book embraces. In particular, Lisa Berger and Susan Berkowitz have worked very diligently in the preparation of this manuscript.

The warm support, encouragement and wisdom of Dr. Philip Felig is genuinely appreciated. We especially thank him for his ongoing counsel as this book was compiled. Finally, sincere gratitude is expressed to H.Y. Pan, M.D., Ph.D. for providing the latitude, guidance, and inspiration for completing this work.

Contents

Contributors

Norman B. Ackerman, M.D.
Department of Surgery
New York Medical College
Metropolitan Hospital Center
New York, New York 10029

Peter B. Alden, M.D.
Department of Surgery
Washington University School of Medicine
St. Louis, Missouri 63110
Current Address:
Parke-Nicollett Medical Center
Minneapolis, Minnesota 55416

Brent T. Allen, M.D.
Department of Surgery
Washington University School of Medicine
St. Louis, Missouri 63110

Charles B. Anderson, M.D.
Department of Surgery
Washington University School of Medicine
St. Louis, Missouri 63110

David J. Ballard, M.D., M.S.P.H.
Department of Internal Medicine; and
Department of Health Sciences Research
Section of Clinical Epidemiology
Mayo Clinic and Mayo Foundation
Rochester, Minnesota 55905

James M. Becker, M.D.
Department of Gastrointestinal Surgery
Harvard Medical School
Brigham and Women's Hospital
Boston, Massachusetts 02115

Vilray P. Blair, III, M.D.
Division of Orthopedic Surgery
Washington University School of Medicine
St. Louis, Missouri 63110

Brian Butler, D.P.M., M.A.
Department of Medicine
New York Medical College
Valhalla, New York; and
Department of Community Medicine
New York, New York 10035

Donald R. Coustan, M.D.
Department of Obstetrics and Gynecology
Brown University Program in Medicine,
and Department of Obstetrics and
*   Maternal-Fetal Medicine*
Women & Infants' Hospital of Rhode
*   Island*
101 Dudley Street
Providence, Rhode Island 02905

Leslie J. Domalik, M.D.
Division of Metabolism, Endocrinology,
*   and Genetic Diseases*
Department of Medicine
Duke University Medical Center and
the Durham Veterans Administration
*   Medical Center*
Durham, North Carolina 27710

Dolores A. Drury, R.N., B.S.N.,
C.D.E.
Division of Orthopedic Surgery
Washington University School of Medicine
St. Louis, Missouri 63110

Jerome M. Feldman, M.D.
Division of Metabolism, Endocrinology,
*   and Genetic Diseases*
Department of Medicine
Duke University Medical Center and the
*   Durham Veterans Administration*
*   Medical Center*
Durham, North Carolina 27710

Philip Felig, M.D.
Lenox Hill Hospital
New York, New York 10021; and
Department of Medicine
New York Medical College
Valhalla, New York 10595

M. Wayne Flye, M.D., Ph.D.
Division of Surgery, Microbiology, and
*   Immunology*
Department of Surgery
Washington University Medical Center
St. Louis, Missouri 63110

Eli A. Friedman, M.D.
Department of Medicine
State University of New York
Health Science Center at Brooklyn
Brooklyn, New York 11203

Todd J. Garvin, M.D.
Division of Urology
University of New Mexico School of
Medicine
Albuquerque, New Mexico 87131

Fredda Ginsberg-Fellner, M.D.
Division of Pediatric Endocrinology and
Metabolism and the
Carole and Michael Friedman and Family
Young People's Diabetes Unit
Department of Pediatrics
Mount Sinai School of Medicine
of the City University of New York
New York, New York 10029

William H. Goodson, III, M.D.
Department of Surgery
University of California Medical Center
San Francisco, California 94143

Dial Hewlett, Jr., M.D.
Infectious Disease Section
Lincoln Medical and Mental Health
Center and
Our Lady of Mercy Medical Center
Bronx, New York, and
Department of Medicine
New York Medical College
Valhalla, New York 10595

Irl B. Hirsch, M.D.
Division of Endocrinology and Metabolism
Department of Medicine
University of Washington
School of Medicine
Seattle, Washington 98144

Kevin T. Jules, D.P.M., F.A.C.F.S.
Department of Surgical Sciences
New York College of Podiatric Medicine
New York, New York 10035

Sonya Jung, R.N., M.S.N.
Diabetes Research and Analysis
Association, Inc.
Lexington, Kentucky 40509

Aaron Kassoff, M.D.
Department of Ophthalmology
Albany Medical College
Albany, New York 12208

Bijoy K. Khandheria, M.D.
Department of Internal Medicine
Division of Cardiovascular Diseases
Mayo Clinic and Mayo Foundation
Rochester, Minnesota 55905

Signe Larson, M.D.
Division of Pediatric Endocrinology and
Metabolism, and the
Carole and Michael Friedman and Family
Young People's Diabetes Unit
Department of Pediatrics
Mount Sinai School of Medicine of the
City University of New York
New York, New York 10029

Carl J. Lavie, M.D.
Department of Internal Medicine
Division of Cardiovascular Diseases
Mayo Clinic and Mayo Foundation
Rochester, Minnesota 55905
Current Address:
Department of Cardiovascular Diseases
and Internal Medicine
Ochsner Clinic and Alton Ochsner Medical
Foundation
New Orleans, Louisiana 70121

Marvin E. Levin, M.D.
Department of Internal Medicine
Washington University School of Medicine
Chesterfield, Missouri 63017

Paula Liguori, B.S.N., C.D.E.
Division of Pediatric Endocrinology and
Metabolism, and the
Carole and Michael Friedman and Family
Young People's Diabetes Unit
Department of Pediatrics
Mount Sinai School of Medicine of the
City University of New York
New York, New York 10029

Dean H. Lockwood, M.D.
Endocrine-Metabolism Unit
University of Rochester
School of Medicine and Dentistry
Rochester, New York 14642

Daniel L. Lorber, M.D., F.A.C.P.
Diabetes Control Foundation
Flushing, New York 11355

Christopher S. McCullough, M.D.
Division of General Surgery
Section of Organ Transplantation
The Islet Transplant Center
Washington University School of Medicine
St. Louis, Missouri 63110

Daniel J. McGraw, M.D.
Department of Surgery
Washington University School of Medicine
St. Louis, Missouri 63110

John S. Munn, M.D.
Department of Surgery
Washington University School of Medicine
St. Louis, Missouri 63110

Kenneth A. Newell, M.D.
Department of Surgery
Loyola University Stritch School of
*   Medicine*
Maywood, Illinois 60153

Pasquale J. Palumbo, M.D.
Department of Internal Medicine and
*   Division of Endocrinology*
Mayo Clinic and Mayo Foundation
Rochester, Minnesota 55905

Michael A. Pfeifer, M.S., M.D.
Diabetes Research and Analysis
*   Association, Inc.*
Lexington, Kentucky 40509

Stephen L. Pohl, M.D.
Diabetes Research and Analysis
*   Association, Inc.*
Lexington, Kentucky 40509

Richard A. Prinz, M.D.
Department of Surgery
Loyola University Stritch School of
*   Medicine*
Maywood, Illinois 60153

Leopoldo Raij, M.D.
University of Minnesota School of
*   Medicine and*
Veterans Administration Medical Center
Minneapolis, Minnesota 55455

Brian G. Rubin, M.D.
Department of Surgery
Washington University School of Medicine
St. Louis, Missouri 63110

David W. Scharp, M.D.
Division of General Surgery
Section of Organ Transplantation
The Islet Transplant Center
Washington University School of Medicine
St. Louis, Missouri 63110

Mary Schumer, M.S.
Diabetes Research and Analysis
*   Association, Inc.*
Lexington, Kentucky 40509

Timothy B. Seaton, M.D.
Department of Medicine
New York Medical College
Valhalla, New York 10595

Charles R. Shuman, M.D.
Department of Medicine
Temple University School of Medicine
Philadelphia, Pennsylvania 19140

Gregorio A. Sicard, M.D.
Department of Surgery
Washington University School of Medicine
St. Louis, Missouri 63110

Nathaniel J. Soper, M.D.
Department of Surgery
Washington University School of Medicine
St. Louis, Missouri 63110

Charles Sweeney, M.D.
University of Minnesota School of
*   Medicine and*
Veterans Administration Medical Center
Minneapolis, Minnesota 55455

Jonathan Tolins, M.D.
University of Minnesota School of
*   Medicine and*
Veterans Administration Medical Center
Minneapolis, Minnesota 55455

Michael J. Trepal, D.P.M., F.A.C.F.S.
Department of Surgical Sciences
New York College of Podiatric Medicine
New York, New York 10035

Jeffrey J. Wang, M.D.
Endocrine-Metabolism Unit
University of Rochester
School of Medicine and Dentistry
Rochester, New York 14642

Paul F. White, M.D.
Department of Anesthesiology
Washington University School of Medicine
St. Louis, Missouri 63110

Surgical Management of the Diabetic Patient

Surgical Management of the Diabetic Patient,
edited by Michael Bergman and Gregorio A. Sicard.
Raven Press, Ltd., New York © 1991.

1

Introduction

Philip Felig

*Lenox Hill Hospital, New York, New York 10021; and Department of Medicine,
New York Medical College, Valhalla, New York 10595*

The past 15 years have witnessed a burgeoning of knowledge regarding diabetes mellitus. While finding a cure for diabetes remains an elusive goal, a far better understanding of the etiology and pathogenesis of diabetes has emerged that is grounded in new insights gained from molecular biology and immunology in addition to physiology and biochemistry. Coupled with these new insights in basic science has been progress in the management of diabetes. The day-to-day care of the motivated and compliant diabetic patient generally involves surveillance of blood glucose levels, assessments of control by glycohemoglobin determinations, and tailoring of insulin doses, oral agents and/or diet to optimize blood glucose level control. What would have been considered unusually meticulous efforts at control of diabetes 15 years ago constitutes a fairly commonplace approach today.

The improvement in the lifespan of the diabetic patient has increased the likelihood that they will encounter conditions requiring surgical intervention. Furthermore, there have been major advances in the surgical management of coronary artery disease and peripheral vascular disease, conditions for which diabetic patients are at increased risk. Renal transplants are now done fairly frequently in diabetic patients and pancreatic transplants are no longer rarities. As a consequence, the management of the diabetic patient in the perioperative period is a circumstance with which the surgeon and internist must deal with increasing frequency.

Surgical intervention is also likely to result in challenging issues of nutritional management in the diabetic patient. When periods of parenteral nutrition or enteral alimentation are required, the decisions regarding choices of fluid regimens, sources of calories, and doses and routes of insulin administration are quite different from the diet and/or insulin regimens employed in the ambulatory, conventionally fed person with diabetes.

It is the premise of this book that the commitment to optimize the metabolic milieu that characterizes current management of diabetes extends to the surgical as well as the medical service of the modern hospital. Implicit in this approach is the concept that successful medical management of the diabetic patient with a surgical condition is a key element in determining the ultimate success of the surgical procedure.

Attention to the details of management of diabetes in the surgical patient is not solely directed at minimizing hyperglycemia, but is also concerned with avoiding hypoglycemia. This is particularly true when the normal waking signals of hypoglycemia become inoperative because of general anesthesia or when normal feeding mechanisms are precluded.

The medical management of the diabetic patient who requires surgery depends, of course, on the nature of the surgical procedure and the comorbid status of the patient as well as the prior status of the diabetic control. The various chapters constituting this book provide the principles and practical details for managing the diabetic patient in a variety of surgical conditions. Guidelines are offered so that management can be individualized, given the inherent variability of diabetes in type I (insulin dependent) as well as type II (noninsulin dependent) patients.

Clearly the diabetic patient requiring surgery is often a challenge to the surgeon as well as the internist. Achieving a successful outcome by applying sound metabolic management is consequently all the more gratifying to the patient as well as the physician.

Surgical Management of the Diabetic Patient,
edited by Michael Bergman and Gregorio A. Sicard.
Raven Press, Ltd., New York © 1991.

2

Carbohydrate Metabolism and Surgery

Leslie J. Domalik and Jerome M. Feldman

*Division of Metabolism, Endocrinology, and Genetic Diseases, Department of
Medicine, Duke University Medical Center and the Durham Veterans Administration
Medical Center, Durham, North Carolina 27710*

In their classic study of the relationship between diabetes and surgery, Galloway and Shuman noted that many diabetic patients undergoing surgery were hyperglycemic, and that the major complication of surgery in this group of patients was an increased incidence of postoperative infection (1). Although there is still debate about the mechanism of this increased susceptibility to infection, hyperglycemia alone can result in a reduction in the phagocytic activity of leukocytes (2). Hyperglycemic diabetic patients may also have impaired healing of their surgical wound, for diabetic animals who are hyperglycemic at the time of surgery have poorer wound healing than diabetic animals whose hyperglycemia is corrected with insulin prior to surgery (3).

General anaesthesia and surgical procedures result in a series of hormonal and metabolic changes that can result in a catabolic state with major tissue protein breakdown and nitrogen loss. Administration of 100 g of glucose to a nondiabetic patient undergoing surgery results in a 30–60% reduction in nitrogen loss during the postoperative period (4). Infusions of amino acid solutions result in a further reduction in the postoperative nitrogen loss (5). When patients with type I diabetes and impaired insulin secretion undergo surgery, there is an increase in the secretion of insulin-antagonistic hormones (such as growth hormone, glucagon, cortisol, norepinephrine, and epinephrine) which in turn increases the problem these patients already have in utilizing glucose and amino acids. Thus, their catabolic state can be even greater than that of nondiabetic patients undergoing surgery.

This chapter describes the pattern of baseline intermediary metabolism and hormonal regulation in nondiabetic and diabetic patients and some of the major changes in intermediary metabolism and hormone secretion that can occur following surgery in these two groups. Further details on intermediary metabolism and hormonal control of homeostasis and their alterations in diabetic subjects can be reviewed for further details (6, 7).

INTERMEDIARY METABOLISM

In any discussion of carbohydrate metabolism, it is prudent to begin with a general discussion of the chemical processes it encompasses. These reactions make it possible to use the energy in carbohydrates as fuel to carry out the physiologic work of cells. Energy is supplied to cells in the form of high-energy intermediary compounds, such as adenosine triphosphate (ATP). These compounds are capable of storing and releasing energy when coupled with the proper enzymes or energy transfer systems. One of the major purposes of biochemical processes of intermediary metabolism is to increase the production of these high-energy phosphate compounds.

Carbohydrate digestion occurs in the gastrointestinal tract prior to absorption. The principal forms of carbohydrate in the human diet are starch, sucrose, and lactose. As outlined in Fig. 1, these disaccharides are broken down into the monosaccharides glucose, galactose, and fructose. Glucose is the major dietary monosaccharide and constitutes approximately 80% of the total monosaccharides that are ingested.

Glucose, galactose, and fructose are rapidly absorbed from the gastrointestinal tract and transported to the liver via the portal system to be further metabolized. Galactose metabolism is outlined in Fig. 2 and fructose metabolism is outlined in Fig. 3.

Fructose does not require insulin for its initial metabolism, and it has therefore been used as a glucose substitute in parenteral alimentation and in dietary supplementation. Fructokinase is very active in the liver; this can result in rapid and substantial depletion of ATP and inorganic phosphate. An increase in purine degradation leads to an increase in liver adenosine monophosphate (AMP), which results in phosphorylase activation and a subsequent increase in glycogenolysis. In addition, fructose metabolism allows metabolites to enter the glycolytic pathway after the metabolic step catalyzed by phosphofructokinase, which allows an important control point to be bypassed.

Because glucose can be used by all cells as a source of energy, the next part of this discussion focuses on the metabolism of glucose. The primary metabolic pathways by which glucose is metabolized, as well as the interrelationships between the

Starch/glycogen $\xrightarrow{\text{Salivary amylase}}$ Maltose + Isomaltose
Pancreatic amylase

Maltose $\xrightarrow{\text{Maltase}}$ Glucose + Glucose

Isomaltose $\xrightarrow{\text{Isomaltase}}$ Glucose + Glucose

Sucrose $\xrightarrow{\text{Sucrase}}$ Glucose + Fructose

Lactose $\xrightarrow{\text{Lactase}}$ Glucose + Galactose

FIG. 1. Digestion of starch, glycogen, and disaccharides to their monosaccharide components in the digestive tract.

Galactokinase

Galactose + ATP ——————————> Galactose-1-Phosphate + ADP

UTP:Galactose-1-Phosphate Uridyl Transferase

Galactose-1-Phosphate + UTP ⇌ UDP - Galactose + PPi

UDP-Galactose ⇌ UDP-Glucose

UDP-Glucose - - - - - - - - - - - - -> Glycogen

FIG. 2. Intermediary metabolism of the monosaccharide galactose.

metabolism of carbohydrate, protein, and fat are outlined in Fig. 4. These metabolic pathways include glycolysis (Cori Cycle), the tricarboxylic acid cycle (Krebs Cycle), the glucuronic acid shunt, and the pentose phosphate shunt (hexosemonophosphate shunt).

Various tissues differ in the way that they metabolize glucose. The erythrocyte and renal medulla cells have an obligate energy requirement for glucose. In times of limited glucose substrate, other cells will switch to other energy substrates to conserve glucose for these cells that absolutely require it. The liver is able to use both fatty acids and glucose. Skeletal muscle utilizes fatty acids for resting metabolism, glucose in the postprandial time when levels are high, and ketone bodies in times of starvation or in those patients with diabetes mellitus. In the immediate postprandial state, the brain uses only glucose. In the fasted state when increased levels of acetoacetate and 3-hydroxybutyrate are present, the brain metabolizes ketone bodies as

Fructokinase

Fructose + ATP ——————————> Fructose-1-Phosphate + ADP

Aldolase

Fructose-1-Phosphate ——————> Glyceraldehyde + Dihydroxyacetone Phosphate

Glyceraldehyde + ATP ————> Glyceraldehyde-3-Phosphate + ADP

Dihydroxyacetone Phosphate - - - - -> Glycolysis

Glyceraldehyde-3-Phosphate - - - - -> Glycolysis

FIG. 3. Intermediary metabolism of the monosaccharide fructose.

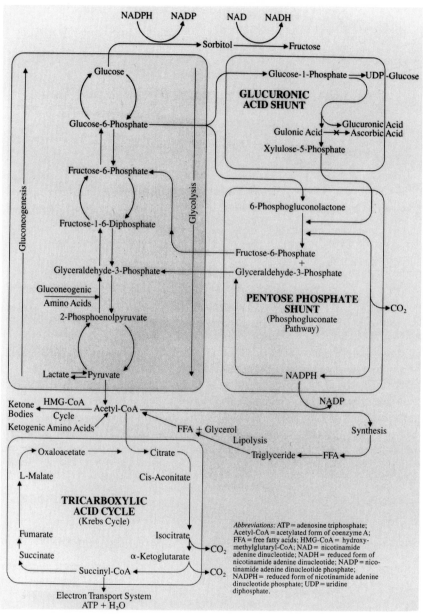

FIG. 4. The primary metabolic pathways and their interrelationships for the metabolism of carbohydrate, protein, and lipid. (From Feldman, ref. 6, used by permission.)

well as glucose. This use of ketone bodies, which is independent of the blood glucose level, is proportional to the level of ketonemia.

The liver is unusual, for glucose diffuses into hepatic cells down a concentration gradient and is phosphorylated by glucokinase. In contrast, most other cells, including muscle and adipose cells, absorb glucose via facilitated diffusion, utilizing a protein carrier molecule, down a concentration gradient (Fig. 5). This process is augmented by the presence of insulin. The glucose is then phosphorylated by a

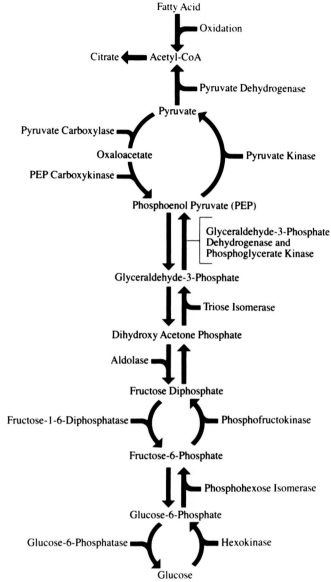

FIG. 5. The reversible and irreversible steps in glycolysis and gluconeogenesis. The reversible steps are depicted by adjacent arrows and irreversible steps are depicted by widely separate arrows. The irreversible steps are major control points for glycolysis and gluconeogenesis. (From Feldman, ref. 6, used by permission.)

Abbreviations: Acetyl-CoA = acetylated form of coenzyme A: PEP = phosphoenol pyruvate.

hexokinase upon entry into the cell. Brain cells do not have insulin-dependent facilitated diffusion of glucose, which allows for a more consistent glucose supply to brain cells. Erythrocytes, too, have insulin-independent facilitated diffusion of glucose into cells, which allows for equilibration of glucose across the membrane. Again, glucose undergoes phosphorylation with a hexokinase immediately upon entering the cell. This phorphorylation is essentially irreversible for most cells. The glucose that is "trapped" by this phosphorylation reaction can be utilized in further pathways of carbohydrate metabolism.

Each enzyme that catalyzes this phosphorylation reaction has unique properties.

Hexokinase has a high affinity for glucose and is the enzyme used for phosphorylation of glucose in most cells. It is inhibited in a negative feedback fashion by glucose-6-phosphate. The second enzyme capable of catalyzing the phosphorylation of glucose is glucokinase. It has a much lower affinity for glucose and its major activity is in liver cells. Its action is of paramount importance in the postprandial state when portal glucose is increased. Although it has no negative feedback loop with glucose-6-phosphate, the levels of available enzyme are affected by insulin. The enzyme activity is increased with increased levels of insulin and decreased in times of fasting or in those patients with diabetes mellitus. Glucokinase also occurs in the pancreatic beta cells. Enzyme activity here is related to the synthesis of proinsulin and the secretion of insulin.

Although the phosphorylation of glucose is essentially an irreversible reaction, there are several cells that have the capacity to dephosphorylate glucose through a separate reaction. Hepatocytes, renal tubular epithelium, and intestinal epithelial cells have a phosphatase enzyme that can catalyze the formation of glucose from glucose-6-phosphate (Fig. 5).

Following its phosphorylation, glucose can enter a variety of pathways. The particular pathway it enters depends on the energy needs of the body and the concentration of insulin in the blood. These pathways of glucose metabolism include glycolysis, the tricarboxylic acid cycle (Krebs Cycle), the pentose phosphate shunt (hexose monophosphate shunt), the sorbitol pathway, the oxidative phosphorylation/electron transport system, glycogen synthesis, glycogenolysis, and gluconeogenesis (Fig. 4).

Glycolysis, the citric acid cycle, and the oxidative phosphorylation/electron transport system provide a means of energy storage and energy release. An outline of the glycolytic pathway is in Fig. 4. All of these reactions take place in the cytosol of the cell. The key regulatory enzymes usually catalyze irreversible reactions. These reactions include those catalyzed by hexokinase/glucokinase, phosphofructokinase, and pyruvate kinase. All of these enzymes are the major control points in glycolysis. The major rate-limiting step is catalyzed by phosphofructokinase. It catalyzes the first "committed step" or step unique to glycolysis. The secondary control points are catalyzed by hexokinase/glucokinase and pyruvate kinase. As discussed previously, insulin increases the activity of hepatic glucokinase. In addition, insulin also stimulates the activity of phosphofructokinase. Pyruvate/lactate are the endproducts of glycolysis under anaerobic conditions. Lactate may be formed when the availability of oxygen is limited, such as when exercising muscle or in cases of inadequate perfusion of heart muscle in those with coronary artery disease. There is no net oxidation-reduction in this case because a nicotinamide-adenine dinucleotide, reduced (NADH) is oxidized in the formation of lactate from pyruvate to regenerate nicotinamide-adenine dinucleotide, oxidized (NAD+).

Glycolysis can be summarized as:

$$\text{Glucose} + 2P_2 + 2NAD + 2ADP \rightarrow 2 \text{ Pyruvate} + 2ATP + 2NADH + 2H + 2H_2O$$

All cells have a glycolytic pathway, which makes glycolysis the fundamental route of carbohydrate metabolism. As can be seen, the oxidation of a molecule of glucose produces a net 2 ATP high-energy phosphate bond. Energy is also provided later by metabolism of the two major products of glycolysis, pyruvate, and lactate.

The first stage of aerobic respiration involves a cyclic series of reactions termed the tricarboxylic acid cycle (TCA), the cirtic acid cycle, or the Krebs' Cycle. The

TCA cycle provides a final common pathway for the oxidation of energy substrates such as amino acids, fatty acids, and carbohydrates. Pyruvate undergoes facilitated transport into the mitochondrial matrix for the conversion to acetyl CoA and the ensuing TCA cycle. This is a very important control step in the continued oxidation of glucose. Pyruvate can be formed from the transamination of alanine and enter the TCA cycle at this point. Acetyl CoA, which can also form in the mitochondria through the beta oxidation of fatty acids or amino acid metabolism, is indistinguishable from that formed in the process of carbohydrate metabolism. This allows for a point of regulation in the selection of energy substrate. Likewise, the fate of acetyl CoA is either oxidation to CO_2 by the TCA cycle or incorporation into lipids. An outline of the reactions that constitute the TCA cycle is shown in Fig. 5. Of note is the fact that amino acid metabolism can be connected with the TCA cycle through deamination or transamination of amino acids, such as glutamic and aspartic acid, to components of the cycle, such as alphaketoglutarate and oxaloacetate. There are two points worth emphasizing. The first is that substrate-level phosphorylation is carried out during the conversion of succinyl-CoA to succinate. A high-energy phosphate bond is thus generated in the form of guanosine triphosphate (GTP). This phosphate group is then transferred to adenosine diphosphate (ADP) to form ATP in the following reaction:

Nucleoside Diphosphate Kinase
$$GTP + ADP \rightleftharpoons GDP + ATP$$

The converse of this process is called oxidative phosphorylation, where the formation of ATP is coupled to the oxidation of NADH or flavin adenine dinucleotide, reduced ($FADH_2$), formed during the conversion of succinate to fumarate by O_2. This process is discussed in the next section.

The net reaction for each molecule of glucose that is metabolized in the TCA cycle is:

$$6NAD + 2FAD + 2GDP + 2P_i + 2Acetyl\ CoA + 4H_2 0 \rightarrow$$
$$4CO_2 + 4H + 2CoA + 2GTP + 6NADH + 2FADH_2$$

The production of NADH and $FADH_2$ during glycolysis and the TCA cycle as well as from fatty acid oxidation provides a substrate for the process of oxidative phosphorylation and the ultimate formation of large quantities of energy in the form of ATP. These energy-rich molecules contain a pair of electrons that are transferred via a series of electron carriers to molecular oxygen to liberate a large amount of energy in the form of ATP.

Oxidative phosphorylation/electron transport is carried out in the inner mitochondrial membrane. There are two shuttles in operation that facilitate the transport of reducing power from the cytosol to the mitochondria. They are the alpha-glycerol phosphate shuttle and the malate-aspartate shuttle. The electrons from NADH can then pass through the electron transport chain in the inner mitochondrial membrane and from up to three ATPs. The oxidative phosphorylation of electrons from $FADH_2$ results in a net production of two ATP molecules. The exact mechanism of how the high-energy phosphate bonds of ATP are formed by this process of electron transport is not clearly understood. The reaction can be summarized as follows:

$$Glucose + 6\ O_2 + 36\ H + 36\ Pi + 36\ ADP \rightarrow 6\ CO_2 + 36\ ATP + 42\ H_2O$$

The ADP provides control for the process of glycolysis, TCA cycle, and oxidative phosphorylation. Its availability dictates the activity of the system. When energy needs are high and there is an abundant supply of ADP, the respiratory process continues. As ADP is converted to ATP and is no longer available for use in these processes, respiration decreases.

Another possible fate for the glucose-6-phosphate is the pentose phosphate shunt (hexose monophosphate shunt). This pathway serves many functions:

1. The formation of nicotinamide-adenine dinucleotide phosphate, reduced (NADPH) as reducing power for fatty acid and steroid synthesis.
2. The conversion of hexoses into pentoses (i.e., ribose-5-phosphate) for nucleotide and nucleic acid synthesis.
3. The conversion of pentoses, in the form of phosphates, into hexose or triose phosphates to enter glycolysis for oxidation.
4. The formation of NADPH to supply reduced glutathione for erythrocytes, to facilitate the hydroxylation of phenylalanine to tyrosine, to promote the reduction of the pteridine nucleus in folic acid, and to participate in the various reactions involving the cytochrome P_{450} system.

In some tissues (i.e., liver, mammary gland, testis, and adrenal cortex) the pentosephosphate shunt is particularly active (Fig. 4). The potent reducing compound NADPH is generated by this pathway. NADPH serves as a hydrogen and electron donor in reductive biosyntheses. This is in contrast to NADH, which is oxidized to generate ATP through the electron transport system. NADPH is an essential intermediate for the biosynthesis of fatty acids, steroids, and the reduced glutathione that is critical in the maintenance of normal red blood cell structure. The most important regulatory factor for the formation of NADPH is the level of cellular NADP+, for this reflects the NADPH requirements of the organism.

Although this discussion concentrates on the formation of energy by the metabolism of glucose, the metabolism of fatty acids is also a very important source of energy. It is of interest to compare the amount of high-energy ATP formed by the metabolism of glucose and fatty acids. When one molecule of glucose is transformed to six molecules of water and six molecules of carbon dioxide, 38 molecules of ATP are formed. Only eight molecules of ATP are formed during glycolysis of glucose to pyruvate; the remaining 30 are formed when pyruvate is metabolized in the TCA cycle. In contrast, the beta oxidation of one molecule of palmitic acid results in the formation of 129 molecules of ATP from oxidation of seven reduced flavoprotein molecules, seven NADH molecules, and eight acetyl-CoA molecules. The acetyl-CoA is then oxidized in the TCA cycle.

GLUCONEOGENESIS

The next major pathway in this examination of carbohydrate metabolism is gluconeogenesis. This pathway allows for the synthesis of glucose from a variety of precursor molecules. These precursors include lactate, amino acids, and glycerol (from the hydrolysis of triacylglycerols in adipose cells). The major site for gluconeogenesis is the liver, with a minor contribution coming from the renal cortex. Two other organs that play a pivotal role in gluconeogenesis are skeletal muscle and intestine. Figure 6 summarizes the interrelationship among these four organs that is so critical for effective gluconeogenesis.

As can be seen in Fig. 5, the mechanism of gluconeogenesis is not a reversal of

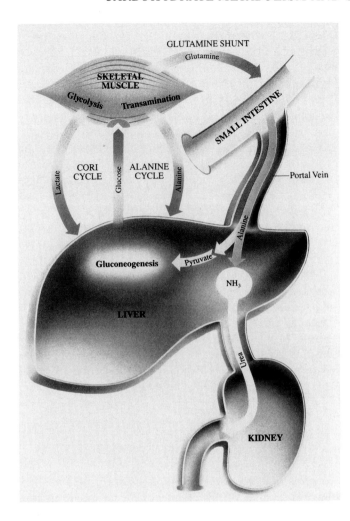

FIG. 6. Interrelationships of skeletal muscle, small intestine, and liver in the production of glucose by gluconeogenesis. In the Cori cycle, lactate furnished by skeletal muscle is converted to glucose by the liver; in the alanine cycle, alanine furnished by skeletal muscle is converted to glucose by the liver; in the glutamine shunt, glutamine furnished by skeletal muscle is converted to alanine in the small intestine and the alanine is subsequently converted to glucose by the liver. (From Feldman, ref. 6, used by permission.)

glycolysis. This is because of the irreversible nature of hexokinase, glucokinase, phosphofructokinase, and pyruvate kinase, the four regulatory enzymes of steps in glycolysis. The important regulatory enzymes in gluconeogenesis are (Fig. 5):

1. The conversion of pyruvate to phosphoenol pyruvate (PEP), which is carried out by a two-step reaction catalyzed by pyruvate carboxylase and phosphoenol-pyruvate carboxykinase.
2. The conversion of fructose 1,6-diphosphate to fructose 6-phosphate, which is catalyzed by fructose 1,6-diphosphatase.
3. The conversion of glucose 6-phosphate to glucose, which is catalyzed by glucose 6-phosphatase.

Because pyruvate carboxylase is a mitochondrial enzyme, the product of its reaction, oxaloacetate, must be transported into the cytosol via a malate shuttle in order for the cytoplasmic-based gluconeogenesis to proceed.

The summary for the reactions of gluconeogenesis is:

$$2 \text{ Pyruvate} + 4ATP + 2GTP + 2NADH + 2H_2O \rightarrow \text{Glucose} + 4ADP + 2GDP + 6Pi + 2NAD+$$

The pathways of glycolysis and gluconeogenesis are active under opposite conditions. Gluconeogenesis is favored when the cell is energy rich and ATP levels are high. Glycolysis is favored under the opposite conditions.

If cells do not require immediate energy, the glucose that is absorbed can be stored in the form of glycogen. The two major sites of glycogen storage are the liver and skeletal muscle. Glucose 6-phosphate is converted into glycogen by a series of reactions requiring various enzymes, uridine 5′ triphosphate (uridine triphosphate) (UTP) (which activates the glucose unit for transfer), and pyrophosphate PP_i. The activated, dephosphorylated form of glycogen synthase is capable of catalyzing the addition of glucose to glucose chain. An alpha 1,4-glucan branching enzyme is necessary to catalyze the transfer of a terminal oligosaccharide fragment from the main chain to create a branch point, thus forming a typical glycogen moiety.

The breakdown of glycogen involves a series of energy-requiring amplification reactions that ultimately lead to the phosphorylation, and thus activation, of glycogen phosphorylase. This enzyme is capable of catalyzing the phosphorolysis of a terminal alpha (1, 4) glucose. This results in a glucose-1-phosphate and a glycogen minus one glucose unit. This process continues until a highly branched core of alpha (1, 6) linkages at the branch points, or a limit dextrin, results. At this point, an amylo-1,6-glucosidase, or debranching enzyme, is necessary to catalyze the hydrolysis of the alpha (1, 6) linkage at the branch point. Another group of alpha (1, 4) linkages are then available for the action of glycogen phosphorylase. The glucose-1-phosphate residues undergo conversion to glucose-6-phosphate by the action of phosphoglucomutase. This glucose-6-phosphate is then available to enter reactions as an energy source for the cell.

HORMONAL REGULATION OF CARBOHYDRATE METABOLISM

Insulin plays a major role in regulating all aspects of metabolism—protein and fat, as well as carbohydrate. Although the focus of this chapter is on carbohydrate metabolism, we discuss the effect of insulin on fat and protein metabolism when it is necessary to have this information to understand the metabolic effect of surgery on patients with diabetes. The effect of insulin on liver, fat cells, and muscle is examined because these are the main tissues whose glucose uptake is dependent on the ambient insulin concentration. In contrast, brain cells and erythrocytes do not have an absolute requirement for insulin in order to take glucose into the cells and utilize it.

Pancreatic insulin secretion is stimulated by elevations of blood glucose levels, certain amino acids such as leucine, arginine, and lysine, and even by ketone bodies. Conversely, the secreted insulin decreases the blood glucose concentration, the plasma-free fatty acid concentration, and the blood amino acid concentration. The insulin also decreases the breakdown of tissue protein and stimulates synthesis of tissue protein. The anabolic effects of insulin are thus of critical importance in surgical wound healing.

In the liver, insulin exerts a major effect on the enzymes glucokinase, glycogen synthase, and glycogen phosphorylase. It increases the activity of glycogen synthase and decreases the activity of glycogen phosphorylase, both of which act to increase the amount of glycogen stored in the liver. It appears that this may be carried out by an insulin-induced increase in activity of a protein phosphatase that acts to dephosphorylate both glycogen phosphorylase and glycogen synthase, which deactivates glycogen phosphorylase and activates glycogen synthase. These alterations facilitate the rapid alterations between glycogen synthesis and breakdown, which maintains the blood glucose within narrow limits under normal conditions. The net effect of these reactions is to increase the amount of glycogen stored by the liver. The maximum concentration of glycogen in the liver is approximately 5–6% of liver weight.

Insulin exerts a delayed effect on glucokinase that may not become evident for several hours. When the synthesis and activity of glucokinase is stimulated by insulin, hepatic glucose uptake increases. Once glucose enters the cell, it is immediately phosphorylated in an irreversible reaction (as previously outlined). The glucose is thus "trapped" inside the cell. This phosphorylated glucose is available for use in the glycolytic pathway, glycogen-synthesis pathway, or pentose-phosphate shunt. As described previously, this effect of insulin on glucose uptake is limited to glucokinase of the liver. In contrast to glucokinase, insulin does not alter the activity of hexokinase, the enzyme that catalyzes glucose phosphorylation in nonhepatic cells.

Insulin stimulates fatty acid synthesis in the liver, especially after the maximal glycogen storage is reached. The mechanism by which this occurs is multifactorial. As described earlier, insulin stimulates glucokinase, which promotes glucose uptake. Part of this effect is manifest in an increase in glycolysis and the TCA cycle. The resulting increase in citrate and isocitrate stimulates the activity of acetyl-CoA carboxylase and, thus, fatty acid synthesis. Another effect of increased glucose uptake is an increase in the activity of the pentose-phosphate shunt. This results in an increase in the availability of NADPH for fatty-acid synthesis. There may also be a direct effect of insulin on acetyl-CoA carboxylase, which would further promote fatty acid synthesis. These fatty acids are then transported to adipose cells where they are stored as triglyceride. As an aside, the ketogenic potential of the liver is reduced as a result of the increased fatty-acid synthesis. The reason for this is that an intermediate in the fatty-acid synthesis pathway, malonyl CoA, is increased. This serves as an inhibitory factor on hepatic carnitine, which is necessary in order to transport fatty acids across the mitochondrial membrane for oxidation.

Insulin also exerts a modest effect to inhibit gluconeogenesis by hepatic tissue. This effect may be mediated by decreasing the quantity and activity of enzymes necessary for gluconeogenesis and/or by decreasing the release of amino acids from extraheptic tissues and the uptake of such precursors of the liver. In the presence of increased insulin activity, the glucose that is produced through the process of gluconeogenesis tends to be directed into increased glycogen synthesis.

In the muscle and adipose tissue, insulin also stimulates glucose uptake by a mechanism that increases facilitated transport of glucose, via a carrier molecule, across the cell membrane. The activity of glycogen synthase, which promotes glycogen storage, and phosphofructokinase, which promotes glycolysis, is increased by insulin. Immediately following a meal, glucose and, subsequently, insulin levels are increased. This stimulates the facilitated transport of glucose into cells and the utilization as an energy source in preference to fatty acids, which are preferentially used in resting muscle that is impermeable to glucose. Muscle is unique with regard to its responsiveness to insulin. Muscle is capable of storing approximately 1–2% of its weight as glycogen. When this threshold is approximated or achieved, muscle cells are less responsive to the circulating levels of insulin. Exercise brings about changes in the muscle membrane that make the muscle cells more permeable to glucose. This helps to maintain an adequate supply of glucose for the continued energy needs of the organism during exercise. The exact mechanism for this exercise-induced permeability to glucose is not known.

Insulin-mediated glucose uptake and metabolism in adipose cells leads to the production of fatty acids and alpha-glycerophosphate. This allows for the formation of triglycerides and the uptake of circulating fatty acids and triglycerides because insulin also has a stimulatory effect on lipoprotein lipase. The overall effect is one of increased lipogenesis.

In response to surgery there is an increased secretion of insulin-antagonist hormones such as glucagon, cortisol, catecholamines, and growth hormone. These hormones promote catabolic reactions that provide cells with increased metabolic substrate for increased energy needs. The action of these hormones contrasts with the anabolic and growth-stimulating effects of insulin. Each of these catabolic hormones can induce hyperglycemia and metabolize lipids and their secretions; thus, there is an exacerbation of hyperglycemia in patients with diabetes.

Glucagon release from pancreatic alpha cells is stimulated by hypoglycemia and certain amino acids, such as arginine and alanine. The close proximity to pancreatic beta cells provides the environment for a close interrelationship between the two hormones. Insulin secretion tends to suppress glucagon release, whereas glucagon secretion tends to stimulate insulin release. It is the relative ratio of insulin to glucagon that contributes to the control of hepatic glucose and fat metabolism. Glucagon's primary effect is on the liver. In contrast to insulin, glucagon stimulates glycogenolysis and gluconeogenesis. Although the mechanism for the stimulation of gluconeogenesis is unclear, glycogenolysis is probably stimulated through the activation of adenylatecyclase, which catalyzes the formation of cyclic AMP from ATP. In a series of amplification reactions, glucagon activates the protein kinase that catalyzes the phosphorylation of phosphorylase kinase. The phosphorylase kinase then catalyzes the phosphorylation with activation of glycogen phosphorylase. The glycogen phosphorylase than catalyzes the breakdown of glycogen, which results in hyperglycemia.

An increased concentration of circulating catecholamines, such as epinephrine and norepinephrine, also increases the concentration of blood glucose. Catecholamines stimulate glycogenolysis through stimulation of beta-adrenergic receptor-mediated activation of adenylate cyclase. This subsequently stimulates the cascade of reactions that lead to glycogen breakdown. Activation of alpha-adrenergic receptor-mediated calcium ion movement may also play a role in the activation of glycogen phosphorylase. Catecholamines also stimulate gluconeogenesis through an inhibitory effect on phosphofructokinase and a stimulatory effect on fructose-1,6-diphosphatase. In addition to the above effects, catecholamines cause a decrease in pancreatic insulin secretion. The result is decreased peripheral glucose uptake and utilization by peripheral tissues, such as muscle, through a decrease in the carrier-mediated glucose uptake of the muscle cells. Catecholamine-induced stimulation of lipolysis makes fatty acids available for peripheral metabolism, which may further decrease peripheral glucose uptake.

Catecholamines also exert an alpha-adrenergic-mediated inhibition of insulin secretion by the beta cells. This explains why there is usually a lack of insulin response to the hyperglycemia induced by catecholamines in nondiabetic patients. Catecholamines also have a modest insulin-like effect of decreasing the circulating levels of amino acids, particularly the branched chain amino acids. This may have the beneficial effect of sparing tissue proteins. However, the net effect of the increased concentration of plasma catecholamines is an increase in the hyperglycemia of postoperative patients with diabetes.

Glucocorticoids such as cortisol also contribute to the development of hyperglycemia by stimulating gluconeogenesis and by increasing the resistance of peripheral tissues to insulin action. Although cortisol ultimately has a potent hyperglycemic effect, the onset of its effect is somewhat delayed in comparison with glucagon and catecholamines. This is probably true because it stimulates gluconeogenesis by inducing the formation of increased amounts of gluconeogenic enzymes. Cortisol induces the formation of gluconeogenic enzymes by producing changes in the nuclear proteins of the cell. The result of these nucleoprotein changes is increased hepatic synthesis and increased activity of gluconeogenic enzymes, such as PEP carboxykinase. In addition to increasing the blood glucose level, there is also an increase in hepatic glycogen production.

Cortisol also stimulates hepatic gluconeogenesis by increasing the transport of gluconeogenic amino acids from the muscle to the liver. This is done by stimulating the degradation of muscle protein, thus increasing the circulating levels of amino acids, particularly branched chain amino acids.

Cortisol also decreases glucose uptake and subsequent glucose utilization by peripheral tissues predominantly at a postinsulin receptor site (8). Cortisol does not appear to have a direct stimulatory effect on other counterregulatory hormones. However, glucose-stimulated insulin secretion may be suppressed because the plasma–insulin concentration does not rise appropriately in response to the increase in blood glucose induced by cortisol. The net effect of the increased cortisol secretion in response to surgery in the diabetic patient is exacerbation of hyperglycemia.

The effects of growth hormone on carbohydrate metabolism are less well defined than those of glucagon, catecholamines, and glucocorticoids. Prolonged exposure to elevated growth hormone is known to stimulate delayed hepatic glucose production and decrease peripheral utilization of glucose. Acromegaly, a disease characterized by chronic elevations of serum growth hormone, is associated with insulin resistance of peripheral tissues and the development of diabetes. Chronic excess of growth hormone may result in hyperglycemia by exerting an antagonistic effect at the levels of the insulin receptor or at a postinsulin receptor site. The deleterious effect of increased growth hormone on the plasma glucose concentration of diabetic patients in the postoperative period is probably not as profound as the effect of glucagon, catecholamines, and cortisol.

Diabetes mellitus is an illness characterized by an absolute or relative insulin deficiency, depending on the type and severity of the disease. Insulin deficiency causes most cells, excluding brain cells and erythrocytes, which have an obligate requirement for glucose as energy substrate, to switch to energy substrates other than glucose. This is secondary to the dependence upon insulin for glucose uptake in those cells. The net effect of this lack of insulin is a switch to catabolism—increased glycogenolysis, lipolysis, proteolysis, gluconeogenesis, and ketogenesis. During times of stress, this effect is further magnified. In addition to lack of insulin, there is an increase of counterregulatory hormones.

Surgery or trauma cause significant stress to nondiabetic patients. Both alter metabolism to an even greater extent in patients with diabetes mellitus. Normally, the counterregulatory hormones, which act synergistically, are elevated in response to this stress. This may be the result of the trauma or surgical procedure, or the pain associated with the procedure, or the effect of anesthesia. This leads to hyperglycemia, which normally stimulates insulin secretion from the pancreatic beta cells. However, patients with diabetes mellitus are unable to appropriately increase pancreatic insulin secretion in response to hyperglycemia, and this leads to a further increase in hyperglycemia. The hyperglycemia and the increased catabolism are detrimental to healing of surgical wounds and may make the postoperative patient with diabetes more susceptible to postoperative wound infections than a nondiabetic patient would be.

REFERENCES

1. Galloway JA, Shuman CR. Diabetes and surgery—a study of 667 cases. *Am J Med* 1963;34: 177–191.
2. Bagdade JB, Root RK, Bulger RJ. Impaired leukocyte function in patients with poorly controlled diabetes. *Diabetes* 1974;23:9–15.
3. Rosenthal S, Lerner B, Dibase F, Enquist IE. Relation of strength to composition in diabetic wounds. *Surg Gynecol Obstet* 1962;437–442.
4. Giddings AEB. The control of plasma glucose in the surgical patient. *Br J Surg* 1974;61:787–792.
5. Greenberg GR, Marlis EB, Anderson GH, et al. Protein-sparing therapy in post operative patients—effects of added hypocaloric glucose or lipid. *N Engl J Med* 1976;294:1411–1416.
6. Feldman JM. Pathophysiology of diabetes Mellitus. In: Galloway JA, Potvin JH, Shuman CR, eds. *Diabetes Mellitus*. Indianapolis, IN: Lilly Research Laboratories, 1988;28–43.
7. Gerich JE. Hormonal control of Homeostasis. In: Galloway JA, Potvin JH, Shuman CR, eds. *Diabetes Mellitus*. Indianapolis, IN: Lilly Research Laboratories, 1988;46–63.
8. Rizza R, Mandarino L, Gerich J. Cortisol-induced insulin resistance in man: Impaired suppression of glucose production and stimulation of glucose utilization due to a postreceptor defect of insulin action. *J Clin Endocrinol Metab* 1982;54:131–136.

Surgical Management of the Diabetic Patient,
edited by Michael Bergman and Gregorio A. Sicard.
Raven Press, Ltd., New York © 1991.

3

Medical Management of Diabetic Patients During Surgery

Charles R. Shuman

*Department of Medicine, Temple University School of Medicine,
Philadelphia, Pennsylvania 19140*

Current estimates of the prevalence of diabetes in the United States indicate that six million persons are known to have diabetes, with an equal number of cases unrecognized. One-third of these persons are in the later years of life, the time when the frequency of surgery is greatest in the general population. Health surveys have shown that among the elderly, 17% have diabetes mellitus or impaired glucose tolerance (1). With the age of the population advancing, it is apparent that the incidence of diabetes mellitus will increase. In addition, recent data have shown a rise in the incidence of diabetes among youth, for reasons as yet obscure. Diabetes mellitus may become clinically apparent with an acute surgical illness or be recognized as a consequence of surgical intervention, as was recorded in one series among 23% of patients (2).

Advances in medical management have improved the quality of life and increased the lifespan of diabetic patients. With prolonged survival has come the increase in the need for surgical intervention for conditions related to diabetes, such as vascular disease, ocular disorders, cholelithiasis, and infections to which are added the usual problems of cardiopulmonary, neoplastic, orthopedic, and other disorders common to aging individuals. Indeed, surgery is the major stress to which the diabetic patient is subjected.

An important issue in the management of the diabetic patient is who has primary responsibility during the perioperative period. When the need for surgical intervention becomes apparent, the practitioner or internist familiar with the medical problems inherent in diabetes plays a salient role as part of a team with the surgeon and anesthetist throughout the entire event. Notable advances in surgical techniques and anesthetic technology have improved the outcome of operative procedures for all high-risk patients. Experience has shown, however, that the management of the diabetic status during the perioperative period requires the careful supervision of the internist familiar with the disease and its complications, not only in the preparation of the patient for surgery but also during the immediate postoperative and recovery periods. Failure to apply the principles of glycemic control with practical methods for intravenous insulin administration, monitored and adjusted with bedside glucose monitoring, can adversely affect the outcome of the most skillful surgery. Therefore, the team approach, including skilled nursing supervision, is mandatory in establishing optimal guidelines for the management of these patients. Under these conditions the diabetic patient has become a candidate for all types of surgical procedures.

CLASSIFICATION OF DIABETES RELATED TO SURGERY

Two major categories of diabetes mellitus, based on interpretations of accumulating clinical and laboratory data, have been defined by the National Diabetes Data Group (3) and by the World Health Organization (4). These are type I, insulin-dependent diabetes mellitus (IDDM) and Type II, noninsulin-dependent diabetes mellitus (NIDDM). Each has distinct, but sometimes overlapping, pathophysiologic features.

Patients with IDDM are identified as insulin deficient and prone to ketosis when insulin therapy is withdrawn. The degree of insulin dependency is affected by many environmental factors, such as physical activity, nutrient loads, emotional or physical stress, and illness. The dependency is caused by an autoimmune process resulting in progressive destruction of pancreatic beta cells, which leads to failure of production and secretion of endogenous insulin (5).

Type II diabetes is a more insidious disorder that is often asymptomatic and frequently associated with obesity in middle-aged or older people. A strong genetic background is ordinarily noted in these patients in whom a reduced insulin response to a rising plasma glucose concentration is a hallmark as is a resistance to the action of insulin in insulin-dependent tissues such as liver, muscle, or fat (6). Because of endogenous insulin supplies, albeit inadequate to suppress basal hepatic glucose output and to maintain tissue uptake of glucose, the patients do not exhibit spontaneous ketosis. During illness or periods of major stress, such as surgery, ketosis and marked hyperglycemia may occur.

During periods of major stress, the clinical distinctions among the major clinical categories of diabetes are obscured by effects of counter-regulatory hormones on insulin secretion and action. Patients with type II diabetes may have decreased insulin activity because of decreased tissue sensitivity to the hormone and a reduction in the secretory activity of pancreatic beta cells (7). Insulin requirements are elevated and may exceed those of the type I patients, particularly in the presence of obesity, sepsis, and stressful conditions, which accelerate insulin resistance. For these reasons, intravenous insulin administration during surgery for patients with IDDM and NIDDM has been emphasized as an effective and safe method for management of the disease, utilizing infusion delivery systems and bedside blood glucose level monitoring (8,9).

INFLUENCE OF STRESS ON DIABETES

The physiologic responses to adverse external stimuli and to disturbing emotional or other endogenous factors constitute the stress reaction. These responses are a series of integrated neural and hormonal signals for adaptation of the organism to stress-related events (7). Activation of the sympathetico-adrenomedullary system stimulates release of catecholamines, epinephrine and norepinephrine, which influence hemodynamic and metabolic responses required for the physiologic counteraction to stress. The pivotal role of epinephrine is manifested in its glycogenolytic and lipolytic activity, in suppressed insulin activity (7), and in stimulation of the pituitary–adrenocortical axis (10). Increased levels of adrenocorticotropic hormone (ACTH), cortisol, and growth hormone occur in more severe gradations of stress. These counterregulatory factors promote further glucose production and decreased glucose clearance. In nondiabetic persons, the raised concentrations of circulating fuels stimulate the release of insulin, which modulates hyperglycemia and inhibits hepatic ketogenesis (8).

In the insulin-deficient state of diabetes, the response to elevated concentrations of counterregulatory hormone is intensified by the increased sensitivity of tissues of the diabetic organism to their actions. A synergistic effect of the catabolic actions of epinephrine, cortisol, and growth hormone in diabetic tissues has been demonstrated (11). Decreased insulin secretory activity by beta cells is a consequence of alpha–adrenergic stimulation of epinephrine, which also decreases tissue sensitivity to insulin (7). Cortisol is active in enhancing hepatic gluconeogenesis from glucogenic precursors, including amino acids and glycerol. The catabolic effect of insulin deficiency and cortisol excess leads to proteolysis and nitrogen losses as amino acids are eliminated in the process of their conversion to glucose and hepatic glycogen (7).

Increments in growth hormone concentration result in decreases in glucose utilization, insulin resistance, and a rise in plasma glucose levels. Liberation of glucose from glycogen stores is sustained by epinephrine, the increased secretion of which can persist for long periods. There are conflicting data concerning the role of glucagon in the stress response (12); its action runs parallel to that of epinephrine in terms of increased glycogenolysis.

The potential consequences of these counterregulatory responses in diabetic subjects are far reaching during the acute operative period as well as during recovery. Sustained hyperglycemia produces an osmotic diuresis with loss of body fluid and electrolytes; a rise in serum osmolality results in hyperosmolar states accompanied by hyperviscosity, thrombogenesis, and central nervous system complications (13). Rising levels of free fatty acids provide substrate for hepatic ketogenesis, which, in the fluid-depleted subject with reduced glucose oxidation, rapidly advances to diabetic ketoacidosis (14). With depletion of tissue protein and amino acids, cellular repair and fibroblastic proliferation in the processes of wound healing are severely retarded (15). In the hyperglycemic milieu, the first line of defense against infection is lost as the phagocytic function of polymorphonuclear leucocytes is severely compromised (16). The long-range consequences of sustained hyperglycemia will involve the accumulation of intracellular sorbitol and the glycosylation of structural and circulating proteins as the principal biochemical alterations that underlie many of the chronic manifestations of diabetes (17).

Effects of Diabetes on Surgical Patients

The prevalence of cardiovascular disorders in patients with diabetes is more than three-fold more common than in the general population. These life-threatening atherosclerotic complications occur prematurely and diffusely in patients with diabetes (18), affect coronary, cerebral, and peripheral vessels, increase the surgical risks, and represent the associated pathologies for which operative procedures are often required for these patients. If the severity and extent of these complications are recognized preoperatively, it facilitates their management during the perioperative period. Hypertension, in nearly half of the diabetic patients, contributes to the gravity of circulatory disorders (19). The hypertensive state and the effects of drugs used in its treatment, such as diuretics and beta blocker therapy, require careful evaluation and correction during the preparation for operation. For example, diuretic-induced hypokalemia that requires potassium replacement is frequently observed in hypertensive diabetic patients referred for surgical procedures.

Diabetic neuropathy is a commonly encountered complication, a component of which is autonomic neuropathy. Involvement of the autonomic nervous system may compromise the neuroreflexive control of cardiovascular and pulmonary function during anesthesia and surgery (20). Orthostatic hypotension and loss of normal variations in cardiac rhythm on deep breathing or during valsalva maneuver are observed in this condition. Visceropathy affecting gastrointestinal or urinary bladder function in autonomic neuropathy can lead to intestinal ileus, gastroparesis or urinary retention. Several of these issues are measured again in Chapter 9 (see Emergency Surgery in the Diabetic Patient).

Microvascular disorders of diabetes are characterized by capillary basement membrane thickening with endothelial cellular changes and lumenal narrowing affecting the renal glomeruli, retinal vessels, and vascular beds of other tissues. Disturbances in renal function with elevations of blood urea nitrogen (BUN) levels, creatinine and proteinuria leading to hypoalbuminemia require careful attention to fluid and electrolyte homeostasis during and after operative procedures. Diabetic nephropathy is a major reason renal transplantation is necessary, accounting for nearly 25% of these procedures in the United States (21).

These complications related to diabetes and others, such as occult infections observed in 17% of patients in one series, require careful preoperative assessment with a thorough medical and diabetic database (2). With appropriate corrective procedures and with efficient surveillance systems for conditions constituting a threat to successful operative interventions, these patients are suitable subjects for any type of surgical procedure.

Preoperative Considerations

A major objective in the medical management of the diabetic patient during surgery is to maintain metabolic homeostasis to prevent fluid imbalance, protein catabolism, and impaired wound healing, and to lessen the risk of infection. The therapeutic strategies used to achieve this goal are usually formulated within a period of 24 hours or less for patients scheduled for elective operations. Among the factors involved in the preliminary evaluation are: the type of diabetes and assessment of previous treatment; the presence or absence of complications; determination of whether the operation is major or minor. Each of these factors has a direct effect upon the estimation of insulin requirements during and after surgery and on the perioperative monitoring procedures required to control diabetes and its complications (22).

The initial doses of insulin required during surgery can be estimated on the basis of the customary total daily insulin needs for type I and for insulin-requiring type II patients. The insulin-sensitive patient maintained on 0.4 units/kg preoperatively is given a lower insulin infusion rate than one receiving 0.6 units/kg daily. Insulin needs are affected by other factors, such as the presence of infection, pain, obesity, or steroid therapy, so that unpredictable individual variations are encountered during the perioperative period. Using the glucose–insulin infusion methods, the insulin requirements in uncomplicated procedures are relatively consistent with those observed in the patients before an operation. Patients undergoing open heart surgery, coronary bypass operations, and transplantation procedures require significantly higher rates of insulin infusion and boluses of regular insulin because of insulin resistance associated with sympathomimetic drug administration, the use of hypothermia, and the priming solutions utilized in the extracorporeal pump. Insulin administration by intravenous methods provides a flexible and readily adjusted rate of infusion to accommodate the anticipated fluctuations in blood glucose concentrations (9,23,24,25).

Anesthesia

Selection of the type of anesthesia is the prerogative of the anesthetist who, during the preoperative visit, has become familiar with the potential risks and disease-related complications that may modify the anesthesia procedures and intraoperative care. Discussions and explanations by the anesthetist with the patient and family are important to allay apprehension and create an atmosphere of reassurance for the patient. The choice of anesthetic agents depends upon the type of surgery, the medical status of the patient, and the surgical risks without primary concern for the presence of diabetes. Modern inhalation anesthetic agents have relatively little effect upon metabolic regulation; regional anesthesia has minimal influence on glycemic control (22). Preoperative medications and muscle relaxants prescribed by the anesthetist do not have significant impact on metabolic regulation. For elderly or debilitated diabetic patients, modest reductions in the doses of these agents are advised to avoid cerebral depressant effects.

The presence of autonomic neuropathy or vascular insufficiency states necessitates careful monitoring of the patient during surgery to avoid cardiorespiratory complications and hypotension. Assisted pulmonary ventilation is utilized where required to maintain oxygenation. Intraoperative determination of blood glucose concentrations may be required during extended procedures or during open heart surgery to avoid marked hyperglycemia or hypoglycemia.

Diabetes Management During Surgery

Surgery for diabetic patients should be scheduled for the morning hours to avoid long periods of preoperative parenteral fluid administration and to provide postoperative time for stabilization. Current methods of insulin glucose infusion, however, permit later timing of operations with good maintenance of glycemic control and hydration. The infusion method is advantageous for hyperglycemic patients because it controls blood glucose levels during the night before surgery that is scheduled for the morning hours.

Control of blood glucose concentrations during surgery can be effectively achieved by several methods of insulin delivery using intravenous routes, two of which have proven effective and satisfactory in a general hospital setting:

1. Combined Dextrose-Insulin Infusion: A selected dose of regular insulin is added to 1000 ml of 5% dextrose 1/2 normal saline solution. The amount of insulin is based on the previous daily insulin requirement and on the level of blood glucose determined preoperatively. The insulin dosage is adjusted according to algorithms based on serial bedside blood glucose determinations during and after operation.

This method was reported initially in 1963 for routine operations by Galloway and Shuman (2) but subsequently extended for use in all patients who require insulin during more difficult procedures (26).

2. Insulin Infusion Pump Method: Insulin is administered by continuous pump infusion inserted into a glucose infusion line, permitting regulation of the rate of insulin delivery (and glucose infusion rate) based on frequent blood glucose level monitoring (9,12,23). This method is advantageous in permitting rapid adjustments in insulin dosage for those with conditions that affect insulin sensitivity such as treatment with sympathomimetic drugs, steroids, and insulin-resistant states. The separate insulin/glucose infusion pump method requires careful surveillance and is used principally in intensive care units and specialized centers. It is the treatment of choice in well-equipped facilities, not only for patients undergoing major surgery but also for diabetic patients with acute medical complications such as sepsis, vascular catastrophes, pneumonia, and ketoacidosis.

Methods for Treatment—Major Surgery

Combined Dextrose-Insulin Infusion

IDDM and Insulin-Requiring NIDDM

In preparation for surgery, an infusion of 1000 ml of 5% dextrose in 1/2 normal saline (D5 ½NS) containing regular insulin is started by intravenous cannulation. The dosage of insulin added to the solution ranges from 10 to 20 units based on the previous daily insulin requirements and the preoperative blood glucose concentration: 10 units for those receiving 40 units or less daily, 15 units for 40–80 units daily, and 20 units for 80 units or more daily. These doses are less than the usual daily requirements due to decreased caloric intake and the withholding of usual feedings. The solution is infused at a rate of 100 ml/h to deliver 1–2 units of insulin with 5 g of dextrose hourly. The infusion rate may be adjusted safely during operation because the amounts of dextrose and insulin are changed simultaneously. Patients with higher insulin needs receive the amount of insulin commensurate with their previously identified resistance to the hormone. If major stress is encountered, the rise in blood glucose level is counteracted by administration of additional insulin either subcutaneously or in the intravenous dextrose-insulin solution or both. Blood glucose concentrations are monitored by the conventional meters used for bedside determinations. These measurements are made preoperatively and postoperatively, in the recovery room, and at 3- to 4-hour intervals thereafter. Accurate results are obtained by trained personnel using calibrated equipment and quality control systems at little expense.

During the perioperative period, adjustments in the insulin dosages may be ordered based on blood glucose level measurements. If the blood glucose level rises above 200 mg/dl, 5 units of regular insulin is added to the dextrose-insulin solution; if >300 mg/dl, give 5 units by intravenous injection and add 5 units to the infusing solution. It is rare that a reduction of blood glucose level occurs; if <90 mg/dl, give 20 ml of D50 dextrose 50% solution intravenously, or change the intravenous dextrose-insulin solution to one providing 5 units/1000 ml (Table 1).

TABLE 1. *Combined dextrose/insulin infusion method for insulin-dependent diabetes*

1. Schedule surgery in the morning if possible. Obtain plasma glucose levels and electrolyte determinations.
2. Start an infusion of 1000 ml 5% dextrose in 0.5% sodium chloride (D5 ½NS) at 100 ml/h with regular insulin added as follows:

Daily insulin requirement (units/24 h)	Insulin (units/L D5 ½NS)	Infusion rate (units/h)
40 or less	10	1.0
40 to 80	15	1.5
Over 80	20	2.0

3. Infusion rate is adjusted during operation if fluid requirements are changed.
4. Test capillary blood glucose level in the recovery room and every 2–4 hours.
5. Adjust insulin dose based on blood glucose level as follows:

Blood glucose level (mg/dl)	Adjust insulin dose
<90	Reduce dose by 5 units (change solution)
90–199	Continue same dose
200–280	Add 5 units to infusion
>280	Add 10 units to infusion and give 5 units subcutaneously or as iv bolus

6. Add potassium chloride, 20 mEq, postoperatively to infusions. If serum potassium level <3.5, increase potassium chloride to 40–80 mEq/l. If serum potassium level >5, no potassium chloride is added.
7. Postoperative management: Administer dextrose-insulin-potassium infusion at rate to maintain hydration, usual 3 l daily in ½ NS; add multivitamin preparation. Adjust insulin and potassium chloride based on daily monitoring data.

With the use of intravenous insulin solutions, adherence of the hormone to the infusion equipment has not caused significant problems. Flushing the first 30 ml of the insulin-containing solution through the tubing has been recommended as the sole precaution. Urine glucose determinations are useless and misleading because the retrospective nature of urinary tests leads to incorrect decisions concerning insulin needs (8).

Patients Treated with Sulfonylurea

In type II patients, major surgery accentuates the pathologic features of the disease—suppression of insulin secretion and decreased tissue response to insulin through the actions of counterregulatory hormones. Administration of exogenous insulin, using the human preparation to avoid antigenicity, is required for blood glucose level control. These patients are maintained on their usual schedule of sulfonylurea therapy until the day of surgery. For major surgery during which the use of intravenous dextrose solution is planned, regular insulin is added to 1000 ml of 5% dextrose solution in doses of 8–10 units (22). The infusion is begun preoperatively at a rate of 100–125 ml/h with adjustments of the infusion rate during the operation, as determined by the anesthetist, to satisfy fluid requirements. The combined dextrose–insulin infusion is continued with adjustments of insulin dosage based on bedside glucose monitoring in the recovery room, and postoperatively at 4-hour intervals until oral feedings are resumed (Table 2).

TABLE 2. *Combined dextrose-insulin infusion method for sulfonylurea-treated patients*

1. On the day of surgery, start the infusion of 1000 ml 5% dextrose in 0.5% saline solution (D5 ½NS) with 8–10 units of human regular insulin at 100 ml/h.
2. Monitor the plasma glucose level in recovery room and every 2–4 hours.

Blood glucose (mg/dl)	Adjust insulin dose
<90	No insulin
90–199	Continue same dose
200–280	Add 5 units to infusion
>280	Add 10 units to infusion and give 5 units subcutaneously

3. Add potassium chloride (20 mEq) to the dextrose–insulin infusion postoperatively.
4. Continue the dextrose-insulin-potassium infusion until oral feedings are resumed. Adjust regular insulin and potassium chloride additions based on monitoring data.
5. Insulin may be required for variable periods during recovery before resuming sulfonylurea or diet alone.

The infusion pump method (*vide infra*) may be used for these patients with regular insulin administered at 0.5–1 units/h by infusion pump piggybacked into the iv line for fluid administration of 5% dextrose solution, the flow rate of which is 125 ml/h. The insulin infusion rate is increased by 0.5 units/h if blood glucose is greater than 200 mg/dl and is decreased by 0.5 units if the blood glucose level is less than 100 mg/dl.

It is interesting to note in some instances of obesity or complicating infection, significant increases in insulin requirements are observed and can be readily accommodated by the application of the previously described algorithm.

For type II patients who do not require intravenous dextrose or who are undergoing minor surgery, exogenous insulin is not usually necessary. Glucose determinations are obtained preoperatively to assure acceptable glycemic control. If the blood glucose concentrations are 180 mg/dl and postoperative hyperglycemia persists, exogenous insulin can be given based on a sliding scale using low doses of regular insulin every 4 hours as long as treatment is required.

Methods for Treatment—Major Surgery

Insulin Infusion Pump Method

This method provides a continuous intravenous infusion of insulin at an adjustable rate to achieve a target glycemic range using a separate infusion pump for insulin delivery. Dextrose solution is administered as D5 ½NS at a fixed (but adjustable) rate to maintain fluid and caloric intake. The rate of insulin infusion is changed in response to blood glucose measurements using bedside monitoring techniques (23,25).

Patients are given 1000 ml of 5% dextrose in 0.45% saline solution at a rate of 100 ml/h administered by infusion pump. A line is inserted into the access of the dextrose line through which an insulin solution is infused, prepared as 250 units of regular insulin in 500 ml saline (0.5 units/ml). The rate of insulin infusion is initiated at 1.5

units (3 ml)/h. Bedside blood glucose level measurements are performed every 2 hours during the perioperative period and the rate of insulin infusion is adjusted depending on the glucose concentration. For blood glucose levels of 100–200 mg/dl, no change is made in insulin infusion rate; if the level is <70 mg/dl, reduce insulin to 0.5 units/h and give 20 ml of D50 solution by iv bolus. For elevated blood glucose levels (201–250 mg/dl), increase insulin to 2 units/h; if >250 mg/dl, increase the infusion rate to 3 units/h and give 6 units of regular insulin by iv bolus. One of the frequent errors in this system is to discontinue insulin when the blood glucose level is <70 mg/dl. Because regular insulin has a half-life of 4 minutes, the effective insulin action can dissipate within 30–40 minutes and marked hyperglycemia may rapidly ensue. Ketosis has been observed with a rise in the anion gap during brief cessation of insulin infusion (Table 3).

An essential precaution with this method is the subcutaneous (SC) administration of a dose of insulin when the insulin infusions are discontinued. In one instance when a patient was transferred from an intensive care unit to another hospital floor, metabolic decompensation occurred when the insulin infusion was stopped and no insulin was given for 2 hours after the transfer. In our experience, problems associated with pump failure have not occurred because of alarm systems and close surveillance by the unit personnel. As with other systems, the insulin infusion method may be used for 72 hours or longer if required.

The insulin infusion pump method is preferred for cardiac surgery and transplantation procedures because a 2–4-fold increase in insulin requirements may be seen in these patients (12,27,28). During the early postoperative period, insulin requirements may have risen to levels of 10–20 units/h, based on blood glucose determinations, particularly in patients receiving anti-insulin drugs (sympathomimetics or glucosteroids) or in the face of sepsis. With the cessation of anti-insulin therapy or with responses in plasma glucose to levels less than 120 mg/dl, the rate of insulin infusion is reduced to avoid hypoglycemia. These adjustments can be made by nurses who are experienced with intensive-care procedures and the management of diabetic patients who require surgery (Table 4).

TABLE 3. *Insulin infusion pump method*

Adjust infusion rates

Blood glucose (mg/dl)	Insulin		Bolus
	units/h	Ml/h	
<70	0.5	1.0	20 ml D50 solution iv
71–99	1.0	2	
100–149	1.5	3.0	
150–199	2.0	4.0	
200–249	3.0	6.0	6 units R insulin iv
250–299	4.0	8.0	10 units R insulin iv
>300	5.0	10.0	10 units R insulin iv

D5 ½NS infusion rate increased to 125 ml/h if blood glucose level is <80 mg/dl and decreased to 80 ml/h if >250 mg/dl.
Dextrose 5% in 0.5 saline (D5 ½NS), 1000 ml
Regular insulin, 250 units in 500 ml saline (0.5 units = 1 ml)
Infusion pump with line inserted into D5 ½NS line
Blood glucose measurement by bedside monitor every 2 hours
Initial infusion rates: D5 ½NS—100 ml/h
                    Insulin—1.5 U/h (3.0 ml/h)

TABLE 4. *Insulin infusion pump method: postoperative management of coronary bypass surgery*

Blood glucose level (mg/dl)	Insulin		Bolus IV regular insulin
	units/h	Ml/h	
100–199	5	10	
200–299	10	20	
300–399	15	25	10 units
>400	20	40	10 units

Hourly rate of insulin infusion is adjusted to maintain blood sugar level in target range of 100–200 mg/dl.

POSTOPERATIVE MANAGEMENT

With intravenous dextrose and insulin treatment (combined in one solution or given by separate infusion pumps), treatment can be continued for several days with satisfactory glycemic regulation.

Because reductions in serum potassium concentrations occur as a consequence of insulin-induced cellular glucose uptake, potassium chloride (KC1) is added to the dextrose solutions after the operation or during prolonged procedures. Potassium levels should be obtained before KC1 is added, and every 12–24 hours until stable. Based on serum potassium level determinations, 20–40 meq of KC1 is added to each liter of the dextrose solution postoperatively (8,22,26). The dextrose/insulin/potassium infusion is often required for ≥48 hours after major surgery. During this period, bedside glucose measurements are obtained at 4–6 hour intervals to maintain glucose concentrations between 90 and 200 mg/dl. Fluid and electrolyte balance is maintained with clinical assessment and daily determination of electrolyte concentrations. Patients who are febrile or have extrarenal fluid loss receive supplementary dextrose–electrolyte solutions with added insulin or SC insulin to replace insensible and measured fluid losses and to maintain metabolic stabilization (22).

With resumption of oral feedings, insulin is given before meals as the regular insulin preparation based on blood glucose level measurement by bedside monitoring at 7:00 AM, 11:00 AM, 4:00 PM and 9:00 PM. Isophane insulin suspension (NPH) is given at bedtime to maintain overnight control of blood glucose levels. The amount of regular insulin varies from 4–10 units depending on the fasting and premeal blood glucose concentrations. The dose of NPH varies from 6–10 units initially and is adjusted on the basis of the 9:00 PM and 7:00 AM glucose levels. To avoid nocturnal hypoglycemia, a 3:00 AM blood glucose determination should be obtained. As the normal feeding schedule ensues during recovery, insulin schedules can be changed conveniently to combined NPH and regular insulins given twice daily, before break-

TABLE 5. *Postoperative change to subcutaneous insulin treatment*

Blood glucose (BG) at 7 AM, 11 AM, 4 PM, 9 PM, 3 AM
Regular insulin—4 units before meals for BG between 100 and 200 mg/dl.
Add 1 unit for each 50 mg/dl above 200 mg/dl.
NPH insulin at 10 PM—10 units ± 4 units based on 9 PM BG; subsequent doses adjusted based on 7 AM BG.
For long-term treatment, change to combined NPH/regular insulin, split-dose schedule.

TABLE 6. *Dextrose/insulin infusions during surgery*

Special considerations
  To reduce fluid volume, use 10% dextrose solution at slower infusion rate.
  Run initial 20–30 ml of dextrose/insulin solution through tubing.
  Avoid filters due to binding of insulin.
  Bedside monitoring performed with calibrated monitors. Check high (<300 mg/dl) or low (>70 mg/dl) in biochemical laboratory.
  Insulin resistance occurs in obese patients or those with infection, or during glucosteroid therapy.
  Cardiopulmonary bypass operations require high insulin doses postoperatively.

fast and before dinner. Blood glucose level monitoring is continued at the same intervals to achieve appropriate adjustments of the individual components of the split–mixed insulin injection schedule. An algorithm is provided for supplementary regular insulin doses for correction of hyperglycemia. When stabilization of the blood glucose level is achieved we have been able to switch many patients to the 70/30 NPH/regular premixed insulin preparation. At this time, the patient is instructed in the dietary program (Table 5) and in the details of ambulatory treatment with self blood glucose level monitoring for adjustments of insulin doses as an outpatient. For type II patients previously controlled on sulfonylurea therapy, these agents are resumed in appropriate dosages. For both type I and type II patients, it may be prudent to modify the postoperative diet to promote wound healing and recovery from surgery (Table 6).

Prolonged Parenteral Therapy

Prompt attention should be given to nutritional requirements for all surgical patients if intravenous fluid administration is continued for more than 48 hours in the absence of oral feedings. Total parenteral nutrition (TPN) formulas using 20–50% dextrose concentrations are employed in conjunction with amino acids and micronutrients as well as separate infusion of lipid solutions. These nutritive solutions are an essential factor in promoting the recovery of the nutritionally depleted patient (29).

For diabetic patients, insulin requirements during TPN therapy are commensurate with the elevated glucose and nutrient load. For those receiving insulin by the separate insulin infusion method, the line from the insulin reservoir is piggybacked into the TPN infusion access site. The rate of insulin infusion is set at 3–5 units/h and is adjusted based on blood glucose level monitoring at 2-hour intervals in a manner similar to that described previously: if the blood glucose level is >250 mg/dl, increase by 1 unit/h; if >300 mg/dl, give a 6-unit bolus and increase the infusion rate by 2 units/h. Most patients receive 6 units/h unless sepsis or other complicating factors are present, in which case the rate of insulin infusion may exceed 10 units/h.

For patients not receiving insulin by separate infusion pump, we have added insulin directly to the TPN solution using between 15 and 40 units/l initially. Supplementary iv insulin boluses may be given if blood glucose concentrations are elevated and additional insulin can be added to subsequent infusions. The maximum dosage of regular insulin required per liter of TPN with 70% dextrose has been 100 units. If a filter is placed in the TPN line, it is recognized that an indeterminate amount of insulin is bound within the filter. Binding of insulin to the other portions of the infusion equipment (plastic bag, etc.) has not been a problem in clinical experience with either separate or combined insulin–dextrose infusion systems.

Hyperalimentation therapy and intravenous dextrose administration are recognized as important predisposing factors that contribute to the development of hyperosmolar, nonketotic coma. This serious complication frequently induces vascular thrombosis in cerebral, mesenteric, or peripheral vessels with potentially fatal postoperative consequences (13). This is "an iatrogenic disease" of increasing significance (30) to which the diabetic patients are particularly susceptible if inadequate amounts of insulin are provided and blood glucose levels are not monitored in the recommended manner.

Other Methods of Management

Several reports have demonstrated the advantages of using the artificial endocrine pancreas (Biostator) to manage the diabetic patient throughout the perioperative period (12,28,31,32). This apparatus permits the maintenance of normoglycemia by means of a feedback system for insulin and glucose administration based on continuous blood glucose level monitoring with computerized control of separate infusion rates. The equipment and its operation are expensive and limited generally to research use.

A more traditional method is that of administering one-third to one-half of the usual insulin dose, NPH and regular insulin or NPH alone, by the SC route before surgery at the time that iv dextrose is initiated (33). The remainder of the usual daily insulin requirement is given postoperatively, with added regular insulin if hyperglycemia prevails. Although patients may respond satisfactorily, wide fluctuations in plasma glucose concentrations can occur, with difficulty in achieving adequate control. It is likely that the SC insulin treatment regimen survives because of tradition and habit rather than effectiveness.

EMERGENCY SURGERY

In one series of surgical procedures in diabetic patients, emergency operations constituted 5% of the cases (2). Eighty percent of the emergent operations were the consequence of severe infections. These acute conditions are frequently conducive to diabetic ketoacidosis (DKA) with severe dehydration, hyperglycemia, metabolic acidosis, and hypodynamic circulation. These metabolic disturbances complicate and confound the diagnosis and management of the underlying surgical problem; for example, DKA can cause abdominal pain mimicking a surgical abdomen. Correction of the metabolic disorder may alleviate the abdominal symptoms of DKA or permit more accurate localization of the causative factors in the surgical abdomen (8,22).

Sufficient rehydration and electrolyte replacement and insulin treatment can be achieved within 4–6 hours to improve hyperglycemia and to suppress ketogenesis. In the presence of DKA, insulin is infused by pump at a rate of 6–10 units/h (0.1 unit/kg) after an iv bolus of 6–10 units. Saline solution is begun with administration of 1000 ml in 1–2 hours followed by 500 ml/h thereafter. Potassium chloride/phosphate frequently needs to be added to the second liter of solution. Plasma glucose concentration should decrease by 80–100 mg/dl hourly as a result of the combined effects of dilution through fluid replacement and insulin-induced glucose uptake and decreased hepatic glucose output. For patients in hyperosmolar nonketotic states, insulin doses are generally lower; obese patients or patients in sepsis have significantly higher insulin requirements. With a decrease in blood glucose values to 250–300 mg/dl, 5% dextrose is given in saline or 1/2 NS solution. If possible, surgery should be delayed until after this initial interval of metabolic correction. During surgery, administration of fluids and insulin is based on the results of glucose and electrolyte concentration monitoring at 2-hour intervals.

At this stage, the insulin pump can be discontinued and insulin added to the dextrose/saline infusion. If the insulin pump is continued, reduce the rate to 3–5 units/h and monitor blood glucose concentration during surgery.

Postoperative management continues with the administration of glucose, insulin, and electrolyte solutions, including potassium replacement, based on bedside and laboratory monitoring of blood glucose levels and electrolyte concentrations. During recovery, the patient resumes oral feedings and is switched to SC-administered insulin. Regular insulin given before meals and at bedtime can be converted to mixed NPH and regular insulin given before breakfast and before dinner, in most instances before dismissal from the hospital.

MORTALITY AND MORBIDITY

Mortality among diabetic patients during surgery has approximated mortality in the nondiabetic population regardless of type of surgery. Cardiovascular diseases associated with atherosclerosis and hypertension have been the leading causes of death, with infection the next most frequent cause. Increased morbidity and length of hospitalization were observed in 17.2% of diabetic patients following surgery; this was the result of the presence of vascular complications, infection, and delayed wound healing (2). These problems occur most frequently in patients with disorders involving the lower extremities. Patients with peripheral vascular disease constituted 37.5% of the total mortality in one series (2), demonstrating that vascular disorders can be widely disseminated in the diabetic patient. Strict attention to blood glucose levels, attention to nutritional needs, and treatment of infection and cardiovascular complications during the immediate postoperative interval continue to improve mortality and morbidity rates in the diabetic population.

DIABETES MANAGEMENT DURING SHORT PROCEDURES

There have been various recommendations for diabetes management during outpatient procedures that require fasting; these procedures include gastrointestinal x-rays, endoscopy, dental work, or minor surgery. With the growth of ambulatory surgery in short-procedure units, there has been an enormous increase in the number of diabetic patients for whom systematic programs of treatment are required. Although these patients are not subjected to the same degree of stress encountered during major operations, it is necessary to avoid the potential loss of blood glucose control that is the result of insulin deficiency over the interventional period.

TABLE 7. *Diabetes management during short procedure*

Blood sugar (mg/dl)	Regular insulin (units)
<199	0
200–299	4–6
300–399	6–8
>400	8–10

IDDM: no breakfast
No AM insulin
Monitor blood sugar level before procedure and every 2–3 hours
If iv access required: D5 ½NS at 60–80 ml/h
Give regular insulin SC for hyperglycemia

At termination of procedure:
Lunch permitted—give ½ AM insulin dose SC
Lunch withheld—monitor blood sugar and resume insulin when feeding permitted using usual PM insulin dose (or ½ AM dose if not on bid)
Blood sugar 90 mg/dl, change iv to D5 ½NS

Recommended Management for Short Procedures

Diabetic patients undergoing minor surgery or other procedures requiring a morning fast are instructed to omit insulin injection or sulfonylurea medication that morning. For patients who need an iv access for operations in the short procedure unit, NS is used at a slow infusion rate (60–80 ml/h). Blood glucose levels are monitored before and after short operations and at 2-hour intervals for those of longer duration. If a blood glucose level lower than 90 mg/dl is obtained either preoperatively or in later testing, the iv solution is changed to 5% dextrose in 1/2 NS. For elevated blood glucose concentrations, regular insulin is given SC: 200–299 mg/dl, 4–6 units; 300–399 mg/dl, 6–8 units; greater than 400 mg/dl, 8–10 units. For procedures terminating in the late morning, one-half of the usual morning dose of insulin is given when the patient is permitted to eat. The usual regimen of treatment is resumed thereafter. Patients treated with sulfonylurea can resume their oral agents following the operation (Tables 5–7).

For procedures not requiring the withholding of breakfast, patients are given their usual morning dose of insulin or sulfonylylurea. Blood glucose levels are monitored with the bedside meter before and after surgery to prevent or correct either hypoglycemia or hyperglycemia with 5% dextrose infusion or SC human insulin, respectively.

During the performance of minor surgical or other procedures it is unusual to

TABLE 8. *Diabetes management during short procedure*

Oral Agents: NPO on Day of Procedure
     Give human regular insulin subcutaneously:

If blood glucose level (mg/dl)	Human regular insulin (units)
250–300	4
300–400	6
>400	8

No oral agent given until after surgery.
If iv access is needed, NS or ½NS at 60–80 ml/h.
Check blood glucose levels before and after procedure.

TABLE 9. *Diabetes management during short procedure*

IDDM or NIDDM: Breakfast permitted
Give usual dose of insulin or oral agent.
Check blood glucose levels before and after procedure.
If blood glucose 250, give human regular (4 units SC)
Resume usual treatment after procedure.

encounter significant glycemic fluctuations. Avoiding hypoglycemia is of paramount importance. In any event, the use of bedside monitoring of blood glucose levels has provided a safe and effective method for all type of surgical procedures.

SUMMARY

The presence of diabetes is considered to be a significant short- and long-term risk factor in patients for whom surgery is required. The insulin-dependent state and its attendant hyperresponsiveness to counterregulatory hormones requires the provision of insulin in a systematic fashion to prevent hyperglycemia, fatty acid mobilization, ketogenesis, and wastage of body protein. Metabolic regulation is needed to sustain homeostasis, to enhance wound-healing, and to decrease infection. Diabetes-related complications must be recognized to forestall problems related to these conditions during the perioperative period.

Control of blood glucose levels during operations can be safely and effectively achieved by the intravenous administration of regular insulin during the perioperative period. Insulin is given either in dextrose solution as a combined insulin–dextrose infusion or by means of a separate insulin-infusion pump. For cardiovascular surgery or other procedures associated with high-insulin requirements, the insulin infusion pump permits rapid dosage adjustments. Frequent capillary blood glucose level determinations are used with both methods to adjust insulin doses to maintain the desired range of blood glucose concentrations. These methods, in the hands of experienced physicians and nurses, can eliminate the hazards of hyperglycemia and the risks of hypoglycemia for diabetic patients during surgery.

REFERENCES

1. Goldberg AP, Andres R, Bierman EL. Diabetes mellitus in the elderly. In: Andres R, Bierman EL, Hazzard WR eds. *Principles of geriatric medicine*. New York: McGraw-Hill, 1985;750–763.
2. Galloway JA, Shuman CR. Diabetes and surgery. *Am J Med* 1963;34:177–191.
3. NDDG National Diabetes Data Group. Classification and diagnosis of diabetes mellitus and other categories of glucose intolerance. *Diabetes* 1979;28:1039–1057.
4. World Health Organization Study Group. Diabetes mellitus. Technical Report Series No. 727. Geneva, Switzerland, 1985.
5. Eisenbarth GS. Type I diabetes mellitus, a chronic autoimmune disease. *N Engl J Med* 1986;314:1360–1368.
6. DeFronzo RA, Ferannini E. The pathogenesis of non-insulin dependent diabetes mellitus—an update. *Medicine* (Baltimore) 1982;61:125–140.
7. Porte D Jr. The role of the neuroendocrine system in the development of diabetes mellitus. In: Fajans SS ed. *Diabetes mellitus*. Bethesda, MD: Department of Health, Education and Welfare, 1976.
8. Alberti KGMM, Thomas DJB. The management of diabetes during surgery. *Br J Anaesth* 1979;51:693–710.

9. Rosenstock J, Raskin P. Surgery! Practical guidelines for diabetes management. *Clin Diabetes* 1987;5:49–61.
10. Axelrod J, Reisine TD. Stress hormones: their interaction and regulation. *Science* 1984;224:452–59.
11. Shamoon H, Hendler R, and Sherwin RS. Synergistic interactions among antiinsulin hormones in pathogenesis of stress hyperglycemia in humans. *J Clin Endocrinol Metab* 1981;52:1235.
12. Crock PA, Ley CJ, Martin IK, Alford FP, Best JD. Hormonal and metabolic changes during hypothermic coronary artery bypass surgery in diabetic and non-diabetic subjects. *Diabetic Med* 1987;5:47–52.
13. Podolsky S. Hyperosmolar nonketotic coma: underdiagnoses and undertreated. In: Podolsky S ed. *Clinical diabetes, modern management.* New York: Appleton-Century-Croft, 1980;209–35.
14. Alberti KGMM. Diabetic Emergencies. In: Galloway JA, Potvin JH, Shuman CR, eds. *Diabetes mellitus,* 9th edition. Indianapolis: Eli Lilly Co, 1988;254–75.
15. Weringer EJ, Kelso JM, Tamai IY, Arguilla ER. The effect of antisera to insulin 2-deoxyglucose induced hyperglycemia and starvation on wound healing in normal mice. *Diabetes* 1981;30:407–10.
16. Wilson RM. Neutrophil function in diabetes. *Diabetic Med* 1986;3:509–12.
17. Greene DA, Lattimer SA, Sima AAF. Sorbitol, phosphinositides, and sodium-potassium-ATPase in the pathogenesis of diabetic complications. *N Engl J Med* 1987;316:599–606.
18. Jarrett RJ, Keen H, Chakrabarti R. Diabetes, hypoglycemia, and arterial disease. In: Keen H, Jarrett J eds. *Complications of diabetes,* Ed 2. London: Edward Arnold, 1982;179–204.
19. Hypertension in the diabetic patient. In: Marble A, Krall LP, Bradley RF, Christlieb AR, Soeldner JS, eds. Joslin's *diabetes mellitus,* 12th Ed. Philadelphia: Lea and Febiger, 1985;583–99.
20. Page MMB, Watkins PJ. Cardiorespiratory arrest with diabetic autonomic neuropathy. *Lancet* 1978;1:14.
21. Friedman EA. Diabetic renal disease: In: Ellenberg M, Rifkin H, eds. *Diabetes mellitus, theory and practice,* 3rd Ed. New Hyde Park, NY: Medical Examination Publishing Co., 1983;759:76.
22. Shuman CR. Medical management of the surgical diabetic patient. In: Levin ME, O'Neal LW eds. *The diabetic foot,* Ed 4. St. Louis: C.V. Mosby, 1988;333–41.
23. Schade DS. Surgery and diabetes. *Med Clin N Am* 1988;72:1531–43.
24. Goldberg NJ, Wingert TD, Levin SR, et al. Insulin therapy in the diabetic surgical patient: metabolic and hormone response to low dose insulin infusion. *Diabetes Care* 1981;4:279–84.
25. Watts NB, Gebhart SSP, Clark RV, Phillips LS. Postoperative management of diabetes mellitus: steady-state glucose control with bedside algorithm for insulin adjustment. *Diabetes Care* 1987;10:722–28.
26. Husband DV, Thai AC, Alberti KGMM. Management of diabetes during surgery with glucose-insulin-potassium solution. *Diabetic Med* 1986;3:69–74.
27. Watson BG, Elliott MJ, Pay DA, Williamson M. Diabetes mellitus and open-heart surgery. *Anaesthesia* 1986;41:250–57.
28. Elliott MJ, Gill GV, Home PD, et al. A comparison of two regimens for management of diabetes during open-heart surgery. *Anesthesiology* 1984;60:364–68.
29. Gaare JM, O'Sullivan-Maillet J. Surgery and surgical nutrition in diabetes. In: Powers MA ed. Handbook of Diabetes Nutritional Management. Rockville, MD: Aspen 1987;398–418.
30. Brenner WI, Lansky Z, Engelman RM, et al. Hyperosmolar coma in surgical patients: an iatrogenic disease of increasing incidence. *Ann Surg* 1973;178:651–58.
31. Kuntschen FR, Taillens C, Galletti PM, Hauf E, Hahn C. Coronary surgery in diabetics: metabolic aspects of glycemic control by an artificial pancreas. *Trans Am Soc Artificial Internal Organs* 1982;28:236–9.
32. Schwartz SS, Horwitz DL, Zehus B, et al. Use of a glucose controlled insulin infusion system (artificial beta cell) to control diabetes during surgery. *Diabetologia* 1979;16:157–60.
33. Wheelock FC, Jr, Gibbons GW, Marble A. Surgery in diabetes. In: Marble A, Krall LP, Bradley RF, Christlieb AR, Soeldner JS eds. *Diabetes Mellitus,* 12th Ed. Philadelphia: Lea and Febiger, 1985;712–15.

Surgical Management of the Diabetic Patient,
edited by Michael Bergman and Gregorio A. Sicard.
Raven Press, Ltd., New York © 1991.

4

Nutritional Support

Timothy B. Seaton

Department of Medicine, New York Medical College, Valhalla, New York 10595

Adequate nutritional support is important for patients recovering from illnesses. The objective of nutritional support is to provide energy and nutrients in amounts that meet the needs of individual patients.

Approximately 30 kcal/kg body weight per day should be sufficient to maintain weight for the relatively unstressed middle-aged patient without fever or other hypermetabolic condition. Nitrogen requirements are 0.8 g/kg/day. In patients with depleted protein stores more calories are necessary, depending on the weight desired. In patients acutely stressed by trauma, burns, or infections, nitrogen requirements per kilogram may have to be doubled and caloric requirements increased to 45 kcal/kg/day.

Solid evidence exists for the nitrogen-sparing effect of carbohydrate in both the absence and presence of amino acids. In patients with an inadequate calorie intake, the effect of added carbohydrate on nitrogen sparing is more pronounced than the effect of an isocaloric amount of fat (1).

Glucose is the most commonly used carbohydrate for caloric replacement and provides 3.4 kcal/g. An individual has a limited ability to oxidize glucose and this limit varies considerably depending on the degree of trauma and presence or absence of sepsis. A reasonably stable patient can oxidize up to 14 mg/kg/min (2), whereas a critically ill patient can oxidize only one-half that amount. Giving glucose above the limiting amount results in conversion to fat, an energy-dependant process. Approximately 25% of the caloric value of the excess carbohydrate is required for conversion to fat (3). Lipogenesis also causes an increase in the respiratory quotient greater than 1. In nondiabetic patients this causes a significant increase in minute ventilation and an increased tidal volume with little or no change in frequency. In patients with compromised lung function, however, the added ventilation stimulus of high glucose levels may aggravate preexisting pulmonary compromise (4).

There are several options for meeting the nutritional goals of the diabetic patient who is undergoing surgery and is unable to take food by mouth. Enteral feeding is preferred in the patient with a functional gastrointestinal tract. Feeding tubes can be placed through the nose or surgically placed in the duodenum, stomach, or jejunum. Percutaneous endoscopic jejunostomy is now replacing the surgical placement of feeding tubes. Enteral feedings are not associated with the risk of sepsis or catheter-related complications and are also cheaper and easier to administer.

Tube feeding is indicated in patients who are unable to meet their daily nutritional requirements with a routine oral diet, including food supplements, or in patients where oral intake is contraindicated. These situations include persistent anorexia, uncooperative patients, odonophagia, mechanical impairment to swallowing, fistula of the abdominal tract which can be bypassed by feeding tubes, and increased or altered metabolic needs that cannot be met by voluntary oral intake.

Tube feedings should not be used in patients with total intestinal obstruction, fistula with drainage, severe diarrhea secondary to malabsorption, or persistent vomiting. Patients at high risk for aspiration are those with unpredictable serious vomiting or with significant pulmonary disease and lack of gag reflex. Patients with pharyngitis may experience pain with tube placement, which may preclude using this modality of nutritional support.

There are several types of enteral formulations available; however, many of these tend to be high in simple sugars and low in fiber and fat. This leads to a rapid absorption and marked hyperglycemic response in diabetic patients.

Enteral formulas differ mainly in their caloric density, protein and carbohydrate content, and osmolarity. Some formulas are oligomeric (Vivonex, Vital HN, Tolerex, or Travasorb HN), which contains free amino acids and/or small peptides, glucose oligosaccharides or monosaccharides, and a small amount of fat. It is assumed that these preparations are absorbed more effectively, as hydrolysis by the gastrointestinal tract is not needed. However, the superiority to complex or polymeric formulations has not been clearly proven in clinical trials (5). The oligomeric formulations tend to be more hyperosmolar and more expensive than other preparations and should be reserved for patients who do not tolerate other forms of gastrointestinal feeding.

Commercially available enteral formulations (Complete Modified, Enrich, Ensure, Isocal, Osmolite) contain protein in the form of isolates (soybean, egg albumin, lactalbumin, or casein) and purified sources of carbohydrates, fats, vitamins, and minerals. In these formulations approximately 50% of calories are from carbohydrate, 15% from protein, and 35% from fat. Some products have been specifically formulated for diabetic patients (Glucerna) and contain less carbohydrate (33%) and soluble fiber. The diabetic formulation does not raise the blood sugar level as high as an equivalent amount of Ensure (6). Each patient's response to an enteral feeding product, however, must be evaluated individually and insulin therapy prescribed as necessary.

A variety of carbohydrates has been included in commercial formulations, all of which are eventually hydrolyzed to glucose in the small intestine. In the individual with normal gastrointestinal function, hydrolysis of short- and long-chain glucose polymers is rapid. With marked pancreatic insufficiency with possible amylase insufficiency, oligosaccharides (4–10 units) are useful because they are hydroylzed by the brush border enzymes.

The osmolarity of the various products ranges from 250 to 900 mOsmol/kg water. The initial rapid infusion into the stomach or jejunum of large volumes of high osmotic solutions should be avoided in patients with vagotomy, gastectrectomy, and intestinal dysfunction because of rapid transit and decreased absorption. Hyperosmolar products can cause nausea, vomiting, reflux esophagitis, and diarrhea. Gastroparesis can be exacerbated by hyperosmolar fluids and rapid infusion of formula in the stomach.

Residual volumes should be checked every 4 hours with continuous feeding and just before the next bolus with bolus feedings. The feeding should be delayed if the residual volume is greater than 150 cc. Dilution of hypertonic fluids to an isotonic level (<350 mOsmol/kg water) might improve gastric emptying. Metaclopropamide can be used either orally or subcutaneously to improve gastric emptying in a patient with gastroparesis. Changing the location of food delivery to the small intestine (feeding jejunostomy) eliminates the problems associated with gastroparesis, but may cause severe diarrhea. Hyperosmolarity of the formula is a common cause of the diarrhea; however, lactose intolerance, fat malabsorption, pseudomembranous colitis, and medication-induced diarrhea (antibiotics, antacids, lactulose) must be considered. The first step to improve the diarrhea is to decrease the osmolarity and the delivery rate of the formula. Adding a product containing fiber can also help.

Isotonic formulas can usually be started at full strength at 50 cc/h and increased every 8–12 hours until the desired infusion rate is reached. Hyperosmolar preparations should be diluted to one-quarter strength and the infusion should be gradually increased.

The insulin requirements of patients receiving tube feedings should be adjusted, as the patients will ultimately be getting more calories than they did before starting the feedings. Patients on continuous feedings often have excellent blood glucose control when given intermediate-acting insulin every 12 hours in equal doses. Type I diabetic patients may need additional regular insulin given every 6 hours, based on a sliding scale. Capillary glucose monitoring of blood sugars should be done every 6 hours with a goal of maintaining blood sugar level in the 100–200 mg/dl range. In neutropenic patients, where it may be undesirable to perform frequent capillary monitoring, urine-glucose monitoring can be used. The goal is to prevent an osmotic diuresis, which ultimately results in fluid and electrolyte imbalances. Patients on bolus feedings should receive intermediate-acting insulin in a fashion similar to their usual regimen, i.e., before breakfast and before the evening meal. A sliding scale of regular insulin should be used to prevent hypoglycemia or hyperglycemia. In the event of an unanticipated interruption of the feeding, an intravenous solution of glucose (5 or 10%) should be started to prevent hypoglycemia. Supplemental water, 30–60 cc, given every 6 hours for continuous feedings or after every bolus feeding ensures adequate water intake (0.2 cc of water for every cc of enteral feeding.) The patient's volume and electrolytes status must be watched. Overhydration is common in patients with cardiac, renal, and hepatic disease.

The amount of fat in the defined-formula diets varies from 2 to 50% of the calories. The lipids are usually corn oil or soya oil; however, some have medium-chain triglycerides. The efficiency of absorption of lipids depends on the rate of infusion, the concentration of the nutrient, and the digestive and absorptive capacity of the alimentary tract. Patients with exocrine pancreatic insufficiency may absorb more than 50% of dietary fat, probably because of lingual and gastric lipases. Administration of pancreatic extract is useful in patients with exocrine pancreatic insufficiency.

Parenteral nutrition is used to maintain an adequate nutritional state or improve the status of a previously undernourished patient when oral or tube feeding are contraindicated or grossly inadequate. A variety of clinical situations exists, such as mechanical obstruction of the gastrointestinal tract, disordered peristalsis, severe malabsorption, hypercatabolic state, persistent nausea or vomiting, and severe mucositis. Serious malnutrition is associated with marked increases in infection, respiratory difficulty, skin breakdown, weakness, edema, and psychological problems.

Peripheral parenteral nutrition, with fat emulsions providing a major source of calories, has been used. The final concentration of glucose in the solution, however, must be 10% to avoid the development of phlebitis. The 10% glucose solution often precludes giving enough carbohydrate calories for fat calories and thus limits the total available calories. Peripheral parenteral nutrition may be useful when the duration of the nutrition is expected to be less than 7 days.

There are no absolute guidelines for initiation of total parenteral nutrition (TPN). Previously well-nourished individuals may be maintained on routine intravenous fluids for 5–7 days without the development of debility. If it is anticipated that the period of food intake will be longer, TPN should be started. Severely catabolic or malnourished patients who will not have a functional gastrointestinal tract in 5 days should be started on total parenteral nutrition. People who are obviously not going to ingest food orally or by tube feeding should be started on TPN.

Parenteral nutrition is generally given via central venous access or when adequate calories cannot be supplied by a peripheral route. The TPN formulation contains hypertonic glucose, which must be delivered into a vessel with high blood-flow rate to allow rapid dilution of the glucose. This minimizes the occurrence of phlebitis and thrombosis.

In standard TPN formulations, 65–75% of the calories are given as carbohydrates (500–700 g/day). In diabetic patients this should be reduced to 45–55% (300–400 g/day) with a proportional increase in fat calories (7). Most patients with diabetes require supplemental insulin while on TPN. The insulin can be added directly to the solution. Up to 40% of the insulin added to the TPN solution is lost, however, because it binds to the bag and tubing and an upward adjustment of the insulin dose must be made. The halflife of intravenous insulin approximates 7 minutes so that insulin levels drop rapidly when there is a change in the rate of delivery of the solution or a sudden interruption.

Patients not on insulin should be started on 250 g/day of glucose and have capillary glucose level monitoring performed every 4–6 hours with a sliding scale of regular insulin. Two-thirds of the total insulin can be added to the following day's TPN solution if the total insulin requirements are found to be greater than 20 units per day. If all the glucose values are below 250 mg/dl, the daily amount of glucose should be increased by 70–100 g/day while maintaining the same insulin:glucose ratio.

Patients already on insulin should be started on 100–150 g/day of glucose and half their usual 24-hour insulin requirements added to the TPN formulation. Insulin may have to be increased up to 1.5 times the usual dosage to allow for insulin binding to the bag and tubing. Capillary glucose monitoring should be done every 4–6 hours with a goal of maintaining glucose values between 100–200 mg/dl. A regular insulin sliding scale should be established to add supplemental subcutaneous insulin every 4–6 hours. Two-thirds of the supplemental insulin required during the previous day should be added to the insulin already in the TPN formulation (8). Many factors, including stress, trauma and sepsis, increase insulin requirements.

Maintaining glucose concentrations between 100 and 200 mg/dl avoids problems with hyperglycemia or hypoglycemia. In neutropenic patients where frequent capillary glucose monitoring may be undesirable, urine testing for glucose allows elevated blood glucose levels to be detected. The insulin dosage in these patients should be adjusted to prevent urinary loss of glucose as these cause electrolyte loss and may lead to hyperosmolar state.

Continuous subcutaneous insulin infusion via an insulin pump has been used with patients on TPN as well as with parenteral nutrition (9,10). This modality, however, depends on the familiarity of the support staff with this technique.

Intravenous fat emulsions consist of tiny droplets of triglycerides. Both 10 and

20% concentrations are available and serve as a source of calories and essential fatty acids. The isotonicity and tolerance of the endothelium of the small vessels to intravenous lipid preparations permit the peripheral infusion of a large number of calories. When the concentration of lipid increases to the level at which binding sites on LPL are saturated, a maximal elimination is reached. This is about 3.8 g of fat/kg/24h (35 kcal/kg/24h) (11). The clearance rate increases with starvation and trauma. Daily infusion of fat emulsion is associated with increased tolerance, as indicated by decreased triglyceride levels. Serum free fatty acids (FFA) are cleared more rapidly when carbohydrate is administered simultaneously. Hypercatabolic states also affect the degree of lipid metabolism. Trauma is associated with increased clearance of exogenous lipids, whereas glucose oxidation is limited in these patients.

Medium-chain triglycerides have an established role in oral and enteral nutrition but recently have been used in TPN formulations on an experimental basis. The medium-chain triglycerides are rapidly oxidized by the liver with the formation of ketones. Medium chain triglycerides (MCT) are utilized by extra hepatic tissues and do not require carnitine to cross the mitochondrial border as do long-chain triglycerides (11).

Complications of fluid and electrolyte abnormalities can be avoided by frequent monitoring of glucose values and obtaining a daily complete chemistry profile. Nonketotic hyperosmolar state occurs more frequently in diabetic patients on TPN; if it does occur, the TPN infusion should be stopped and insulin and hypotonic fluids administered until the condition is resolved. Phosphate depletion can be a significant problem. There is increased phosphate metabolism in malnourished patients started on TPN because of glucose metabolism and protein synthesis. Glucose intolerance caused by chromium deficiency has been reported in long-term administration of TPN. Nutrient deficiencies or excesses, metabolic problems, including abnormal plasma amino acid levels, liver dysfunction, bone abnormalities, hyperglycemia or hypoglycemia, infection, problems with insertion of catheters or ports, and psychological problems. Cholestasis has been reported in a large number of patients receiving TPN formulations. There is often a mild to moderate rise in alkaline phosphatase and aminotransferase. Catheter and ports should be placed by experienced physicians under aseptic conditions. Close supervision, good technique, and aggressive and rational antibiotic coverage bring about excellent results. Infection must be considered in any unexplained sudden increase in the blood glucose levels. Contamination of the line must be avoided. Clotted lines can be treated with urokinase infusion.

Adequate nutritional support is important for recovery from illness. The nutritional management of the diabetic patient is generally similar to other surgical patients; however, frequent blood-glucose level monitoring must be done and patients should be started on nutritional supplements containing lower amounts of carbohydrate. The carbohydrate content is gradually increased depending on the blood glucose values. Insulin dosage must be adjusted on the basis of the measured glucose concentrations and may vary from day to day as the diet is advanced and as surgical stress diminishes.

REFERENCES

1. Shaw SN, Elwyn DH, Askanazi J, Iles M, Schwarz Y, Kinney JM. Effects of increasing nitrogen intake on balance and energy expenditure in nutritionally depleted adult patients receiving parenteral nutrition. *Am J Clin Nutr* 1983;37:930–940.

2. Wolfe RR, Alsop JR, Burke JF. Glucose metabolism in man: response to intravenous glucose infusion. *Metabolism* 1979;28:210–220.
3. Elwyn DH, Grump FE, Munro HN, Isles M, Kinney JM. Changes in nitrogen balance of depleted patients with increasing infusions of glucose. *Am J Clin Nutr* 1979;32:1597–1601.
4. Askanazi J, Nordenstrom J, Rosenbaum SH, et al. Nutrition for the patient with respiratory failure: glucose versus fat. *Anesthesiology* 1981;54:373–377.
5. Koretz RL, Meyer JH. Elemental diets—facts and fantasies. *Gastroenterology* 1980;78:383–410.
6. Peters AL, Davidson MB, Issac RM. Lack of glucose elevation after simulated tube feeding with a low-carbohydrate high fat enteral formula in patients with type I diabetes. *Am J Med* 1989;87:178–182.
7. Clouse RE, Sandrock M. Intensive nutritional support. *Diabetes Spectrum* 1989;2:329–384.
8. Mascioli EA, Bistrian BR. Total parenteral nutrition in the patient with diabetes. *Nutr Support Services* 1983;3:12–16.
9. Beau P, Marechaud R, Matuchansky C. Cyclic total parenteral nutrition, diabetes mellitus, and subcutaneous insulin pump. *Lancet* 1986;1:1272–1273.
10. Bergman M, RaviKumar S, Auerhahn C, DelSavio N, Savino J, Felig P. Insulin pump therapy improves glucose control during hyperalimentation. *Arch Int Med* 1984;144:2013–2015.
11. Adamkin DH, Gelke KN, Andrews BF. Fat emulsions and hypertriglyceridemia. *J Parenter Enteral Nutr* 1984;8:563–567.
12. Bach AC, Babayan VK. Medium-chain triglycerides: an update. *Am J Clin Nutr* 1982;36:950–962.

Surgical Management of the Diabetic Patient,
edited by Michael Bergman and Gregorio A. Sicard.
Raven Press, Ltd., New York © 1991.

5

Wound Healing in Diabetes

William H. Goodson, III

*Department of Surgery, University of California Medical Center,
San Francisco, California 94143*

Today, surgery is performed in diabetic patients with the expectation that wounds will heal and there will not be excess mortality. This is a significant change from the turn of the century when mortality approached 25% for elective surgery in diabetic patients. The improved surgical outcome has been achieved by understanding the pathophysiology of diabetes and by improvements in general and perioperative care of diabetic patients.

When we reviewed wound healing and diabetes 10 years ago (1) the major conclusion was that better control produced lower mortality and better healing. In the past decade there have been major increases in understanding the biology of wound healing, and the general pathophysiology of diabetes. This discussion, therefore, brings together experimental studies of wounds in diabetic patients and animal models of diabetics, and studies of various aspects of diabetic pathophysiology that are relevant to pivotal aspects of wound healing, both understood in the context of improved clinical understanding of diabetes.

ANIMAL STUDIES OF WOUND HEALING IN DIABETES

Animal studies consistently show a decrease in wound parameters in experimental diabetes. The majority of studies have been in animals with diabetes induced by alloxan or streptozotocin, both of which selectively destroy pancreatic beta cells and cause an insulin-deficient, type I or insulin-dependent diabetes.

Animals with induced diabetes have decreased wound strength and decreased wound collagen (2). The effects of diabetes can be seen very early in healing. For example, at 8 hours there is a decrease in wound capillaries, fibroblasts, polymorphonuclear leukocytes, and collagen, and an increase in edema in diabetic animals (Fig. 1) (3). Animals treated with insulin are closer to controls, but are not totally normal. The importance of insulin in these early phases of healing is shown in a complementary study by the same authors in which an antibody to insulin also caused reduced capillaries, collagen, fibroblasts, and polymorphonuclear leukocytes and increased edema (4). Hyperosmolarity with a metabolically inert sugar did not alter healing. Similar results have been obtained with Chinese hamsters that are spontaneously diabetic (5). Thus wound healing defects can be detected in dermal wounds as early as 8 hours; these defects seem directly related to a decreased effect of insulin. (There is one study with conflicting results, in that three days after wound-

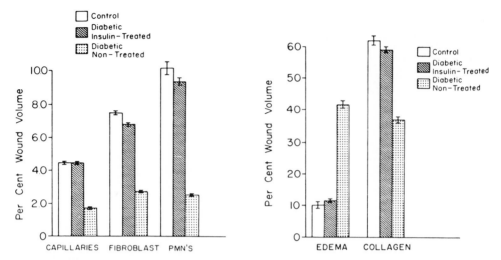

FIG. 1. Morphometric analysis of the volume of wounds occupied by various elements 8 hours after a puncture wound of the ear in diabetic mice compared with controls. Untreated diabetic mice have fewer capillaries, fewer fibroblasts, fewer polymorphonuclear leukocytes and less collagen, but more edema. After Weringer et al., ref. 3.

ing, diabetic animals were healing ahead of the control animals (6). However these studies were carried out in animals with defects in bowel mesentery and therefore may not relate to effects in cutaneous wounds).

The importance of an early defect in diabetic wounds was further evaluated in an experiment in which wound chambers were implanted in streptozotocin diabetic animals for three weeks (7). One and one-half weeks of insulin therapy begun at the time of injury gave results comparable to controls: when the same amount of insulin was begun a week and a half after injury however, there was no benefit at all. As with puncture wounds in animals, these authors concluded that the importance of early insulin indicated that uncontrolled diabetes had an effect on early healing events, quite possibly inflammation.

Andreassen and Oxlund (8) added measurements of standard engineering parameters and found that, 7, 10, and 20 days after wounding, diabetic animals had less maximum stress and decreased relative failure energy in incised wounds. Healing improved only when the animals were started on insulin at the time diabetes was induced. Healing was best in diabetic animals with some long-term effort at control. Yue et al. (9) refined the relationship of long-term control even further when they showed an inverse relationship of wound healing strength to levels of glycosylated hemoglobin (Fig. 2). Thus control is not only an issue of initiation of healing after surgery, but it is also part of preparation for surgery.

Seifter et al. (10) tested the importance of early insulin treatment data to inflammatory effects by treating streptozotocin diabetic animals with vitamin A—a known stimulant of wound inflammation. They found that vitamin A produced an increase in wound-breaking strength and collagen accumulation, but more important was their observation that the vitamin A achieved improvement in healing without lowering hyperglycemia or reducing the polyuria, polydipsia, polyphagia triad seen in diabetic animals. As with the work of Weringer, this suggested that the defect is not the

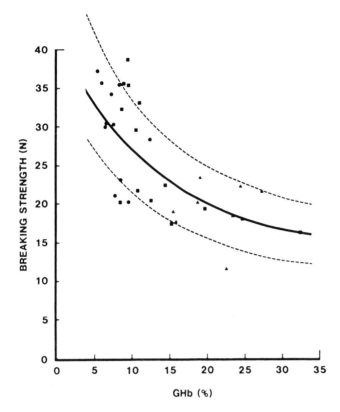

FIG. 2. Wound-breaking strength versus glycosylated hemoglobulin levels. Circles equal normal rats, triangles equal diabetic rats without insulin, squares equal diabetic rats with insulin. This relationship supports the importance of better control, including long-term preoperative control. After Yue et al., ref. 9.

hyperglycemia but rather the absence of growth factors or other growth stimulants related to insulin that cause the defect in healing. Grotendorst et al. (11) evaluated platelet-derived growth factor (PDGF) in wounds in diabetic animals and found improved healing, especially if the PDGF was combined with insulin applied locally in the wound. The local insulin by itself did not have benefit. These results again suggest the importance of local insulin and mediators associated with early inflammatory response in diabetes. Other studies with basic fibroblast growth factor and transforming growth factor have not shown results that are as beneficial (12). Related *in vivo* animal studies have also examined fracture healing and infection. Macey et al. (13) found a 29% decrease in callus and a 50% decrease in stiffness in closed femoral fractures in diabetic animals as compared with controls. Insulin corrected the defects in physical measurement and also the 50% reduction in collagen in callus.

There have been several *in vivo* studies of infection of diabetic animals. These are not direct studies of wound healing, but because inflammation is necessary for normal healing they are relevant. Two studies are presented by way of illustration.

Herbert and Coil (14) demonstrated increased susceptibility of diabetic mice to an inspired aerosol of type III *streptococcus pneumoniae*. This was corrected with insulin. Bessman et al. (15) evaluated persistence of bacteria in abscesses created with *Escherichia coli* (E. coli), enterococcus, and bacteroides fragilis. Diabetic animals have more persistent bacteria at two weeks; of special note, is that by two weeks nondiabetic animals had eliminated *Bacteroides fragilis* (*B. fragilis*) while it persisted in many diabetic animals. In a follow-up study with combinations of bacteria, these authors observed that pH ranged from 6.28 to 6.79 in infected wounds in diabetic animals compared with 7.17 to 7.30 in infected controls (16). Even uninfected wounds in diabetic animals are somewhat more acidic [pH 7.23 compared to 7.36 in controls (2)]. But the extreme drop in the infected diabetic animal probably reflects an additional compromise in resistance to infection, which may be due to local inflammatory processes. It may also reflect decrease perfusion because of poor capillary growth (3) or there may be decreased perfusion because of dehydration. Either way, wounds are more susceptible to infection in diabetic patients, and the wound environment is more adverse in the presence of infection in diabetics.

There have been only limited studies of models of noninsulin-dependent, insulin-resistant, or type II diabetes. Goodson and Hunt (17) have studied wounds in obese mice. Such animals are insulin resistant, obese, hyperglycemic (though rarely ketotic) and they heal poorly (Fig 3). Unlike insulin-dependent diabetes, however, these animals do not improve healing with insulin treatment. In fact, studies of individual animals studied before and after development of the obese phenotype and studies of diet restriction in genetically obese mice led these authors to conclude that poor healing develops as the animal becomes obese and may be related equally or perhaps more to the physical properties of skin and subcutaneous tissue of obese individuals than to the hyperglycemia in these animals.

Animal studies conclude universally that diabetes has an adverse effect upon healing. These effects relate to the early events of healing; in most individual studies of insulin-dependent diabetes, the adverse effects are reversible. The limited studies of non-insulin dependent diabetes do not indicate an improvement after insulin control of hyperglycemia and suggest that the physical presence of adipose tissue may con-

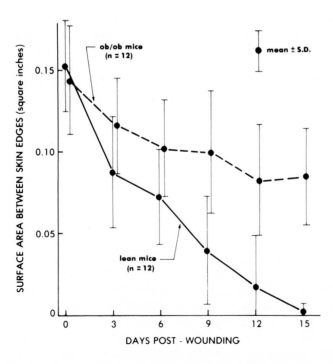

FIG. 3. Surface area (measured by planimetry) of open wounds in obese hyperglycemic mice and their lean litter mates. Wounds close much slower in these animals with a model of type II insulin-resistant diabetes. Insulin treatment did not improve healing in these animals. After Goodson et al., ref. 17.

tribute to wound complications in this type of diabetes that is often associated with excess adipose tissue in humans.

CLINICAL STUDIES OF HEALING IN DIABETIC PATIENTS

As reviewed elsewhere (1), the improvement in surgical care of diabetes has been parallel with understanding of diabetic care in general. In 1902, Phillips reported his results on surgery in 90 diabetic patients: 24% suffered wound complications and there was a 24% mortality. This was in comparison to 6.3% mortality rate for gastric surgery at the Mayo Clinic at the same time. Preoperative treatment with dietary restriction, popularized by Allen in 1914, led to decreased mortality; within a few years of the clinical introduction of insulin therapy, surgery could occur without major complications in diabetic patients.

Nevertheless, complications are seemingly more frequent among diabetic patients. In their monumental study of 23,649 wounds, Cruse and Foord found a 10.7% infection rate in patients with diabetes compared with a 1.8% rate in nondiabetic patients. The results of studies of lower extremity amputations indicate there has been, in the past, a trend toward more wound failure in diabetic patients, but in six of seven studies the difference was not significant (1). Because of this trend, care of the lower extremities is an area that has been studied closely to summarize the implications of clinical wound healing in persons with diabetes.

Because of their chronic disease, diabetic patients are at greater risk of vascular disease and may have more problems as a result; with proper care, these are not overwhelming problems.

When vascular disease is present it is more likely to progress to more serious complications in diabetic than in nondiabetic patients. Jonasson and Ringqvist followed 47 persons with diabetes with intermittent claudication for six years (18). Gangrene developed in 31% and rest pain and/or gangrene developed in 40%, compared with 5% and 18%, respectively, in nondiabetic persons. This progression of disease is also reflected in their 6-year study in which mortality was 50% in diabetic patients compared with 26% in nondiabetic patients. This agrees with the high incidence of end-organ disease (kidney, heart, etc.) in diabetic patients who undergo surgery (19).

The risk of progression of disease, however, does not mean that diabetic patients cannot heal when they have adequate blood flow. Christensen et al. (20) demonstrated a direct relationship between skin perfusion pressure and healing of above-knee or below-knee amputations. Among these patients, there was a higher below-knee perfusion pressure, an average that reflects the patient population. However, when they matched patients in corresponding categories of skin perfusion pressure, diabetic patients were as likely to heal as nondiabetic patients. Thus, when present, the vascular occlusive disease restricted healing but not the diabetes *per se,* i.e., diabetic patients may require more intensive wound and general care, but they can heal. A more recent report by Rubinstein and Pierce (21) indicates what can be accomplished with intense therapy. Twelve of 15 patients with neuropathy and foot ulcers were healed with intensive wound care and diabetic control.

It is not always necessary to hospitalize a patient to provide proper care to prevent amputation. Malone et al. (22) randomly selected 100 diabetic patients to receive education on self-care. After a mean of 12 months follow-up, 96% of the patients still had intact limbs compared with 88% of a control group followed for a mean of only 8 months. Thus, care and prompt attention to problems can prevent complications. Because nicks and scratches are almost unavoidable aspects of life, this suggests that with care and control of disease, healing can be achieved in diabetes. This conclusion is supported by what limited clinical experimental data are available. Goodson and Hunt (23), using a small invasive tube device to measure human healing in the upper arm of volunteers, found that well-controlled diabetic men (mean HbA1C of 9% and an average of 37 units of insulin per day in three or four divided doses) healed as well as control patients despite a mean duration of disease of 11 years. In the other clinical study of diabetic wounds, Olerud et al. (24) did find a decrease in fibroblasts and collagen in test wounds in the lower extremities of diabetic patients compared to controls. However, those with diabetes were indistinguishable from patients with peripheral vascular disease but without diabetes, and there were no healing problems in the amputations in either group.

Although animal studies can sometimes be interpreted to indicate poor healing in diabetic patients, those who have used insulin therapy usually see a return nearly to normal. Combined with the successful care of the limbs of diabetic patients, the success of clinical surgery, and the experimental data showing restoration of healing with insulin, it seems more accurate to conclude that a person with well-controlled diabetes can heal well. The problem of wound healing in diabetes is therefore not an obstacle that has yet to be mastered. It is, fortunately, a reality that usually occurs without a problem. The questions that remain concern how to understand what can go wrong and cause poor healing if diabetes has not been successfully managed. The list of potential causes of poor healing is growing.

POSSIBLE MECHANISMS OF HEALING FAILURE IN DIABETES

Successful healing of wounds results from the interaction of a complex series of local and systemic factors. The process requires recognition of injury, which generally is triggered by local events such as damage of endothelium or skin and/or exposure of bare collagen to clotting factors and other inflammatory mediators normally found in blood. Clotting factors, along with circulating cells—most notably platelets, polymorphonuclear leukocytes (PMN), macrophages, and to a lesser extent lymphocytes—quickly collect in wounds and initiate the next phases of healing as well as contribute to hemostasis, resistance to infection, and removal of dead or damaged tissue and foreign bodies. These cells (and damaged endothelium) release various growth factors that act locally and systemically to attract other inflammatory cells, register pain, and initiate collagen repair. As has long been recognized, collagen synthesis by fibroblasts is a central requirement for tissue repair, but the refinements in understanding are what control the function of fibroblasts. It must also be understood that, in order to function, fibroblasts and other cells require adequate circulation to bring the oxygen, nutrients, and necessary inflammatory cells as well as to remove toxic wastes from the wound environment and to carry them to the liver, kidneys, and lungs for disposal.

When there is poor healing, questions should address how diabetes might effect factors that control healing and/or how diabetes might limit the ability of cells, circulation, or growth factors to produce normal healing. There are almost as many possible mechanisms for poor healing in diabetes as there have been experimental studies. In all probability, when healing problems occur in persons with diabetes, the etiologies are as diverse as the causes of the various other complications that beset diabetics.

Almost at the moment of injury, platelets arrive alive in a wound. They participate in the initial processes of hemostasis and also release potent factors that influence healing, e.g., platelet-derived growth factor (PDGF) which stimulates angiogenesis, fibroblast growth, and collagen synthesis; thromboxane A_2 (a potent vasoconstrictor); and prostaglandins, which mediate pain and vascular permeability. In poorly controlled diabetes, platelets are hypersensitive to aggregating agents but there is disagreement whether this occurs if diabetes is well controlled (25). For example, Hendra et al. (26) found normal function in platelets from diabetic patients, but Gisinger (27) found that thromboxane A_2 release was increased in all diabetic patients (their report was in the context of studies showing that therapeutic doses of vitamin E normalize thromboxane A_2 release). Trovati et al. (28) have strengthened the argument that control restores normal aggregation by showing in normal volunteers that insulin leads to a reduction in platelet aggregation, i.e., control seems likely to restore normal function resulting from a reduction in aggregation. Sugimoto et al. (29) have approached the problem directly from the standpoint of function. Using a crude extract applied to explanted endothelial cells, they measured growth-promoting activity in platelets from diabetic patients. With conventional control there was an increase in 3H-thymidine uptake by fibroblasts exposed to platelet extract from diabetic subjects, but after three months of tight control, the response of 3H-thymidine uptake was similar to nondiabetic controls. Sugimoto et al. agree with the postulate that this growth activity, which probably involves PDGF, may contribute to intimal growth in atherosclerotic lesions. If this occurs, as seems likely, the increased platelet function could also occur in wounds. Because the addition of PDGF in fact enhances healing (11), it seems unlikely that the platelet dysfunctions described so far in diabetes would adversely affect healing.

The next cells to arrive in a wound are polymorphonuclear leukocytes (PMN), which are responsible for primary nonspecific resistance to infection by ingesting and killing bacteria. PMNs have been studied extensively. In the presence of hyperglycemia there is a decrease in phagocytosis and killing of various bacteria (30,31). Mowat and Baum (32) showed that PMNs from diabetic individuals had a decreased chemotactic response and Molenaar et al. (33) showed that there was also a decreased response in first degree relatives of diabetic persons. Bagdade and Walters (34) showed that granulocyte adhesiveness was decreased in outpatients whose only sign of disease was hyperglycemia. After 4 weeks of therapy, granulocyte adhesion improved if hyperglycemia responded to treatment. Recently Neilson and Hindson (35) have shown that the respiratory burst that accompanies normal phagocytosis is decreased in the presence of high glucose concentration. This occurs both with the D and L isomers so it is probably not related to the metabolism of glucose, but rather to a direct effect of the hypertonic solution.

Although it is clear that PMNs may function poorly in diabetes, this probably has minimal effect on healing unless there is heavy contamination with the inherent risk of infection. The reason for this is that healing can proceed normally in the absence of PMNs; the *necessary* inflammatory cell for healing is the macrophage.

The pivotal role of the macrophage in wound healing has been the subject of much wound-healing research in the last two decades. Macrophages are a major source of chemotactic, angiogenic, mitogenic, and collagen-stimulating factors. Without macrophages, wounds do not heal. Much of the literature on diabetes has considered macrophages immune agents in the development of diabetes via isletitis, although there have been few studies of general macrophage function in diabetes. The available studies, however, do suggest decreased function. Jones et al. (36) found they could elicit fewer peritoneal macrophages in diabetic animals and Van Rees et al. (37) found evidence of a general decrease in cellular immune function in BB diabetic rats. In this regard, the increased metabolic parameters reported by Kitaham et al. (38) in blood monocytes are puzzling. As was evident with enhanced platelet activity, it is difficult to understand how increased function can impair healing. On the other hand, if macrophages are less responsive to chemical stimuli in diabetes, a similar defect in wounds could significantly retard healing. Macrophage function in diabetic wounds deserve more study.

The fibroblast is the final common cellular pathway in healing. It synthesizes collagen, which is the basis for the restoration of tissue continuity. In extensive studies of fibroblasts from diabetic patients consistent alterations in function have not been demonstrated (39). Insulin has a direct effect on collagen formation as does glucose, but this seems to be true in fibroblasts from both diabetic and nondiabetic persons. For example, among the Pima Indians (a population with high risk of developing diabetes) no difference in thymidine labeling could be detected between diabetic and nondiabetic individuals (40). Both groups, however, have significantly lower labeling than Caucasian controls. It is possible that the decrease seen in the entire population is somehow related to the predisposition to diabetes, but at this time a mechanism is speculative. In two Scandinavian studies (41,42), however, which included controls as well as insulin-dependent and insulin nondependent diabetic persons, the authors found that the resting rate of collagen formation was similar. When insulin was added, normal cells increased collagen production by about 50% while fibroblasts from both types of diabetes increased collagen production by nearly 100%. Thus, an inability to respond to insulin does not seem to be present in fibroblast obtained from diabetic subjects.

The work of Spanheimer (43) indicates a more likely explanation for limited fibroblast function: a high molecular weight substance in serum from diabetic animals inhibits collagen formation in culture. An alternative explanation might also be that ascorbic acid, a necessary cofactor for collagen formation, is reduced in plasma and tissue in diabetic persons (44).

Study of fibroblasts may give some clues to healing, but as noted above, collagen formation is nearly normal in well-controlled diabetic animals and humans. The collagen in diabetes is, like hemoglobin, exposed to higher glucose concentrations. This means that the process of passive (nonenzymatic) glycation (formerly called glycosylation) may occur more rapidly. This situation, similar to the aging process (45), makes collagen more insoluble (46) changes its molecular structure (47), and may interact with a macrophage system, which specifically seems to remove glycated proteins (48). Recently, Vishwanath et al. have shown that complications of diabetes (e.g., retinal, renal, and arterial disease) were directly related to increased amounts of glycated collagen in skin biopsies from diabetic subjects (Fig. 4) (49). There is no obvious relationship of this to healing, since glycation occurs in collagen even as it is being formed (45); possible structural differences in collagen formed during poor control of diabetes should be studied further. For example, a possible clinical effect of collagen abnormalities is supported by the observation of limited joint mobility in diabetic persons, and correlates with the development of microvascular disease (50), which probably correlates with control of diabetes (see below).

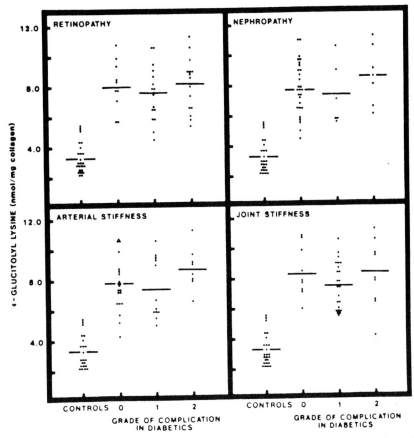

FIG. 4. The relationship of glycated collagen (reflected as glycated lysine in collagen) to the development of complications of diabetes. After Vishwanath et al., ref. 49.

The final possible mechanism of healing failure is microvascular and/or macrovascular diseases. As noted above, major vessel occlusion is common and usually progressive with diabetes. Arterial occlusion is an unambiguous impediment to healing even in the absence of diabetes and will not be considered further in this discussion. The role of microvascular disease is less clear.

Electronic microscopy study of many tissues indicates diabetic individuals do have visible thickening of the capillary basement membrane, especially skin and kidneys. Capillary basement membrane thickening (CBMT) increases with the duration of diabetes and is present in first degree relatives of diabetic persons, but is probably not genetic in origin because it also develops in animals with induced-insulin dependent diabetes (e.g., streptozotocin) (51). The ubiquitous presence of this change makes it a likely component of diabetic pathophysiology. It can be shown that surgical complications are more common in diabetic patients with CBMT than in nondiabetic subjects, although it is difficult to control these studies by evaluation of diabetes in the absence of CBMT (52). Thus, the effect of CBMT on healing is not defined. The cause of CBMT is also not defined, but it seems to relate to abnormal glycation and possibly increased permeability. Glycated lysine residues are more common in diabetic basement membranes (53). This may contribute to the decrease in the proteoglycan component of the basement membrane (54,55). Proteoglycans have major functional roles in other tissues and it is expected that they also have a significant role in capillary function, which may relate to ion permeability. In addition to possible secondary effects of protein glycation on proteoglycan content, there is also evidence of reduced proteoglycan synthesis in diabetic individuals (56). The passive nature of the etiology of CBMT is further suggested by studies that show a relation of CBMT to the duration of the disease (57). Conditions associated with CBMT (e.g., nephropathy and retinopathy) improve with enhanced control subsequent to insulin use (58) and, more important, CBMT decreases with the use of oral hypoglycemic agents (59). Thus, CBMT seems to reflect the disease process rather than cause it.

Whatever the mechanism, increased permeability does occur in capillaries of diabetic individuals (60,61). Although increased vascular permeability is a normal part of healing, the role of increased permeability in diabetes is unclear. It is also possible that small vessels function abnormally in ways not related to CBMT. For example, autonomic vasoconstriction in response to cold is reduced in diabetic persons (62), pulse-wave form is flattened and abnormalities in minute blood flow response to exercise have been noted as well (63).

CONCLUSION

Experimental studies and clinical experience have shown that patients with well-controlled diabetes can heal normally. There are, however, many known aspects of diabetic pathophysiology that might adversely affect healing. These include increased platelet aggregation, decreased white cell function, recently confirmed impaired opsonic efficacy (64), direct or indirect effects on fibroblast synthesis of collagen, nonenzymatic changes in collagen or capillary structures secondary to exposure to high levels of glucose, and possible alterations in vasomotor control.

REFERENCES

1. Goodson WH III, Hunt TK. Wound healing and the diabetic patient. *Surg Gynecol Obstet* 1979;149:600–608.
2. Goodson WH III, Hunt TK. Studies of wound healing in experimental diabetes mellitus. *J Surg Res* 1977;22:221–227.
3. Weringer EJ, Kelso JM, Tamai IY, et al. Effects of insulin on wound healing in diabetic mice. *Acta Endocrinol* 1982;99:101–108.
4. Weringer EJ, Tami IY, Arquilla ER. The effect of antisera to insulin, 2-deoxyglucose-induced hyperglycemia, and starvation on wound healing in normal mice. *Diabetes* 1981;30:407–410.
5. Weringer EJ, Arqilla ER. Wound healing in normal and diabetic Chinese hamsters. *Diabetologia* 1981;21:394–401.
6. Franzen L, Norrby K. Mitogenesis in wound-healing cells in diabetic rats. *APMIS* 1988;519–524, 1988.
7. Goodson WH III, Hunt TK. Wound healing in experimental diabetes mellitus: importance of early insulin therapy. *Surg Form* 1978;29:95–98.
8. Andreassen TT, Oxlund H. The influence of experimental diabetes and insulin treatments on the biomechanical properties of rat skin incisional wounds. *Acta Chir Scand* 1987;153:405–409.
9. Yue DK, McLennan S, Marsh M, et al. Effects of experimental diabetes, uremia, and malnutrition on wound healing. *Diabetes* 1987;36:295–299.
10. Seifter E, Rettura G, Padawer J, et al. Impaired wound healing in streptozotocin diabetes. Prevention by supplemental vitamin A. *Ann Surg* 1981;194:42–50.

11. Grotendorst GR, Martin GR, Pencev D, et al. Stimulation of granulation tissue formation by platelet-derived growth factor in normal and diabetic rats. *J Clin Invest* 1985;76:2323–2329.

12. Broadley KN, Aquino AM, Hicks B, et al. Growth factors bFGF and TGBB accelerate the rate of wound repair in normal and in diabetic rats. *Int J Tissue React* 1988;10:345–353.

13. Macey LR, Kana SM, Jingushi S, et al. Defects of early fracture-healing in experimental diabetes. *J Bone Joint Surg* 1989;71-A:722–733.

14. Herbert JC, Coil JA Jr. Increased susceptibility to pulmonary infection in alloxan diabetic mice. *J Surg Res* 1981;31:337–342.

15. Bessman AN, Sapico FL, Tabatabai M, et al. Persistence of polymicrobial abscesses in the poorly controlled diabetic host. *Diabetes* 1986;35:448–453.

16. Bessman AN, Page J, Thomas LJ. *In vivo* pH induced soft-tissue abscess in diabetic and nondiabetic mice. *Diabetes* 1989;39:659–662.

17. Goodson WH III, Hunt TK. Wound collagen accumulation in obese hyperglycemic mice. *Diabetes* 1986;35:491–495.

18. Jonasson T, Ringqvist I: Diabetes mellitus and intermittent claudication. Relation between peripheral vascular complications and location of the occlusive atherosclerosis in the legs. *Acta Med Scand* 1985;218:217–221.

19. MacKenzie CR, Charlson ME. Assessment of perioperative risk in the patient with diabetes mellitus. *Surg Gynecol Obstet* 1988;167:293–299.

20. Christensen KS, Falstie-Jensen N, Christensen ES, et al. Results of amputation for gangrene in diabetic and non-diabetic patients. *J Bone Joint Surg* 1988;17-A:1514–1519.

21. Rubinstein A, Pierce CE Jr II. Rapid healing of diabetic foot ulcers with meticulous blood glucose control. *Acta Diabetol Lat* 1988;25:25–32.

22. Malone JM, Snyder M, Anderson G, et al. Prevention of amputation by diabetic education. *Am J Surg* 1989;158:520–524.

23. Goodson WH III, Hunt TK. Wound healing in well-controlled diabetic men. *Surg Form* 1984;35:614–616.

24. Olerud J, Odland G, Burgess E, et al. The systematic study of partial thickness wounds in normal elderly adults and patients with peripheral vascular disease (PVD) and diabetes mellitus (DM). *J Invest Dermatol* 1989;92:494.

25. Mustard JF, Packham MA. Platelets and diabetes mellitus. *N Engl J Med* 1984;311:665–667.

26. Hendra TJ, Oughton J, Smith CCT, et al. Platelet function in uncomplicated insulin-dependent diabetic patients at rest and following exercise. *Diabetic Med* 1988;5:469–473.

27. Gisinger C, Jeremy J, Speiser P, et al. Effect of vitamin E supplementation on platelet thromboxane A_2 production in type I diabetic patients. *Diabetes* 1988;37:1260–1264.

28. Trovati M, Anfossi G, Cavalot F, et al. Insulin directly reduces platelet sensitivity to aggregating agents. Studies *in vitro* and *in vivo*. *Diabetes* 1988;37:780–786.

29. Sugimoto H, Franks DJ, Lecavalier L, et al. Therapeutic modulation of growth-promoting activity in platelets from diabetics. *Diabetes* 1987;36:667–672.

30. van Oss CJ. Influence of glucose levels on the in vitro phagocytosis of bacteria by human neutrophils. *Infect Immun* 1971;4:54–59.

31. Bagdade JD, Root RK, Bulger RJ. Impaired leukocyte function in patients with poorly controlled diabetes. *Diabetes* 1974;23:9–15.

32. Mowat AG, Baum J. Chemotaxis of polymorphonuclear leukocytes from patients with diabetes mellitus. *N Engl J Med* 1971;284:621–627.

33. Molenaar DM, Palumbo PJ, Wilson WR, et al. Leukocyte chemotaxis in diabetic patients and their nondiabetic first-degree relatives. *Diabetes* 1976;25(Suppl 2):880–883.

34. Bagdade JD, Walters E. Impaired granulocyte adherence in mildly diabetic patients. Effects of tolazamide treatment. *Diabetes* 1980;29:309–311.

35. Nielson CP, Hindson DA. Inhibition of polymorphonuclear leukocyte respiratory burst by elevated glucose concentrations *in vitro*. *Diabetes* 1989;38:1031–1035.

36. Jones CA, Seifert MF, Dixit PK. Macrophage migration inhibition in experimental diabetes (41434). *Proc Soc Exp Biol Med* 1982;170:298–304.

37. van Rees EP, Voorbij HAM, Dijkstra CD. Neonatal development of lymphoid organs and specific immune responses *in situ* in diabetes-prone BB rats. *Immunology* 1988;65:465–472.

38. Kitahara M, Eyre HJ, Lynch RE, et al. Metabolic activity of diabetic monocytes. *Diabetes* 1980;29:251–256.

39. Rowe DW, Starman BJ, Fujimoto WY, et al. Abnormalities in proliferation and protein synthesis in skin fibroblast cultures from patients with diabetes mellitus. *Diabetes* 1977;26:284–290.

40. Howard BV, Helds RM, Mott DM, et al. Diabetes and cell growth—lack of differences in growth characteristics of fibroblasts from diabetic and nondiabetic Pima Indians. *Diabetes* 1980;29:119–124.

41. Kjellstrom T, Malmquist J. Effects of heparin and dextran sulphate on the production of collagen and protein in diabetic and non-diabetic human skin fibroblast cultures. *Med Biol* 1983;61:186–190.

42. Kjellstrom T, Malmquist J. Insulin effects on collagen and protein production in cultured human skin fibroblasts from diabetic and non-diabetic subjects. *Horm Metab Res* 1984;16:168–171.
43. Spanheimer RG. Direct inhibition of collagen production *in vitro* by diabetic rat serum. *Metabolism* 1988;37:479–485.
44. McLennan S, Yue DK, Fisher E, et al. Deficiency of ascorbic acid in experimental diabetes. Relationship with collagen and polyol pathway abnormalities. *Diabetes* 1988;37:359–361.
45. Monnier VM, Sell DR, Abdul-Karim FW, et al. Collagen browning and cross-linking are increased in chronic experimental hyperglycemia. *Diabetes* 1988;37:867–872.
46. Chang K, Uitto J, Rowold EA, et al. Increased collagen cross-linkages in experimental diabetes. Reversal by B-aminopropionitrile and D-penicillamine. *Diabetes* 1980;29:778–781.
47. Tanaka S, Avigad G, Brodsky B, et al. Glycation induces expansion of the molecular packing of collagen. *J Mol Biol* 1988;203:495–505.
48. Vlassara H, Brownlee M, Cerami A. Specific macrophage receptor activity for advanced glycosylation end products inversely correlates with insulin levels *in vivo*. *Diabetes* 1988;37:456–461.
49. Vishwanath V, Krank KE, Elmets CA, et al. Glycation of skin collagen in type I diabetes mellitus. *Diabetes* 1986;35:916–921.
50. Rosenbloom AL, Silverstein JH, Lezotte DC, et al. Limited joint mobility in childhood diabetes mellitus indicates increased risk for microvascular disease. *N Engl J Med* 1981;305:191–194.
51. Sipperstein MD. Diabetic microangiopathy. *West J Med* 1974;121:404–412.
52. Kihara S-I, Mori K, Masanobu A. Electron microscopic observation of gastric mucosal capillaries in diabetics. Relationship between diabetic micro-angiopathy and complications following gastrectomy. *Gastroenterol Jpn* 1983;18:181–196.
53. Garlick RL, Bunn HF, Spiro RG. Nonenzymatic glycation of basement membranes from human glomeruli and bovine sources. *Diabetes* 1988;37:1144–1150.
54. Tarsio JF, Reger LA, Furcht LT. Molecular mechanisms in basement membrane complications of diabetes. Alterations in heparin, laminin, and type IV collagen association. *Diabetes* 1988;37:532–539.
55. Parthasarathy N, Spiro RG. Effect of diabetes on the glycosaminoglycan component of the human glomerular basement membrane. *Diabetes* 1982;31:738–741.
56. Brown DM, Klein DJ, Michael AF, et al. $_{35}$-S-glycosaminoglycan and $_{35}$S-glycopeptide metabolism by diabetic glomeruli and aorta. *Diabetes* 1982;418–425.
57. Sosenko JM, Miefttinen OS, Williamson JR, *et al.* Muscle capillary basement-membrane thickness and long-term glycemia in type I diabetes mellitus. *N Engl J Med* 1984;311:694–698.
58. The Kroc Collaborative Study Group: Blood glucose control and the evolution of diabetic retinopathy and albuminuria. A preliminary multicenter trial. *N Engl J Med* 1984;311:365–372.
59. Camerini-Davalos RA, Velasco C, Glasser M, et al. Drug-induced reversal of early diabetic microangiopathy. *N Engl J Med* 1983;309:1551–1556.
60. Alpert JS, Coffman JD, Balodimos MC, et al. Capillary permeability and blood flow in skeletal muscle of patients with diabetes mellitus and genetic prediabetes. *N Engl J Med* 1972;286:454–460.
61. Bollinger A, Frey J, Jager K, Furrer J, Sesglias J, Siegenthaler W. Patterns of diffusion through skin capillaries in patients with long-term diabetes. *N Engl J Med* 1982;307:1305–1310.
62. Scott AR, MacDonald IA, Bennett T, et al. Abnormal thermoregulation in diabetic neuropathy. *Diabetes* 1988;37:961–968.
63. Cunningham LN, Labrie C, Soeldner JS, et al. Resting and exercise hyperemic pulsatile arterial blood flow in insulin-dependent diabetic subjects. *Diabetes* 1983;32:664–669.
64. Hostetter MK. Perspectives in diabetes. Handicaps to host defense effects of hyperglycemia on C_3 and Candida albicans. *Diabetes* 1990;39:271–275.

Surgical Management of the Diabetic Patient,
edited by Michael Bergman and Gregorio A. Sicard.
Raven Press, Ltd., New York © 1991.

6

Surgery in Diabetic Nephropathy

Eli A. Friedman

*Department of Medicine, State University of New York Health Science Center at
Brooklyn, Brooklyn, New York 11203*

Performance of both minor and major surgery in patients with diabetic nephropathy is a common event. For most major operations, diabetes increases the chance of morbidity and the risk of dying. Diabetic individuals exhibit retarded wound healing (1,2) and a greater susceptibility to operative wound and systemic infection (3) than do nondiabetic persons with similar demographic background. Nephropathy imposes further risks in terms of drug toxicity (especially aminoglycoside antibiotics) when renal function is impaired, and the sequelae of poor nutrition when proteinuria induces hypoproteinemia. Substantive concerns in planning surgery for a diabetic person with renal disease are generated because of usually concurrent disorders in other organ systems, particularly the eyes, heart, and extremities. Awareness of hazards and provision of reasonable comprehensive medical management permits even extensive surgery in diabetic patients who lack any renal function without inordinate—though increased—mortality and morbidity; for example, despite the extent of surgery, in most series, fewer than 5% of diabetic kidney and/or pancreas transplant recipients die during surgery or in the perioperative period (4).

RACIAL DISPARITY IN INCIDENCE OF DIABETES

Approximately 5% of Americans have been diagnosed as having diabetes mellitus (5). An additional 5% of the population have undetected diabetes although they are exposed to its attendant risks, including microvasculopathy expressed as retinopathy and nephropathy (6). Recognition and description of differences in the course and clinical expression of renal involvement in insulin-dependent diabetes (IDDM, type I) and noninsulin-dependent diabetes (NIDDM, type II) are the subject of multiple ongoing investigations (7,8). There is demographic variation in incidence of diabetes by type: Some subsets of the population, [(e.g., black women over the age of 55 years, and adult Pima Indians (9)] manifest a prevalence of diabetes greater than 25% (10,11). Whites have a higher rate of IDDM than do blacks, Hispanics (12) or Asians (13,14), although blacks (15) and Hispanics (16) have a higher rate of NIDDM than do whites or Asians (17).

FAMILIAL PREDISPOSITION TO NEPHROPATHY

Several recent reports indicate that in addition to racial differences in the rate of diabetes and nephropathy, familial clusters of diabetic nephropathy can be identified. Seaquist et al. (18), to illustrate the point, found that diabetic siblings of probands with diabetic nephropathy severe enough to lead to kidney transplantation had a higher frequency of nephropathy than did diabetic siblings of diabetic persons with no evidence of nephropathy (18). Furthermore, studies at the Joslin Clinic suggest that associated with a genetic predisposition to diabetic nephropathy is a genetic risk of hypertension (19). Parents of patients with IDDM and proteinuria have a higher blood pressure than do parents of individuals with IDDM without proteinuria (20). Also sustaining the argument that familial factors are involved in the pathogenesis of diabetic nephropathy is the report that erythrocyte lithium-sodium countertransport, a marker for the risk of essential hypertension, is increased in diabetic patients with microalbuminuria (21), a finding that suggests broad genetic differences between diabetic individuals who will and will not develop nephropathy. Tollins and Raij (22) speculate that diabetic patients *destined* to develop nephropathy have a genetic predisposition to hypertension coupled with defective regulation of preglomerular resistance vessels. In this context, slight increases in systemic blood pressure may be directly transmitted to the glomerulus, which undergoes hemodynamic injury.

RENAL SYNDROMES IN DIABETES

Among the more than ten million Americans who have diabetes, there exist individuals within the diabetic population who contract each of the renal disorders afflicting the nondiabetic population. Prudence, therefore, dictates that before ascribing kidney malfunction in a diabetic patient to diabetic nephropathy, other diagnoses (polycystic kidney disease, poststreptococcal glomerulonephritis, heroin-associated nephropathy) must be considered and, where possible, excluded. Listed in Tables 1 and 2 are the main renal syndromes that have been attributed to diabetes. Urinary

TABLE 1. *Renal disorders associated with diabetes*

Infectious
  Bacteriuria
  Pyelonephritis
  Renal carbuncle
  Renal papillary necrosis
Toxic
  Contrast media-induced nephropathy
Neurogenic
  Cystopathy (hydronephrosis)
Vascular
  Nephrosclerosis
  Atheromatous embolic disease
  Renal artery stenosis
Microvasculopathic
  Diffuse intercapillary glomerulosclerosis
  Nodular intercapillary glomerulosclerosis

TABLE 2. *Renal syndromes in diabetic surgical patients*

Previously normal renal function with superimposed acute insult
    Radiocontrast media
    Drug toxicity (aminoglycoside antibiotics)
    Nonsteroidal antiinflammatory drugs
Nephrotic, hypoproteinemic patients with superimposed acute injury
Azotemic patients with further renal injury
    Radiocontrast media
    Drug toxicity (aminoglycoside antibiotics)
    Nonsteroidal antiinflammatory drugs
    Prerenal azotemia
Uremic patients requiring support during intercurrent surgery
    Maintenance hemodialysis
    On peritoneal dialysis
    On a protein restricted diet
    Kidney transplant recipients in rejection or cyclosporine nephrotoxicity
Urosepsis with or without renal insufficiency
    Acute pyelonephritis
    Renal papillary necrosis
    Renal carbuncle

tract infection in diabetes can, without obvious reason, evolve into a life-threatening unilateral renal carbuncle or bilateral renal papillary necrosis. Renal abscesses may be ominously silent, yet their presence must be considered when evaluating a diabetic patient for occult sepsis.

Diabetic Nephropathy

Diabetic nephropathy is a mixed micro- and macrovasculopathy culminating in intercapillary glomerulosclerosis and nephrosclerosis. The incidence of diabetic nephropathy in the United States has risen each year over the past decade to its current first place among disorders causing end-stage renal disease (ESRD) (23). Throughout Europe, Japan, and South America, a similar progressive increase has been recorded in the proportion of new uremic diabetic patients begun on renal replacement therapy—ranging from 12 to 28%, depending on the country—who are diagnosed as having diabetic nephropathy (24).

There is much ambiguity in the literature of diabetic nephropathy as to precisely which type of diabetes (IDDM, NIDDM, or both) is being discussed. Compounding this confusion is the use of terms such as "insulin requiring" to rationalize a physician's decision to treat an individual with insulin who is thought to have *resistant* type II diabetes. With the exception of carefully studied small series of patients from individual centers, the majority of registry reports detailing outcome in large numbers of ESRD patients who have diabetes have not sorted patients by diabetes type. Data to assess nephropathy are listed in Table 3. It had been thought that renal disease leading to ESRD was relatively rare in NIDDM (25). Recent recognition of the high prevalence of proteinuria and azotemia in individuals with NIDDM who have been carefully followed (26), however, has blurred its distinction from IDDM in terms of ultimate rate of renal failure (27). Our 1986 point-prevalence survey of 232 adult diabetic individuals—both IDDM and NIDDM—undergoing hemodialysis in Brooklyn (28) supports Knuiman *et al.'s* (29) contention that there are "very few

TABLE 3. *Assessment of presence of nephropathy in diabetic patients*

Urine color	Dark red-brown suggests myoglobinuria. Orange red suggests hepatic failure.
Urine specific gravity	When >1.020 in an azotemic patient, prerenal azotemia highly probable. A constant 1.010 is found in chronic renal failure.
Urinary sodium concentration	Acute renal failure is associated with a concentration >30 mEq/l in a spot measurement. Prerenal azotemia (and hepatorenal syndrome) is likely when <10 mEq/l. Prior administration of diuretics may induce natriuresis, blunting diagnostic specificity of low urinary sodium measurement.
Daily urinary protein excretion	Minute amounts of proteinuria (daily albumin excretion >30 mg and <200 mg/day) is termed microalbuminuria. Larger amounts of proteinuria, due to diabetic nephropathy, signal extensive anatomic glomerular damage and precede azotemia. Nephrotic-range (>3.5 g/24 h) proteinuria is present months to several years before the onset of renal functional decline.
Azotemia	An elevated serum creatinine concentration indicates a reduction in renal function to approximately less than 30% of normal. When resulting from diabetic nephropathy, an increased serum creatinine level is reason for concern in prescribing drugs that are mainly excreted by the kidney, as extensive prolongation of serum half-life may occur (aminoglycoside antibiotics, for example) necessitating a dose reduction.
Renal size	Early in the course of type I diabetes an increased renal size, as well as raised glomerular filtration rate and renal plasma flow, are characteristic findings. Normal or reduced renal size is noted in the later stages of type I diabetes and in all phases of type II diabetes.

differences in the risk-factor profiles for complications for IDDM compared with NIDDM patients."

Without reflection, it may appear paradoxical that dialysis units are filled mainly with patients manifesting NIDDM, although IDDM patients *as a group* face a proportionately greater threat of uremia. As a generalization, approximately 30% of those manifesting IDDM (30) and 5–10% of patients with NIDDM (31) eventually become uremic (32). From population surveys in the United States, it is estimated that the prevalence ratio of NIDDM to IDDM is about 9.5:1, and that the majority of diabetic patients undergoing maintenance hemodialysis or peritoneal dialysis have NIDDM. A simple computation explains this finding:

1. Of 100 American diabetic persons, about 95 have NIDDM and five have IDDM
2. About 5% of the 95 individuals with NIDDM will become uremic (approximately five)
3. Assume 30–40% of those with IDDM will become uremic (approximately two)
4. The ESRD patient ratio expressed by diabetes type is, therefore, five NIDDM (72%) to two IDDM (18%).

PATHOPHYSIOLOGY OF RENAL MANIFESTATIONS OF DIABETES

Postulated mechanisms that may contribute to development of diabetic microvasculopathy (nephropathy and retinopathy) include metabolic (hyperglycemia, glycation, sorbitol pathway (33)), hemodynamic (glomerular hyperfiltration, increased glomerular and renal tubular pressure), and/or rheologic (34) (increased blood viscosity (35), decreased erythrocyte deformability (36)) perturbations. Although evidence substantiates the contribution of each of the abnormalities mentioned above to the pathogenesis of nephropathy in one or more animal models of diabetes, no single explanation covers all of the clinical findings in patients with nephropathy. Translation of experimental and clinical studies into interventive protocols designed to retard or prevent glomerular injury, however, demands application of undigested and fragmentary knowledge during the "silent" years of diabetes. At the onset of diabetes, individuals with IDDM manifest a "supernormal" glomerular filtration rate (GFR), a phenomenon termed hyperfiltration that has been linked in its pathogenesis to hyperglycemia (37,38). Support for the hyperglycemia explanation for hyperfiltration is deduced from the reduction of a greater than normal GFR to normal by continuous infusion of insulin. Glomerular hyperfiltration is accompanied by intraglomerular hypertension that, in addition to denaturation of glomerular proteins by glycation, results in morphologic change (39). Hostetter (40) and his associates foster the view that glomerular hyperfiltration and associated intrarenal hypertension are the main causes of continuing glomerular pathological injury in diabetes (and some other chronic kidney disorders) (40). Consonant with this view are experiments in which normal rats, after an 80% nephrectomy, undergo compensatory functional changes in the remaining nephrons, which are similar to those observed in rats with streptozotocin-induced diabetes. Increased single-nephron GFR and intraglomerular pressure have been measured in rats with reduced nephron mass (41). These increases in pressure and flow, it is reasoned, alter glomerular permselectivity (solute handling properties), initially causing proteinuria, and later morphologic changes.

Hyperglycemia, in our opinion, is the major cause of diabetic microvasculopathy (nephropathy). Multiple reports document the prevention of nephropathy in streptozotocin-induced diabetic rats through the establishment of euglycemia. As examples, control of hyperglycemia in streptozotocin-induced diabetic rats by insulin treatment, or islet of Langerhans transplants, completely interdicts subsequent glomerulopathy. Similar experiments have not been done in humans with diabetes. To delineate the role of hyperglycemia in the genesis of diabetic complications, a multicenter trial of the effect of strict glucose control on the subsequent development of diabetic vasculopathy, including glomerulopathy, is now in progress (42). This is the largest such study ever funded by the National Institutes of Health. Elevated blood glucose concentrations in diabetes lead to irreversible chemical changes (glycation) in vital proteins including albumin, globulin, glomerular basement membrane (GBM), collagen and those in nerve axons and the lens of the eye. Glycated collagen (and other glycated proteins) then polymerizes into advanced glycosylated endproducts (AGE). According to Brownlee and others (43), one avenue of therapy to avoid development of diabetic nephropathy is to block formation of AGE by either sustaining euglycemia or by administering substances such as aminoguanidine (44), which block its synthesis. First- and second-stage clinical trials of the safety and efficacy of aminoguanidine in adult diabetic persons are now in progress in the author's clinic.

The glomerulus in the streptozotocin-induced diabetic rat has an expanded mesangium and a thickened GBM. Months after the onset of GBM thickening and a reduced filtration surface area, development of focal and segmental glomerular sclerosis follows; this is a lesion atypical of human glomerulosclerosis, the characteristic abnormality of diabetic nephropathy. Extrapolation of findings generated in the streptozotocin-induced diabetic rat to human diabetes, therefore, may be misleading. Glomerular lesions of mesangial expansion, GBM thickening, and segmental sclerosis in streptozotocin-induced diabetic rats do not progress to nodular and diffuse intercapillary glomerulosclerosis typical of human diabetic nephropathy. Furthermore, rats made diabetic with streptozotocin do not become uremic.

Protein feeding acutely increases renal function in healthy individuals as a prelude to digestion. GFR in normal volunteers rises by a maximum of about 40% two and a half hours after a large protein meal. Subtracting baseline GFR from the maximal GFR after protein loading yields what has been termed the renal reserve (45). In contrast to nondiabetic individuals, diabetic persons do not have a rise in GFR after protein loading, suggesting that they may be functioning at a level that utilizes their renal reserve all of the time (46). Based on the finding that a restricted dietary protein intake slows progression of glomerulosclerosis in the streptozotocin-induced diabetic rat (47), a low-protein diet has been advocated as therapy for human diabetic nephropathy (48,49).

Results of kidney transplantation in uremic diabetic recipients permit the inference (by those favoring the importance of hyperglycemia in the genesis of vasculopathy) that hyperglycemia is a major, if not the sole, determinant of diabetic glomerulopathy. Favoring this view are observations by Maryniak et al. (50) of recurrent intercapillary glomerulosclerosis causing renal failure in kidneys obtained from a nondiabetic donor when transplanted into a diabetic recipient and Abouna et al. (51) that morphologic improvement in diabetic glomerulopathy may follow transplantation of a kidney from a diabetic donor to a nondiabetic recipient.

CLINICAL MANIFESTATIONS

Diabetic persons in whom clinically expressed nephropathy is developing experience a silent phase lasting months to a decade or longer, before the onset of nephrotic-range proteinuria. During this silent phase, small amounts of urinary albumin (microalbuminuria, described immediately below) are detectable in both IDDM (52) and NIDDM (53). Subsequently, there is a progressive increase in the quantity of urinary protein leakage. Years of urinary protein loss amounting to as much as 40 or more g/day precede a continuous loss of renal function. After 20 or more years in IDDM, and 5–15 years in NIDDM, renal reserve falls below 5% and the diabetic individual is said to be in ESRD.

MICROALBUMINURIA AND PROTEINURIA

According to a Consensus Committee attempting to delineate diagnostic criteria for diabetic nephropathy, proteinuria of 300 mg/day is a reliable and consistent sign of renal damage (54). Healthy adults excrete between 2.5 and 26 mg of albumin per day with a geometric mean of about 9.5 mg/24 h; almost all values (92%) fall below 18 mg/24 h (55). Clinical measures of proteinuria (such as Albustix or sulfosalicylic acid) do not detect excess urinary protein until daily protein excretion amounts to 250 mg, of which about 50% is albumin (56). With the advent of sensitive tests for small amounts of urinary albumin, there is now a preproteinuric interval during which previously undetectable amounts of albuminuria have been discovered. Albumin excretion rates between 26 and 250 mg/24h, now termed microalbuminuria, have been identified in diabetic persons who subsequently are at higher risk for proteinuria and azotemia. The predictive value of microalbuminuria in NIDDM was shown by Jarrett et al. (57) in their report of 44 Albustix-negative diabetic British adults who were found to be microalbuminuric in 1966/67. By the end of 1980, 17 of these 44 patients (39%) had died, all but two from cardiovascular causes.

Once urinary albumin excretion reaches about 1 g/day, anatomically advanced diabetic nephropathy with near-term renal insufficiency is highly probable (58); the risk of renal insufficiency developing is approximately 20 times greater in diabetic persons with gross proteinuria. Typically, progression to renal failure follows in 3 to 20 years (median 10 years) after the onset of proteinuria (59). Characteristic of the nephropathic diabetic individual with declining renal function is a nephrotic syndrome—lasting for months to years—during which daily urinary protein excretion ranges from 3 to 40 or more g/day. Nephrotic diabetic persons differ from other nephrotic patients because of the presence of substantive comorbid conditions, especially coronary artery disease (60). A challenge in total patient care is presented when surgery is required for a diabetic person who has fluid overload, marginal cardiac compensation, and wide excursions in plasma glucose concentration.

As renal insufficiency worsens, decreasing renal catabolism of insulin is responsible in some individuals with IDDM for frequent and profound hypoglycemic episodes; normally about one-third of secreted insulin is metabolized by the kidney. As GFR falls below 10 ml/min, uremic signs including anemia, acidosis, lethargy, nausea, and severe hypertension dictate the end of conservative care and signal the need for dialysis or renal transplantation. Any surgical procedure at this stage of nephropathy is likely to be complicated by excessive bleeding, retarded healing, and a greater than usual incidence of infection.

Coincident with deterioration of renal function is worsening visual acuity, intensifying neuropathy, and cardiac failure, which create a series of seemingly insurmountable impediments to rehabilitation. Lacking an overall plan, the patient faces fragmented, often contradictory, approaches to correcting organ or systemic disease. Multiple consultants offer sometimes conflicting advice and independently prescribe activity level, proscribed behavior, diet, and drugs. Successful rehabilitation of uremic diabetic patients by peritoneal dialysis (61), hemodialysis (62), or renal transplantation (63) requires a team approach in which a single physician—the patient's doctor—integrates needed consultants' services, including collaborating ophthalmologist and nephrologist. In selecting a specific option in uremia therapy for an individual patient, what had been the clearly established superiority of kidney transplantation as a means of effecting rehabilitation must now be reassessed in light of the extraordinary improvement in well-being induced in dialysis patients whose hematocrit has been raised by recombinant erythropoietin (64).

A policy of full disclosure to the patient of available options in therapy, including the statistical chances of success for each, has been enthusiastically received by our patients. We encourage patient participation in selecting and scheduling each aspect of management, which means that we permit free access to hospital charts and office records. Regular performance of finger-stick glucose monitoring, or hemodialysis, or peritoneal dialysis at home, promotes a feeling of accomplishment and maintains the patient's self-esteem.

RENAL-RETINAL SYNDROME

Diabetic patients experiencing deteriorating renal function must also cope with declining vision due to progressive proliferative diabetic retinopathy. Newly diagnosed individuals who have ESRD due to diabetes risk a greater than 95% probability of retinopathy; indeed, half of newly evaluated uremic diabetic patients are blind or have reduced visual acuity. In the mid-1970s, early trials of hemodialysis and peritoneal dialysis in ESRD caused by diabetic nephropathy were associated with an inordinately high incidence (50%) of blindness or severe vision loss in what has been termed a renal–retinal syndrome (65). Subsequently, an appreciation for the importance of controlling hypertension and improved regulation of blood glucose concentration have sharply reduced the rate of visual decline in patients who have undergone hemodialysis and renal transplant (66). Retention of usable vision for most uremic diabetic persons can be accomplished by cooperative planning between nephrologist and ophthalmologist (67).

HYPERTENSION

Hypertension is without question a major risk factor for progression of kidney, eye, and heart disease in diabetes. Hypertension accelerates the rate of decline of renal function in diabetic nephropathy (68). Conversely, normalization of hypertensive blood pressures to a target blood pressure of 130/70 mmHg or below will slow—and in some individuals, arrest—further renal functional deterioration (69). One hypothesis as to how hypertension injures the glomerulus, and which fits these observations, is that in diabetic patients, systemic hypertension is freely transmitted to the glomerulus where proteinuria and morphologic injury result. In the absence of renal insufficiency, both mild diastolic hypertension (90–105 mmHg) and systolic hypertension (above 160 mmHg) can be initially managed by a reduction in plasma volume using a thiazide diuretic (hydrochlorothiazide 50–150 mg/day). The latter medication, however, may cause undesirable change in glucose and lipid levels.

Drugs that lower both systemic and intraglomerular pressure, such as the angiotensin converting enzyme (ACE) inhibitors (enalapril, captopril, lisinopril) have received wide attention from those studying diabetic nephropathy. Parving et al. (70) found that after two years of treatment with captopril combined with a diuretic, individuals with IDDM had a reduction in urinary albumin excretion as well as a decrease in the rate of renal functional loss. Similar results have been obtained in carefully constructed studies employing enalapril (71). Calcium channel blockers, especially their long-acting forms, are well tolerated and highly efficacious in patients with diabetic nephropathy and have tolerable adverse effects on lipid and glucose metabolism (72,73). Beta-blocking drugs, by contrast, may cause hyperglycemia and often exacerbate and prolong insulin-induced hypoglycemia in IDDM. Alpha-blockers, central agonists, and vasodilators have neutral effects on carbohydrate metabolism in hypertensive diabetic individuals.

No single drug sequence for management of hypertension in diabetic nephropathy has been uniformly recognized as superior to other approaches. We first use an ACE inhibitor, and in nephrotic patients add one or two diuretics (furosemide and metolazone). A calcium channel blocker (nifedipine) is added next; in only rare instances is it necessary to use other drugs, such as sympathetic inhibitors (clonidine); vasodilators (hydralazine); and alpha-adrenergic blockers (prazosin) in unresponsive moderate hypertension (diastolic pressure 105–114 mmHg) as advocated by the Joint National Committee on the Detection, Evaluation, and Treatment of High Blood Pressure (74). Our therapeutic objective is to achieve a standing blood pressure of about 120–130/60–80 mmHg. For about one in fifty azotemic diabetic patients who manifest severe hypertension (diastolic pressure above 115 mmHg), minoxidil is uniformly effective in controlling hypertension. The side effects of minoxidil including fluid retention, tachycardia, and intense facial hair growth, complicate its acceptance and long-term use. For the past eight years, a combination of diuretics plus other antihypertensive drugs has eliminated the desperate need to resort to binephrectomy as a means of controlling intractable hypertension in our program.

Unusual or particularly severe complications from antihypertensive drugs can develop in diabetic hypertensive persons. These include: worsened hyperglycemia from diuretics; muted or altered signs and symptoms of hypoglycemia from beta-blockers; and intensified fluid retention from sympathetic inhibitors and vasodilators. Hyperkalemia and worsening azotemia are troublesome reactions to ACE inhibitors in about 20% of patients. Weekly measurements of serum potassium levels and creatinine concentrations should be obtained during the first month of treatment with an ACE inhibitor. Furthermore, about 10% of patients (more women than men) discontinue treatment with an ACE inhibitor because of a persistent dry cough (75).

CREATININE CLEARANCE BELOW 20 ML/MIN

Until about five years ago, it was possible to predict—with reasonable precision—by plotting creatinine clearance or the reciprocal of the serum creatinine concentration against time—the date when renal failure would supervene in a diabetic individual with declining renal function. Contemporary interventive regimens that stress euglycemia, normalization of blood pressure, restriction of dietary protein ingestion, and correction of anemia with erythropoietin have sharply blunted the slope of the curve of renal functional decline. Several patients in our own program have remained relatively stable for three or more years with serum creatinine concentrations above 4 mg/dl, an occurrence unseen a decade earlier. There is sufficient opportunity in most instances to inform and prepare each patient for the ultimate and still inevitable need for uremia therapy. Panic and surprise over the need for dialytic therapy or a kidney transplant can be largely avoided by sensitive planning and repeated review of the course of treatment with the patient.

Initiation of uremia therapy has been recommended early (creatinine clearance of 10–25 ml/min) or later (creatinine clearance of 5–10 ml/min), although few would disagree that a creatinine clearance of less than 5 ml/min is an absolute indication for switching from conservative to more aggressive treatment. Conversion from *conservative* management to dialytic treatment or a kidney transplant in patients whose serum creatinine level has reached 8 mg/dl is mandated by: development of uremic bleeding due to gastritis or colitis; pericarditis; convulsions; or nonspecific deterioration characterized by weight loss, worsening hypertension, and lethargy. Relative indications for starting dialysis or performing a renal transplant when the serum creatinine concentration increases to 4–8 mg/dl were based on clinical judgment in the preerythropoietin era. Patients who are unable to work, concentrate, or enjoy any substantial portion of their life should be started on dialysis, even though their creatinine clearance may be as high as 15 ml/min. Massry et al. (76), reflecting on the question of when to start dialysis, observed that: "Early dialysis will lead to early amelioration of uremia, control of fluid overload, normalization of blood pressure and reduction of bleeding tendencies." Lacking either prospective or retrospective studies of the ideal time to start dialysis, it is reasonable to select that point in a patient's course at which further deterioration, especially of visual acuity and the cardiovascular system, appears inevitable.

CO-MORBID RISK FACTORS

Clinical expression of renal disease, starting with a nephrotic syndrome through advanced renal insufficiency, induces more stress in a diabetic individual than in a nondiabetic person with equivalent renal malfunction because of the impact of usually symptomatic, concurrent, extrarenal disease (Table 4). For example, in preparation for maintenance hemodialysis, creation of a vascular access, which in a nondiabetic patient is relatively minor surgery, may, in a diabetic patient, induce major morbidity due to limb swelling, infection, or deranged glucose regulation. Cardiac decompensation, stroke, and the risk of limb amputation hang as a dark cloud over the head of all long-term diabetic patients with renal insufficiency. During initial nephrologic evaluation, therefore, an inventory of coincident extrarenal vascular disease (especially ophthalmic, cardiovascular, cerebrovascular, and of the extremities) should be conducted to construct an appropriate treatment regimen for an illness afflicting the entire patient (Table 5).

Before recommending dialytic therapy or a kidney transplant, we request consultations with collaborating team members including an ophthalmologist, cardiologist, and podiatrist familiar with management of diabetic patients in renal failure. Before a kidney transplant is scheduled, the urgency of laser photocoagulation and/or vitreous surgery is weighed to preserve ambulatory vision. Toward the same objective of maximizing rehabilitation during uremia therapy, cardiac evaluation, including coronary angiography, is performed prior to transplantation to detect those patients who might benefit from prophylactic coronary artery angioplasty or bypass surgery. This evaluation is also performed on asymptomatic patients. More than 95% of diabetic individuals who begin maintenance dialysis or receive a renal allograft, in our experience, have been treated for retinopathy by laser photocoagulation and/or vitrectomy. Scheduling repetitive visits with a podiatrist as a component of routine

TABLE 4. *Co-morbid risk factors in diabetic patients evaluated for uremia therapy*

Cystopathy resulting in urinary retention. Cystometrogram, urine culture, residual volume.
Coronary artery or other cardiac disease. Electrocardiogram, exercise stress test, coronary angiography.
Gastrointestinal disease. Gastroparesis interfering with glucose regulation, obstipation, diarrhea. Abdominal radiography. Radionuclide test meal.
Respiratory disease likely to progress or induce infection. Vital capacity.
Eye disease (cataracts, retinopathy, vascular occlusion). Visual acuity, sonography, electroretinography, fluorescein angiography.
Bone consequences of uremia. Metabolic radiographic bone survey, plasma aluminum level, bone scan.
Disease of the extremities (lower limb arterial insufficiency, venous stasis, Charcot's joint, neuropathic insensitivity). Podiatric assessment including prescription footwear, Doppler flow studies of limb perfusion. Pentoxifylline.
Gum and other dental disorders. Dental assessment and corrective care.
Limited social support system preventing home or continuing care. Social worker and nurse educator's assessment of potential for self-care.

TABLE 5. *Variables influencing morbidity in diabetic kidney transplant recipients: The co-morbidity index*

Coronary artery disease inducing persistent angina and/or myocardial infarction.
Other cardiovascular problems, hypertension, congestive heart failure, cardiomyopathy.
Respiratory disease unrelated to diabetes (asthma, emphysema).
Autonomic neuropathy (gastroparesis, obstipation, diarrhea, cystopathy, orthostatic hypotension).
Macrovascular disease of the brain with neurologic deficit due to cerebrovascular accident or
    reduced blood flow to the brain.
Musculoskeletal disorders that limit motion and/or activity, including renal bone disease caused by
    hyperparathyroidism and aluminum intoxication.
Infections including AIDS, but excluding vascular access-site or peritonitis.
Hepatitis, hepatic insufficiency, enzymatic pancreatic insufficiency.
Hematologic problems other than anemia.
Spinal abnormalities, lower back problems, or arthritis.
Vision impairment (minor to severe—decreased acuity to blindness).
Limb amputation (minor to severe—finger, toe, portion of foot, entire lower extremity).
Mental or emotional illness (neurosis, depression, psychosis).

To obtain a numerical Co-Morbidity Index for an individual patient, rate each variable from 0 to 3 (0 = absent; 1 = mild, of minor import to patient's life; 2 = moderate; 3 = severe). By proportional hazard analysis, the relative significance of each variable can be isolated from the others.

care in diabetic patients on dialysis or after a renal transplant sharply reduces the need for lower limb amputations, a complication noted in about 20% of uremic diabetic persons who do not receive podiatric care.

AUTONOMIC NEUROPATHY AND DIABETIC NEPHROPATHY

Among diabetic azotemic patients referred to our service, the presence and morbid impact of autonomic neuropathy (77)—especially gastropathy and cystopathy (78)—are frequently overlooked. Visceral autonomic neuropathy (79), a ubiquitous complication of diabetes after a decade, may confound every aspect of management of the nephrotic, azotemic, or uremic diabetic individual by:

1. Inconsistently retarding timely food digestion (gastroparesis), thereby preempting careful glucose regulation
2. Inducing functional urinary obstruction simulating renal transplant rejection (cystopathy) and
3. Interfering with normalization of blood pressure by inducing orthostatic hypotension-limiting ambulation.

Unrecognized cystopathy may simulate worsening diabetic nephropathy and is sometimes misdiagnosed as renal allograft rejection in diabetic kidney transplant recipients. We evaluated bladder function in 22 diabetic patients in whom renal failure developed, including 14 men and eight women of mean age 38 years (19 with type I diabetes and 3 with type II diabetes). Cystopathy had not been previously diagnosed in any patient. Testing included an air cystogram, maximal pressure, and capacity measurements. Cystopathy was detected in eight patients (36%), manifested as detrusor paralysis in one patient, severe malfunction in five patients (24%), and mild impairment in one patient.

Gastroparesis, thought to be an expression of autonomic neuropathy, can be detected in one-quarter to one-half of azotemic diabetic persons during their first nephrologic evaluation. Clues to the presence of gastroparesis include:

1. Patient complaints of abdominal fullness and vomiting of undigested food hours after a meal
2. Erratic metabolic control of the plasma glucose level due to an inability to link insulin doses with the timing of food ingestion and
3. Unexplained intermittent severe hypoglycemia in the midst of inadequately regulated hyperglycemia.

Abdominal radiography confirms the diagnosis of gastroparesis by showing a distended stomach containing a large air bubble or by abnormalities in gastric emptying studies. Symptomatic improvement can be attained in about one-half of patients by increasing the frequency and reducing the size of meals and administering metoclopramide 5–20 mg 30 minutes before meals and at night.

Alternating obstipation and explosive nighttime diarrhea often coexist with gastroparesis. More than half of the diabetic patients evaluated by us for renal insufficiency report embarrassing, clothes-soiling diarrhea as a life-compromising complication. Treatment is empiric and consists of cathartics for obstipation with as much as 120 ml of castor oil required in difficult cases. Of our referred diabetic patients, about half of those reporting diarrhea respond to a psyllium seed dietary supplement (Metamucil or generic equivalent) taken one to three times daily.

ANTIBIOTIC PROPHYLAXIS FOR SURGERY

Antimicrobial prophylaxis in surgery has not been reported as different for diabetic individuals in comparison with nondiabetic persons. As carefully reviewed in the Medical Letter (80), prophylactic antibiotics decrease the incidence of infection after open heart surgery, vascular reconstruction of the abdominal aorta, limb amputations, total hip replacement, intestinal and oral pharyngeal surgery, and vaginal hysterectomy. For most procedures, cefazolin, which has a moderately long serum half-life (1 g intravenously) is advised, although vancomycin (1 g intravenously) is also widely used. Renal insufficiency prolongs the serum half-life but does not increase peak concentration values for either of these antibiotics; thus no change in dosage is required for the uremic patient.

CONTRAST MEDIA NEPHROTOXICITY

The majority of our nephrology consultations for diabetic patients originate from our surgical and neurosurgical services and are concerned with the risk and avoidance of renal injury induced by contrast media. In one study, radiocontrast agents accounted for 12% of acute renal failure acquired during the hospital stay (81). Well-documented reports of both reversible and irreversible acute renal failure followed increasing use of synthetic, triiodinated compounds (sodium or meglumine salts of diatrizoate) following drip-infusion urography, excretory urography, and arteriography (82). Evidence suggests that contrast media nephrotoxicity is mediated by renal ischemia and resultant hypoxia combined with direct cellular toxicity of the iodinated molecule. Risk factors in patients with contrast-associated nephropathy include baseline renal insufficiency (serum creatinine ≥1.5 mg/dl), albuminuria (≥2 g/dl), and hypertension. Diabetes was found to be a risk factor in both prospective and retrospective studies (83,84), but this inference was drawn from patients with advanced renal insufficiency. In a study conducted by our group at an Alabama diabetes center, only three of 49 (6%) diabetic individuals with normal or only mildly impaired renal function had an increase in basal serum creatinine concentration (<2 mg/dl) of at least 25% after intravenous exposure to radiocontrast media (85). Another study addressing the same issue determined that renal failure did not develop in 85 diabetic patients without renal insufficiency (mean serum creatinine concentration 1.0 mg/dl) after intravenous injection of radiocontrast media (86). Current consensus holds that diabetes is a risk factor only when azotemia is present (serum creatinine >2.5 mg/dl). The hope that newer iodinated contrast agents (nonionic monomers and dimers as well as ionic dimers) are less nephrotoxic, has not been born out in studies in which patients were randomly assigned to ionic or nonionic contrast media (87).

Prevention of contrast-associated nephrotoxicity has generally been unsuccessful. Although mannitol infusion (500 ml of 5% mannitol) (88), intravenous injection of furosemide (100 mg for each mg/dl of serum creatinine) (89), and a brisk saline infusion (550 ml of 0.9% saline per hour) (90), have been advocated as renal-protective measures, evidence of their efficacy is far from compelling. In the absence of proof, we nevertheless advise that maintenance of urine flow at a rate of at least 100 ml/h and infusion of mannitol are appropriate steps that are unlikely to be in themselves harmful and may proffer some protection.

EXTRACORPOREAL SOLUTE AND WATER EXTRACTION

Whether from sepsis, or worsening of preexisting renal insufficiency, diabetic patients can deteriorate in the perioperative period in a syndrome of combined cardiac, pulmonary, and renal failure with a mortality rate greater than 80%. Barzilay et al. (91) applied continuous arteriovenous hemofiltration (CAVH), plus hemodialysis, and/or hemofiltration to small groups of patients with multiple organ failure, decreasing their mortality rate to 36% from 50%. A similar study of 100 consecutive patients with multiorgan failure and acute renal failure during and after major surgery evaluated CAVH applied for several hours to as long as 90 days, with a mean of 8 days, in which the survival rate was 45% (92). CAVH was termed "safe and effective" in a study comprising treatment of 61 patients with surgery-related acute renal failure (93).

One disadvantage of CAVH as compared with peritoneal dialysis or hemodialysis is its requirement for either an arterial cannula or a blood pump in a continuously heparinized patient. The need for vascular access for hemodialysis has been simplified by the introduction of thin diameter double-lumen catheters such as the Permcath (94). The choice among peritoneal dialysis, hemodialysis, or CAVH must be governed by local expertise and the extent of skilled nursing support. Outside an intensive-care environment, CAVH is difficult to monitor and hemodialysis may be preferable. Patients undergoing peritoneal dialysis or maintenance hemodialysis who require perioperative uremia therapy can be managed by continuing their established means of treatment. As an illustration, a maintenance hemodialysis patient given a renal transplant is usually treated with intermittent hemodialyses until the transplanted kidney begins to function.

METABOLIC REGULATION DURING SURGERY

Preoperative management of diabetic patients has improved to the extent that the risks of major surgery have been minimized. Modern inhalation anesthetic agents cause but minor metabolic effects, which can be monitored by intraoperative determination of blood glucose concentration, thus avoiding the extremes of hyperglycemia and hypoglycemia. Glucose regulation is easily maintained intraoperatively by adding a selected dose of insulin to a liter of 5% dextrose in 0.45% saline solution. The amount of insulin is derived from the previous daily requirement and the preoperative blood glucose level. The dose of insulin ranges from 10 to 20 units/l for patients who require insulin; an infusion rate of 100 ml/h delivers 1 to 2 units of insulin with 5 g of dextrose hourly. Guidelines for adding hourly bolus doses of insulin are discussed in chapter 3. For patients treated with sulfonylurea (NIDDM), a similar approach is begun with an infusion of 100 ml/h of a 5% dextrose in 0.45% saline solution to which 10 units of regular insulin have been added. When serum potassium concentration falls below normal levels, 20–40 mEq of KCl are added to each liter of the glucose-insulin-saline infusion. When surgery is necessary, there are no special restrictions imposed by the presence of diabetic nephropathy other than striving to remove a bladder catheter as soon as the patient is able to void spontaneously to avoid an iatrogenic urinary tract infection. Should total parenteral nutrition (TPN) be required, insulin can be added to the infusion at a rate of 3–5 units/h, which may be adjusted based on results obtained from repeated finger-stick blood glucose level measurements.

GENERAL REMARKS ON SURGERY FOR DIABETIC PATIENTS

For not entirely explicable reasons, it has proven to be virtually beyond the ability of several university hospital-affiliated surgical ward staffs, directly observed by the author, to proffer reasonable comprehensive diabetic management. Starting with provision of an appropriate mattress and heel guards to prevent decubitus ulcers, and extending to faulty interpretation of capillary blood glucose reagent strips, almost every aspect of diabetic care was noted to be inconstant and often faulty. Nurse-induced hypoglycemic and hyperglycemic episodes were daily events for several patients with IDDM who were not practicing self-monitoring of glucose levels. Patients were injected with long-acting insulin and then maintained without food for protracted radiologic studies that precipitated profound hypoglycemic reactions. Coordination between the dietary service's delivery of meals and injection of insulin by the nurses was far from optimal. Postoperatively confined to bed in a ward short of nurses, the diabetic convalescent patient may not have been given a bedside snack, which may result in an insulin reaction. Without a team approach, the patient is at the center of a jurisdictional tug-of-war between several specialists, none of whom accepts responsibility for overall patient care. To facilitate the review of pertinent items in the care of patients with diabetic nephropathy, a check list is presented as Table 6.

The long-duration ESRD patient with diabetes has probably learned to deal with an imprecise medical–surgical interface during hospitalizations for vascular or peritoneal access. During surgery for a first access, or in preparation for a renal transplant, however, the surgeon's extra moment of empathy and warmth eases the bur-

TABLE 6. *Pre-surgery check list for nephropathic diabetic patients*

Quantify renal function
  Serum creatinine concentration
  Blood urea nitrogen concentration
Measure proteinuria
  24-hour urinary protein excretion
  If no measurable protein, test for microalbuminuria
Quantitative urine culture
Hemoglobin and hematocrit measurements
Anticipate need for extracorporeal solute and water extraction
  If radiocontrast agents given when serum creatinine concentration $\geqslant 3$ mg/dl
  Where renal function is marginal pre-operatively—serum creatinine concentration $\geqslant 5$ mg/dl
  In active urosepsis
  During renal allograft rejection
  Prepare for peritoneal or hemodialysis or continuous arteriovenous hemofiltration (CAVH)
Review each medication to modify dosage according to renal function if reduced.

den for a frightened and lonely patient caught in the midst of what is so often, unnecessarily, an enervating, bewildering, and stressful experience.

REFERENCES

1. Pearl SH, Kanat IO. Diabetes and healing: a review of the literature. *J Foot Surg* 1988;27:268–270.
2. McMurry JF Jr. Wound healing with diabetes mellitus. Better glucose control for better wound healing in diabetes. *Surg Clin North Am* 1984;64:769–778.
3. MacKenzie CR, Charlson ME. Assessment of perioperative risk in the patient with diabetes mellitus. *Surg Gynecol Obstet* 1988;167:293–299.
4. Heino A. Operative and postoperative non-surgical complications in diabetic patients undergoing renal transplantation. *Scand J Urol Nephrol* 1988;22:53–58.
5. National Diabetes Data Group. Diabetes in America. NIH Publication No. 85-1468, August 1985.
6. Herman WH, Teutsch SM, Geiss LS. Closing the gap: The problem of diabetes mellitus in the United States. *Diabetes Care* 1985;8:391–406.
7. Mauer SM, Chavers BM. A comparison of kidney disease in type I and type II diabetes. *Adv Exp Med Biol* 1985;189:299–303.
8. Melton LJ, Palumbo PJ, Chu CP. Incidence of diabetes mellitus by clinical type. *Diabetes Care* 1983;6:75–86.
9. Knowler WC, Bennett PH, Hamman RF, Miller M. Diabetes incidence and prevalence in Pima Indians: a 19-fold greater incidence than in Rochester Minnesota. *Am J Epidemiol* 1978;108:497–505.
10. Hadden WC, Harris MI. Prevalence of diagnosed diabetes, undiagnosed diabetes, and impaired glucose tolerance in adults 20–74 years of age. *Vital Health Stat* 1987;11:1–55.
11. Harris MI, Hadden WC, Knowler WC, Bennett PH. Prevalence of diabetes and impaired glucose tolerance and plasma glucose levels in U.S. population aged 20–74 yr. *Diabetes* 1987;36:523–534.
12. Lorenzi M, Cagliero E, Schmidt NJ. Racial differences in incidence of juvenile-onset type 1 diabetes: epidemiologic studies in southern California. *Diabetologia* 1985;28:734–738.
13. Mustaffa BE. Diabetes mellitus in peninsular Malaysia: ethnic differences in prevalence and complications. *Ann Acad Med Singapore* 1985;14:63–67.
14. Urakami T, Miyamoto Y, Fujita H, Kitagawa T. Type 1 (insulin-dependent) diabetes in Japanese children is not a uniform disease. *Diabetologia* 1989;32:312–315.
15. Cowie CC, Port FK, Wolfe RA, Savage PJ, Moll PP, Hawthorne VM. Disparities in incidence of diabetic end-stage renal disease according to race and type of diabetes. *N Engl J Med* 1989;321:1074–1079.
16. Pugh JA, Stern MP, Haffner SM, Eifler CW, Zapata M. Excess incidence of treatment of end-stage renal disease in Mexican Americans. *Am J Epidemiol* 1988;127:135–144.
17. King H, Zimmet P. Trends in the prevalence and incidence of diabetes: non-insulin-dependent diabetes mellitus. *World Health Stat Q* 1988;41:190–196.
18. Seaquist R, Goetz FC, Rich S, Barbosa J. Familial clustering of diabetic kidney disease. Evidence for genetic susceptibility to diabetic nephropathy. *N Engl J Med* 1989;320:1161–1165.

19. Krowelewski AS, Canessa M, Warram JH, Laffel LM, Christlieb AR, Knowler WC, Rand LI. Predisposition to hypertension and susceptibility to renal disease in insulin dependent diabetes mellitus. *N Engl J Med* 1988;318:146–150.
20. Viberti GC, Keen H, Wiseman MJ. Raised arterial pressure in parents of proteinuric insulin-dependent patients. *Br Med J* 1987;295:575–577.
21. Mangili R, Bending JJ, Scott G, Lai LK, Gupta A, Viberti G. Increased sodium–lithium counter-transport activity in red cells of patients with insulin-dependent diabetes and nephropathy. *N Engl J Med* 1988;318:140–145.
22. Tollins JP, Raij L. Concerns about diabetic nephropathy in the treatment of diabetic hypertensive patients. *Am J Med* 1989;87:(Suppl 6A) 29S–33S.
23. U.S. Renal Data System, USRDS 1989 Annual Data Report. Bethesda MD: The National Institutes of Health, National Institute of Diabetes and Digestive and Kidney Diseases, August 1989.
24. Brunner FP, Fassbinder W, Broyer M, et al. Survival on renal replacement therapy: data from the EDTA Registry. *Nephrol Dial Transplant* 1988;3:109–122.
25. Schmitz A, Vaeth M. Microalbuminuria: a major risk factor in non-insulin-dependent diabetes. A 10-year follow-up study of 503 patients. *Diabetic Med* 1988;5:126–134.
26. Krolewski AS, Warram JH, Christlieb AR. Onset, course, complications, and prognosis of diabetes mellitus. In: Marble A, Krall LP, Bradley RF, Christlieb AR, Soeldner JS, eds. *Joslin's diabetes mellitus,* 12th ed. Philadelphia: Lea & Febiger, 1985; 251–277.
27. Tung P, Levin SR. Nephropathy in non-insulin-dependent diabetes mellitus. *Am J Med* 1988;85(Suppl 5A):131–136.
28. Lowder GM, Perri NA, Friedman EA. Demographics, diabetes type, and degree of rehabilitation in diabetic patients on maintenance hemodialysis in Brooklyn. *J Diabetic Complications* 1988;2:218–226.
29. Knuiman MW, Welborn TA, McCann VJ, Stanton KG, Constable IJ. Prevalence of diabetic complications in relation to risk factors. *Diabetes* 1986;35:1332–1339.
30. Physician's guide to insulin-dependent (Type I) diabetes: Diagnosis and treatment. Alexandria, Virginia: American Diabetes Association, Inc., 1988.
31. Physician's guide to non-insulin-dependent (Type II) diabetes. Diagnosis and treatment, second edition. Alexandria, Virginia: American Diabetes Association, Inc., 1988.
32. Grenfell A, Bewick M, Parsons V, Snowden S, Taube D, Watkins PJ. Non-insulin-dependent diabetes and renal replacement therapy. *Diabetic Med* 1988;5:172–176.
33. Stribling D, Armstrong FM, Harrison HE. Aldose reductase in the etiology of diabetic complications: 2. Nephropathy. *J Diabetic Complications* 1989;3:70–76.
34. Feher MD, Rampling MW, Sever PS, Elkeles RS. Diabetic hypertension—the importance of fibrinogen and blood viscosity. *J Hum Hypertension* 1988;2:117–122.
35. Van Acker K, Xiang DZ, Rillaerts E, Van Gaal L, De Leeuw I. Blood rheology during an intensified conventional insulin treatment (ICIT) in insulin-dependent diabetes. *Diabetes Res Clin Pract* 1989;6:259–264.
36. Vague P, Juhan I. Red cell deformability, platelet aggregation, and insulin action. (Review). *Diabetes* 1983;32(Suppl 2):88–91.
37. Anderson S, Brenner BM. Pathogenesis of diabetic glomerulopathy: Hemodynamic considerations. *Diabetes Metab Rev* 1988;2:163–177.
38. Chiumello G, Beccaria L, Meschi F, Mistura L, Brambilla P, Bognetti E. Etiology, diagnosis, and prevention of renal involvement in insulin-dependent diabetes mellitus. *Pediatrician* 1983;85:12:199–207.
39. Winegrad AI: Banting lecture 1986. Does a common mechanism induce the diverse complications of diabetes? *Diabetes.* 1987;36:396–406.
40. Hostetter TH, Olson JL, Rennke HG, Venkatachalam MA, Brenner BM. Hyperfiltration in remnant nephrons: A potentially adverse response to renal ablation. *Am J Physiol* 1981;24:F85–F93.
41. Meyer TW, Rennke HG. Progressive glomerular injury after limited renal infarction in the rat. *Am J Physiol* 1988;254:(6 Pt 2)F856–F862.
42. The DCCT Research Group. The diabetes control and complications trial DCCT. Design and methodologic considerations for the feasibility phase. *Diabetes* 1986;35:530–545.
43. Brownlee M. Pharmacological modulation of the advanced glycosylation reaction. *Prog Clin Biol Res* 1989;304:235–248.
44. Nicholls K, Mandel TE. Advanced glycosylation end-products in experimental murine diabetic nephropathy: effect of islet isografting and of aminoguanidine. *Lab Invest* 1989;60:486–491.
45. Robertson JL, Goldschmidt M, Kronfeld DS, Tomaszewski JE, Hill GS, Bovee KC. Long-term responses to high dietary protein in dogs with 75% nephrectomy. *Kidney Int* 1986;29:511–519.
46. Bosch JP, Lew S, Glabman S, Lauer A. Renal hemodynamic changes in humans. Response to protein loading in normal and diseased kidneys. *Am J Med* 1986;81:809–815.
47. von-Herrath D, Saupe J, Hirschberg R, Rottka H, Schaefer K. Glomerular filtration rate in response to an acute protein load. *Blood Purif* 1988;6(4):264–268.

48. Zatz R, Meyer TW, Nodding JL, et al. Dietary protein restriction limits glomerular hyperfiltration in experimental diabetes. *Kidney Int* 1984;25:225.
49. Evanoff G, Thompson C, Brown J, Wienman E. Prolonged dietary protein restriction in diabetic nephropathy. *Arch Intern Med* 1989;149:1129–1133.
50. Maryniak RK, Mendoza N, Clyne D, Balakrishnan K, Weiss MA. Recurrence of diabetic nodular glomerulosclerosis in a renal transplant. *Transplantation* 1985;39:35–38.
51. Abouna GM, Adnani MS, Kumar MSA, Samhan SA. Fate of transplanted kidneys with diabetic nephropathy. *Lancet* 1986;1:622–623.
52. Viberti GC, Jarrett RJ, Mahmud U, Hill RD, Argyropoulos A, Keen H. Microalbuminuria as a predictor of clinical nephropathy in insulin-dependent diabetes mellitus. *Lancet* 1982;1:1430–1432.
53. Mogensen CE. Microalbuminuria predicts clinical proteinuria and early mortality in maturity-onset diabetes. *N Engl J Med* 1984;310:356–360.
54. Consensus Statement. *Am J Kidney Dis* 1989;13:2–6.
55. Viberti CG, Pickup JC, Jarrett RJ, Keen H. Effect of control of blood glucose on urinary excretion of albumin and B2-microglobulin in insulin-dependent diabetes. *N Engl J Med* 1979;300:638–641.
56. Mogensen CE. Microalbuminuria and incipient diabetic nephropathy. *Diabetic Nephropathy* 1984;3:75–78.
57. Jarrett RJ, Viberti CG, Argyropoulos A, Hill RD, Mahmud U, Murrels TJ. Microalbuminuria predicts mortality in non-insulin-dependent diabetics. *Diabetic Med* 1984;1:17–19.
58. Noth RH, Krolewski AS, Kaysen GA, Meyer TW, Schambelan. Diabetic nephropathy: Hemodynamic basis and implications for disease management. *Ann Intern Med* 1989;110:795–813.
59. Anderson AR, Christiansen JS, Andersen JK, Kreiner S, Deckert T. Diabetic nephropathy in Type I (insulin-dependent) diabetes: an epidemiologic study. *Diabetologia* 1983;25:496–501.
60. Borch-Johnsen K, Kragh-Andersen P, Deckert T. The effect of proteinuria on relative mortality in type I (insulin dependent) diabetes mellitus. *Diabetologia* 1985;28:590–596.
61. Berisa F, McGonigle R, Beaman M, Adu D, Michael J. The treatment of diabetic renal failure by continuous ambulatory peritoneal dialysis. *Diabetic Med* 1989;6:67–70.
62. Zander E, Schultz B, Gums G, Lorenz G, Warzok R. Causes of death in insulin-dependent diabetic patients treated with hemodialysis. *J Diabetic Complications* 1989;3:163–166.
63. Larsson O, Attman PO, Blohme I, Nyberg G, Brynger H. Morbidity and mortality in diabetic and non-diabetic recipients of living related donor kidneys. *Nephrol Dialysis Transplant* 1987;2:109–116.
64. Statement on the clinical use of recombinant erythropoietin in anemia of end-stage renal disease. Ad Hoc Committee for the National Kidney Foundation. *Am J Kidney Dis* 1989;14:163–169.
65. Friedman EA, L'Esperance FA. Improved outlook for diabetic renal-retinal syndrome. In: Friedman EA, L'Esperance FA, eds. *Diabetic renal-retinal syndrome*. New York: Grune & Stratton; 1980:1–4.
66. Friedman EA, Chou LM, Beyer MM, Butt KMH, Manis T. Adverse impact of hyptertension on diabetic recipients of transplanted kidneys. *Hypertension* 1985;76(2):1131–1134.
67. Ramsay RC, Cantrill HL, Knobloch WH, Goetz FC, Sutherland DER, Najarian JS. Visual parameters in diabetic patients following renal transplantation. *Diabetic Nephropathy* 1983;2:26–9.
68. Mogensen CE. Progression of nephropathy in long term diabetics with proteinuria and effect of initial antihypertensive treatment. *Scand J Clin Lab Invest* 1976;36:383–388.
69. Parving H-H, Andersen AR, Smidt UM, Hommel E, Mathiesen ER, Svendsen PA. Effect of antihypertensive treatment on kidney function in diabetic nephropathy. *Br Med J* 1987;294:1443–1447.
70. Parving HH, Hommel E, Smidt UM. Protection of kidney function and decrease in albuminuria by captopril in insulin-dependent diabetics with nephropathy. *Br Med J* 1988;297:1086–1091.
71. Marre M, Chateillier G, Leblanc H, Guyenne TT, Menard J, Passa P. Prevention of diabetic nephropathy with enalapril in normotensive diabetics with microalbuminuria. *Br Med J* 1988;297:1092–1095.
72. Trost BN, Weidman P, Beretta-Piccoli C. Anti-hypertensive therapy in diabetic patients. *Hypertension* 1985;7:102–108.
73. Zawada ET, Jr. Metabolic considerations in the approach to diabetic hypertensive patients. *Am J Med* 87 1989;(Suppl 6A):34S–38S.
74. Final Report. The Working Group on hypertension in diabetes. Statement on hypertension in diabetes mellitus. *Arch Intern Med* 1987;147:830–842.
75. Gibson GR. Enalapril-induced cough. *Arch Intern Med* 1989;149:2701–2703.
76. Massry SG, Feinstein EI, Goldstein DA. Diabetic nephropathy: Clinical course and effect of hemodialysis. *Nephron* 1978;20:286–296.
77. Quadri R, Veglio M, Flecchia D, Tonda L, DeLorenzo F, Chiandussi L, Fonz D. Autonomic neuropathy and sexual impotence in diabetic patients: Analysis of cardiovascular reflexes. *Andrologia* 1989;21:346–352.

78. Norden G, Granerus G, Nyberg G. Diabetic cystopathy—a risk factor in diabetic nephropathy? *J Diabetic Complications* 1988;2:203–206.
79. Nompleggi D, Bell SJ, Blackburn GL, Bistrian BR. Overview of gastrointestinal disorders due to diabetes mellitus: emphasis on nutritional support. *Jpn Parenter Enteral Nutr* 1989;13:84–91.
80. Abramowicz M. Antimicrobial prophylaxis in surgery. *Med Letter* 1989;31:105–108.
81. Hou SH, Bushinsky DA, Wish JB, Cohen JJ, Harrington JT. Hospital-acquired renal insufficiency: A prospective study. *Am J Med* 1983;74:243–248.
82. Berns AS. Nephrotoxicity of contrast media. *Kidney Int* 1989;36:730–740.
83. Byrd L, Sherman RL. Radiocontrast-induced acute renal failure. A clinical and pathophysiologic review. *Medicine* 1979;58:270–279.
84. Harkonen S, Kjellstrand CM. Exacerbation of diabetic renal failure following intravenous pyelography. *Am J Med* 1977;63:939–946.
85. Shieh SD, Hirsch SR, Boshell BR, Pino JA, Alexander LI, Witter DM, Friedman EA. Low risk of contrast media-induced acute renal failure in nonazotemic type-2 diabetes mellitus. *Kidney Int* 1982;21:739–743.
86. Parfrey PS, Griffiths SM, Barrett BJ, et al. Contrast media-induced renal failure in patients with diabetes mellitus, renal insufficiency or both. *N Engl J Med* 1989;320:143–149.
87. Schwab SJ, Hltaky MA, Pieper KS, et al. Contrast nephrotoxicity: A randomized controlled trial of a nonionic and an ionic radiographic contrast agent. *N Engl J Med* 1989;320:149–153.
88. Anto HR, Chou SY, Porush JG, Shapiro WB. Infusion intravenous pyelography and renal function: Effects of hypertonic mannitol in patients with chronic renal insufficiency. *Arch Intern Med* 1981;141:1652–1656.
89. Berkseth RO, Kjellstrand CM. Radiologic contrast induced nephropathy. *Med Clin North Am* 1984;68:179–181.
90. Eisenberg RL, Bank WO, Hedgcock MW. Renal failure after major angiography can be avoided with hydration. *Am J Roentgenol* 1981;136:859–861.
91. Barzilay E, Kessler D, Berlot G, Gullo A, Geber D, Ben Zeev I. Use of extracorporeal supportive techniques as additional treatment for septic-induced multiple organ failure patients. *Crit Care Med* 1989;17:634–637.
92. Weiss L, Danielson BG, Wikstrom B, Hedstrand U, Wahlberg J. Continuous arteriovenous hemofiltration in the treatment of 100 critically ill patients with acute renal failure: Report on clinical outcome and nutritional aspects. *Clin Nephrol* 1989;31:184–189.
93. Mault JR, Dechert RE, Lees P, Swartz RD, Port FK, Bartlett RH. Continuous arteriovenous filtration: An effective treatment for surgical acute renal failure. *Surgery* 1987;101:478–484.
94. Pourchez T, Morinière P, Fournier A, Pietri J. Use of Permcath (Quinton) catheter in uraemic patients in whom the creation of conventional vascular access for haemodialysis is difficult. *Nephron* 1989;53:297–302.

Surgical Management of the Diabetic Patient,
edited by Michael Bergman and Gregorio A. Sicard.
Raven Press, Ltd., New York © 1991.

7

Diabetes and Cardiovascular Disease

*Carl J. Lavie, *Bijoy K. Khandheria, †David J. Ballard, and
‡Pasquale J. Palumbo

*Department of Internal Medicine, *Division of Cardiovascular Diseases, and
†Department of Health Sciences Research, Section of Clinical Epidemiology, and
‡Division of Endocrinology, Mayo Clinic and Mayo Foundation,
Rochester, Minnesota 55905*

Diabetes is one of the leading causes of death in the United States, and cardiac disease is the major cause of mortality among diabetic patients. The prevalence of risk factors for ischemic heart disease is high among diabetic individuals, and premature and accelerated coronary artery disease develop in diabetic patients, even independently of other risk factors. Coronary heart disease is often asymptomatic in diabetic patients; when cardiac events occur, complications occur more frequently and morbidity and mortality rates are higher in diabetic patients when compared with nondiabetic patients. In addition, clinical, epidemiologic, and pathologic data indicate that diabetes is associated with a specific cardiomyopathy, even in the absence of macrovascular coronary artery disease. Not surprisingly then, cardiac complications after major surgical procedures are common among individuals with diabetes.

Patients with diabetes often require detailed evaluation before major noncardiac surgery. Guided by a careful history, physical examination, and selective preoperative testing, the physician can estimate the potential risk for diabetic patients. In this chapter, we review the evidence that diabetes is an independent risk factor for cardiac complications associated with major surgical procedures, the preoperative cardiac assessment of these high-risk patients, and the perioperative management of those with evidence of ischemic heart disease.

BACKGROUND AND EPIDEMIOLOGY

Association of Diabetes and Perioperative Cardiac Complications

The association of diabetes and cardiac complications following major surgical procedures has been addressed in numerous studies that encompass a wide variety of surgical procedures. Studies with sufficient power to demonstrate an increased independent risk of perioperative cardiac complications associated with diabetes have found such an elevated risk. For example, with respect to the placement of coronary artery bypass grafts (CABG), perioperative mortality was greater for individuals with noninsulin-dependent diabetes (5.1%, $N = 250$) or insulin-dependent diabetes (4.5%, $N = 162$) than for nondiabetic CABG patients (2.5%, $N = 3,295$) at Good Samaritan Hospital and Medical Center, Portland, Oregon, from April 1969 to May 1982 (1). Similarly, Lawrie et al. (2) reported a 7.1% perioperative mortality rate in diabetic patients contrasted with a 4.5% rate among nondiabetic patients undergoing CABG. In contrast, however, the perioperative mortality rate was reported to be only 1.8% among 384 diabetic individuals undergoing CABG at Bay State Medical Center, Springfield, Massachusetts, from January 1979 to December 1985, contrasted with a rate of 2.5% for 396 randomly sampled nondiabetic patients undergoing CABG at the same institution (3).

With respect to noncardiac surgery, in a study of all first operations for cholelithiasis at the North Carolina Memorial Hospital from 1973 to 1982, individuals with diabetes had an approximately two-fold increased risk of a major perioperative cardiovascular complication (4). Diabetes was also independently associated with a two and one-half-fold increased risk of postoperative cardiac ischemic events among 200 patients undergoing major vascular surgery at Massachusetts General Hospital (5). Among patients undergoing first kidney transplantation at Helsinki University Central Hospital from September 1981 to September 1987, six of 81 (7.4%) diabetic patients died within one month of surgery; the rate among nondiabetic patients was 1.2%, or four of 330. Four of the deaths among patients with diabetes were cardiac in origin (6). In summary, although all studies do not provide consistent results because of inadequate statistical power, there is substantial evidence that diabetes is, in general, an independent risk factor for perioperative cardiac complications associated with both cardiac and major noncardiac surgery.

PREOPERATIVE ASSESSMENT

When estimating cardiac risk, the magnitude of the surgical procedure and the surgical and anesthetic expertise in one's own institution must be considered, as well

TABLE 1. *Goldman's preoperative cardiac risk index*

Variable	Point Score
History	
Age > 70 years	5
Preoperative MI within 6 months	10
Physical examination	
S_3 gallop or elevated jugular venous pressure (>12 cm H_2O)	11
Significant aortic stenosis	3
Electrocardiogram (ECG)	
Rhythm other than sinus or atrial ectopy	7
Documentation of >5 PVCs/min	7
General medical status	3
P_aO_2 < 60 or P_aCO_2 > 50 torr	
K < 3.0 or HCO_3 < 20 mEq/l	
BUN > 50 or creatinine > 3.0 mg/dl	
Chronic liver disease or debilitated patient	
Operation	
Intraperitoneal, intrathoracic, or aortic surgery	3
Emergency operation	4
Total possible =	53

Modified from Goldman L, et al. (7).

as the characteristics of the patients undergoing the operation. By using a multivariable analysis of 39 variables in 1,001 surgical patients, Goldman and colleagues (7) identified nine variables as independent predictors of perioperative cardiac events; from these data, a point score system was derived that correlated with subsequent cardiac events (Table 1). Other studies have validated these initial findings (8,9). The applicability of the Goldman cardiac risk index to major surgical procedures (intrathoracic, upper abdominal, vascular, and major orthopedic), however, has been questioned (10), and the presence and severity of angina or remote myocardial infarction (MI) are conspicuously absent from this index. Others, however, have incorporated these important additional factors into a modified cardiac risk index (11,12). In our practice, we incorporate all of these factors (discussed below) into our preoperative assessment.

History

A thorough cardiovascular history is vital in the preoperative assessment of diabetic patients, particularly regarding history and time of prior MI; presence, severity and pattern of angina; symptoms of left ventricular (LV) dysfunction; and transient cerebral ischemia. In patients with prior MI, the risk of perioperative infarction is substantial during the first three to six months (30 and 15%, respectively) but reaches about 5% thereafter (13,14). The presence of unstable angina (rest angina or rapidly progressive anginal pattern) requires vigorous preoperative medical stabilization and often coronary angiography and revascularization procedures, even prior to fairly low-risk surgical procedures. Likewise, active cerebral ischemia requires preoperative assessment and management. Although dyspnea can occur as the result of a number of etiologies (pulmonary parenchymal disease, pulmonary vascular disease, poor conditioning, and systolic and/or diastolic dysfunction), close attention should be paid to this symptom because, in a number of diabetic patients, dyspnea may be an "anginal equivalent" and require aggressive preoperative assessment.

Physical Examination

The role of the physical examination in the assessment of known or presumed ischemic heart disease is limited. An apical holosystolic murmur that develops only during chest pain or with exertion suggests ischemic-induced papillary muscle dysfunction. On cardiac auscultation, S_4 and S_3 gallops (both diastolic sounds) indicate diastolic and systolic ventricular dysfunction, respectively; but these are not specific findings for ischemic heart diease. Patients with evidence of vascular disease (reduced peripheral pulses or bruits) have a high prevalence of significant coronary disease, and certain cutaneous signs (especially tendon xanthomas) suggest familial hypercholesterolemia and a high prevalence of premature coronary atherosclerosis. Otherwise, the major purpose of the physical examination is to assess ventricular function and to rule out uncompensated congestive heart failure. An elevated jugular venous pressure, hepatic congestion, and peripheral edema all suggest right-sided congestive heart failure. Pulmonary crackles, a soft S_1, S_3 gallop, and paradoxic splitting of the second heart sound all suggest LV dysfunction. In particular, an S_3

gallop, wet-sounding pulmonary crackles, and evidence of right-sided failure indicate *decompensated* congestive heart failure, suggesting that further medical therapy is required before an elective operation.

Resting Electrocardiogram (ECG)

The resting ECG is helpful in ruling out prior or recent MI, and several ECG findings are associated with an increased risk of ischemic heart disease, including LV hypertrophy (especially with repolarization abnormalities or strain), intraventricular conduction defects, and nonspecific ST-T wave abnormalities (15). The resting ECG also provides valuable information regarding resting LV function. In a recent study of 874 patients from our Nuclear Cardiology Laboratory, the ejection fraction (EF) was greater than 50% in 90–95% of those with a normal or near normal ECG and only 2% had an EF less than 40%. On the other hand, of those with nonspecific ST-T wave changes and a "history" of MI, nearly 30% had an EF less than 50%, and half of these had EF less than 40% (16).

LV Function

Clinical evidence of LV dsyfunction is predictive of cardiac events in patients undergoing noncardiac surgery, but these remain indirect and imperfect estimates of LV function. As discussed above, in patients with normal or near normal resting ECG, the prevalence of significant LV dysfunction is low; in the absence of cardiomegaly on chest roentgenogram or evidence of cardiac enlargement on physical examination, no further evaluation of LV function is required in these patients. In patients with congestive heart failure or clinical evidence of LV dysfunction, an assessment of LV function with radionuclide angiography or echocardiography is useful for predicting perioperative cardiac morbidity and mortality and for tailoring postoperative medical management. This approach can be particularly applicable for diabetic patients with a high prevalence of systolic and diastolic (including restrictive abnormalities in some patients and relaxation abnormalities in others) ventricular abnormalities (17), even in the absence of macrovascular coronary disease. In some patients with significant congestive heart failure with normal systolic function, assessment of diastolic function with echocardiography (digitized M-mode or preferably pulsed-wave Doppler evaluation of mitral valve inflow) or radionuclide angiography may be indicated.

Stress Testing

In diabetic patients who have no definite history of ischemic heart disease, routine stress testing is not required prior to low-risk surgical procedures. Data from our institution and elsewhere indicate that the classic cardiac risk index of Goldman et al. (7) and other historical parameters (18) are quite insensitive for predicting perioperative cardiac events in patients undergoing high-risk operations (intrathoracic, upper abdominal, vascular surgery, or other major orthopedic procedures). We therefore believe that preoperative stress assessment is indicated in diabetic patients who are scheduled to undergo a high-risk elective surgical procedure. Our general preoperative approach is illustrated in Figure 1. Contraindications for stress assessment include unstable angina, uncontrolled hypertension, uncompensated congestive heart failure, active cerebral ischemia, recent aortic dissection, and inability to exercise for whatever reason.

Exercise ECG

The hallmark for the noninvasive assessment of ischemic heart disease is exercise ECG testing (treadmill or bicycle ergometry). Previous studies evaluating the preoperative ECG response to exercise in patients undergoing high-risk operations have had mixed results, with some finding the ECG response to be predictive of subsequent events while others do not (8,18). In a study from our Nuclear Cardiology Laboratory of 148 patients who did supine bicycle exercises prior to major vascular surgery, major cardiac events occurred in nine of 91 patients (12%) who were unable to exercise beyond 400 kg-m/min compared with no major cardiac events among 57 patients who exercised beyond this workload (18). Other recent studies corroborate the ability of modest levels of exercise (>400 kg-m/min by bicycle ergometry or >5 metabolic equivalents (METS) by treadmill exercise) to identify patients who are at low risk for perioperative cardiac events. Diabetic patients who can perform modest

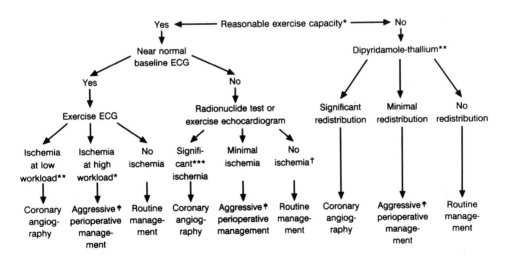

*5 METS on treadmill and/or 400 kg-M/min on supine bicycle ergometry
**Or other alternative to leg exercise
***See text for definitions
†Or mild ischemia only at high workload
*See text for details

FIG. 1. General algorithm for the preoperative assessment of high-risk diabetic patients, including those with ischemic heart disease undergoing any surgery as well as all those undergoing major surgical procedures (intrathoracic, upper abdominal, vascular, or major orthopedic).

exercise without angina or an ischemic ECG can safely undergo a major surgical procedure with no additional preoperative assessment.

Nuclear Testing

In certain patients, exercise assessment with radionuclide techniques may be indicated (Table 2), including exercise radionuclide angiography or thallium scintigraphy. In many situations, decisions regarding which nuclear imaging procedure to perform depends on the expertise of the particular institution. In settings where significant expertise in both techniques is available, several factors can influence the decision regarding what modality to use in a given patient (Table 3).

Exercise radionuclide angiography performed with 99-^{m} technetium ^{99m}Tc-DTPA labeling of red blood cells allows for assessment of LV regional and global function at rest and at different stages of exercise. As mentioned earlier, assessment of resting LV function may provide important information regarding perioperative and long-term prognosis and provides information helpful in tailoring postoperative medical management. Mechanical evidence of ischemia can be assessed by a significant fall in LVEF with exercise (usually $\geq 5\%$) or the development of new regional wall motion abnormalities. A fall in LVEF $\geq 10\%$ or a peak LVEF $< 50\%$ suggests severe ischemia. Exercise echocardiography is an alternative technique to assess mechanical evidence of ischemia, which is being increasingly used in many institutions.

Myocardial perfusion is assessed by thallium perfusion imaging. Thallium 201 is injected near the peak of exercise; imaging is performed soon after exercise, and then approximately 4 hours later. A persistent defect on both the post exercise and delayed image usually represents scar, and reversible defects indicate ischemia. In patients with a persistent thallium defect at 4 hours who have no history of MI or Q-waves on ECG, often 24–48-hour imaging is performed because delayed redistribution often occurs in patients with severe coronary obstructive lesions. Indicators of severe ischemia by thallium criteria include increased LV cavity size with exercise, increased pulmonary uptake of thallium with exercise, and redistribution in several vascular territories.

In patients who are unable to adequately exercise (usually as a result of vascular

---

TABLE 2. *Indications for exercise radionuclide testing as opposed to exercise ECG*

High-risk of false–positive ECG results
    Certain drugs (e.g. digitalis, phenothiazines, type I antiarrhythmic drugs)
    Wolf-Parkinson-White syndrome
    Mitral valve prolapse
    Left ventricular hypertrophy
    Significant resting ST-T wave abnormalities
    Significant valvular heart disease
ECG not interpretable for ischemia
    Left bundle branch block
    Pacemaker dependency
    Marked resting ST-T wave abnormalities
Information desired regarding anatomic area of ischemia
    After revascularization procedure
    To correlate with catheterization
Increased sensitivity and/or specificity is necessary

TABLE 3. *Comparison of exercise radionuclide testing with radionuclide angiography (RNA) or thallium scintigraphy*

Advantages of RNA	Advantages of thallium
Lower cost	When mechanical abnormalities may occur without coronary disease[a]
Ejection fraction (major prognostic indicator)	Better anatomic correlation
Time onset of ischemia	Better sensitivity with tomographic imaging
Diastolic function	
Quantify valvular regurgitation	

[a]Left bundle branch block (LBBB), hypertrophic cardiomyopathy (HCM), severe hypertension or severe valvular heart disease.
Note: In both LBBB and HCM, exercise ECG, RNA, and thallium perfusion may be abnormal without macrovascular coronary disease.

disease or orthopedic limitations), several alternatives to exercise testing are available, including pacing nuclear studies and pharmacologic stimulation (dobutamine, adenosine, dipyridamole) combined with either thallium scintigraphy or echocardiography. Of these techniques, dipyridamole thallium testing has emerged as the most commonly used alternative to exercise testing. With this technique, dipyridamole (given intravenously in experimental protocols or orally) causes significant coronary vasodilation, increasing coronary perfusion to areas supplied by nonstenotic vessels with limited increase in perfusion in regions supplied by stenotic vessels (with limited coronary flow reserve). Dipyridamole also causes redistribution of perfusion from the endocardium to the epicardium. In some patients, a "coronary steal syndrome" is produced, causing wall motion abnormalities, ECG changes, and angina pectoris.

Leppo and colleagues (19) performed dipyridamole-thallium imaging in 100 consecutive patients prior to aortic or peripheral vascular surgery. Major perioperative cardiac events (MI or death) occurred in 33% of those with redistribution on a dipyridamole–thallium study in comparison with only 2% in those with no redistribution. Sensitivity for the procedure for predicting major cardiac events was excellent (93%), but the specificity was 62% and the positive predictive accuracy only 33%. Positive predictive value of the test was markedly increased in the diabetic patients; in those patients with both diabetes and ST depression with dipyridamole, 60% had perioperative cardiac events.

In a recent large study by Eagle and colleagues (5) of 254 consecutive patients having vascular surgery, dipyridamole–thallium imaging and clinical parameters helped predict early postoperative cardiac events. Logistic regression analysis identified five clinical predictors (Q-wave on ECG, ventricular ectopy, diabetes, age over 70, and angina) and two dipyridamole–thallium predictors (redistribution and ischemic ECG changes) of postoperative events. These data indicate that dipyridamole–thallium testing was not useful for patients who had none of the clinical variables (cardiac event rate only 3%) or in those with three or more clinical variables (cardiac event rate 50%). Dipyridamole–thallium testing was very useful in those patients with one or two clinical variables (one being diabetes); of those with no thallium redistribution, only two of 62 (3.2%) had cardiac events in comparison with 16 of 54 (29.6%) with thallium redistribution.

In our experience at Mayo Clinic, dipyridamole–thallium testing has also proven to be very useful in predicting major events prior to major noncardiac surgical procedures (20). Of 116 consecutive patients who underwent dipyridamole-thallium testing prior to a major operation, 46 had reversible defects and 69 had either normal perfusion or nonreversible defects. Of those with redistribution, nine (19.6%) had a perioperative MI in comparison with only one (1.5%) of those patients without redistribution. Recent data from our institution indicate that the presence of ischemic ECG changes during dipyridamole study is a particularly poor prognostic sign, indicating both severe ischemia and a very high prevalence of either severe three-vessel coronary disease or left main coronary disease (21).

Cardiac Catheterization

Some physicians advocate routine preoperative coronary angiography and prophylactic coronary artery bypass grafting in high-risk patients scheduled to undergo major surgical procedures, particularly vascular surgery. There is often, however, considerable discrepancy between coronary anatomy and the functional significance of coronary lesions. Therefore, we believe that noninvasive testing prior to coronary angiography is preferred in most situations. Coronary angiography is reserved for those with high-risk parameters on noninvasive testing (Fig. 1) and those with at least three of the five major clinical criteria of Eagle and colleagues (diabetes, Q-wave on ECG, angina, age over 70, and significant ventricular arrhythmia). In those patients with severe coronary artery disease and suitable coronary anatomy, consideration should be given to a revascularization procedure, either percutaneous transluminal coronary angioplasty or coronary artery bypass grafting, before elective major noncardiac operation. The benefit of the coronary revascularization procedures must be carefully weighed against the potential risks (which at times may be higher) in an effort to reduce potential cardiac morbidity or mortality associated with high-risk noncardiac surgery. The presence of cardiac risk index factors, severity of ischemic heart disease, functional limitation, presence and degree of LV function, age, sex, medical therapeutic options, and other associated medical conditions are all factors that could have a significant impact on the individual patient's preoperative management.

PERIOPERATIVE MANAGEMENT

The perioperative management of diabetic patients with definite or high likelihood of ischemic heart disease includes special attention given to management of plasma glucose concentrations as well as measures to decrease cardiac complications.

Diabetes Management

The goal of diabetes management is to maintain the plasma glucose level between 80 and 120 mg/dl before, during, and after surgery, to decrease the catabolism of carbohydrate, fat, and protein, and minimize ketogenesis, fluid and electrolyte disturbances, and the risk of hypoglycemia. The plasma glucose level can be maintained within the desirable range by the use of insulin infusion pumps or the artificial pancreas, such as the Biostator, or through careful titration of insulin in intravenous solutions. The use of insulin infusion pumps is preferable for diabetes control in the perioperative period.

For patients on insulin treatment, such therapy will need to be adjusted in the perioperative period, as indicated by glucose measurements, either plasma or capillary. Random urine glucose measurements have no place in the intensive management of diabetes mellitus. For patients on diet alone or oral agents, insulin treatment will usually be necessary to maintain adequate control of hyperglycemia in the perioperative period. Diet and oral agents can usually be restarted when the patient resumes and maintains oral intake.

For short (less than one hour) and/or minor surgical procedures (such as excision biopsy) or diagnostic invasive procedures (such as endoscopy) for which food intake may be resumed within 6 hours postoperatively, monitoring of plasma or capillary glucose levels and the judicious use of insulin in intravenous fluid infusions should suffice. For such short-term or minor procedures, the patient may or may not be required to fast. If the patient is fed, the usual morning insulin dose can be given before breakfast. Blood glucose levels should be determined every 2 to 4 hours and supplemental regular insulin as indicated provided. When the patient's condition is stable and the patient has fully recovered from the procedure and is ready for dismissal, the usual diabetes program can be resumed with the instruction to monitor capillary glucose levels every 4 hours for 24 hours and then the usual capillary glucose monitoring thereafter. Supplemental regular insulin can be used to control glucose levels equal to or greater than 150 mg/dl according to the algorithm in Table 4. If the patient has no food for more than 6 hours after surgery, the patient will need to continue with subcutaneous supplemental regular insulin to control rising glucose levels. The patient should be able to resume the usual insulin program within 24 hours. The major precaution with such algorithms is the development of hypoglycemia and the need to avoid the same by adequate blood glucose monitoring and providing supplemental feeding or other treatment should hypoglycemia develop.

There is no known long-term risk to patients whose glucose levels are above 150 mg/dl and who will be undergoing minor surgical procedures that will last no longer than 1 hour and for whom the usual diabetes management will be resumed within 6 hours or less postoperatively.

For major surgical procedures, such as abdominal exploration, cancer removal surgeries, revascularization procedures, etc., that last more than one hour, more careful monitoring of blood glucose levels and the use of insulin to maintain the goal range of 80 to 120 mg/dl will be necessary. A glucose and insulin solution allows for titration of both substances to maintain the desirable glucose level. For major surgery, the patient continues the usual diabetes management program until the day of

TABLE 4. *Algorithm for control of glucose levels*

Blood glucose (mg/dl)*	Subcutaneous regular insulin (units)
≤150	0
151–200	6
201–300	10
301–400	20

*Add 10 units per 100 mg/dl glucose level over 400 mg/dl.

surgery. A glycosylated hemoglobin level should be obtained the day before surgery. On the day of surgery, the patient should fast and not be given insulin until the blood glucose level and the most recent glycosylated hemoglobin results are available and reviewed. Blood glucose level should be measured preoperatively and an intravenous solution containing dextrose should be started after the blood has been drawn for a glucose determination. An insulin solution should be prepared by placing 25 units of regular insulin in 250 cc of 0.45% normal saline for infusion at a constant rate for control of glucose levels. The initial insulin infusion rate of regular insulin is determined on the basis of the preoperative glucose level according to the guidelines listed in Table 5. The major precaution is the risk of hypoglycemia. The blood glucose level is checked at hourly intervals perioperatively and the insulin infusion rate stabilized so as to maintain the desirable blood glucose levels of 80 to 120 mg/dl. The insulin infusion should be given separate from the other intravenous solutions but may be piggybacked at a constant rate into the other intravenous fluid solutions.

When the blood glucose concentration and insulin infusion rate are stabilized, the frequency of blood glucose level monitoring can be decreased to every 2 hours and then every 4 to 6 hours. Ideally, diabetic patients should be admitted to a diabetes intensive-care unit while they recover from anesthesia and surgery over a 24-hour period. When the blood glucose level drops below 80 mg/dl, the insulin infusion may need to be stopped in order to avoid hypoglycemia. It may be necessary to continue the dextrose solution or to provide 50% dextrose to control symptoms of hypoglycemia. A 50% dextrose solution should be considered for blood glucose levels less than 50 mg/dl.

If the blood glucose level fails to decrease at 4 units/h of insulin infusion, it may be necessary to double the insulin infusion rate at glucose concentrations of 300 mg/dl or more. The other insulin infusion rates at lower concentrations of blood glucose will need to be proportionately adjusted. The algorithm for glucose concentrations less than 150 mg/dl should be maintained. When subcutaneous insulin is to be resumed, the intravenous insulin infusion should be discontinued approximately 2 hours after the first injection of subcutaneous insulin.

Within one week of major surgery if there have been no complications, the patient should be able to resume the usual diabetes program. The program of self-monitoring of capillary glucose levels and adjustment of insulin dosage accordingly should be reviewed with the patient before dismissal.

TABLE 5. *Algorithm for control of glucose levels by insulin infusion*

Blood glucose (mg/dl)	Insulin /nfusion rate (units/h)
≤80	0.2
80–99	0.5
100–119	1.0
120–149	1.5
150–199	2.0
200–249	2.5
250–300	3.0
≥300	4.0

This algorithm is appropriate for the average 70 kg person; infusion rates may have to be modified proportionately for larger or smaller individuals.

Diabetic patients on total parenteral nutrition (TPN) usually require insulin added to the TPN solution starting with an initial dose of 0.1 unit of regular insulin per gram of dextrose in the solution so that for 150 g of dextrose in 1 liter of TPN, 15 units of regular insulin would be added. The amount of insulin added to the TPN solution may need to be increased to maintain the plasma glucose level within the desirable range. Usually the addition of insulin to the concentrated dextrose solutions of TPN is quite safe and has not been associated with hypoglycemia, even in nondiabetic patients. Once nutritional support is established, it should be easier to maintain the desirable blood glucose range.

Blood glucose levels should be measured at least every 6 hours in patients with diabetes receiving TPN. Once glycemic control is in an acceptable or desirable range, an alteration in the frequency of monitoring may be appropriate. Some unstable patients, particularly those with insulin-dependent diabetes mellitus or those receiving other infusions or other medications, may initially require more frequent monitoring. Blood glucose levels in excess of 200 mg/dl should be managed by increasing the insulin coverage in the TPN solution to 0.15 units of regular insulin per gram of dextrose up to a maximum of 0.2 units of regular insulin per gram of dextrose. If the blood glucose remains greater than 200 mg/dl with insulin coverage of 0.2 units per gram of dextrose, intravenous insulin infusion may be considered as outlined above. This level of hyperglycemia may indicate insulin resistance induced by illness, glucocorticoids, or overfeeding. In general, the TPN dextrose load should not be increased until the blood glucose levels of the previous 24 hours are less than 200 mg/dl. Insulin in the TPN may need to be adjusted appropriately. Hypoglycemia, that is blood glucose levels less than 50 mg/dl, should be treated by immediate dextrose supplements added directly to or piggybacked to the TPN admixture. If there is no explanation for the hypoglycemia, a significant (30 to 50%) reduction of insulin in the following day's TPN admixture should help decrease the chance of recurrent hypoglycemia. The rate of the TPN solution can be tapered or decreased by 50% for 1 hour before its cessation. The incidence of symptomatic hypoglycemia after sudden or inadvertent cessation of TPN is very low, provided there has been no recent increase in TPN infusion rate.

Patients on enteral nutrition can be managed by either subcutaneous insulin administration or insulin infusion (as outlined above) to maintain the glucose levels in the desirable range mentioned above.

Cardiac Management

In all patients with definite or probable ischemic heart disease who are scheduled to undergo general anesthesia, the administration of topical nitrates (for example, one-half to one inch of nitrol paste) immediately prior to surgery and every 4–6 hours after surgery for the first 24–48 postoperative hours provides reasonable prophylactic protection against myocardial ischemia. Efforts should be made not to begin nitrate therapy too early, because tolerance to continuous nitrate administration has been noted within the first 24 hours of therapy. In addition, an ECG soon after surgery and at 24 hours, and testing of cardiac enzymes (creatine phosphokinase MB fraction every 8 hours over a 24-hour period) is indicated in most cases.

In many diabetic patients, special cardiac management is indicated in efforts to decrease perioperative cardiac morbidity and mortality. Although some controversy still exists regarding the type of anesthesia to use, most studies suggest that the method (general versus spinal) and specific type of anesthesia administered do not significantly contribute to perioperative risk (8). In this regard, there may be considerable variability among different institutions, depending on particular local expertize. In patients with ischemic heart disease who are undergoing major surgical procedures, continuous blood-pressure monitoring is necessary, usually with intraarterial techniques. In high-risk diabetic patients (Table 6), more aggressive management is indicated, including pulmonary arterial catheterization to monitor LV filling (or pulmonary capillary wedge) pressure intraoperatively and during the first 24–48 postoperative hours. In addition, prophylactic low-dose intravenous nitroglycerine is indicated in these patients, with the wedge pressure, intraarterial blood pressure, and cardiac output helping guide the dose of intravenous nitrates as well as intravenous fluids, inotropes, and need for arterial vasodilators. Benefit of such monitoring could continue well into the postoperative period, where major extravascular fluid mobilization could precipitate pulmonary edema, particularly in patients with severe LV dysfunction. In certain patients undergoing particularly high-risk surgery (e.g., patients undergoing major abdominal aortic aneurysm surgery with recent unstable angina and revascularization not possible), consideration should be given to monitoring cardiac function intraoperatively with transesophageal echocardiography.

There are several specific points pertinent to the preoperative and postoperative management of diabetic patients with ischemic heart disease, which are summarized in Table 7. In general, diabetic patients have more severe ischemia and their ischemia is more often silent compared with ischemia in nondiabetic patients (22); when ischemic complications occur in diabetic patients (e.g., MI or other acute coronary syndromes), their morbidity and mortality is higher. Therefore, the index of suspicion for myocardial ischemia needs to be heightened in diabetic patients, and more vigorous medical management is required. In addition, factors are present that affect the type of medical management for diabetic patients. It is well known that a heart-muscle disease often accompanies diabetes (diabetic cardiomyopathy), and diabetic patients usually have a lower LVEF at any given levels of coronary disease and myocardial ischemia. Therefore, it is necessary to closely assess postoperative fluid status of diabetic patients, who often require higher doses of nitrates; many diabetic patients require inotropes and other intravenous vasodilators. Because beta blockade reduces myocardial contractility and cardiac output and inhibits both the symptoms and signs of hypoglycemia and gluconeogenesis, these agents are often not ideal for diabetic patients. When beta blockade is required, cardioselective agents (metoprolol or atenolol) or the short-acting intravenous agent (esmolol) should be used in low doses. Numerous studies have demonstrated that diastolic ventricular

TABLE 6. *Diabetic patients requiring aggressive perioperative cardiac management*

Major emergency operation without preoperative cardiac assessment
Abdominal aortic aneurysm surgery
High-risk patients with significant ischemia without revascularization preoperatively
High-risk surgical procedure with minimal ischemia or ischemia at high workloads
Myocardial infarction $\leq$ 6 months
Relatively low-risk surgical procedure in patients with significant ischemia
Patients with significant left ventricular dysfunction or valvular heart disease

TABLE 7. *Factors affecting management of diabetic patients with myocardial ischemia*

Factor	Impact
More ischemia and worse prognosis	Need more aggressive management
More silent ischemia	Need more aggressive preoperative assessment and postoperative management
More diastolic dysfunction	Calcium-channel blockers are ideal agents (possibly in combination with low doses of cardioselective beta-blockers)
More systolic dysfunction with similar coronary disease	Need close management of fluid status perioperatively and often vasodilators (possibly with inotropic support)
Beta-blockers inhibit symptoms and signs of hypoglycemia and inhibit gluconeogenesis	Calcium blockers and nitrates are ideal agents; use cardioselective beta blockers at low doses

dysfunction is a very early manifestation of diabetic heart disease; calcium channel blockers, particularly diltiazem and verapamil, should be ideal agents for treating ischemia and hypertension in diabetic patients, particulary in those with relatively preserved LV systolic function.

CONCLUSION

We believe that rigorous assessment of preoperative cardiac risk in conjunction with aggressive preoperative and postoperative diabetic and cardiac management results in reduction of cardiac morbidity and mortality in diabetic patients undergoing noncardiac surgical procedures. It is important to emphasize that cardiac disease is the leading cause of premature death in diabetic patients. Therefore, long-term follow-up of the diabetes and cardiac status is necessary with these patients, particularly those with early, mild cardiac abnormalities detected during the preoperative assessment and postoperative management.

ACKNOWLEDGMENT

Supported in part from research grants from the National Institutes of Health (HL24326 AR30582). The authors thank Ms. Sondra Buehler for manuscript preparation.

REFERENCES

1. Salomon NW, Page US, Okies JE, Stephens J, Krause AH, Bigelow JC. Diabetes mellitus and coronary artery bypass—Short-term risk and long-term prognosis. *J Thorac Cardiovasc Surg* 1983;85:264–71.
2. Lawrie GM, Morris GC Jr, Glaeser DH. Influence of diabetes mellitus on the results of coronary bypass surgery—Follow-up of 212 diabetic patients ten to 15 years after surgery. *JAMA* 1986;256:2967–71.
3. Clement R, Rousou JA, Engelman RM, Breyer RH. Perioperative morbidity in diabetics requiring coronary artery bypass surgery. *Ann Thorac Surg* 1988;46:321–3.
4. Sandler RS, Maule WF, Baltus ME. Factors associated with postoperative complications in diabetics after biliary tract surgery. *Gastroenterology* 1986;91:157–62.
5. Eagle KA, Coley CM, Newell JB, et al. Combining clinical and thallium data optimizes preoperative assessment of cardiac risk before major vascular surgery. *Ann Intern Med* 1989;110:859–66.

6. Heino A. Operative and postoperative non-surgical complications in diabetic patients undergoing renal transplantation. *Scand J Urol Nephrol* 1988;22:53–8.

7. Goldman L, Caldera DL, Nussbaum SR, et al. Multifactorial index of cardiac risk in noncardiac surgical procedures. *N Engl J Med* 1977;297:845–50.

8. Freeman WK, Gibbons RJ, Shub C. Preoperative assessment of the cardiac patients undergoing noncardiac surgical procedures. *Mayo Clin Proc* 1989;64:1105–17.

9. Zeldin RA. Assessing cardiac risk in patients who undergo noncardiac surgical procedures. *Can J Surg* 1984;27:402–4.

10. Jeffrey CC, Kunsman J, Cullen DJ, Brewster DC. A prospective evaluation of cardiac risk index. *Anesthesiology* 1983;58:462–4.

11. Detsky AS, Abrams HB, Forbath N, Scott JG, Hilliard JR. Cardiac assessment for patients undergoing noncardiac surgery—A multifactorial clinical risk index. *Arch Intern Med* 1986; 146:2131–4.

12. Detsky AS, Abrams HB, McLaughlin JR, et al. Predicting cardiac complications in patients undergoing non-cardiac surgery. *J Gen Intern Med* 1986;1:211–19.

13. Tarhan S, Moffitt EA, Taylor WF, Giuliani ER. Myocardial infarction after general anesthesia. *JAMA* 1972;220:1451–4.

14. Steen PA, Tinker JH, Tarhan S. Myocardial reinfarction after anesthesia and surgery. *JAMA* 1978;239:2566–70.

15. Kannel WB. Detection and management of patients with silent myocardial ischemia. *Am Heart J* 1989;117(1):221–6.

16. O'Keefe JH Jr, Zinsmeister AR, Gibbons RJ. Value of normal electrocardiographic findings in predicting resting left ventricular function in patients with chest pain and suspected coronary artery disease. *Am J Med* 1989;86:658–62.

17. Zarich SW, Arbuckle BE, Cohen LR, Roberts M, Nesto RW. Diastolic abnormalities in young asymptomatic diabetic patients assessed by pulsed Doppler echocardiography. *J Am Coll Cardiol* 1988;12:114–20.

18. Kopecky SL, Gibbons RJ, Hollier LH. Preoperative supine exercise radionuclide angiogram predicts perioperative cardiovascular events in vascular surgery. *J Am Coll Cardiol* 1986;7:226A.

19. Leppo J, Plaja J, Gionet M, Tumolo J, Paraskos JA, Cutler BS. Noninvasive evaluation of cardiac risk before elective vascular surgery. *J Am Coll Cardiol* 1987;9:269–76.

20. Lapeyre AC, Gibbons RJ, Forstrom LA. Prediction of cardiac complications of non-cardiac surgery by intravenous dipyridamole thallium tomography (abstract). *J Nucl Med* 1988;29:838.

21. Spittell PC, Gibbons RJ. ECG changes during dipyridamole infusion are a marker for severe coronary disease (abstract). *Circulation* 1989;80(Suppl II):247.

22. Hammill SC, Khandheria BK. Silent myocardial ischemia. *Mayo Clin Proc,* 1990;65:374–83.

Surgical Management of the Diabetic Patient,
edited by Michael Bergman and Gregorio A. Sicard.
Raven Press, Ltd., New York © 1991.

8

Syndromes of Infection in Diabetic Patients

Dial Hewlett, Jr.

*Infectious Disease Section, Lincoln Medical and Mental Health Center and Our Lady
of Mercy Medical Center, Bronx, New York, and Department of Medicine, New York
Medical College, Valhalla, New York 10595*

The effects of infection upon diabetes are well known. Infections have been shown to be the most common precipitating factors for both diabetic ketoacidosis and the nonketotic hyperosmolar state (1,2). Over 15 years ago, Arieff (2) noted that approximately 66% of the patients in his review of hyperosmolar state carried the diagnosis of sepsis. The majority of these individuals had gram-negative bacteremia secondary to a urinary tract focus. The issue of whether infections occur more frequently among diabetic persons or merely follow an altered clinical course in a setting of immunological impairment remains controversial. A variety of defects in leukocyte function have been described by a number of investigators (3–5).

In some of the patients, defects have been linked to extrinsic/correctable factors such as hyperglycemia, acidemia, or uremia; in other patients the defects appear to be intrinsic and irreversible (6). Recently, congenital factors have been linked to myeloperoxidase deficiency among diabetic children with persistent refractory periodontal infections (7).

In this chapter, an overview of the major syndromes of infection that occur in diabetic persons are provided. Special emphasis is placed upon those syndromes in which there are unique features uncommonly encountered among nondiabetic patients. The reader is referred to standard texts of internal medicine, surgery, or infectious diseases for a more thorough discussion of the disease processes.

PATHOGENESIS OF INFECTION IN DIABETIC PATIENTS

Acute infections can affect carbohydrate metabolism adversely in two major ways. Direct destruction of the pancreatic islet tissue occurs by agents such as coxsackie virus, adenovirus, mumps virus or similar pathogens. Damage to the islet cells can also occur during the course of therapy for infection such as during the administration of pentamidine in the treatment of pneumocystosis. More commonly, however, carbohydrate metabolism is affected indirectly through the antagonism of insulin action by hormones secreted in excessive amounts during septic episodes (cortisol, glucagon, growth hormone). Acute infection may unmask diabetes that under ordinary circumstances would go unrecognized. Infections are the most frequent causes of diabetic ketoacidosis and the nonketotic hyperosmolar state (Table 1).

TABLE 1. *Metabolic and endocrinologic responses to infection*

Factor/hormone	Alteration during infection
Adrenal glucocorticoids	Increased cortisol production
Glucose	Fasting hyperglycemia/hypoglycemia in neonates and during fulminant hepatitis
Insulin	Hypoinsulinemia in *E. coli* sepsis/animal model
Growth hormone	Increased levels during febrile stage of infections
Glucagon	Elevated levels
Catecholamines	Increased norepinephrine and epinephrine levels

DEFECTS IN HOST-DEFENSE MECHANISMS IN DIABETIC PATIENTS

During the past several years, a variety of defects in host-defense mechanisms has been described in diabetic patients. Defects in neutrophil chemotaxis and phagocytosis have been studied extensively. In most studies, the defective chemotaxis can be corrected by placing the cells into a euglycemic media. Similarly, defects in phagocytosis can also be corrected. The intracellular cidal function of neutrophils has also been a focus of study. Decreased intracellular killing of staphylococci has been documented with improvement induced via stringent control of blood glucose. In contrast to the reversible defects in neutrophil function, defects in the ability of lymphocytes to respond to staphylococcal phage lysate appear to be intrinsic and are not corrected with euglycemia. Likewise, it is generally believed that diabetic patients exhibit an overall irreversible defect in cell-mediated immune function. Antibody production and function, however, appear to be intact along with complement system functions (Table 2).

The precise role contributed by each of the aforementioned defects remains an engima at this juncture. It is likely, however, that these defects act synergistically with other multiple factors such as carbohydrate metabolism and nutritional status to produce the sometimes unfavorable response to systemic infection.

CLINICAL SYNDROMES OF INFECTION IN THE DIABETIC PATIENT

Head and Neck Infections in Diabetes

Rhinocerebral Mucormycosis and Diabetes

Mucormycosis is an acute fungal infection that is often fatal. The causative organisms belong to four families of the order Mucorales. Mucormycosis is a relatively rare condition; however, the incidence may actually be increasing. Fortunately, the prognosis in some centers appears to be improving. The manifestations of mucormycosis can be divided into six clinical categories: rhinocerebral, pulmonary, cutaneous, gastrointestinal, central nervous system, and miscellaneous (Table 3). Rhinocerebral mucormycosis is the type encountered most often among diabetic patients. In general, patients presenting with diabetic ketoacidosis should improve in level of consciousness within 24–48 hours. Patients with a persistence in mental status change should be evaluated for the possibility of rhinocerebral mucormycosis. Patients usually complain of headache or facial pain. Fever and signs of orbital cellulitis may also be noted. As the disease advances, conjuctival edema, proptosis,

TABLE 2. *Defects in host defense mechanisms in diabetics*

Mechanism	Impaired	Reversal with euglycemia
Cell-mediated immunity [CMI]	Yes	No
Neutrophil function chemotaxis	Yes	Yes
Phagocytosis	Variable	Yes
Intracellular cidal activity	Yes	Yes
Antibody production/function	No	No
Complement system	No	No
Serum opsonic activity	Yes	Variable
Lymphocyte transformation/staphylococcal phage lysate	Yes	No

and loss of extraocular muscle movement develops. Loss of vision may occur as the result of retinal artery thrombosis. Cerebral abscess formation, cavernous sinus thrombosis, and thrombosis of the carotid artery are well known complications of mucormycosis.

Tissue necrosis and invasion of blood vessels are the most reliable markers for disease caused by Mucorales. Black eschars, black discharges from the nares, or dark, necrotic lesions on the soft palate or nasal mucosa, should prompt an immediate diagnostic evaluation for mucormycosis. The diagnosis of mucormycosis is based upon the identification of the organism on tissue biopsy specimens from suspicious lesions. Swabs or scrapings are usually not adequate and may lead to an erroneous diagnosis. Plain roentgenographs of the sinuses may reveal thickening of the mucosa and, as the disease progresses, erosion of bone. Computerized tomography of the brain may also be helpful in delineating bone destruction and abnormalities in the adjacent soft tissue. In addition to histopathology, tissue obtained from biopsies should be sent for fungal cultures.

Therapy for suspected rhinocerebral mucormycosis should begin at once with the correction of ketoacidosis and hyperglycemia (Table 4). Amphotericin B in high doses of between 1–1.5 mg/kg bw/24 h. Unfortunately, the imidazoles and triazoles have not been effective in the treatment of mucormycosis; however, during the past several years, earlier recognition of the syndrome combined with earlier aggressive antifungal therapy have improved the prognosis.

Periodontal Disease

A severe form of periodontal disease has been described among young diabetic patients whose disease is poorly controlled. These patients usually lack plaque formation. Recently, it has been shown that links exist between myeloperoxidase deficiency and periodontal disease. Moreover, in recent years, a bacterium known as capnocytophagia has been isolated from individuals with advanced periodontal infections. The presence of capnocytophagia has been linked to defective neutrophil chemotaxis. Close control of blood glucose is the mainstay of treatment.

Malignant External Otitis

Malignant external otitis (MEO) is a syndrome that occurs most commonly in diabetic patients. It is most likely to be encountered during warm humid summer

TABLE 3. *Syndromes of infection related to diabetes*

Infection or syndrome	Common clinical manifestations
Head and neck infections	
Mucormycosis [Rhinocerebral]	Altered mentation/ketoacidosis facial pain/periorbital cellulitis conjunctival edema/sinusitis/bone erosion
Malignant external otitis	Persistent otalgia/otorrhea/edematous erythematous external ear/ patient often nontoxic/usually secondary to pseudomonas aeruginosa/rarely aspergillus
Periodontal disease	Correlates with hyperglycemia, i.e., glucose levels exceeding 200 and duration of diabetes
Pulmonary infections	
Gram-negative pneumonia	*Klebsiella* Pneumoniae/Necrotizing Pneumonitis/cavitary lesions/ effusions empyema/fulminant course
	Bacteremic *E. coli* pneumonia lobar consolidation/sputum culture usually positive for *E. coli*/often community acquired
Legionaire's disease	Wide range of roentgenographic findings
	Ill-defined patchy infiltrates to dense lobar infiltrates/ nondiagnostic sputum/prominent cough/high fever/hyponatremia/ markedly elevated Esr/delerium with normal CSF/failure to improve on beta lactam and or aminoglycoside antibiotics
Tuberculosis	Reactivated disease/apical densities/primary disease/lower lung infiltrates sometimes with adenopathy/effusion/pneumonitis which fails to clear on standard antibiotics/primary disease may be seen in elderly exposed to open cavitary cases within institutions/+/→PPD sputum acid-fast smear often positive
Genitourinary tract infections	Definitely increased incidence among diabetic women/onset may be insidious/Candida vaginitis may predispose/urinary tract infections are among the most common precipitating factors in diabetic ketoacidosis and hyperosmolar state
Papillary necrosis	Diabetes is the most frequent predisposing cause/onset of symptoms may be abrupt with severe flank pain, fever, hematuria/evidence for unilateral obstructive uropathy/shock/ tissue in urine/insidious onset/patient may be asymptomatic/may be incidental finding on excretory urography
Emphysematous pyelonephritis	Acute onset/often critically ill diabetic with fever, flank pain/ costovertebral angle tenderness/abdominal mass/crepitus/gas in renal parenchymal on roentgenograph/*E. coli* in blood and urine/ 50% mortality/unilateral nephrectomy indicated
Emphysematous cystitis	Gas filled bladder visualized on roentgenograph/often due to infection of bladder with clostridial species or other gas forming organisms/pneumaturia present
Torulopsis glabrata	Form of cystitis seen predominantly in elderly diabetics/most often asymptomatic/heavy infections may lead to obstructive uropathy/ antimicrobials are predisposing factors
Candidiasis	Cystitis/vaginitis/dysuria/vaginal discharge/persistent glycosuria and poor control of glucose levels are precipitating factors
Fournier's disease of scrotum	Form of necrotizing fasciitis/begins as small necrotic eschar on scrotum that spreads insidiously/usually caused by strep pyogenes and anaerobes/extensive débridement essential; similar syndrome involving labia seen in middle-aged and elderly diabetic women
Soft-tissue infections	
Nonclostridial gas infections	Mixture of aerobic gram negatives, anaerobes sometimes strep species and staph./crepitus often noted on exam/gas visible on soft-tissue roentgenograph/débridement usually indicated
Foot ulcerations	Often chronic/patients usually nontoxic/often no pain detected despite extensive tissue destruction/usually mixed infection staph aureus/anaerobes/gram-negative aerobics; commonly evolve to osteomyelitis
Bone and joint infections	Osteomyelitis of the axial skeleton more common among diabetics/ persistent back pain and elevated ESR may be only clue to vertebral osteomyelitis/septic arthritis is more common among diabetics patients

(*Table continues*)

TABLE 3. *Continued*

Infection or syndrome	Common clinical manifestations
Intraabdominal infections Emphysematous cholycystitis	Associated with clostridia and gas forming *E. coli.* Definite correlation with diabetic control lacking
Sepsis/endovascular infection Endocarditis	Diabetic patients are more likely to have endocarditis secondary to staph aureus bacteremia eminating from a known focus than nondiabetic patients. Diabetes is often the most common predisposing factor for group B streptococcal endocarditis
Mycotic aneurysms	Salmonella species/staph aureus/persistent fever/positive blood cultures/pulsatile abdominal mass/preexisting atherosclerosis of aorta/Sonography-CT helpful/arteriograms and surgical resection will be indicated

weather or in warm climates. The patients are usually middle aged or elderly who present with a painful erythematous edematous ear. Occasionally, there is a history of irrigating the external canal, swimming, or use of a hearing aid.

MEO is believed to be the result of a suppurative vasculitis that is nearly always due to pseudomonas aeruginosa. Very recently, a case of MEO secondary to *aspergillus* was reported in a middle-aged woman. The authors emphasized the need for establishing a definitive diagnosis and noted that clinically the patient could not be easily distinguished from individuals with the far more common pseudomonas. The patient responded to Itraconazole. Failure to treat both forms of MEO results in the

TABLE 4. *Selected syndromes of infection in the diabetic patient*

Syndrome	Most likely pathogens	Antibiotic
Malignant external otitis	*Pseudomonas aeruginosa*	Ceftazidime with an aminoglycoside Ureidopenicillin and aminoglycoside/ ciprofloxacin $+/-$ Rifampin
Periodontal disease	Oral flora/capnocytophagia	Clindamycin or penicillin
Lower respiratory tract [pneumonia]	Strep Pneumoniae/H. Influenza Branhamella/Staph/*Klebsiella* Nosocomial [mixed] severe	2nd or 3rd gen. cephalosporin Imipenem or ticarcillin-clavulanate and aminoglycoside
Urinary tract infections	*E. coli*/proteus/klebsiella simple UTI	Trimethoprim/ sulfamethoxazole
	complicated nosocomial	Quinolone 3rd generation cephalosporin or quinolone
Endocarditis	Staph aureus/group B strep	Nafcillin/ampicillin/ gentamicin
Mycotic aneurysms	Salmonella/staph aureus	ampicillin and nafcillin or ceftriaxone or quinolone
Diabetic foot ulcers	Mixed/aerobic and anaerobic staph aureus	Cefoxitin/or ceftizoxime/or ticarcillin-clavulanate or clindamycin and ciprofloxacin

extension of infection into the adjacent parietal bone, sinuses, and, rarely, meninges. Despite the disasterous consequences, the patients are usually nontoxic, and for that reason, there may be a tendency to underestimate the severity of the condition. In addition to tenderness, erythema, and edema of the external ear, there is often a granular discharge. External ear cultures are nearly always positive for pseudomonas aeruginosa. There is usually no evidence of otitis media. MEO is a medical emergency. Patients should be hospitalized at least for the initial management of infection and tight control of glucose. An otolaryngologist is often the primary physician for patients with MEO; however, aside from the removal of necrotic material from the external canal, the management is primarily medical. Traditionally, extended spectrum penicillins such as ticarcillin, piperacillin, or mezlocillin have been combined with an aminoglycoside: gentamicin, tobramycin, amikacin. More recently, cephalosporins with activity against pseudomonas (ceftazidime) have been utilized both in combination with aminoglycosides or as monotherapy. During the past two years, favorable results have been achieved with high doses of the quinolone ciprofloxacin, which is sometimes combined with rifampin. Recommendations regarding length of therapy are controversial. With the use of oral quinolones, 6–12-week courses have been offered.

Despite the advances in antibiotic therapy, Rubin and Yu noted a 20% mortality rate (9).

Pulmonary Infections

In most clinical situations, community-acquired pneumonia among diabetic patients is quite similar to the pneumonia that occurs in nondiabetic patients. A major difference, however, is the increased likelihood for fulminant necrotizing pneumonitis secondary to *Escherichia coli* or *Klebsiella* to develop in the diabetic patient. Tillitson and Lerner (10) reported 20 cases of *E. coli* pneumonia at the Detroit General Hospital in 1967. Of the 16 patients for whom a complete history was obtainable, 11/16 [69%] were diabetic. The association between diabetes and infections with *K. pneumoniae* has been extensively reviewed. Ayvazian (11) noted the occurrence of diabetes in 43% of patients with extrapulmonary involvement with klebsiella: bacteremia, liver abscess, and meningitis. Diabetes was present in 12% of the patients with extrapulmonary involvement and in 23% of those with all types of klebsiella infections. Although these infections occur infrequently, early recognition and institution of the appropriate antibiotic therapy significantly decreases the mortality rates. Berk (12) reported a 71% survival rate among 17 patients presenting to the Johnson City, Tennessee VA Hospital in 1982. Sputum gram stains may be useful in establishing a tentative diagnosis in gram-negative pneumonia; therapy with third generation cephalosporins or augmented penicillins parenterally should prove efficacious in most situations.

Atypical pneumonia secondary to *Legionella* species is more likely to occur in diabetics (13). The patient may present with evidence for pneumonia—persistent cough with nondiagnostic sputum, high fever sometimes with delerium, markedly elevated erythrocyte sedimentation rate, hyponatremia, and failure to improve on betalactam agents. Serology may be helpful in establishing the diagnosis. In some laboratories, special charcoal yeast extract is available for culturing the organism. High dose erythromycin, i.e., 3–4 g/24 h should be given intravenously if the patient is toxic.

Another diagnosis to consider in the diabetic patient with lower lobe infiltrates that fail to clear is primary tuberculosis. A 5-tuberculin unit skin test and acid-fast smears of the sputum are often helpful. Apical infiltrates may signal reactivated disease in the elderly diabetic patient with underlying neoplastic or other immunosuppressive disorders.

Genitourinary Tract Infections in Diabetic Patients

Infections of the urinary tract are a frequent cause of morbidity among diabetic patients. It appears that covert urinary tract infections among diabetic women are common, and the subsequent development of renal parenchymal involvement can occur insidiously. In contrast, the prevalence of urinary tract infections in diabetic and nondiabetic men is essentially equal. The presence of *Candida vaginitis* in diabetic women is undoubtedly a predisposing factor. Both *Candida* and *Torulopsis* have been observed more commonly in the setting of glucosuria.

Infections in the urinary tract are among the most common precipitating factors in the hyperosmolar state and diabetic ketoacidosis.

Because covert infections of the urinary tract commonly occur in the diabetic woman, physicians must maintain a high index of suspicion. Moreover, the diabetic woman with a lower urinary tract infection is less likely to respond to single-dose therapy such as two double-strength tablets of trimethoprim-sulfa metoxazole or a single 3 g dose of amoxacillin. Longer courses for the management of lower urinary tract infections in this patient group seem warranted. Bacterial isolates among diabetic patients are more likely to be non-*E. coli* and therefore more difficult to eradicate.

Acute pyelonephritis occurs with greater frequency among diabetic patients. In some instances, classic manifestations of upper urinary tract infection may be lacking.

Emphysematous pyelonephritis is a rare albeit unusually fulminant form of acute pyelonephritis caused by gas-forming bacteria, most often *E. coli* (14). Recent case reports, however, have implicated candida species as a cause of emphysematous pyelonephritis in a diabetic drug addict. This syndrome is seen nearly exclusively in diabetic patients who very frequently also have a history of ethanol abuse. The patients may present initially with findings suggestive of a typical urinary tract infection and suddenly severe flank or back pain develops, sometimes with a palpable flank or abdominal mass. Crepitance may be present and gas within the renal parenchyma is visible on plain roentgenographs of the abdomen. The patient will deteriorate rapidly despite appropriate antibiotic therapy unless surgical measures are immediately taken. Nephrectomy is believed by most to be the only alternative in cases of emphysematous pyelonephritis. In some instances, the disease has been known to recur in the remaining kidney. It is for this reason that questions regarding the potential benefits of long-term antibiotic prophylaxis have occasionally been raised.

Acute papillary necrosis is a distinct syndrome characterized by focal or diffuse ischemic necrosis of segments of the renal medulla (15). Clinically, patients may present with an acute, devastating illness that leads to rapid death, or an illness characterized by worsening back and flank pain often accompanied by manifestations of obstructive uropathy. Diabetes mellitus was the leading cause of papillary necrosis in two large reviews. Frequent symptoms and signs upon presentation include: fever/chills, flank pain, dysuria, gross hematuria, proteinuria, leukocytosis, and azotemia. Oliguria and progressive uremia were uncommon in a recent review despite the fact that papillary necrosis was bilateral in 74% of the 27 cases.

The diagnosis of renal papillary necrosis can be established on roentgenographs or on excretory urography. In some patients, sloughed papillae may cause intense lumbar and flank pain accompanied by gross hematuria. Portions of the papilla may sometimes be found in the urine and are diagnostic.

Early diagnosis, effective antibiotic therapy, and maintenance of ureteral drainage are essential. Surgical intervention can improve the prognosis. Nephrectomy has been performed during rare episodes of exsanguinating hemorrhage from ruptured papillae.

Candidiasis

Colonization of the bladder with *Candida* is common among diabetic patients with indwelling catheters. Although in most instances colonization is evident, if there is true invasion of the bladder, cystitis, therapy is indicated. Treatment can consist of bladder irrigation with amphotericin B, 50 mg/1000 cc fluid, administered continuously every 24 h via triple port catheter for 3–5 days. Another approach has been a single dose of systemic amphotericin B (.3 mg/kg bw) following the standard test dose of 1 mg. Patients with renal parenchymal involvement may present with evidence of obstructive uropathy and require systemic amphotericin B. The new triazole agent Fluconazole is excreted into the urine and shows promise as a possible less toxic alternative.

Soft-Tissue Infections in Diabetic Patients

Infections involving the soft tissue, especially of the lower extremities are among the most feared complications in diabetic patients (16). Diabetic foot ulcers are the leading cause for hospitalization of diabetic patients in the United States, and complications arising from diabetic foot infections are the leading cause of lower extremity amputations. Other soft-tissue syndromes, such as streptococcal gangrene, synergistic necrotizing cellulitis, and necrotizing fascitis, have a predilection for occurring in diabetic patients. Early recognition of these conditions combined with prompt initiation of antimicrobial therapy and aggressive surgical débridement may be life saving. Control of blood glucose levels also exerts a favorable effect upon the patient's recovery. In a study conducted on patients with infected diabetic foot ulcerations, it was noted that the rates of healing were rapid when blood glucose levels were maintained at or below 150 mg/dl via continuous insulin pump infusion, regardless of the antibiotics utilized (17). Conversely, patients with poorly controlled glucose levels had unsatisfactory healing rates independent of the antibiotics chosen.

Foot Infections in the Diabetic Patient

Infections of the foot may develop in the diabetic patient in a number of ways; however, the predisposing factors include:

1. Peripheral neuropathy, which results in significant impairment in sensory function, thereby predisposing towards occult injury.

2. Autonomic neuropathy, which leads to decreased perspiration resulting in a dry cracked/fissured foot, which, in turn fascilitates the entry of pathogenic bacteria.
3. Angiopathy resulting from longstanding diabetes. Areas of thrombosis result in regions of tissue ischemia.

Infections of the foot in diabetic patients usually involve a mixture of organisms that include: staph aureus, anaerobes, and aerobic gram negatives. Evolution into osteomyelitis is common (18). Control of blood glucose levels, surgical débridement, and a broad-spectrum antimicrobial are essential (19). Cultures from the wounds commonly yield two or three potential pathogens. Soft-tissue roentgenographs may reveal the presence of soft-tissue gas, which indicates the necessity of prompt surgical débridement. Technetium bone scans and in some instances CT scans give clues to the presence of early osteomyelitis that would not be visualized on the routine roentgenograph until 50% of the bone matrix is destroyed (usually 3 weeks). Enthusiasm for bone biopsy in cases of osteomyelitis of the diabetic foot has decreased over the last several years. Prevention of infection in the diabetic patient should be emphasized. The feet of diabetic patients should be examined by the physician on each visit. Nail care should be supervised, especially in the elderly or visually impaired. Diabetics should be instructed to test the temperature of water prior to bathing. Moisturizing agents should be used to prevent fissuring of the skin. Dermatophytic infections of the nails result in brittle toenails which facilitate entry of pathogenic bacteria. Twice daily application of clotrimazole cream to the toenails may prove helpful for some patients. These applications may have to continue for three months or longer. Bathroom surgery must be condemned and patients must be instructed to avoid plastic or poorly constructed footwear and to purchase leather footwear.

Streptococcal Gangrene

This rare form of gangrene can be due to group A, C or G streptococci, and usually develops at sites of trauma on an extremity; however, in some cases, a portal of entry cannot be identified (20). The infection begins as a local painful area of erythema and edema followed by the development of dark discoloration and bullous formation. The bullae contain fluid that is yellow or dark red. A necrotic eschar forms. Blood and wound cultures are often positive for streptococci. Aqueous penicillin G in doses of 2–3 million units iv every 4 hours should be administered. If questions regarding etiologic agent arise, concurrent utilization of nafcillin 2 g iv every 4 hours is warranted. Surgical excision of all necrotic tissue is essential as is control of underlying diabetes. Figure 1 illustrates the result of wide excision of necrotic tissue in a previously healthy 28-year-old woman with adult onset diabetes who presented with diabetic ketoacidosis and presumed streptococcal cellulitis of the foot. *Streptococcus pyogenes* was cultured from the wounds initially and at the time of surgical débridement. Blood cultures were also positive for streptococci. Despite aggressive antibiotic therapy with high-dose penicillin, nafcillin, and, later in her course, imipenem, a below the knee amputation was necessary. The patient subsequently underwent a slow recovery that was complicated by renal failure.

Synergistic Gangrene/Necrotizing Fascitis

These infections are also observed more commonly among diabetic patients. They can follow trauma or surgery, especially colon resections. Commonly within 24–72

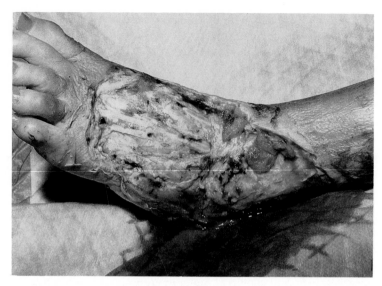

FIG. 1. Left foot of a 29-year-old woman with diabetes mellitus and streptococcal gangrene. The patient eventually required a below knee amputation.

hours of surgery, the wound will appear intensely erythematous. A raised, palpable border may become apparent and erythema will follow the fascial plains sometimes into the adjacent flank, groin, and upper thigh. Crepitance may be present and soft-tissue films may reveal subcutaneous gas formation. Broad-spectrum antibiotics and prompt surgical débridement are the life-salvaging procedures when this syndrome is suspected. Antibiotics alone are ineffective. *S. pyogenes* often plays a prominent role in the pathogenesis of this syndrome when extremities are involved; however, aerobic gram negatives and anaerobic bacteria such as bacteroides play a prominent role in the abdomen.

Fournier's Disease of the Scrotum

A unique form of necrotizing fasciitis known as Fournier's disease of the scrotum can occur more frequently among diabetic patients. The pathogenesis for the syndrome is not completely known; however, it is believed that bacteria gain entry via Buck's fascia of the penis and spread along dartos fascia of the scrotum, into the perineum and onto the abdominal wall. The patient usually notes severe pain and a discolored area on the under surface of the scrotum. The organisms responsible are probably a mixture of anaerobes, streptococci, and possibly aerobic-gram negatives. Surgical débridement must be undertaken and a variety of antimicrobial regimens could be employed such as: ampicillin, clindamycin, and gentamicin; ampicillin, gentamicin and metronidazole; imipenem or ticarcillin-clavulanate and gentamicin.

Intraabdominal Infections in Diabetic Patients

Associations between diabetes and a variety of intraabdominal infections are not well defined. Although some investigators have found higher rates of morbidity and mortality among diabetic patients with cholecystitis, a review of 311 patients at the Cleveland Clinic Hospital by Ransohoff (21,22) suggests that the natural history of gall bladder disease among diabetic patients does not differ significantly from that seen in nondiabetic patients. The need for prophylactic removal of so-called silent gall stones in diabetic patients is therefore questioned.

Sepsis/Endovascular Infection/Endocarditis

Bacteremia secondary to *Staphylococcus aureus* occurs at a greater frequency among diabetic patients when compared with the general population (23). The daily use of injectable insulin undoubtedly plays a significant role in many individuals. As a result of preexisting atherosclerotic disease, a diabetic with *S. aureus* bacteremia is much more likely to have an endovascular lesion such as endocarditis or a mycotic aneurysm. Patients presenting with ketoacidosis, hyperosmolar states, or unexplained hyperglycemia should be evaluated for the possibility of occult bacteremia. Tachypnea can occur before the onset of fever in some bacteremic patients. Blood cultures must always be drawn before antibiotic therapy is begun for suspected sepsis. Combinations of nafcillin and gentamicin have been utilized in the management of community-acquired sepsis from an unknown source. Diabetic patients who present with gastroenteritis, fever, and fecal leukocytes should be treated for the possibility of salmonellosis (24). It is believed that diabetic patients are at significant risk for the development of endarteritis and mycotic aneurysms as complications of salmonella bacteremia possibly resulting from gastroenteritis (25). Parenteral ampicillin, ceftriaxone, trimethoprim sulfamethoxazole or ciprofloxacin have been utilized in the management of salmonella bacteremia. It appears, however, that the quinolone antibiotics may be more effective in the eradication of intestinal carriage. Doses of 500 mg po every 12 hours 5–7 days have been effective for gastroenteritis. Persistent salmonella bacteremia despite effective parenteral antibiotic treatment is highly suggestive of endovascular seeding. A meticulous search for a vascular lesion should be undertaken with special attention being paid to the abdominal exam for the presence of bruits over the aorta or femorals, a pulsatile mass, cardiac murmurs, or bruits over the great vessels. An echocardiogram, abdominal plain film with lateral view, and abdominal sonogram may prove helpful. Surgical resection is the only effective treatment for mycotic aneurysms of the great vessels.

SUMMARY

Although the relationship between diabetes mellitus and infection is not completely understood, it has been well established that numerous syndromes of infection involving a variety of organisms occur either exclusively or with a marked increased frequency in diabetic patients. It has also become abundantly clear that tight control of blood glucose level serves to at least partially prevent the occurrence of many of the syndromes of infection and often favorably alters the course of infections that have already occurred. Poor blood supply with resultant tissue ischemia and necrosis point out the need for surgical débridement in the management of entities such as necrotizing fascitis, diabetic foot ulcers, and mycotic aneurysms. Antibiotic regimens often must cover a wide range of pathogens in the treatment of such infections as fascitis and the diabetic foot. The role played by anaerobic organisms in these syndromes and to the better known pathogens (staphylococci and streptococci), should enter into the antibiotic selection process and, it is hoped, lead to improved clinical outcomes for the diabetic patient.

ACKNOWLEDGMENTS

The author thanks Dr. Julius Weber for providing Figure 1, and the members of the medical and surgical housestaff and attending staff for their cooperation in the management of the patient discussed in this chapter.

REFERENCES

1. Rayfield EJ, Ault MJ, Keusch GT, Brothers MJ, Nachemias C, Smith H. Infection and diabetes: The case for glucose control. *Am J Med* 1982;72:439.
2. Arieff AI, Carroll HJ. Nonketotic hyperosmolar coma. *Medicine* 1972;51:73.
3. Mowat AG, Baum J. Chemotaxis of polymorphonuclear leukocytes from patients with diabetes mellitus. *N Engl J Med* 1971;284:621.
4. Bagdade JD, Root RK, Bulger RJ. Impaired leukocyte function in patients with poorly controlled diabetes. *Diabetes* 1974;23:9.
5. Drachman RH, Root RK, Wood WB Jr. Studies on the effect of experimental nonketotic diabetes mellitus on antibacterial defenses. Demonstration of a defect in phagocytosis. *J Exp Med* 1966;124:227.
6. Casey JI, Heeter BJ, Klyshevich KA. Impaired response of lymphocytes of diabetic subjects to antigen of staphylococcus aureus. *J Infect Dis* 1977;136:495.
7. Chow AW. Infections of the oral cavity neck and head. In: Mandell GL, Douglas RG, Bennett JE, eds, Principles and Practice of Infectious Diseases. 3rd ed. New York: Churchill-Livingston 1990.
8. Parfrey NA. Improved diagnosis and prognosis of mucormycosis. A clinicopathologic study of 33 cases. *Medicine* 1986;65:113.
9. Rubin J, Yu VL. Malignant external otitis. Insights into pathogenesis clinical manifestations diagnosis and therapy. *Am J Med* 1988;85:391.
10. Tillotson JR, Lerner AM. Characteristics of pneumonia caused by *Escherichia coli*. *N Engl J Med* 1967;277:115.
11. Ayuazian LF. Friedlander's bacillus meningitis successfully treated with streptomycin: Consideration of Friedlander's bacillus infections in diabetes. *Am J Med* 1948;5:470.
12. Berk SL, Newmann P, Holtsclaw S, Smith JK. *Escherichia coli* pneumonia in the elderly. *Am J Med* 1982;72:899.
13. England AG, Fraser DW, Plikaytis BD, et al. Sporadic legionellosis in the United States: The first thousand cases. *Ann Intern Med* 1981;94:164.
14. Spagnola AM. Emphysematous Pyelonephritis. Report of two cases. *Am J Med* 1978;64:840.
15. Eknoyan G, Qunibi WJ, Grissom RT, et al. Renal papillary necrosis: An update. *Medicine* 1982;61:55.
16. Bamberger DM, Daus GP, Gerding DN. Osteomyelitis of the feet of diabetic patients. *Am J Med* 1987;83:653.
17. Rubinstein A, Pierce CE, Bloomingarden Z. Rapid healing of diabetic foot ulcers with continuous insulin infusion. *Am J Med* 1983;75:161.
18. Wheat LJ, Allen SD, Henry M, et al. Diabetic foot infections: Bacteriologic analysis. *Arch Intern Med* 1986;146:1935.
19. Scher KS, Steele FJ. The septic foot in patients with diabetes. *Surgery* 1988;104(4) 661.
20. Swartz MN. Cellulitis and superficial infections. In: Mandell GL, Douglas RG, Bennett JE, eds. third ed. Principles and Practice of Infectious Diseases, New York: Churchill Livingston, 1990.
21. Ransohoff DF, Miller GL, Forsythe SB, et al. Outcome of acute cholecystitis in patients with diabetes mellitus. *Ann Intern Med* 1987;106:829.

22. Hickman MS, Schwesinger WH, Page CP. Acute cholecystitis in the diabetic. A case control study of outcome. *Arch Surg* 1988;123:404.
23. Cooper G, Platt R. Staphylococcus aureus bacteremia in diabetic patients. *Am J Med* 1982;73:658.
24. Cohen OS, O'Brien TF, Schoenbaum SC, et al. The risk of endothelial infection in adults with salmonella bacteremia. *Ann Intern Med* 1978;89:931.
25. McIntyre KE Jr, Malone JM, Richards E. Mycotic aortic pseudoaneurysm with aortoenteric fistula caused by arizona hinshawii. *Surgery* 1982;91:173.

Surgical Management of the Diabetic Patient,
edited by Michael Bergman and Gregorio A. Sicard.
Raven Press, Ltd., New York © 1991.

9

Emergency Surgery in the Diabetic Patient

Brian G. Rubin and Gregorio A. Sicard

*Department of Surgery, Washington University School
of Medicine, St. Louis, Missouri 63110*

In 1896, Sir Frederick Treves warned that "Diabetes offers a serious bar to any operation" (1). Since then, the discovery and routine use of insulin, as well as improvements in surgery, anesthesia, and perioperative care have made his statement no longer true. Nonetheless, the diabetic patient presents special perioperative management problems that can be morbid or lethal if incorrectly handled. This is particularly true in diabetic patients who require emergency surgery. Although several principles contained in this chapter have been alluded to previously (see Chapter 3, General Medical Care Operations), repetition of vital points is worthwhile.

It has been estimated that one-half of all diabetic patients will require surgery (2). They are at only a slightly increased operative mortality risk overall (3.4%) versus their nondiabetic counterparts (2.5%) (3,4). Of all these cases, about 5% are performed on an emergency basis. It is unclear whether diabetic patients whose glucose levels are under control represent an increased operative risk due to the emergent nature of their surgery. Unfortunately, surgeons often encounter either metabolic catastrophe, such as profound hypoglycemia, diabetic ketoacidosis (DKA), or hyperosmolar hyperglycemic nonketotic dehydration (HHND) and coma accompanying an acute surgical condition. It is this subgroup whose metabolic condition alone carries significant risk in addition to that of the emergent surgical problem (Table 1) (5). It should be noted that not all diabetic patients requiring surgery have the diagnosis made prior to the perioperative period. In a study of 667 patients, 20% had the diagnosis of diabetes made for the first time during the operative process (6). This group as well is at high risk if this disorder is not recognized early.

The frequent association of combined surgical and metabolic derangements makes diagnosis and management of diabetes difficult; unfortunately this simultaneous presentation is not uncommon. The surgical problem may be the etiology of an uncontrolled hyperglycemic state (e.g., ruptured viscus with sepsis exacerbating glucose intolerance), or the result of disordered glucose regulation (e.g., hypoglycemic coma while operating a motor vehicle that results in an accident.) Caution needs to be exercised regarding the reliability of physical findings in the diabetic patient. A paucity of symptoms in diabetic patients with intraabdominal pathology is seen frequently by general surgeons (7), a fact attributed to sensory neuropathy involving peritoneal efferent fibers. Physicians must avoid a cavalier approach to patients with few symptomatic complaints yet who have objective evidence of disease (e.g., high fever, tachycardia, hypotension). To complicate matters further, signs or symptoms usually indicative of a "surgical abdomen" with pain, tenderness, distention, nau-

TABLE 1.

Metabolic state	Mortality (%)
Hypoglycemic coma	3–6
Hyperosmolar hyperglycemia nonketotic coma	40–70
Diabetic ketoacidosis	1–5

sea, vomiting, and rigidity have been recognized in up to 50% of patients in diabetic ketoacidosis; these signs and symptoms resolve completely with only correction of the underlying metabolic abnormality (8). Laboratory determinations may be misleading in this setting as well, with an elevated amylose level without an elevated lipase level or pancreatitis (9). A marked leukocytosis with a white blood cell (WBC) count of 20,000/mm³ and an accompanying left shift in the differential is common in diabetic ketoacidosis. Furthermore, serum ketones interfere with several laboratory tests including determination of serum glutamic oxaloacetic transaminase (SGOT), serum glutamic pyruvic transaminase (SGPT) and creatinine. ·

The presence of neuropathy as a complication of diabetes has an impact in three additional ways on perioperative patient care. First, gastroparesis may be present and in order to prevent emesis and aspiration pneumonitis timely nasogastric decompression should be considered. Second, neuropathy of the urinary bladder can lead to difficulty in voiding requiring catheterization in order to monitor urine output and prevent urinary retention. The third major problem is inherent to cardiac autonomic neuropathy. Patients with this problem are at risk for perioperative cardiorespiratory arrest (10), and have a 50% mortality rate at 2.5 years (11). They are characterized clinically by persistent tachycardia, unaffected by vagal tone (valsalva) or positional changes, and can be diagnosed by a lack of change in the R-R interval on electrocardiogram (ECG) before or after these maneuvers. These patients often have significant postural hypotension as well, resulting from autosympathectomy (8).

PREOPERATIVE MANAGEMENT

For the diabetic patient undergoing elective surgery, there is no consensus as to which of the many widely used management schemes is preferable. Because there is no significant difference in the outcome of any of the more widely used methods, they are probably all equivalent (2,12–14). A management plan that can be initiated preoperatively by the surgeon or internist and continued intraoperatively by the anesthesiologist should be agreed upon in advance. Most authors agree that the diabetic patient requiring emergency surgery and whose glucose level is under control should be managed by whichever method would have been chosen for an equivalent elective surgical procedure. Detailed description of patient management can be found in chapter 3. To summarize, the main options include either subcutaneous administration of part (usually one-half) of the usual daily NPH and regular insulin dose before surgery, or continuous intravenous infusion of insulin, closely monitoring glucose and potassium levels. Whichever technique is chosen, it should be familiar to all members of the care team. When glucose levels are poorly controlled, an intravenous insulin infusion technique is preferable. A normal saline (0.9%) solution with 0.1 units/ml of regular insulin is prepared, the tubing flushed with 25–50 ml and the infusion administered by a pump delivery system. Infusion is begun at 0.1 units/kg/h with hourly monitoring of blood glucose levels. When the blood glucose level decreases to 250 mg/dl, a 5% dextrose-containing solution is begun at 100 ml/h, and the insulin drip is lowered to 1–2 units/h. The goal should be to decrease blood glucose levels 10% per hour, with doubling of the insulin infusion rate as necessary to achieve this goal (8,15).

Careful monitoring of capillary blood glucose levels, preferably using a reflectance meter, is essential. This should be done at least every 2 hours, but hourly or more frequent testing is preferable during periods of glucose lability. The goal should be to maintain a glucose level of 150–200 mg/dl with minimal or no glycosuria. In the preoperative, perioperative, and immediate postoperative periods, very tight control of the glucose level (80–120 mg/dl) should be avoided because it may lead to hypoglycemic problems (see Chapter 3). There is no longer a role for basing insulin therapy on urinary glucose levels alone, since the fingerstick capillary glucose testing technique is more accurate. This technique, commonly available in hospitals, provides immediate results, is relatively cost effective and results with visual interpretation can be obviated with the use of a reflectance meter (2,13). Correlation of the fingerstick capillary and whole blood glucose levels is suggested, but changes in therapy should not be delayed until laboratory results are available. The ability to make frequent adjustments in glucose or insulin therapy is the chief advantage of an intravenously administered insulin regimen, and results in better glucose control during the perioperative period (4). Towards this end, a computerized system for monitoring glucose levels and titrating insulin dosage has been successfully employed (16).

The primary function of insulin is to allow cellular use of glucose, thereby inhibiting the release of ketone bodies. In the adequately insulinized individual approximately 50 g of glucose every 8 hours is required to prevent ketoacidosis. Stress associated with the perioperative period results in an increase in counter-regulatory hormones, notably epinephrine and glucagon, which serve to inhibit insulin-dependent glucose metabolism. Therefore, this period is marked by heightened insulin requirements to prevent ketogenesis. As urine ketone levels parallel those in the blood, the presence of ketonuria indicates a lack of metabolizable glucose in the insulin-deficient patient.

Management of ketonuria and hyperglycemia involves an increase in the insulin dosage; concurrent ketonuria and normoglycemia in a patient receiving glucose infusion necessitates that insulin be infused with an increase in glucose infusion as well to prevent subsequent hypoglycemia. Ketonuria may become more marked despite decreasing blood glucose levels, before improvement is noted. This is due to the conversion of β-hydroxybutyrate to acetoacetate during resolution of the ketonemic state, the latter measured in urine ketone tests. Other than for minor surgical cases, essentially all diabetic patients, whether type I or II, require insulin in the perioperative period. In patients who have not previously received insulin, human insulin should be used to avoid antibody formation associated with administration of animal-derived insulin preparations.

Changes in blood glucose levels result in substantial alterations in blood volume and electrolyte composition. Careful but adequate hydration during the perioperative period cannot be overemphasized. The kidney's disposal of glucose is compromised in the presence of reduced intravascular fluid volume and renal perfusion. With adequate circulating volume, it is difficult to sustain glucose levels in excess of

350 mg/dl (2). A normal saline-based solution represents the crystalloid infusion of choice, as lactate-containing solutions (e.g., Ringer's lactate) are a source of ketones. Many physicians are cognizant of the assocation of diabetes and cardiovascular disease, and are fearful of infusing the large crystalloid volumes required during the perioperative period. Nonetheless, third-space, evaporative, and glycosuric osmotic diuretic losses are often substantial. Tenuous cardiac status is an indication for invasive monitoring including pulmonary artery catheterization. Because potassium flux between intracellular and extracellular pools is parallel to that of glucose, frequent determinations of potassium levels are also necessary.

The patient presenting in metabolic crisis who requires immediate surgery represents a substantial operative risk. There are two advances, however, that can improve outcome. The first is the ability to temporize or delay the surgical procedure, most often through the use of radiologic or endoscopic intervention. Examples of this include endoscopic or percutaneous transhepatic drainage of the biliary tree in

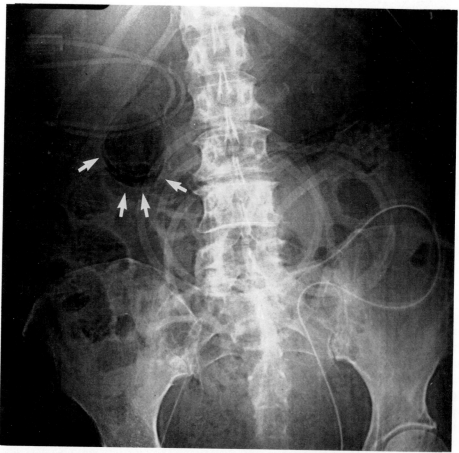

FIG. 1. Obstructive series of a 62-year-old diabetic patient on chronic ambulatory peritoneal dialysis with acute myocardial infarction and severe right upper quadrant pain. Note air in wall of gallbladder (arrows) consistent with emphysematous cholecystitis.

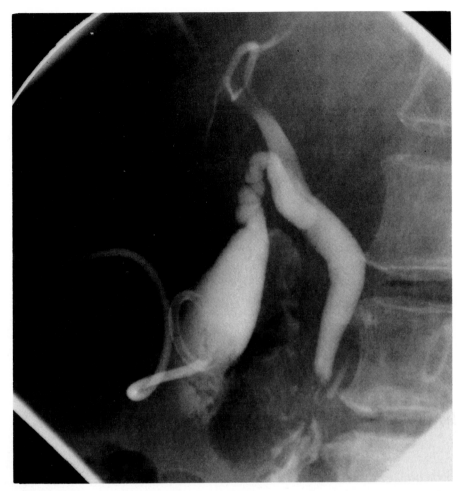

FIG. 2. Transcatheter cholecystogram in patient described in Figure 1. Percutaneous drainage permitted resolution of cholecystitis. Patient underwent uneventful cholecystectomy six months later.

the patient with cholangitis or cholecystitis (Figs. 1 and 2), colonoscopic detorsion of a sigmoid volvulus, or CT scan-guided drainage of an abdominal abscess (Figs. 3 and 4). These initial procedures may not be definitive; however, they can be done quickly, with minimal patient stress or trauma. The value of temporizing therapy lies in the second advance: a well-defined, successful protocol for treating the metabolic disorders. A complete review of the appropriate treatment regimens is beyond the scope of this chapter, and has been recently reviewed (5). Significant hyperglycemia should be treated as outlined above. Briefly, the patient in hypoglycemic coma is treated with either glucagon and/or glucose; those with DKA or HHND are treated with low-dose, intravenous insulin infusions, and crystalloid volume reexpansion. These protocols are best performed in the intensive care unit, with frequent monitoring of vital signs and appropriate laboratory parameters. If it becomes apparent that the metabolic situation is secondary to a surgical problem and the patient is

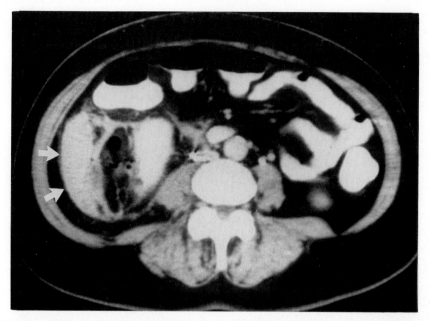

FIG. 3. Computerized tomographic scan of severe diabetic patient with a one-week history of fever, difficult to control glucose levels, and right flank pain. Large perinephric abscess from perforated retrocecal appendix is demonstrated (arrows).

responding poorly despite appropriate therapy, surgery should not be delayed further. Adequate glucose level control cannot easily be obtained until the underlying surgical problem has been rectified.

INTRAOPERATIVE MANAGEMENT

In the past, it had been suggested that local or regional anesthetic techniques were preferred whenever possible. This view was due, in large measure, to the fact that the anesthetic agents of the day resulted in substantial stimulation of the sympathetic nervous system. Because epinephrine is a potent counter-regulatory hormone, its effects aggravated the preexisting hyperglycemia. Hyperglycemia, inhibition of endogenous insulin, and fatty acid mobilization were reported (17). Newer anesthetic agents and techniques no longer result in sympathetic outpouring, and general anesthesia is therefore no longer the least preferable choice (2).

The responsibility for intraoperative regulation of glucose levels typically resides with the anesthesiologist. The anesthesiologist must beware of hypoglycemia in the eventuality that the patient took the usual morning dose of insulin or oral hypoglycemic agent but has missed meals since then. Hypoglycemia can be unrecognized in the anesthetized patient. Alternatively, the combination of a 5% dextrose-containing intravenous solution in the presence of elevated catecholamine levels can result in

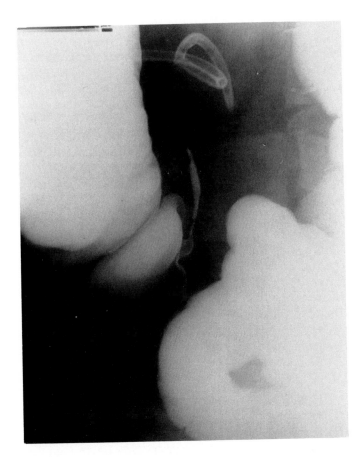

FIG. 4. Barium enema performed five days later demonstrated contrast from appendix communicating with perinephric catheter. (Patient described in Figure 3.)

frequently elevated glucose levels. Thus, frequent intraoperative determinations of blood glucose levels and electrolytes is therefore mandatory to diagnose the presence of either hypoglycemia or hyperglycemia.

If emergency surgery is necessary in the presence of significant hyperglycemia, intraoperative management is parallel to the usual protocols for handling severe hyperglycemia, DKA, or HHND, with the additional replacement of volume losses from bleeding, evaporation, or anesthesia-related vasodilation. Chapter 3 details the management of this situation.

POSTOPERATIVE MANAGEMENT

Optimal postoperative care includes an awareness of the association between diabetes and accelerated cardiovascular disease. Cardiac mortality is the leading cause of postoperative death in diabetic patients. In an emergent setting, the usual preoperative cardiac evaluation of a patient is not possible; in cases involving elderly diabetic patients, or those with a previous history of cardiac disease, or in the presence of suggestive physical findings, invasive monitoring (e.g., pulmonary artery catheterization, arterial line, Foley catheter) is advisable.

Once metabolic derangements have been corrected, the postoperative state is often uncomplicated. Reinstitution of normal preoperative insulin regimen is usually possible within a few days. In fact, failure to see marked metabolic improvement, or a recurrence of hyperglycemia, often signals a recrudescence of the primary pathology (e.g., recurrent infection). In patients whose blood glucose levels are difficult to control with the use of oral agents, the postoperative recovery period provides an excellent time to commence insulin therapy. It should be noted though, that many type II patients requiring insulin during the perioperative period may be able to discontinue insulin administration after discharge. Clearly, this decision needs to be arrived at on an individual basis. Predischarge planning is further discussed in Chapter 16.

CONCLUSION

The care of the diabetic patient needing emergency surgery requires the expertise and cooperation of multiple disciplines. The primary effort should be concentrated in the correction of glucose and electrolyte level abnormalities in a planned, controlled manner. The use of percutaneous drainage techniques can be extremely helpful in diabetic patients with undrained septic foci during the period of metabolic imbalance. In patients who require surgical intervention expeditiously, the presence of an experienced anesthesiologist in the setting of intraoperative cardiovascular monitoring can provide the patient with the best opportunity for a speedy and less complicated recovery.

REFERENCES

1. Treves FA. *System of surgery*. London: Cassell & Company, 1896.
2. Schade DS. Surgery and diabetes. *Med Clini North Am*. 1988;72(6):1531–1543.
3. Olson OC. Surgical considerations. In: *Diagnosis and management of diabetes mellitus*. New York: Raven Press, 1987;157–161.
4. Thomas DJB. Diabetes and surgery. In: Besser I, Bodansky GM, Jonathan H, Cudworth AG, eds. *Clinical diabetes*. Philadelphia: J.B. Lippincott Company, 1988;19.1–19.8.
5. Kitabchi AE, Rumbak M. The management of diabetic emergencies. *Hosp Pract* 1989;24;129–160.
6. Galloway JA, Schuman CR. Diabetes and surgery: A study of 667 cases. *Am J Med* 1963;34:177.
7. Wheelock FC, Gibbons GW, Marble A. Surgery in diabetes. In: Marble A, Krall LP, Bradley RF, Christlieb AR, Soeldner JS, eds. *Joslin's diabetes mellitus*, 12th ed. Philadelphia: Lea & Febiger, 1985;730–731.
8. Caldwell MD. Diabetes mellitus. In: Wilmore DW, Brennan MF, Harken AH, Holcroft JW, Meakins JL, eds. *Care of the surgical patient*, vol 2. New York: Scientific American, Inc., 1988;p1–12.
9. Knight AH, Williams DN, Ellis G, et al. Significance of hyperamylasaemia and abdominal pain in diabetic ketoacidosis. *Br J Med* 1973;3:128.
10. Page MM, Watkins PJ. Cardiorespiratory arrest and diabetic autonomic neuropathy. *Lancet* 1978;1:14.
11. Ewing DJ, Campbell IW, Clarke BF. Mortality in diabetic autonomic neuropathy. *Lancet* 1976;1:601.
12. Reynolds C. Management of the diabetic surgical patient: A systematic but flexible plan is the key. *Diabetic Surg Patient* 1985;77(1):265–279.
13. Davis JH. Surgical aspects of diabetes mellitus. In: *Textbook of surgery*. Philadelphia: W.B. Saunders Company, 1981;172–177.
14. Mahvi DM. Endocrinology. In: Lyerly HK, ed. *The handbook of surgical intensive care: Practices of the surgery residents at the Duke University Medical Center*, 2nd ed. Chicago: Year Book Medical Publishers, Inc., 1989;409.
15. Podolsky S. Management of diabetes in the surgical patient. *Med Clin North Am* 1982;66(6):1361–1372.
16. Schwartz SS, Horowitz DC, Zehfus B, et al. Use of a glucose controlled insulin infusion (artificial beta cell) to control diabetes during surgery. *Diabetologia* 1979;16:157–164.
17. Allison SP, Tomlin PJ, Chamberlain MJ. Some effects of anesthesia and surgery on carbohydrate and fat metabolism. *Br J Anaesth* 1969;41:588–593.

Surgical Management of the Diabetic Patient,
edited by Michael Bergman and Gregorio A. Sicard.
Raven Press, Ltd., New York © 1991.

10

Medical Considerations for Diabetic Patients Undergoing Outpatient Surgery

*Irl B. Hirsch and †Paul F. White

*Division of Endocrinology and Metabolism, Department of Medicine, University of
Washington School of Medicine, Seattle, Washington 98144, and †Department of
Anesthesiology, Washington University School of Medicine,
St. Louis, Missouri 63110

The optimal perioperative management of diabetic outpatients presenting for elective ambulatory (outpatient) surgery remains controversial. Indeed, it has recently been shown the actual management practices of these patients had not been changed in the last 30 years despite many improvements in their ambulatory care (1). Although home blood glucose level monitoring, glycated hemoglobin measurements, and insulin regimens that better mimic physiologic demands are considered routine aspects of diabetes care today, these modalities have only recently been developed. Just as the trends in diabetes care have changed, operative procedures, which in the past would have only been considered inpatient operations, are now routinely being performed on an outpatient basis. Although the procedures may be considered "minor" by the patients and their surgeons, general anesthesia is still required in a majority of the cases (2).

The definition of "minor surgery" is not only changing but differs markedly among surgeons. Currently available intravenous and inhalation anesthetics result in varying degrees of hyperglycemia and impaired insulin secretion (3) as well as increases in cortisol (4) and catecholamine (5) concentrations. Because "major" changes in counterregulatory hormones can occur during "minor" procedures under general anesthesia, it is more logical to simply classify patients as inpatient versus outpatient. Chapter 3 (Medical Management of Diabetic Patients During Surgery) touches upon several concepts discussed within this chapter. Nonetheless, as increasingly larger numbers of diabetic patients undergo ambulatory surgical procedures, a separate section describing this particular topic is timely.

Metabolic treatment strategies differ for patients with insulin-dependent diabetes mellitus (IDDM) compared to those with noninsulin-dependent diabetes mellitus (NIDDM); it is therefore important to understand the basic difference between these two entities. IDDM is characterized by autoimmune pancreatic islet β-cell destruction resulting in insulin deficiency. The absolute lack of insulin eventually leads to ketosis; therefore, these patients must be treated with insulin. With the widespread availability of home blood glucose level monitoring, more physiologic strategies for insulin administration have been devised (6).

NIDDM, on the other hand, is characterized by insulin resistance and a decreased insulin secretory response (7). Many of these patients are taking insulin although they are not "insulin dependent" in the true sense. Some of these patients, especially the nonobese group, behave metabolically like the classic patient with IDDM and therefore should be treated in an analogous fashion during surgery. Indeed, it is not uncommon for IDDM to present in adulthood, as the age of onset has been shown to be bimodal (8). Finally, IDDM can present in patients with NIDDM who have "pancreatic exhaustion" and "conversion" to IDDM (9).

AMBULATORY SURGERY IN THE PATIENT WITH IDDM

General Principles

Preoperative evaluation and treatment of hyperglycemia and electrolyte abnormalities is imperative because of the potential for deleterious metabolic effects from surgery. All physicians caring for these patients during the perioperative period need to be familiar with the sophisticated insulin regimens that are being used by an increasing number of patients with diabetes. Furthermore, the introduction of intermediate and long-acting human insulins, with differing pharmacokinetic profiles (10), have further complicated the perioperative management of diabetic patients scheduled for ambulatory surgery.

The therapeutic strategy for patients with IDDM who are having surgery involves the mimicking of normal metabolism as closely as possible. This includes avoidance of hypoglycemia, excessive hyperglycemia, lipolysis, ketogenesis, protein catabolism, and electrolyte disturbances. The catabolic responses were due to the elevation in counterregulatory hormones that are seen with surgery, especially with general anesthesia (11). Elevations in blood levels of growth hormone, cortisol, epinephrine, and glucagon result in an increase in hepatic glucose production and a state of general insulin resistance (Table 1). Furthermore, as the catabolic events are promoted, there is a reduction in the anabolic processes. In the situation of insulin deficiency, these catabolic and antianabolic events have the potential for leading to metabolic decompensation. Therefore, the insulinopenic patient needs to be provided with enough insulin to counterbalance the catabolic response to the surgical procedure itself. In addition, an adequate glucose supply is required to meet the patient's basal

TABLE 1. *Metabolic effects of anabolic and catabolic hormones*

	Anabolic effects			Catabolic effects			
	Glyco-genesis	Lipo-genesis	Protein synthesis	Glyco-genolysis	Gluco-neogenesis	Lipo-lysis	Proteo-lysis
Insulin	+	+	+	−	−	−	−
Epinephrine	−	0	0	+	+	+	−
Glucagon	−	0	0	+	+	?[a]	+
Cortisol	+/−	+/−	−	−	+	+	+[b]
Growth hormone	0	0	+	−	+	+	+[b]

[a]Effects increased with nonphysiologic concentrations
[b]Effects important in the absence of insulin
+, stimulatory effect
−, inhibitory effect
0, no effect
+/−, stimulatory in the presence of insulin, inhibitory in the absence of insulin

caloric requirements and the added requirements related to elevations in stress hormone levels.

Insulin

Numerous factors affect the serum insulin concentrations following subcutaneous injection, including site of injection (12), depth of injection (12,13), and concentration of insulin (13). In addition, there are marked intra- and intersubject variations in insulin absorption following subcutaneous insulin injection (12). Although the effects of surgery on subcutaneously injected insulin have not been studied, it seems reasonable to assume that the fluid shifts and hemodynamic changes that occur during and after an operation would alter cutaneous blood flow and result in highly unpredictable variations in serum insulin concentrations. Therefore, use of a continuous intravenous (iv) insulin infusion is the most rational way to manage a patient with IDDM during surgery.

Only a few investigators have studied the blood glucose concentration differences following iv compared to subcutaneous (sc) insulin administration. Pezzarossa et al. (14) demonstrated that iv insulin administration offered improved glycemic control in comparison with the "standard" sc insulin administration during the intraoperative period, whereas it did not offer advantages over the sc route during the preoperative and postoperative periods. In another study, Watts and colleagues (15) showed more stable blood glucose level control 12–24 hours after surgery with a variable-rate iv insulin infusion compared to a conventional sc sliding scale or fixed-rate iv insulin infusion. Two other studies (16,17) have shown that the use of fixed-rate insulin infusion provides glucose control similar to that achieved by sc sliding scale insulin.

To initiate an insulin infusion, a separate saline-insulin mixture should be "piggy-backed" into the patient's existing iv line. The insulin-glucose-potassium infusion proposed by Alberti (18) has the disadvantage of having a fixed insulin-to-glucose concentration ratio. Thus, the entire bag has to be changed each time the plasma glucose is outside of targeted values. This problem is resolved with the separate infusion. In addition, if the amount of fluid administration is a concern, the insulin concentration can be increased.

Initial rates of insulin infusion on the morning of an outpatient procedure vary depending on initial blood glucose levels, serum-free insulin levels from previously injected sc insulin, and the presence of a significant "dawn phenomenon" (19). The dawn phenomenon is characterized by abrupt increases in fasting levels of plasma glucose or insulin requirements or both between 5 and 9 AM. This is generally thought to be the result of dissipation of insulin plus the effects of nocturnal growth hormone (20). Because the usual dose required for optimal control during surgery can vary (15), the usual starting dose is 1.0 units·h^{-1}, although it is reasonable to start thin women, who tend to be more sensitive to insulin, at a rate of 0.5 units·h^{-1}. Similarly, lower initial doses of insulin should be used for those patients who take their intermediate-acting insulin at bedtime. Once the insulin infusion is started, the blood glucose level should be measured at the bedside hourly intervals.

Patients using ultralente insulin at home who are scheduled for ambulatory surgery with general anesthesia present a special problem. The animal preparations of this insulin have a sluggish onset with a peakless action profile with a duration of action in excess of 36 hours (21,22). Human ultralente insulin has a shorter duration with an onset of action in 4–6 hours and a very broad peak lasting approximately 12–16 hours, and duration of action that persists up to 24 hours (22). Although the pharmacokinetics of the ultralente insulins have not been studied during surgery (indeed, there have been no studies examining the pharmacokinetics of any sc insulin preparation during surgery), this insulin should be given in the usual dose at the usual time. If the ultralente insulin was omitted on the day of surgery, basal insulin levels (especially for the animal insulins) would be minimally affected during the operation and blood glucose concentrations would be expected to be higher the next day. Stopping the ultralente insulin 2 or 3 days before the procedure, an option some physicians use if the patient is to be admitted before surgery (18), seems unnecessarily complicated for brief ambulatory procedures. Therefore, patients who take ultralente insulin at home should be given their usual dose before surgery, but any hyperglycemic response should be treated with an insulin infusion or sc regular insulin as discussed below.

Another advantage of using an insulin infusion concerns the patient who is not scheduled for surgery in the early morning. For late morning or afternoon outpatient procedures, it is inappropriate to withhold insulin in the insulinopenic individual. If sc insulin is administered, unpredictable absorption can be expected during the perioperative period and glucose requirements will change depending on plasma glucose and serum insulin levels. However, a variable-rate insulin infusion based on measured blood glucose concentrations used in conjunction with a continuous glucose infusion (see below) alleviates these problems.

Watts et al. (15) have proposed a useful insulin-infusion algorithm (Table 2). For a capillary glucose level less than 4.4 mmol/liter (80 mg/dl), the insulin infusion should be discontinued, 20 ml of 50% dextrose (10 g) should be administered, and the glucose concentration rechecked in 30 minutes. The insulin infusion may be restarted between 0.3 and 0.6 units·h^{-1} if the blood glucose level is greater than 6.7 mmol (120 mg/dl). However, if the glucose level is between 4.5–6.7 mmol/liter (81–120 mg/dl), it is reasonable to wait another 30 minutes before restarting the insulin infusion. A common etiology for perioperative hypoglycemia is high-plasma insulin levels from previously injected sc insulin.

For blood glucose concentrations between 4.5–6.7 mmol/liter (81–120 mg/dl), the insulin infusion should be decreased by 0.3 units·h^{-1}. For glucose levels between 6.7–10.0 mmol/liter (121–180 mg/dl), no change is necessary in the rate of the insulin infusion. For glucose concentrations between 10.1–13.3 mmol/liter (181–240 mg/dl), the infusion should be increased by 0.3 units·h^{-1}, and for levels greater than 13.3 mmol/liter (240 mg/dl), it may be increased by 0.5 units·h^{-1}. In addition to the in-

TABLE 2. *Intravenous insulin infusion algorithm*

<4.4 mmol/liter	Turn infusion off for 30 minutes, give 20 ml of 50% dextrose; remeasure glucose level in 30 minutes*
4.5–6.7 mmol/liter	↓ insulin infusion by 0.3 units·h^{-1}
6.7–10.0 mmol/liter	No change in insulin infusion rate
10.1–13.3 mmol/liter	↑ insulin infusion by 0.3 units·h^{-1}
>13.3 mmol/liter	↑ insulin infusion by 0.5 units·h^{-1}

Adapted from Watts et al., ref. 15.

*Restart insulin infusion between 0.3 and 0.6 units·h^{-1} only after blood glucose level is > 6.7 mmol/liter

creased rate of insulin infusion, an iv bolus dose of 5 units of regular insulin should be administered if the glucose concentration is greater than 16.6 mmol/liter (300 mg/dl). If the glucose level decreases by more than 5.6 mmol·liter^{-1}·h^{-1} (100 mg·dl^{-1}·h^{-1}), the insulin infusion should be decreased by 50% and the blood glucose level rechecked in 30 min.

Glucose

The average nondiabetic adult needs a minimum of 100 to 125 g (400–500 calories) of exogenous glucose each day for protein sparing and ketosis prevention (23,24). In addition, excessive lipolysis with resulting free fatty acid (FFA) accumulation has been shown to increase myocardial oxygen consumption (25) and may increase the risk of arrhythmias (26). Thus, sufficient glucose needs to be administered to prevent these catabolic processes, in addition to preventing hypoglycemia.

The exact quantity of glucose needed during an operation is not known. Both 10 g (14,27) and 5 g (28) of glucose per hour has been suggested, but further studies are needed to determine the most important factors affecting energy requirements during surgery to prevent undesirable fat and protein catabolism.

Potassium and Other Fluids

Serum potassium levels are dependent on free insulin concentrations (29), blood tonicity (30), and acid-base balance (31). Furthermore, because only 2% of the total body potassium is extracellular, a normal serum potassium level does not necessarily reflect a normal total body potassium. Therefore, a volume-depleted, insulin-deficient, acidemic patient with diabetes who is admitted with a normal serum-potassium level has a risk of severe hypokalemia when administered fluids and insulin. These patients, therefore, should not be scheduled to undergo an elective outpatient operation until their metabolic status is corrected. In the normokalemic diabetic patient with normal renal function, potassium chloride, 20 mEq/liter should be added to each liter of fluid. All diabetic patients should have their glucose and electrolyte concentrations rechecked while in the recovery room.

If a patient is receiving adequate insulin, glucose, and potassium, any additional fluids given during surgery should not contain glucose. In general, a standard solution of 5% dextrose in 0.45% saline is used. Finally, it is probably best to avoid lactated ringers (LR) in the diabetic population because lactate, a gluconeogenic precursor, is rapidly metabolized in a catabolic state. Although one study showed a deterioration of glucose control in a group of patients with NIDDM receiving LR (32), a more recent investigation showed no change in glucose production with lactate infusion (33). Further studies regarding the perioperative effects of LR in the diabetic population are clearly needed.

Other Concerns for the Outpatient with IDDM

Despite the increasing emphasis on ambulatory surgery, there are few studies examining the metabolic effects after common outpatient operations in patients with IDDM. Christiansen et al. (34) recently compared two groups of insulin-dependent diabetic patients having minor surgery under general anesthesia. One group received an insulin-glucose infusion, the other conventional sc insulin therapy. The former group had significantly better control of blood glucose levels, although there were no differences between the two groups when lactate, β-hydroxybutyrate, and glycerol levels were determined (FFAs were not measured). Unfortunately, C-peptide measurements were not made. The mean age of both groups was 52 years (with patients older than 70 years in both groups), so it is likely that some of these subjects were actually patients with NIDDM. This could, at least in part, explain why there were no differences in the measured metabolites. Nevertheless, insulin-deficient patients are optimally managed with variable-rate insulin infusions during surgery because of the erratic absorption of sc insulin.

There are many situations where it is acceptable to deviate from iv insulin infusion regimen for brief outpatient surgical procedures. The decision not to begin an insulin infusion depends upon:

1. the outpatient's current metabolic status (e.g., the individual with marked hyperglycemia and/or acidemia should be placed on an insulin infusion)
2. preoperative insulin regimen (e.g., it would be easier to continue with sc insulin for those patients using ultralente insulin
3. the type of diet the outpatient will be allowed to eat after the operation
4. the physician's ability to handle a metabolic crisis related to protracted postoperative nausea and vomiting, a common complication after outpatient anesthesia (Table 3) (35). Indeed, it was recently reported that 18% of unanticipated hospital admissions following ambulatory surgery in a general patient population were due to intractable vomiting (36). Furthermore, nausea and vomiting can be early harbingers to diabetic ketoacidosis (DKA). Thus, close monitoring of blood glucose, electrolyte, and urinary ketone levels is necessary for any diabetic patient with postoperative vomiting.

TABLE 3. *Common etiologies of nausea and vomiting in outpatients*

Predisposing factors
  Female gender
  Motion sickness
  Morbid obesity
  Early pregnancy
Increased gastric volume
  Excessive anxiety (air swallowing)
  Noncompliance with NPO instructions
Premedicants
  Narcotic analgesics (e.g., morphine, meperidine, fentanyl)
Anesthetic agents
  Inhaled drugs (e.g., isoflurane, N_2O)
  Intravenous drugs (e.g., etomidate, ketamine)
Surgical procedures
  Dilatation and extraction
  Laparoscopy
  Strabismus correction
  Insertion of PE tubes
  Orchiopexy
Postoperative factors
  Hypotension
  Pain

Adapted from White PF, Shafer A, ref. 35.

Gastroparesis occurs in 20–30% of diabetic patients (37). Although often asymptomatic, gastroparesis presents clinically as nausea, postprandial fullness, early satiety, epigastric pain, and occasionally as protracted vomiting. Although there are no data that diabetic patients, with or without gastroparesis, have an increased risk of perioperative nausea and vomiting, this complication can lead to regurgitation and aspiration (38) as well as unexpected admissions. In the patient with IDDM who is receiving sc insulin, the inability to eat after surgery complicates postoperative medical management. Glucose infusions may be titrated for a targeted glycemic goal. However, if the serum-insulin levels are declining while the glucose infusion is increasing, the patient can be placed at an unnecessary risk of excessive hyperglycemia and ketosis. The alternative approach, utilizing a variable-rate insulin infusion, diminishes the metabolic risks during the postoperative period.

Metoclopramide, a gastrokinetic agent that increases gastric motility and possesses antiemetic properties (39), may be effective in patients with gastroparesis (40,41). Thus, metoclopramide, 10 mg iv, appears to be the drug of choice for initial therapy of postoperative vomiting in patients with diabetes. Other effective antiemetics include iv droperidol, 0.5–1 mg, and iv hydroxyzine, 10–25 mg. In fact, a combination of metoclopramide and droperidol may be more effective than either drug alone (42).

Specific SC Insulin Regimens

All sc insulin regimens must achieve adequate plasma insulin concentrations to prevent excessive gluconeogenesis, glycogenolysis, lipolysis, and ketogenesis. There are several strategies that can be used to accomplish this goal. If the patient normally takes neutral protamine Hagedorn (NPH) and regular insulin before breakfast and supper, one-third to two-thirds of the usual dose of each type of insulin dose can be given in the morning unless there is evidence for fasting hypoglycemia [blood glucose level less than 4.4 mmol/liter (80 mg/dl)]. In the latter case, the regular insulin dose can be held until the capillary glucose concentration rises above 6.7 mmol/liter (120 mg/dl). The lower dose of NPH insulin reduces the risk of afternoon hypoglycemia if the surgery is delayed or postoperative emetic sequelae develops. Because supplemental regular insulin can be given later in the day, the full dose of NPH insulin is not necessary. The patient is administered a glucose infusion (5 g·h^{-1}) and the capillary glucose levels should be measured hourly.

If oral intake is tolerated immediately after the procedure, the remainder of the morning regular insulin should be given 20–30 minutes before resuming a regular diet. However, additional regular insulin should be given if the capillary glucose level is above 11.1 mmol/liter (200 mg/dl). The NPH insulin given in the morning will take effect approximately 4 hours after injection while its peak will occur in approximately 8–10 hours; therefore, it is not necessary to be overly aggressive with supplemental regular insulin if the patient is capable of eating between 2 and 4 PM. This regimen depends on a degree of guesswork and may be associated with misjudgment.

A second option for outpatients who take their insulin before breakfast and supper is to give the NPH insulin (from the second injection) at bedtime on the night before surgery. If NPH insulin is usually taken at bedtime, no changes need to be made. On the morning of the procedure, one-half to two-thirds of the usual dose of NPH insulin can be administered and little or no regular insulin needs to be given because plasma insulin levels should be adequate from the NPH insulin administered the night before. As suggested previously, a glucose infusion is started and the capillary glucose levels should be checked hourly. Blood glucose concentrations above 11.1 mmol/liter (200 mg/dl) require treatment with supplemental regular insulin. However, the "peaking" NPH insulin given the night before needs to be considered because serum-insulin levels will be highest between 6 and 9 AM. If the patient is capable of eating immediately after surgery, one-half to two-thirds of the usual dose of regular insulin can be given before the meal.

The patient taking ultralente insulin should be given the usual dose of this insulin. Regular insulin is only necessary for capillary glucose concentrations greater than 11.1 mmol/liter (200 mg/dl). Due to the long duration of action of ultralente insulin (21,22), the patient should have adequate insulin levels from the insulin given during the previous few days. Increasing the ultralente insulin dose on the morning of surgery has no effect on the plasma glucose concentrations during the procedure, and changing to a different type of insulin several days before the procedure is unnecessarily complicated for patients undergoing brief ambulatory surgical procedures.

AMBULATORY SURGERY IN THE PATIENT WITH NIDDM

General Principles

The majority of patients undergoing surgery have NIDDM. As opposed to the microvascular complications that are predominant in patients with IDDM, those with NIDDM have a much higher prevalence of macrovascular disease (43). Many of these patients, therefore, undergo angiographic studies, angioplasties, ulcer débridements, and abscess drainage procedures, which often can be performed as an outpatient procedure. In addition, this population frequently presents for cataract extraction (44).

Insulin Regimens during Ambulatory Surgery for Patients with NIDDM

Most agree that patients with NIDDM treated with diet or oral hypoglycemic agents (OHA), whose disease is well controlled, do not require special treatment before and during surgery. If the fasting plasma glucose level for the diet-treated patient is less than 7.8 mmol/liter (140 mg/dl), the patient may be treated initially with observation alone. Patients with this degree of glycemic control treated with OHA may be given their medication and started on a glucose infusion at the usual time (around 7 AM). Treatment decisions for higher glucose concentrations are more controversial for this outpatient population. Perioperative insulin therapy, however, should be considered when blood glucose concentrations (fasting or random) exceed 11.1 mmol/liter (200 mg/dl), and definitely initiated when they are in excess of 13.9 mmol/liter (250 mg/dl). These values are chosen for these reasons: First, patients with fasting plasma glucose concentrations exceeding 11.1 mmol/liter tend to manifest absolute deficiency with respect to insulin secretion (45). Second, the renal threshold for glucose is approximately 10.0–11.1 mmol/liter (180–200 mg/dl) in most patients with normal renal function (46). Osmotic diuresis with resulting water and electrolyte losses occurs when this glucose level is exeeded. Finally, there are data indicating impaired wound strength and wound healing with plasma glucose levels greater than 11.1 mmol/liter (47–50).

Although the decision to begin an insulin infusion should depend on the patient and type of operative procedure, the initial infusion rate should not exceed 1.0 units·h^{-1}. If an infusion is not started, sc regular insulin should be given. It is difficult to give a precise recommendation regarding the optimal amount of insulin required to maintain euglycemia during and after the procedure. Four to 6 units of sc regular human insulin is a reasonable initial dose for a surgical patient not previously treated with insulin. More significant hyperglycemia [≥ 19.4 mmol/liter (350 mg/dl)] should be treated with an intravenous insulin infusion.

Malling and colleagues (51) recently studied two groups of patients with NIDDM before ambulatory surgical procedures. The patients were treated with either an infusion of glucose-insulin-potassium or sc insulin followed by an infusion of glucose. Mean fasting glucose levels were less than 8 mmol/liter (144 mg/dl) and all patients were taking an OHA at home. There was no difference in blood glucose levels and metabolic (β-hydroxybutyrate, lactate, glycerol, alanine) or hormonal (insulin, glucagon, growth hormone) parameters between the two groups. Therefore, both treatment options are reasonable for this outpatient surgical population.

Patients with NIDDM previously taking insulin at home also have the option of receiving either an intravenous insulin infusion or sc insulin during the perioperative period. The same principles of insulin strategy discussed for the patient with IDDM apply to this population. Furthermore, some of these patients are insulinopenic and thus are prone to ketosis. Finally, for any patient who requires insulin therapy, there is less guesswork when an insulin infusion (versus sc insulin) is used during the operation, particularly for patients at risk to developing postoperative nausea and vomiting (Table 3) (35).

HYPOGLYCEMIA

Hypoglycemia is a frequent complication from the treatment of diabetes. Indeed, it has been estimated that during 40 years of IDDM, the average patient can experience 2000–4000 episodes of symptomatic hypoglycemia (20). Furthermore, patients with NIDDM treated with an OHA and diet were recently found to have a 20% incidence of hypoglycemia during a 6-month period (52). Although the true incidence of hypoglycemia during the perioperative period is not known, a recent report found that 13% of patients with IDDM had a blood glucose level measurement less than 3.3 mmol/liter (60 mg/dl) (1). However, this very well could be an underestimate due to the infrequency of blood glucose level monitoring. It is therefore important for health-team members to be suspicious of hypoglycemia in their diabetic patients.

Symptoms of hypoglycemia can be classified as neurogenic or neuroglycopenic (Table 4). The old terminology of "adrenergic" symptoms is now referred to as neurogenic because some of these symptoms (e.g., sweating) are cholinergic, albeit sympathetic (20). The most common of these neurogenic symptoms are sweating, palpitations, and anxiety. Because these symptoms can mimic several other entities, including anxiety attacks and hyperventilation (53), it is critical not to confuse the usual preoperative anxiety with hypoglycemia. Thus, blood glucose measurements should be routine before surgery in all patients with diabetes. Furthermore, because

TABLE 4. *Symptoms of hypoglycemia*

Neurogenic	Neuroglycopenic
Anxiety	Headache
Nervousness	Blurred vision
Tremulousness	Paresthesia
Sweating	Weakness
Hunger	Tiredness
Palpitations	Confusion
Pallor	Dizziness
Nausea	Amnesia
Angina	Abnormal mentation
	Behavioral change
	Feeling cold
	Transient hemiplegia
	Transient aphasia
	Seizures
	Coma

plasma glucose levels can change very quickly, the suspicious physician will monitor blood glucose concentrations frequently during the perioperative period (eg., hourly) because symptoms can be misleading. Finally, Boyle and colleagues have shown that in poorly controlled patients with IDDM, glycemic thresholds for the symptoms of hypoglycemia were 4.3 ± 0.3 mmol/liter (78 ± 5 mg/dl) compared with 2.9 ± 0.1 mmol/liter (53 ± 2 mg/dl) in nondiabetic controls (54). Thus, in this group of outpatients, it is even more difficult to separate preoperative anxiety from hypoglycemic symptoms. Because it is not always possible to differentiate between these two entities [e.g., when neurogenic symptoms are present with a blood glucose level between 3.9–5.0 mmol/liter (70–90 mg/dl)], glucose should be administered.

Headaches, changes in vision, alterations in behavior and higher intellectual functions are characteristic of neuroglycopenia. Seizures and coma are the most severe forms. Unfortunately, some diabetic patients lose their ability to recognize developing hypoglycemia (neurogenic symptoms) and therefore fail to eat. Thus, these individuals present with severe hypoglycemia and resultant neuroglycopenia. Although there is some degree of individual variation, the threshold for neuroglycopenia is approximately 2.0 mmol/liter (36 mg/dl) (55). Although never studied, one would expect the early neuroglycopenic symptoms to be blunted if the outpatient is excessively sedated with premedication drugs.

Because there are only a few signs suggestive of hypoglycemia in the anesthetized patient, hourly blood glucose concentrations should be measured in all patients receiving insulin or an OHA. These signs during anesthesia are nonspecific, but include electrocardiograph changes (ischemia) (56), diminished alpha waves and increased delta waves on electroencephalogram (EEG) (57), hypothermia (58), and hyperthermia (59,60).

Although there is considerable controversy regarding the biochemical definition of hypoglycemia, it is clear that iv glucose needs to be administered as blood glucose levels fall below normal to protect the central nervous system. Although permanent neurological deficits resulting from episodes of hypoglycemia appear to be uncommon, the issue has not been well studied. Changes in EEG have been found to persist for at least 1 month after an episode of hypoglycemia in some patients (61). Because capillary blood glucose measurements at the bedside risk considerable error, the consequences of prolonged hypoglycemia may be devastating, and the usual symptoms of hypoglycemia will be blunted (in the sedated patient) or absent (with general anesthesia), 20 ml of 50% dextrose (10 g) should be administered iv if glucose concentrations fall below 4.4 mmol/liter (80 mg/dl). If the patient is receiving insulin from an iv infusion, this should be turned off for 30 minutes. In the patient with IDDM, however, this results in a rapid decline in serum-insulin levels and increases the risk for ketosis, even if the plasma glucose concentration is not markedly elevated. Indeed, 17% of all episodes of DKA occur with plasma glucose levels less than 16.7 mmol/liter (300 mg/dl) (62). Therefore, the iv insulin infusion should be restarted between 0.3 and 0.6 units·h^{-1} after the blood glucose level is greater than 6.7 mmol/liter (Table 2). If after 30 minutes the glucose is between 4.4–6.7 mmol/liter (80–120 mg/dl), the iv insulin infusion should not be restarted, and the blood glucose level measured 30 minutes later. If the blood glucose level is still below 6.7 mmol/liter, a low-dose iv insulin infusion should be started (0.3 units·h^{-1}) because there is the risk of ketosis in the patient with IDDM. The potential for ketosis is lessened when sc insulin in administered.

These same principles apply for patients with NIDDM who are receiving an iv insulin infusion, although the risk for ketosis is generally not present. Hypoglycemia in patients receiving an OHA should similarly be treated with iv dextrose, and blood glucose levels should be remeasured after 30 minutes.

CONCLUSIONS

Because it is becoming necessary to make health-care delivery more cost efficient, it is obvious that many elective surgical procedures, which were traditionally performed on the day after the diabetic patient had been admitted to the hospital, are now being performed on the same day or as an outpatient. Therefore, it is important for the diabetes treatment team to be familiar with current management practices for diabetic patients who are scheduled for elective outpatient operations. The metabolic treatment goals for these individuals in the perioperative period include avoiding hypoglycemia, excessive hyperglycemia, lipolysis and ketogenesis, protein catabolism, and electrolyte disturbances. If these goals are achieved, the diabetes *per se* should not add any further risk to those already associated with the surgery and anesthesia. With further advances in the treatment of surgically related stress (63) and postoperative pain (64), it should be possible to optimize the care provided for both IDDM and NIDDM patients undergoing ambulatory surgical procedures.

ACKNOWLEDGMENTS

Supported in part by *U.S.P.H.S.* grants DK07102, RR0036, and 20579.

REFERENCES

1. Farkas-Hirsch R, Boyle PJ, Hirsch IB. Glycemic control of the surgical patient with IDDM. *Diabetes* 1989;38(Suppl 2):39A.
2. White PF. Outpatient anesthesia—an overview. In: White PF, *Outpatient anesthesia.* New York: Churchill Livingston, 1990.
3. Halter JB, Pflug AE. Relationship of impaired insulin secretion during surgical stress to anesthesia and catecholamine release. *J Clin Endocrinol Metab* 1980;51:1093–1098.

 4. Gordon NH, Scott DB, Persey-Robb JW. Modification of plasma corticosteroid concentrations during and after surgery by epidural blockage. *Br Med J* 1973;1:581–583.
 5. Brown FF, Owens WD, Felts JA, Spitznagel EL, Cryer PE. Plasma epinephrine and norepinephrine levels during anesthesia: Enflurane-N_2O-O_2. *Anesth Analog* 1982;61:366–370.
 6. Schade DS, Santiago JV, Skyler JS, Rizza RA. Intensive concentional therapy. In: *Intensive insulin therapy,* first ed. Amsterdam:Excerpta Medica, 1983;129–148.
 7. Reaven GM. Role of insulin resistance in human disease. *Diabetes* 1988;37:1595–1606.
 8. Karjalainen A, Salmela P, Ilonen J, Surgel H, Knip M. A comparison of childhood and adult type I diabetes mellitus. *N Engl J Med* 1989;320:881–886.
 9. Morley JE, Mooradian AD, Rosenthal MS, Kaiser FE. Diabetes mellitus in elderly patients: Is it different? *Am J Med* 1987;83:533–544.
10. Skyler JS. Insulin pharmacology. *Med Clin N Am* 1988;72:1337–1354.
11. Hirsch IB, McGill JB, Cryer PE. Role of insulin in management of surgical patients with diabetes mellitus. *Diabetes Care* 1990;13:980–991.
12. Galloway JA, Apradlin CT, Nelson RL, Wentworth SM, Davidson JA, Swarmer JL. Factors influencing the absorption, serum insulin concentration and blood glucose responses after injections of regular insulin and various insulin mixtures. *Diabetes Care* 1981;4:366–376.
13. Hildebrant P, Sestoft L, Nielson SL. The absorption of subcutaneously injected short-acting soluble insulin: Influence of injection technique and concentration. *Diabetes* 1983;6:459–462.
14. Pezzarossa A, Taddei F, Cimicchi MG, et al. Perioperative management of diabetic subjects: Subcutaneous vs intravenous insulin administration during glucose-potassium infusion. *Diabetes Care* 1988;11:52–58.
15. Watts NB, Gebhart SP, Clark RV, Phillips LS. Perioperative management of diabetes mellitus: Steady-state glucose control with bedside algorithm for insulin adjustment. *Diabetes Care* 1986;9:40–45.
16. Taitelman U, Reese EA, Bessman AN. Insulin in the management of the diabetic surgical patient. *JAMA* 1977;237:658–660.
17. Goldberg NJ, Wingert TD, Levin SSR, Wilson SD, Vilgoen JF. Insulin therapy in the diabetic surgical patient: Metabolic and hormone responses to low-dose insulin infusion. *Diabetes Care* 1981;4:279–284.
18. Alberti KGMM, Gill GV, Elliot MJ. Insulin delivery during surgery in the diabetic patient. *Diabetes Care* 1982;5(Suppl. 1):65–77.
19. Bolli GB, Gerich JE. The "dawn phenomenon"—a common occurrence in both non-insulin dependent and insulin-dependent diabetes mellitus. *N Engl J Med* 1984;310:746–750.
20. Cryer PE, Binder C, Bolli GB, et al. Hypoglycemia in IDDM. *Diabetes* 1989;38:1193–1199.
21. Rizza RA, O'Brien PC, Service FJ. Use of beef ultralente for basal insulin delivery: Plasma insulin concentrations after chronic ultralente administration in patients with IDDM. *Diabetes Care* 1986;9:120–123.
22. Seigler DE, Reeves ML, Goldberg RB, et al. Pharmacokinetics of ultralente insulin preparations. *Diabetes* 1985;34(Suppl. 1):61A.
23. Elwyn DH. Nutritional requirements of adult surgical patients. *Crit Care Med* 1980;8:9–20.
24. Gamble JL. Physiological information gained from studies on the life raft ration. *Harvey Lect* 1947;42:247–273.
25. Challoner DR, Steinberg D. Effect of free fatty acid on the oxygen consumption of perfused rat heart. *Am J Physiol* 1966;210:280–286.
26. Tansey MJ, Opie LH. Relation between plasma free fatty acids and arrhythmias within the first twelve hours of acute myocardial infarction. *Lancet* 1983;2:419–421.
27. Husband DJ, Thai AC, Alberti KGMM. Management of diabetes during surgery with glucose-insulin-potassium infusion. *Diabetic Med* 1986;3:69–74.
28. Clarke RSJ. The hyperglycemic response to different types of surgery and anesthesia. *Br J Anaesth* 1970;42:45–52.
29. DeFronzo RA, Tobin JD, Andres R. Glucose clamp technique: a method for quantifying insulin secretion and resistance. *Am J Physiol* 1979;237:E214–229.
30. Bratusch-Marrain R, DeFronzo RA. Impairment of insulin-mediated glucose metabolism by hyperosmolality in man. *Diabetes* 1983;32:1028–1034.
31. Adler S, Fraley DS. Potassium and intracellular pH. *Kid Int* 1977;11:433–442.
32. Thomas DJB, Alberti KGMM. Hyperglycemic effects of Hartmann's solution during surgery in patients with maturity onset diabetes. *Br J Anaesth* 1978;50:185–187.
33. Jenssen T, Nurjhan N, Consoli A, Gerich J. Increased supply of lactate which increases gluconeogenesis three-fold does not affect overall glucose production in normal man. *Diabetes* 1989;38(Suppl 2):11A.
34. Christiansen CL, Schurizek BA, Malling B, Knudsen L, Alberti KGMM, Hermansen K. Insulin treatment of the insulin-dependent diabetic patient undergoing minor surgery. *Anaesthesia* 1988;43:533–537.
35. White PF, Shafer A. Nausea and vomiting: causes and prophylaxis. *Sem Anesth* 1987;6:300–308.

36. Gold BS, Kitz DS, Lecky JH, Neuhaus JM. Unanticipated admission to the hospital following ambulatory surgery. *JAMA* 1989;262:3008–3010.
37. Glyal RK, Spiro H. Gastrointestinal manifestations of diabetes mellitus. *Med Clin North Am* 1971;55:1031–1044.
38. Malhall BP, O'Fearghail M. Diabetic gastroparesis. Case report and review of the literature. *Anesthesia* 1984;39:468–469.
39. Pinder R, Brogden R, Sawyer P, Speight TM, Avery GS. Metochlopramide: a review of its pharmacological properties and clinical use. *Drugs* 1986;12:81–131.
40. Snape WJ Jr, Battle WM, Schwartz SS. Metochlopramide to treat gastroparesis due to diabetes mellitus. A double-blind controlled trial. *Ann Intern Med* 1982;96:444–446.
41. Trapnell BC, Mavko LE, Birskovich LM, Falko JM. Metochlopramide suppositories in the treatment of diabetic gastroparesis. *Arch Intern Med* 1986;146:2278–2279.
42. Doze VA, Shafer A, White PF. Nausea and vomiting after outpatient anesthesia—effectiveness of droperidol alone and in combination with metoclopramide. *Anesth Analg* 1987;66:S41.
43. Marble A. Late complications of diabetes. A continuing challenge. *Diabetologia* 1976;12:193–199.
44. Bradley RF, Ramos E. The eyes and diabetes. In: Marble A, White P, Bradley RF, and Krall LP, eds. *Joslin's diabetes mellitus,* 11th ed. Philadelphia: Lea & Febiger, 1971;478–525.
45. DeFronzo RA, Ferrannini E, Kovisto V. New concepts in the pathogenesis and treatment of non-insulin-dependent diabetes mellitus. *Am J Med* 1983;74(Suppl 1A):52–81.
46. Elsas L, Rosenberg L. Renal glycosuria. In: Earley L, Gottschalk C, eds. *Strauss and Welt's diseases of the kidney,* 3rd ed, Boston: Little, Brown and Co, 1979;1021–1028.
47. McMurray JF. Wound healing with diabetes mellitus: better glucose control for better healing in diabetes. *Surg Clin North Am* 1984;64:769–778.
48. Goodson WH, Hunt TK. Status of wound healing in experimental diabetes. *J Surg Res* 1977;22:221–227.
49. Rosen RB, Enquist IF. The healing wound in experimental diabetes. *Surgery* 1961;50:525–528.
50. Yue DK, Mclennan S, Marsh M, et al. Effects of experimental diabetes, uremia, and malnutrition on wound healing. *Diabetes* 1987;36:295–299.
51. Malling B, Knudsen L, Christiansen BA, Schurizek BA, Hermansen K. Insulin treatment in non-insulin-dependent diabetes mellitus undergoing minor surgery. *Diab Nutr Metab* 1989;2:125–131.
52. Jennings AM, Wilson RD, Ward JD. Symptomatic hypoglycemia in NIDDM patients treated with oral hypoglycemic agents. *Diabetes Care* 1989;12:203–208.
53. Rice RL. Symptom of patterns of the hyperventilation syndrome. *Am J Med* 1952;8:691–700.
54. Boyle PJ, Schwartz NS, Shah SD, Clutter WE, Cryer PE. Plasma glucose concentrations at the onset of hypoglycemic symptoms in patients with poorly controlled diabetes and in nondiabetics. *N Engl J Med* 1988;318:1487–1492.
55. Siesjo BK. *Brain energy metabolism.* Chicester, England: John Wiley and Sons, 1979.
56. Loyd-Mostyn RH, Oram S. Modification by propranolol of cardiovascular effects of induced hypoglycaemia. *Lancet* 1975;1:1213–1215.
57. Himwich HE, Hadidian Z, Fazekas JF, Hoagland H. Cerebral metabolism and electrical activity during insulin hypoglycemia in man. *Am J Physiol* 1939;125:578–585.
58. Kedes LH, Field JB. Hypothermia: A clue to hypoglycemia. *N Engl J Med* 1964;271:785–789.
59. Chochinov R, Daughaday WH. Marked hyperthermia as a manifestation of hypoglycemia in long-standing diabetes mellitus. *Diabetes* 1975;24:859–860.
60. Ramos E, Zorilla E, Hadley WB. Fever as a manifestation of hypoglycemia. *JAMA* 1968;205:590–592.
61. Anghelescu L, Otetea G, Varadeanu A, et al. Hypoglycaimic encephalopathy—experimental, clinical and electroencephalographic study [Abstract]. *Diabetes Res Clin Pract.* 1985;1(Suppl 1): S19.
62. Monro JF, Cambell IW, McCuish AG, Duncan LJP. Euglycemic diabetic ketoacidosis. *Br Med J* 1973;2:578–580.
63. Monk TG, White PF, Mueller M, Kothapa V. Stress response during balanced anesthesia-optimal therapy (Abstract). *Anesthesiology* 1989;71:A128.
64. White PF. Pain management after day-case surgery. *Cur Opin Anaesth* 1988;1:70–75.

Surgical Management of the Diabetic Patient,
edited by Michael Bergman and Gregorio A. Sicard.
Raven Press, Ltd., New York © 1991.

11

Diabetic Neuropathy

Michael A. Pfeifer, Mary Schumer, Sonya Jung, and Stephen L. Pohl

Diabetes Research and Analysis Association, Inc., Lexington, Kentucky 40509

Neuropathy is a concern to the surgeon operating on any diabetic patient. No definitive study of the prevalence of diabetic neuropathy has been completed; however, the largest epidemiological study found that 12% of diabetic patients have clinical neuropathy at the time of diagnosis. Prevalence increases linearly with the duration of diabetes to almost 50% after 25 years. Therefore, the presence of neuropathy should be considered in the preoperative screening of each diabetic patient. Diabetic neuropathy is of concern to the surgeon in several regards: it can certainly affect the method of anesthesia, anesthesia risk, and cardiovascular lability during surgery; and it can affect postoperative recovery as far as cardiovascular, bladder, and gastrointestinal (GI) function.

There are few papers in the literature concerned with surgical experience in diabetic patients with neuropathy. Of those studies available, most are case reports describing only a few patients. There are only a few well-designed research studies. Our information was drawn from these papers as well as surgical experience in patients with nondiabetic neuropathies. This chapter briefly describes the surgical complications and management of diabetic patients with neuropathy.

PREOPERATIVE MANAGEMENT

Appropriate preoperative preparation can ameliorate many of the complications encountered during surgery. Preoperative care should include: adequate hydration, reducing hypotension, decreasing gastric secretions, and controlling apprehension.

Patients with autonomic neuropathy often do not have the normal cardiovascular responses to volume depletion and hypotension induced by some forms of anesthesia. There should be a careful preoperative assessment of fluid status, especially in patients with postural hypotension. Intravenous hydration for at least 12 hours before anesthesia has been suggested (1). The pharmacologic agent of choice is oral 9-alpha-fludrocortisone (2–4). Fludrocortisone increases plasma volume and peripheral resistance. Furthermore, accurate monitoring of blood loss during surgery is important (5).

In patients with nondiabetic autonomic neuropathy, apprehension frequently aggravates or causes an autonomic crisis in patients about to undergo surgery. An autonomic crisis is characterized by intractible vomiting, hypertension, cardiac arrhythmias, erythematous skin blotching, and diaphoresis. Diazepam administered the night before surgery and then iv on call to the operating room is often helpful

(1). Premedication with narcotics should be avoided because patients with autonomic neuropathy have blunted responses to hypercarbia and hypoxia.

Gastric secretions can be minimized by the use of cimetidine (5mg/kg) the night before and just prior to anesthesia in surgical patients.

INTRAOPERATIVE MANAGEMENT

Diabetic neuropathy can present two major problems with anesthesia. In patients with severe motor neuropathy, the use of succinylcholine may cause hyperkalemia (6). Motor neuropathy may also make the evaluation of neuromuscular blockade difficult. In general, neuromuscular and skeletal muscle relaxants should be avoided in patients with severe motor neuropathy. A nondepolarizing relaxant may be more appropriate. A careful preoperative examination can detect the presence of significant motor neuropathy.

Autonomic neuropathy can create severe problems with cardiovascular lability in diabetic patients (7–9). The problems encountered in patients with autonomic neuropathy can vary from bradycardia and hypotension (7,8) to hypertension and tachyarrhythmias (9,10) to gastric emptying difficulties, respiratory depression due to decreased sensitivity to carbon dioxide (11,12), and bladder dysfunction.

Patients with autonomic neuropathy commonly experience severe hypotension and bradycardia that is unresponsive to the usual pharmacologic agents (7,8). Bradycardia and hypotension may not respond predictably to atropine and epinephrine and their judicious use is therefore advisable. Episodes of bradycardia and hypotension in diabetic patients with renal failure have been reported (8). These episodes occurred suddenly and were unresponsive to iv atropine or usual doses of ephedrine. Epinephrine and/or external cardiac massage were required for resuscitation.

There are two reports that suggest that defective respiratory reflexes may be an adjunct feature of autonomic neuropathy (11,12). It is clear that many patients do not respond normally to hypercarbia or hypoxia. In both reports of cardiorespiratory arrest, profound respiratory depression occurred.

Hypertension during surgery can occur in diabetic individuals (3) and is also common in individuals with autonomic neuropathy of other etiologies (1,2,5,11–19). Occasionally, tachyarrhythmias may occur that respond to propranolol. Hypertension can be treated with an alpha-blockade. Sympathetic nervous system activation by surgical trauma can produce arrhythmias and myocardial ischemia. Afferent blockade may prevent these cardiac complications.

Inhalation analgesics such as nitrous oxide with halothane (0.5%) or enflurane (1%) are often used in these patients. Other studies have found that fentanyl is quite useful (19–21). Patients with autonomic neuropathy have diminished sympathetic innervation potentially resulting in exaggerated responses to direct-acting sympathetic stimuli or agonists and erratic responses to indirect-acting sympathomimetic agents. Furthermore, general anesthesia is associated with a release of epinephrine from the adrenal medulla (10). Every effort should be made to avoid the use of autonomic drugs and to minimize the release of epinephrine in the presence of autonomic dysfunction.

Clearly, a preoperative estimate of autonomic function would be of help to the anesthesiologist. Simple noninvasive tests are often helpful for determining high-risk individuals. They include RR-variation, the Valsalva maneuver, and postural testing. In combination, these three tests have an 83% sensitivity and an 82% specificity for identifying patients who are at risk for intraoperative lability (7).

POSTOPERATIVE MANAGEMENT

The stress associated with pain may produce an autonomic crisis which can be treated with diazepam (1).

Autonomic neuropathy may also impair gastrointestinal motility. Ridetadine should be avoided as this causes a decrease in gastric emptying and may actually aggravate biliary function postoperatively. Stomach decompression and diazepam may be useful to prevent nausea, retching, and hypertension. Urocholine enhances gastric emptying and should be used cautiously as it may also result in increased diapheresis, apprehension, and nausea.

The degree of activation of the sympathetic nervous system is elevated for at least 2 hours after surgery and positively correlates with rises in mean arterial pressure (10). These patients should be closely monitored for occurrence of a hypertensive crisis.

Postoperative urinary retention is often a problem in the diabetic patient as they may be predisposed to bladder neuropathy which can be aggravated by anesthesia.

Cardiovascular autonomic neuropathy may also predispose the patient to a greater incidence of painless myocardial ischemia. Surgeons should be advised that patients may have atypical symptoms of cardiac ischemia resulting from the denervated heart syndrome (22,23). As such, prudent use of cardiac drugs and a high index of suspicion is important in postoperative management of these patients. Again, simple, non-invasive, preoperative procedures (e.g., RR-variation, Valsalva, and postural testing) may identify patients at risk for this complication. Patients at risk for painless myocardial ischemia should have a thorough cardiovascular evaluation before surgery, if at all possible. A treatment algorithm has been recently published (23). As discussed above, treatment with autonomic drugs can have unexpected effects. Patients may be highly sensitive to sympathetic stimulants and unresponsive to parasympathetic antagonists (atropine). Pain management is of paramount importance in patients with autonomic dysfunction and a denervated cardiovascular system.

SURGICAL TREATMENT OF NEUROPATHY

Patients with severe diabetic neuropathy may require surgical treatment. Diabetic gastroparesis can be treated initially with bethanechol and metoclopramide. Gastro-jejunostomy has been used successfully in some patients with severe gastroparesis (24). This is obviously a measure resorted to only in the most severe, refractory patient with unrelenting gastroparesis.

Carpal tunnel syndrome and tarsal tunnel syndrome occur more frequently in diabetic individuals than in the nondiabetic population. These syndromes are amenable to surgical correction which should be instituted prior to the development of muscle atrophy.

SURGICALLY INDUCED NEUROPATHY

Reflex sympathetic dystrophy is occasionally found following surgery. The reflex sympathetic dystrophy syndrome is characterized by pain, swelling, and limited range of motion of an extremity with an associated sign of vasomotor instability, trophic skin changes, and patchy bone demineralization. The onset of pain may occur within a few days or may be delayed for several months following surgery (25–29). This can be particularly problematic when this occurs at the sight of a scar. In the past this condition has been treated with sympathectomy. However, the causalgia may also be treated with capsaicin, which depletes the nerve of a chemical called Substance P. Substance P is often associated with the neuropathic pain along suture lines in these patients. Capsaicin is available at 0.25% and 0.075% concentrations. The 0.075% concentration seems to be more effective. Patients should be instructed to use a very thin amount on the affected area as larger quantities can result in aerolization and irritation of mucus membranes. Capsaicin is derived from hot chili peppers and as a result, initially increases the burning before symptoms improve. Patients should be advised that the increased burning persists for only 2 to 3 days with a subsequent decline reaching its maximum effect in approximately two to six weeks. This treatment of the neuropathic pain associated with surgery can greatly improve the quality of life for these individuals.

SUMMARY

The presence of diabetic neuropathy places patients at increased risk during anesthesia and the postoperative recovery period. Careful preparation for surgery and prudent use of appropriate medications, anesthesia, and adrenergic drugs can prevent many problems. General anesthesia should be avoided in patients who can undergo regional (without epinephrine) or spinal anesthesias. Adequate hydration, reduction of apprehension, and management of pain and gastric secretions, special attention to motor neuropathy, and prudent use of analgesics can prevent serious complications when general anesthesia is indicated. Patients who are at risk may be identified with simple preoperative testing procedures. Patients who have bradycardia and are hypotensive may not respond to atropine and patients with tachyarrhythmias and/or hypertensive crisis may require α and β adrenergic blocking agents. Diazepam is especially useful in treating preoperative apprehension. Although general anesthesia presents unique problems in diabetic patients with autonomic neuropathy, it can be managed successfully and should not be contraindicated for these patients.

Surgery may also help relieve some forms of diabetic neuropathy. Neuropathic pain along suture lines can frequently occur, but it can be treated with capsaicin.

ACKNOWLEDGMENTS

We gratefully acknowledge Krista Crump for her fine secretarial skills. We also acknowledge support from Diabetes Associates and the Diabetes Center of Excellence, Humana Hospital-Lexington, Lexington, Kentucky.

REFERENCES

1. Axelrod FB, Donenfeld RF, Danziger F, Turndorf H. Anesthesia in familial dysautonomia. *Anesthesiology* 1988;68:631–635.
2. Hutchinson RC, Sugden JC. Anaesthesia for Shy-Drager syndrome. *Anaesthesia* 1984;39:1229–1231.

3. Lewis RK, Haselrig CG, Fricke FJ, Russell RO: Therapy of idiopathic postural hypotension. *Arch Intern Med* 1972;129:943–949.
4. Bannister R, Ardill L, Fentem P. An assessment of various methods of treatment of idiopathic orthostatic hypotension. *Q J Med* 1969;38:377–395.
5. Freeman TT, Shelby J, Becker KE. Riley-Day syndrome. *J Kansas Med* 1983;84:446–447.
6. Schonwald G, Fish KJ, Perkash I. Cardiovascular complications during anesthesia in chronic spinal cord injured patients. *Anesthesiology* 1981;55:550–558.
7. Burgos LG, Ebert TJ, Asidao C, et al. Increased intraoperative cardiovascular morbidity in diabetics with autonomic neuropathy. *Anesthesiology* 1989;70:591–597.
8. Ciccarelli LL, Ford CM, Tsueda K. Autonomic neuropathy in a diabetic patient with renal failure. *Anesthesiology* 1986;64:283–287.
9. Takeshima R. Abnormal hemodynamic responses. *Masui* 1988;37:1249–1254.
10. Halter JB, Pflug AE, Porte D. Mechanism of plasma catecholamine increases during surgical stress in man. *J Clin Endocrinol Metabol* 1977;45:936–944.
11. Sweeney BP, Jones S, Langford RM. Anaesthesia in dysautonomia: further complications. *Anaesthesia* 1985;40:783–786.
12. Page McB, Watkins PJ. Cardiorespiratory arrest and diabetic autonomic neuropathy. *Lancet* 1978;1:14–16.
13. Stirt JA, Frantz RA, Gunz EF, Conolly ME. Anesthesia, catecholamines, and hemodynamics in autonomic dysfunction. *Anesth Analg* 1982;61:701–704.
14. Vinograd I, Udassin R, Beilin B, Neuman A, Maayan C, Nissan S: The surgical management of children with familial dysautonomia. *J Pediatr Surg* 1985;20:632–636.
15. Foster JMG. Anaesthesia for a patient with familial dysautonomia. *Anaesthesia* 1983;38:391.
16. Cox RG, Sumner E. Familial dysautonomia. *Anaesthesia* 1983;38:293.
17. Saarnivaara L, Kautto UM, Teravainen H. Ketamine anaesthesia for a patient with the Shy-Drager syndrome. *Acta Anaesthesiol Scan* 1983;27:123–125.
18. Stenqvist O, Sigurdsson J. The anaesthetic management of a patient with familial dysautonomia. *Anaesthesia* 1982;37:929–932.
19. Beilin B, Maayan C, Vatashsky E, Shulman D, Vinograd I, Aronson HB: Fentanyl anesthesia in familial dysautonomia. *Anesth Analg* 1985;64:72–76.
20. Kritchman MM, Schwartz H, Papper EM. Experiences with general anesthesia in patients with familial dysautonomia. *JAMA* 1959;170:529–533.
21. Meridy HW, Creighton RE. General anesthesia in eight patients with familial dysautonomia. *Can Anaesth Soc J* 1971;18:563–570.
22. Pfeifer MA, Peterson H. Cardiovascular autonomic neuropathy in diabetic neuropathy. In: Dyck P, et al., eds. Philadelphia: W.B. Saunders, 1987.
23. Pfeifer M, ed. Cardiovascular autonomic neuropathy. *Diabetes Spectrum* 1990;3(1):17–48.
24. Guy RJC, Dawson JL, Garrett JR, et al. Diabetic gastroparesis from autonomic neuropathy: Surgical considerations and changes in vagus nerve morphology. *J Neurol Neurosurg Psych* 1984;47:686–691.
25. Schwartzman RJ, McLellan TL. Reflex sympathetic dystrophy. *Arch Neurol* 1987;44:555–561.
26. Headley B. Historical perspective of causalgia: Management of sympathetically maintained pain. *Physical Therapy* 1987;67:1370–1374.
27. Schutzer SF, Gossling HR. Current concepts review the treatment of reflex sympathetic dystrophy syndrome. *J Bone Joint Surg* 1984;66:625–629.
28. Rowlingson JC. The sympathetic dystrophies. *Int Anesth Clin* 1983;21(4):117–129.
29. Carlson T, Jacobs AM. Reflex sympathetic dystrophy syndrome. *J Foot Surg* 1986;25:149–153.

Surgical Management of the Diabetic Patient,
edited by Michael Bergman and Gregorio A. Sicard.
Raven Press, Ltd., New York © 1991.

12

Hypertension in Diabetes

Principles and Therapeutics

Charles Sweeney, Jonathan Tolins, and Leopoldo Raij

*University of Minnesota School of Medicine and Veterans Administration Medical
Center, Minneapolis, Minnesota 55455*

Hypertension is common in patients with diabetes, and its management requires special consideration by the practitioner. Hypertension generally develops in individuals with insulin-dependent diabetes (IDDM), after the onset of diabetic nephropathy. In noninsulin-dependent diabetes (NIDDM) hypertension is seen earlier and may even precede the development of glucose intolerance. When hypertension occurs in diabetic individuals, it worsens many of the complications of this disease, particularly the vascular ones. For this reason, control of hypertension in diabetes assumes added importance, since effective blood pressure control may delay the onset, or slow the progression, of the devastating systemic complications of this disease.

DIABETES AND HYPERTENSION

Epidemiology of Hypertension and Relation to Diabetic Nephropathy

In IDDM, hypertension occurs coincident with, and as an integral part of, the onset of nephropathy. Diabetic nephropathy ultimately develops in a subset of patients with IDDM (40–50%), usually becoming clinically manifest 15–20 years after the diagnosis of diabetes is made (1,2). The onset of this complication is heralded by the appearance of increased urinary albumin excretion rates (3,4). Once this occurs, the subsequent progression to end-stage renal failure may be inevitable. Diabetic individuals with normal renal function usually have normal blood pressure; however, even the very early stages of diabetic nephropathy, characterized by so-called microalbuminuria (urinary albumin excretion rate of 30–250 mg/24 h) are frequently associated with increased blood pressure (5). In patients with established nephropathy, hypertension is ubiquitous (6).

Individuals with NIDDM have been shown to have a greater prevalence of hypertension than nondiabetic persons matched by age and sex, even when the obesity frequently associated with this disorder is taken into account (7). Hypertension in this type of diabetes occurs independently of the development of diabetic renal disease. In many patients, hypertension is present before NIDDM develops (8).

NIDDM, hypertension, and obesity are commonly associated with aging populations. For instance, approximately 75% of individuals with NIDDM and 66% of individuals with hypertension are overweight (9). Evidence indicates that insulin resistance and hyperinsulinemia may be pathogenetic in both conditions. Certain subsets of individuals with essential hypertension given an oral glucose load respond with prolonged periods of hyperinsulinemia compared with normotensive age-matched controls (10). Population studies from Israel, where there is a high rate of NIDDM, demonstrate a significant correlation between insulin levels, blood pressure, and body-mass index (11). The pathophysiology of these associations is not clear; however, possible mechanisms include insulin-induced changes in renal sodium handling, increased sympathetic tone, insulin-related alterations in ion transport at the cellular level, and finally genetic differences in muscle fiber composition, which could account for differential responses to insulin (9).

Effects of Hypertension on the Complications of Diabetes

Patients with diabetes mellitus (DM) who are also hypertensive have a higher rate of morbidity and mortality as a result of diabetic complications. Many prospective studies have shown that hypertension is an important risk factor for diabetic macrovascular disease (12–14). The morbid effects of hypertension in NIDDM are primarily a result of accelerated atherosclerosis and the corresponding lesions that develop in the affected organ systems: coronary artery disease (CAD), stroke, and peripheral vascular disease. The Whitehall Study revealed a significant increase in CAD mortality in diabetic patients with increased systolic blood pressure at 10-year follow-up. Age and systolic blood pressure were demonstrated to be the major contributors to this higher mortality (13). In a study of Finnish men, those individuals who were hypertensive and diabetic had a relative risk of CAD mortality of 4.69 compared with normotensive diabetic individuals (14). Data from the Framingham Study show that glucose intolerance alone was not associated with an increased risk for development of CAD. When elevated systolic blood pressure occurred along with glucose intolerance, however, the risk increased to 81 per 1000 patients. If an elevation in serum cholesterol levels was present along with glucose intolerance and an elevated systolic blood pressure, the risk increased to 326 per 1000 in nonsmokers and 459 per 1000 in smokers (15). These studies clearly demonstrate that when diabetes is complicated by hypertension the risk for CAD increases.

Microvascular complications of diabetes, such as nephropathy and retinopathy, are also affected by hypertension. The incidence of retinal exudates was doubled in Pima Indians with diabetes who were hypertensive, compared with nonhypertensive patients over a 6-year period (16). Similar findings have been reported in other groups (17). Nephropathy develops in IDDM 15–20 years after diabetes begins, and presents clinically with a triad of hypertension, proteinuria, and decreased glomerular filtration rate (GFR). Nephropathy develops almost exclusively in individuals who also have retinopathy, most likely reflecting generalized microvascular disease. Uncontrolled hypertension accelerates the rate of progression of diabetic nephropathy. Two studies have suggested that effective antihypertensive therapy can slow the rate of progression of established nephropathy (18,19). From the above discussion, a clear association can be seen between systemic hypertension and the development and progression of the macrovascular and microvascular complications of diabetes. Consequently, rigorous blood-pressure control is an important objective in these patients.

PATHOGENESIS OF HYPERTENSION IN DIABETES

Hypertension is seen in both IDDM and NIDDM, but different mechanisms underly this condition in the two types of diabetes. In IDDM, hypertension is not seen until proteinuria occurs and diabetic nephropathy is established. Hypertension in this case is associated with definite structural changes in the glomerulus (5). The elevated systemic blood pressure accelerates the progressive decline in renal function seen in diabetic nephropathy (20). Consequently, a vicious cycle is created where the intrinsic renal damage due to diabetic nephropathy triggers elevations in systemic blood pressure, and the elevated blood pressure accelerates the decline in renal function. Elevated blood pressure (although not to the degree we customarily define as hypertensive) is seen in the very earliest stages of diabetic nephropathy, when only microalbuminuria is present (5). Furthermore, recent studies have suggested that a genetic predisposition to hypertension may be present in that subset of diabetic individuals at risk for the development of diabetic nephropathy (21). Seaquist et al. (22) reported familial clustering of diabetic nephropathy, independent of glycemic control or hypertension. Other environmental factors that could contribute to nephropathy were not controlled in this study. Increased activity of the red blood cell (RBC) sodium-lithium (Na-Li) countertransport system has been reported in individuals with essential hypertension, as well as in patients with IDDM and nephropathy (23). Carr et al. (24) have recently shown RBC Na-Li countertransport to be elevated in a subset of patients with IDDM in whom microalbuminuria or nephropathy have not developed, but who do have elevated GFRs. In this study, 33% of the patients with IDDM exhibited elevations in both the sodium-lithium countertransport system and GFR, a percentage that is similar in magnitude to the proportion of the IDDM population in whom nephropathy will eventually develop. Given the proposed role of abnormal renal hemodynamic alterations (hyperfiltration due to glomerular capillary hypertension and hyperperfusion) in the progression of diverse forms of chronic renal failure, including diabetic nephropathy, this study suggests that determinations of Na-Li countertransport may be useful in identifying, at a very early stage, those patients with renal hemodynamic abnormalities that may develop into diabetic nephropathy. If the findings of this study hold true, identifying this population at an early stage by abnormalities in RBC countertransport would be a first step in developing therapeutic interventions that could have an impact on the natural history of diabetic nephropathy.

In NIDDM, the relationship between hypertension and nephropathy is not as clear. Approximately 40–50% of patients with NIDDM are hypertensive (25); however, as discussed above, the onset and time course of hypertension is different from that seen in IDDM. Microalbuminuria is found in 15–20% of individuals with NIDDM at the time of diagnosis and may eventually develop in up to 60% (26). In this population, the presence of microalbuminuria does not correlate with the onset of hypertension (27). Furthermore, proteinuria in NIDDM does not necessarily serve as an indicator of the development of nephropathy, although its presence is correlated with an increased frequency of cardiovascular disease (26). Albuminuria is frequently seen with systemic hypertension in nondiabetic individuals (28); consequently, in NIDDM it may be a manifestation of hypertension and not a complication of diabetes *per se* (8). Compared with the nephropathy of IDDM, the renal disease in NIDDM is seen earlier, becoming evident approximately 10 years after the diagnosis of diabetes. It also, on average, occurs in fewer than 15% of individuals with NIDDM, is generally seen in an older population with ages ranging from 60–70 years, and progresses to end-stage renal disease over a shorter time period, approximately 10 years on average (26).

DIABETIC NEPHROPATHY: HEMODYNAMIC AND METABOLIC FACTORS

Diabetic nephropathy in IDDM begins with a prolonged subclinical phase during which time the GFR may actually be elevated above normal and the affected kidneys demonstrate significant hypertrophy (29). Hyperfiltration peaks between 5 and 7 years after the diagnosis of DM. During this time systolic blood pressure is normal and the urinary albumin excretion rate is also normal (less than 20–30 mg/24 h). Microalbuminuria (30–250 mg/24 h) is the first clinical sign that the nephropathy of DM has developed (3). This occurs approximately 10–15 years after DM is first diagnosed, often progressing to end-stage renal disease within 7 to 10 years (29). There are both metabolic and hemodynamic features peculiar to the diabetic state that seem to contribute to the development and progression of diabetic nephropathy. Therapeutic interventions aimed at arresting or at least slowing the progression of diabetic nephropathy have evolved around efforts to normalize the metabolic milieu by maintaining tight control of blood glucose levels and normalizing renal hemodynamics with antihypertensive agents.

In experimental diabetic animals, strict regulation of blood sugar prevents the development of diabetic vascular complications (30), but this has not consistently proven to be the case in humans. When strict control of blood sugar is established prior to the onset of microalbuminuria, progression to overt nephropathy can be halted, at least temporarily (31). Even if strict control is established during the earliest stages of microalbuminuria (30–300 mg/24 h), progression of diabetic nephropathy can be slowed (32). After clinically detectable proteinuria is established, however, no degree of strict glycemic control, including continuous insulin infusion, slows the progression of nephropathy (33). Consequently, it seems that metabolic factors may be important in the initial stages of diabetic nephropathy. Once renal function begins to deteriorate, however, even the strictest metabolic control cannot halt the progression of renal failure.

Micropuncture studies in experimental animals have confirmed that glomerular hyperfiltration is seen early in the course of experimental diabetic nephropathy, a result of increased pressures and flows within the glomerular capillaries (34). Hostetter studied glomerular hemodynamics in rats with streptozotocin-induced diabetes, maintained in a moderately hyperglycemic state by daily insulin injections (35). Diabetic rats demonstrated elevations in glomerular capillary plasma flow and glomerular capillary pressure associated with preglomerular or afferent arteriolar vasodilatation. In diabetic nephropathy, the ability to autoregulate blood flow by varying afferent arteriolar resistance is impaired. Consequently, elevations in systemic blood pressure are transmitted directly to the glomerulus resulting in simultaneous glomerular capillary hypertension (36).

Genetic influences on the hemodynamics and metabolic milieu of the diabetic may affect the development of nephropathy. Cowie (37) studied the incidence of diabetic nephropathy in a large population of patients who acquired end-stage renal disease over a 10-year-period. She found a 2.6-fold higher incidence of end-stage renal disease among black patients, compared with white patients. In this study, most black patients with renal failure caused by diabetes had NIDDM. Some of the factors that may account for the higher incidence of end-stage renal disease in diabetic black patients compared with white patients include: increased diastolic blood pressure in black patients compared with white patients prior to the onset of renal disease (37), an increased tendency for renal disease to develop in black patients when hypertension is present (38,39), and socioeconomic factors relating to the delivery and quality of health care to this segment of the population.

The renal hemodynamics observed in experimental diabetic nephropathy may have therapeutic implications. Diets high in protein have been shown to increase renal blood low and intraglomerular pressure in diabetic rats (40). In these rats, dietary protein restriction results in normalization of glomerular capillary pressures and protection from progressive glomerular injury. Similarly, angiotensin-converting enzyme (ACE) inhibitors have been shown to favorably affect glomerular hemodynamics in experimental animals (41). These antihypertensive agents that inhibit the formation of the potent vasoconstrictor angiotensin II (AII), reduce intraglomerular pressure by preferentially decreasing efferent arteriolar vascular tone. This action results in maintenance of glomerular blood flow and GFR despite a fall in intraglomerular pressure. It is not clear at this time whether ACE inhibitors exert their protective effects in experimental diabetic nephropathy solely by alterations in hemodynamic responses of the glomerulus, or if other effects also play a role (42).

TREATMENT

It seems clear that control of hypertension in diabetes is a desirable goal. Normalizing blood pressure slows the development of diabetic complications, decreasing the morbidity and mortality of this progressive disease. In light of the complexities involved in the clinical management of most diabetic patients, it is important that any antihypertensive therapy used in this patient population have a minimum of side effects. Properties that must be considered include effects on glycemic control, serum-lipid metabolism, renal function, and mental status, as well as how the intervention affects the patient's quality of life.

Nonpharmacologic Approaches

Most diabetic patients require pharmacologic therapy to control blood pressure. There are, however nonpharmacologic interventions that may suffice to control blood pressure, particularly in NIDDM, and may at least improve the response to drug therapy. Weight loss can effectively lower blood pressure in obese individuals with NIDDM (43). It has also been demonstrated that increased physical activity in NIDDM helps to lower blood pressure (44). Specific dietary interventions can serve to decrease blood pressure. One study compared the effects of a high-fiber, low-fat, low-sodium diet with thiazide diuretic therapy in diabetic patients with mild hypertension (45). Similar decreases in blood pressure were seen in both groups; however, the dietary group showed improvement in glycemic control and lipid profiles, while these worsened in the patients treated with thiazide. Restricting sodium in the diet to 3–5 g per day lowers blood pressure and enhances the action of diuretics and other antihypertensive agents (46). Patients with renal disease who are on salt-restricted diets and diuretics may have impairment of normal sodium homeostasis and must be followed carefully for extremes of sodium depletion or overload with the corresponding derangements in volume status. A reasonable plan for nonpharmacologic management of hypertension in diabetic individuals, particularly those with NIDDM, should include a weight reduction diet and exercise along with modest salt restriction. Although blood pressure may not become normalized with these measures, they may enhance the efficacy and minimize the need for drug therapy.

Thiazide Diuretics

Thiazide diuretics have proven to be effective antihypertensive agents. Due to the low activity of plasma renin in diabetic individuals with hypertension and the relative volume expanded state, thiazides seem to be ideal agents to control blood pressure in these patients (47). Widespread use of these agents over time, however, has revealed many undesirable side effects. Prerenal azotemia along with other metabolic abnormalities are frequently seen in patients treated with thiazides. These abnormalities include hyponatremia, hypokalemia, hypomagnesemia, and hyperuricemia (48). Worsening of glycemic control is frequently seen in diabetic individuals, manifested by increases in fasting blood sugar, glucosuria, and elevated glycosylated hemoglobin (49). Hypokalemia may not only increase the risk for ventricular ectopic activity, but may also impair insulin release and increase insulin resistance, accounting for the thiazide-induced impairment of glycemic control (50). Thiazides also have unfavorable effects on serum lipids, increasing total serum triglycerides and cholesterol (51). This effect could add to the already increased risk of artherosclerosis in hypertensive diabetic individuals. Consequently, in diabetic patients the undesirable side effects of thiazides may outweigh their benefits.

Agents That Interact with Adrenergic Receptors

Beta-adrenergic agonists are accepted implements in the antihypertensive armamentarium. Like thiazides, however, there is also the potential for drawbacks when used in patients with diabetes. The beta-blockers exert their antihypertensive actions by decreasing cardiac output through both a decrease in heart rate and contractility. Although diabetic patients frequently display a baseline tachycardia due to loss of vagal suppression and therefore may not manifest a negative chronotropic effect, contractility is often already compromised in these patients, and the negative ionotropic effect can further decrease the cardiac output, precipitating congestive heart failure.

Beta-blockers can also mask the adrenergic response to the insulin-induced hypoglycemic episodes to which diabetic individuals are prone. However, this theoretical disadvantage has not been confirmed in clinical studies. Blohm compared the beta-one selective blocker metoprolol to a placebo given to five insulin-dependent diabetic patients with hypertension, all of whom were prone to hypoglycemic attacks (52). During treatment with the beta-blocker no increase in the number of severe hypoglycemic episodes was observed. Only one patient noted slight masking of hypoglycemic symptoms.

Like thiazides, beta-blockers may also have an adverse effect on serum lipids causing a decrease in the high-density lipoprotein (HDL) fraction of cholesterol (53). In the peripheral circulation, nonselective beta-blockers can cause vasoconstriction triggered by unopposed alpha-receptor stimulation (54). This can worsen preexistent peripheral vascular disease. For this reason when beta-blockers are used in diabetic patients, beta-one selective agents are preferable to nonselective ones.

Prazocin and other alpha-one adrenergic blockers have been shown to be effective in the control of hypertension in diabetic individuals with no adverse effects on glucose tolerance (55). Furthermore, these agents reduce total peripheral resistance, maintain cardiac output, and have a favorable impact on serum-lipid profiles. Some diabetic patients with peripheral neuropathy are prone to orthostatic hypotension, both after the first dose and with ongoing treatment with these agents (47).

Centrally acting sympatholytic agents such as alpha-methyl-dopa and clonidine effectively control blood pressure in diabetic patients (56) through a centrally mediated reduction in sympathetic outflow. They have no effect on glucose tolerance. The major drawback of these drugs is the side effects they produce in nondiabetic as well as in diabetic individuals: sexual dysfunction, sedation, and other adverse central nervous system (CNS) effects, as well as rebound hypertension when discontinued (56).

Calcium Channel Blockers

Calcium channel blockers (CCB) have proven to be useful antihypertensive agents in diabetic patients (57). They decrease peripheral resistance with a minimum of systemic side effects. Some drugs in this group are safe to use in patients with congestive heart failure, unlike the beta-blockers, which are contraindicated in these individuals. Serum glucose and lipids are unaffected by these drugs (57). Whether the effects of this class of agents confers a specific hemodynamically mediated protection from the progression of renal failure is as yet unanswered. In the kidney CCB act predominantly at the afferent arteriole, causing vasodilation. Consequently the net effect on glomerular capillary pressure depends on the balance between the reduction in systemic blood pressure and the reduction in preglomerular or afferent arteriolar vascular resistance (58). In laboratory experiments and in clinical trials, CCB have been reported to have variable effects: some studies show a protective effect against the progression of chronic renal failure (59,60) and others do not (61). Furthermore, it is unclear whether protection is achieved through hemodynamic mechanisms alone. CCB have a spectrum of metabolic actions that have the potential to protect against the progression of renal failure. These actions include a decrease in renal metabolic demands (62), reduction in mesangial trafficking of macromolecules (42), inhibition of mesangial cell proliferation (63), and decreased synthesis of endogenous inflammatory mediators (64).

ACE Inhibitors

ACE inhibitors have emerged as the drugs of choice for the treatment of hypertension in diabetic patients, for many reasons. These drugs are efficacious in controlling blood pressure, they have relatively few side effects, and they exhibit favorable effects on renal function, slowing the progression of diabetic nephropathy. The most common side effects include a persistent nonproductive cough of unclear etiology, which occurs in fewer than 10% of patients, and a tendency toward hyperkalemia, which is probably due to the inhibition of aldosterone release by these drugs. ACE inhibitors are contraindicated in individuals with bilateral renal artery stenosis and in unilateral stenosis when only one kidney is present. In such individuals, elevated plasma levels of AII, which acts preferentially at the glomerular efferent arteriole, contribute to maintenance of GFR. Inhibition of the synthesis of this vasoconstrictor with an ACE inhibitor can cause a reversible, functional decline in GFR reflected in elevated serum creatinine values (65).

ACE inhibitors have proven efficacy in blood pressure control in diabetic patients. D'Angelo et al. (66) studied 20 hypertensive diabetic patients (IDDM and NIDDM) treated with captopril for 12 weeks. All patients achieved adequate blood pressure control, with four requiring the addition of a thiazide diuretic. No deterioration in metabolic control of diabetes was seen. Dominguez et al. (67) showed captopril alone or captopril plus a thiazide diuretic established effective blood pressure control in 16 patients with NIDDM. In this study and in others, captopril was shown to have a beneficial effect on glucose tolerance (67). Ferriere et al. (68) demonstrated improved glucose tolerance with captopril therapy using the glucose clamp technique to measure insulin sensitivity. The rate of peripheral glucose disposal in these trials was significantly increased during captopril treatment. Pollare et al. (69) showed that captopril increased, while hydrochlorothiazide decreased, insulin sensitivity in non-diabetic patients with essential hypertension.

The beneficial effects of ACE inhibitors on the progression of renal disease have been demonstrated in experimental and clinical diabetes. Anderson et al. (41) showed that rats with nondiabetic chronic renal failure responded favorably to treatment with ACE inhibitors. Those rats treated with enalapril had similar blood pressure control but decreased proteinuria and intraglomerular pressure compared to similar rats treated with triple therapy (reserpine, hydralazine, and hydrochlorothiazide). In diabetic rats, ACE inhbition also decreased glomerular capillary pressure and proteinuria. Hommel et al. (70) gave captopril (twice per day for 1 week) to 16 hypertensive diabetic humans with early nephropathy and showed a decrease in blood pressure and urinary albumin excretion rate, without a significant change in GFR. Parving et al. (71) have shown that long-term administration of an ACE inhibitor and a diuretic (2 1/2 years) to hypertensive diabetic patients with nephropathy results in a decreased albumin excretion rate and a slowing of the decline in GFR. ACE inhibitors also appear to have beneficial effects for nonhypertensive insulin-dependent diabetic patients. Marre et al. (72) demonstrated that treating diabetic patients with enalapril who have microalbuminuria but are normotensive causes the urinary excretion of albumin to decrease. Finally Ruliope et al. (73) compared two different antihypertensive regimens, propranolol-hydralazine-furosemide and captopril alone, in 10 hypertensive patients with various types of renal failure. Patients who had been on triple therapy for at least 6 months were switched to captopril for 12 months. Despite similar degrees of blood-pressure control, renal function actually improved during the first 3 months of captopril treatment and remained stable thereafter; on the triple therapy it had been deteriorating.

ACE inhibitors can slow the progression of renal failure in diabetic patients through metabolic as well as hemodynamic mechanisms. Reduced levels of AII might decrease the mesangial traffic of macromolecules, reducing the mesangial injury in DM (44). If this is the case, the beneficial effects of ACE inhibitors in slowing the progression of renal failure can be explained, at least in part, on the basis of inhibition of the deleterious effects of glomerular hypertrophy.

The optimal therapeutic regimen for hypertension in diabetes has yet to be formulated. ACE inhibitors may slow the progression of nephropathy once it has begun by alternating the hemodynamic and metabolic environment of the glomerulus. Whether early intervention before the onset of clinical hypertension and/or nephropathy in IDDM is of any added benefit in arresting the development of diabetic nephropathy, remains to be seen. Given the favorable metabolic effects of the CCB, it may be that these drugs in combination with an ACE inhibitor currently provide the most prudent therapy for the treatment of hypertension in diabetes particularly for patients in whom single-drug therapy is ineffective.

REFERENCES

1. Andersen JR, Christiansen JS, Andersen JK, et al. Diabetic nephropathy in type I diabetes: an epidemiological study. *Diabetologia* 1983;25:496–501.
2. Knowles HC, Guest GM, Lampe J. The course of juvenile diabetes treated with a measured diet. *Diabetes* 1975;14:239–273.
3. Viberti GC, Heen H. The patterns of proteinuria in diabetes mellitus: relevance to pathogenesis and prevention of diabetic nephropathy. *Diabetes* 1984;33:686–692.
4. Bennett PH. Microalbuminuria and diabetes: a critique-assessment of urinary albumin excretion in its role in screening for diagnostic nephropathy. *Am J Kid Dis* 1989;13:29–34.
5. Mogensen CE. Microalbuminuria as a predictor of clinical diabetic nephropathy. *Kidney Int* 1987;31:673–689.
6. Parving HH, Smidt UM, Friisberg B. A prospective study of glomerular filtration rate and arterial blood pressure in insulin dependent diabetics with diabetic nephropathy. *Diabetologia* 1981;20:457–461.
7. Pell S, D'Alonzo CA. Some aspects of hypertension in diabetes mellitus. *JAMA* 1967;202:10–16.
8. Daniels BS. Hypertension and renal disease in non-insulin dependent diabetes mellitus. *Kidney* 1989;22:13–17.
9. Ferrannini E, Defronzo RA. The association of hypertension, diabetes, and obesity: a review. *J Nephrol* 1989;1:3–15.
10. Manicardi V, Camellini L, Bellodi G, Coscelli C, Ferrannini E. Evidence for an association of high blood pressure and hyperinsulinemia in obese men. *J Clin Endocrinol Metab* 1986;62:1302–1304.
11. Modan M, Halkin H, Almog S, et al. Hyperinsulinemia. A link between hypertension, obesity, and glucose intolerance. *J Clin Invest* 1985;75:809–817.
12. Fuller JH. Blood pressure and diabetes. In: Birkenhager WH, Reid JL eds. *Epidemiology of hypertension*, vol 6. New York: Elsevier, 1985;319.
13. Fuller JH, Shipley MJ, Rose G et al. Mortality from coronary heart disease and stroke in relation to degree of glycemia: the Whitehall Study. *Br Med J* 1983;287:867–870.
14. Aromaa A, Reunanen A, Pyorala K. Hypertension and mortality in diabetic and nondiabetic Finnish men. *J Hypertension* 1984;2:S205–S207.
15. Dawber TR. The Framingham Study: the epidemiology of atherosclerotic disease. Cambridge MA: Harvard University Press, 1980; chapter 12.
16. Knowler WC, Bennett PH, Ballintine EJ. Increased incidence of retinopathy in diabetics with elevated blood pressure. A six year follow up in Pima Indians. *N Engl J Med* 1980;302:645–650.
17. Lombrail P, Thibult N, DiConstanzo P. Influence of arterial hypertension in diabetic retinopathy. *Diabetes Metab* 1983;9:297–302.
18. Mogensen CE. Long term antihypertensive therapy reduces the rate of decline in kidney function in diabetic nephropathy. *Lancet* 1983;1:1175.
19. Parving HH, Smidt UM, Anderson AR, et al. Diabetic nephropathy and arterial hypertension. *Diabetologia* 1983;24:10–12.
20. Mogensen CE. Progression of nephropathy in long term diabetics with proteinuria and effect of initial antihypertensive treatment. *Scan J Clin Lab Invest* 1976;36:383–388.
21. Krolewski AS, et al. Predisposition to hypertension and susceptibility to renal disease in insulin dependent diabetes mellitus. *N Engl J Med* 1988;318:140–145.

22. Seaquist ER, Goetz FC, Rich S, Barbosa J. Familial clustering of diabetic kidney disease. Evidence for genetic susceptibility to diabetic nephropathy. *N Engl J Med* 1989;320:1161–1165.
23. Mangili R, Bending JJ, Scott G, Lai LK, Gupta A, Viberti G. Increased sodium-lithium countertransport activity in red cells of patients with insulin dependent diabetes and nephropathy. *N Engl J Med* 1988;318:146–150.
24. Carr S, Mbanya J, Thomas T, et al. Increase in glomerular filtration rate in patients with insulin dependent diabetes and elevated erythrocyte sodium-lithium countertransport. *N Engl J Med* 1990;322:500–505.
25. Turner RC. United Kingdom prospective diabetic survey II: Prevalence of hypertension and hypotensive therapy in patients with newly diagnosed diabetes. *Hypertension* 1985;7:118–123.
26. Tolins JP, Raij L. Concerns about diabetic nephropathy in the treatment of diabetic hypertensive patients. *Am J Med* 1989;87(Suppl 6A):29S–33S.
27. Uusitupa M, Sutonen O, Pentila I, Aro A, Pyorala K. Proteinuria in newly diagnosed type II diabetic patients. *Diabetes Care* 1987;10:191–194.
28. Mogensen CE, Gjode P, Christensen CK. Albumin excretion in operating surgeons and in hypertension. *Lancet* 1979;1:774.
29. Mogensen CE, Christiansen CK. Predicting diabetic nephropathy in insulin dependent patients. *N Engl J Med* 1984;311:89–93.
30. Mauer S, Steffes MW, Sutherland D, et al. Studies of the rate of regression of the glomerular lesions in diabetic rats treated with pancreatic islet transplantation. *Diabetes* 1974;24:280–285.
31. Wiseman M, Saunders A, Keen H, Viberti G. Effect of blood glucose control on increased glomerular filtration rate and kidney size in insulin dependent diabetes. *N Engl J Med* 1985;312:617–621.
32. Feldt-Rasmussen R, Mathiesen ER, Deckert T. Effect of two years of strict metabolic control on progression of renal failure in insulin dependent diabetes. *Lancet* 1986;2:1300–1304.
33. Viberti GC, Bilous RW, Makintosh D, et al. Long term correction of hyperglycemia and progression of renal failure in insulin dependent diabetes. *Br Med J* 1983;286:589–602.
34. Hostetter TH, Rennke HG, Brenner BM. The case of intrarenal hypertension in the initiation and progression of diabetes and other glomerulopathies. *Am J Med* 1982;72:375–380.
35. Hostetter TH, Troy JL, Brenner BM. Glomerular hemodynamics in experimental diabetes mellitus. *Kidney Int* 1981;19:410–415.
36. Tolins JP, Shultz PJ, Raij L. Mechanisms of hypertensive glomerular injury. *Am J Cardiol* 1988;62:54G–58G.
37. Cowie CC, Port FK, Wolfe RA, Savage PJ, Moll PP, Hawthorne VM. Disparities in incidence of diabetic end-stage renal disease according to race and type of diabetes. *N Engl J Med* 1989;321:1074–1079.
38. Rostand SG. Diabetic renal disease in blacks—inevitable or preventable? *N Engl J Med* 1989;321:1121–1122.
39. Rostand SG, Brown G, Kirk KA, Rutsky EA, Dustan HP. Renal insufficiency in treated essential hypertension. *N Engl J Med* 1989;320:684–688.
40. Zatz R, Meyer TW, Rennke HG, Brenner BM. Predominance of hemodynamic rather than metabolic factors in the pathogenesis of diabetic glomerulopathy. *PNAS* 1985;82:5963–5967.
41. Anderson S, Myer T, Rennke HG, Brenner BM. Control of glomerular hypertension limits glomerular injury in rats with reduced renal mass. *J Clin Invest* 1985;76:612–619.
42. Raij L, Keane W. Glomerular mesangium: its function and relationship to angiotension II. *Am J Med* 1985;79(Suppl 3C):24–30.
43. Heyden S. The workingman's diet II. Effect of weight reduction in obese patients with hypertension, diabetes, hyperuricemia, and hyperlipidemia. *Nutr Metab* 1978;22:141–159.
44. Siscovick DS, Laporte RE, Newman JM. The disease specific benefits and risks of physical activity and exercise. *Pub Health Rep* 1985;100:180–188.
45. Pacy PJ, Dodson P, Kubicki AJ, et al. Comparison of the hypotensive and metabolic effect of bendrogluazide therapy and a high fiber, low fat, low sodium diet in diabetic subjects with mild hypertension. *J Hypertension* 1984;2:215–220.
46. Parijs J, Van der Linden L, et al. Moderate sodium restriction and diuretics in the treatment of hypertension. *Am Heart J* 1973;85:22–34.
47. Raij L, Tolins JP. Diabetes and hypertension: consideration for therapy. In: Hollenberg NK, ed. *Management of hypertension: a multifactorial approach*. Stoneham, MA: Butterworths, 1987;121–134.
48. Tuck ML, Griffiths R, Johnson L, Stern N, Morley J. UCLA geriatric grand rounds: Hypertension in the elderly. *J Am Ger Soc* 1988;36:630–643.
49. Goldner MG, Zarowitz H, Akgun S. Hyperglycemia and glucosuria due to thiazide derivatives administered in diabetes mellitus. *N Engl J Med* 1960;262:403–405.
50. Struthers AD, Whitesmith R, Reid JL. Prior thiazide diuretic treatment increased adrenalin-induced hypokalemia. *Lancet* 1983;1:1358–1361.

51. Ames RP. Coronary heart disease and the treatment of hypertension: impact of diuretics on serum lipids and glucose. *J Cardiovasc Pharmacol* 1984;6:S466–S473.
52. Blohm G, Lager I, Lonroth P, et al. Hypoglycemic symptoms in insulin dependent diabetics. A prospective study of the influence of beta blockade. *Diabetes Metab* 1981;7:235–238.
53. Leren P. Comparison of effects on lipid metabolism of antihypertensive drugs with alpha and beta adrenergic antagonistic properties. *Am J Med* 1987;82(Suppl 1A):31.
54. Barnett AH, Leslie D, Watkins PJ. Can insulin treated diabetics be given beta adrenergic blocking drugs? *Br Med J* 1980;280:976–978.
55. Shionoir H, Noda K, Miyamoto K, et al. Glucose tolerance during chronic prazocin therapy in patients with essential hypertension. *Curr Ther Res* 1986;40:171–180.
56. Guthrie GP, Miller RE, Kotchen TA, et al. Clonidine inpatients with diabetes and mild hypertension. *Clin Pharmacol Ther* 1983;34:713–717.
57. Trost BN, Weidman P, Beretta-Piccoli C. Antihypertensive therapy in diabetic patients. *Hypertension* 1985;7:102–108.
58. Loutzenhiser R, Epstein M. Effects of calcium antagonists on renal hemodynamics. *Am J Physiol* 1985;249:F619–F629.
59. Harris DCH, Hammond WS, Burke TJ, Schorier RW. Verapamil protects against progression of experimental chronic renal failure. *Kidney Int* 1987;31:41–46.
60. Tolins JP, Ha B, Hartich L, Raij L. Effect of antihypertensive therapy on glomerular injury in the Dahl rat. Comparisons of calcium channel blockers and converting enzyme inhibitors. (Abstract) *Clin Res* 1989;37:503A.
61. Brunner F, Thiel G, Hermle M, Bock A, Mihatsch M. Long term enalapril and verapamil in rats with reduced renal mass. *Kidney Int* 1989;36:969–977.
62. Harris DCH, Chan L, Schrier RW. Remnant kidney hypermetabolism and progression of chronic renal failure. *Am J Physiol* 1988;254:F267–F276.
63. Shultz PJ, Raij L. Role of calcium channels in human mesangial cell proliferation. (Abstract) *Kidney Int* 1989;35:183.
64. Tolins JP, Melemed A, Sulcimer D, Gustafson KS, Vercellotti G. Calcium channel blockade inhibits platelet activating factor production by human umbilical vein endothelial cells. (Abstract) *Clin Res* 1989;37:503A.
65. Anderson S. Converting enzyme inhibitors. In: Bennett WM, McCarron PA, Brenner BM, Stein JH, eds. Pharmacotherapy of renal disease and hypertension. New York: Churchill Livingstone, 1987;277–297.
66. D'Angelo A, Sartori L, Gambaro G, et al. Captopril in the treatment of hypertension in type I and type II diabetes patients. *Postgrad Med J* 1986;62(Suppl 1):69–72.
67. Dominguez JR, de La Calle H, Hurtado A, et al. Effect of converting enzyme inhibitors in hypertensive patients with non-insulin dependent diabetes mellitus. *Postgrad Med J* 1986;62(Suppl 1):66–68.
68. Ferriere M, Lachkar H, Richard JL, et al. Captopril and insulin sensitivity. *Ann Intern Med* 1985;102:134–135.
69. Pollare T, Lithell H, Berne C. A comparison of the effects of hydrochlorothiazide and captopril on glucose and lipid metabolism in patients with hypertension. *N Engl J Med* 1989;321:868–873.
70. Hommel E, Parving HH, Mathiesen E et al. Effect of captopril on kidney function in insulin dependent diabetic patients with nephropathy. *Br Med J* 1986;293:467–470.
71. Parving HH, Hommel E, Smidt U. Protection of kidney function and decrease in albuminuria by captopril in insulin dependent diabetics with nephropathy. *Br Med J* 1988;297L:1086–1091.
72. Marre M, Chatellier G, LeBlanc H, Guyenne T, Menard J, Passa P. Prevention of diabetic nephropathy with enalapril in normotensive diabetics with microalbuminuria. *Br Med J* 1988;297:1092–1095.
73. Ruliope LM, Miranda B, Morales JM, Rodicio JL, Romero JC, Raij L. Converting enzyme inhibition in chronic renal failure. *Am J Kidney Dis* 1989;13:120–126.

Surgical Management of the Diabetic Patient,
edited by Michael Bergman and Gregorio A. Sicard.
Raven Press, Ltd., New York © 1991.

13

Pancreatitis and Diabetes Mellitus

Kenneth A. Newell and Richard A. Prinz

*Department of Surgery, Loyola University Stritch School of Medicine,
Maywood, Illinois 60153*

ACUTE PANCREATITIS

Inflammatory diseases of the pancreas can be divided into acute and chronic forms. Acute pancreatitis is characterized by an attack of acute abdominal pain associated with increased blood or urinary levels of pancreatic enzymes such as amylase and lipase. In 60 to 75% of patients, acute pancreatitis is the result of gallstones or ethanol abuse. The relative frequency of these two major etiologies varies with patient population. In 10 to 20% of patients, the etiology of acute pancreatitis is never found. A complete list of possible etiologies is shown in Table 1.

Acute pancreatitis most frequently runs a benign course and resolves completely with supportive medical management. By definition, the clinical symptoms, morphologic and functional changes seen in acute pancreatitis return to normal after or between attacks. In a minority of patients, acute pancreatitis may run a fulminant course with life-threatening complications including shock, respiratory failure, renal failure, and death. The medical therapy of acute pancreatitis is primarily supportive care. Massive amounts of fluid can be sequestered in the retroperitoneum and fluid and electrolyte management is extremely important. Respiratory and nutritional support must be instituted when appropriate. Inhibition of pancreatic secretion has been attempted by a variety of means but none has proven effective. Surgical management of acute pancreatitis is needed when the diagnosis is uncertain or when complications arise. Diagnostic laparotomy may be necessary because nonpancreatic lesions such as ulcer perforation, gangrenous cholecystitis, and mesenteric infarction may mimic pancreatitis.

There is no evidence that diabetes mellitus increases the risk of acute pancreatitis developing. Likewise, acute pancreatitis does not cause diabetes mellitus. However, attacks of acute pancreatitis may make diabetic management more difficult, and diabetes is a factor in measuring the risk of any inflammatory process. Transient hyperglycemia does occur in acute pancreatitis. In fact, most prognostic criteria evaluating the severity of acute pancreatitis include hyperglycemia. Decreased insulin secretion, increased glucagon secretion, and increased insulin resistance are possible causes of this hyperglycemia. Insulin resistance is the most likely explanation because of stress effects such as increased circulating catecholamines and steroids.

TABLE 1. *Etiology of acute pancreatitis*

Gallstones
Alcohol
Postoperative/and post ERCP
Traumatic
Hypercalcemia
Hyperlipidemia—Frederickson types I, IV, and V
Drugs—chlorothiazide, furosemide, corticosteroids, azathioprine, asulfidine
Hereditary
Viral
Idiopathic

CHRONIC PANCREATITIS

Unlike acute pancreatitis, chronic pancreatitis is a relentless disease characterized by repeated or persistent attacks of abdominal or back pain and progressive endocrine and exocrine deterioration. Like acute pancreatitis, only a minority of patients with chronic pancreatitis require surgery. When surgery is necessary, preservation of pancreatic tissue and thus pancreatic function should be a major factor in determining the type of procedure performed. The choice of operation in chronic pancreatitis directly influences the likelihood of diabetes mellitus developing. Although this is a progressive disease in terms of loss of endocrine and exocrine function, major resections of the pancreas are associated with a much greater frequency of diabetes mellitus as well as a greater likelihood of insulin dependence. Resection of pancreatic tissue may also increase the difficulty of blood sugar management in patients who are already diabetic. Management of insulin-dependent diabetes in patients with little or no pancreatic endocrine function requires a great deal of patient cooperation and compliance. The typical patient with chronic pancreatitis who is addicted to alcohol and/or narcotic drugs often lacks the reliability and stability for this rigorous management.

The etiology and pathogenesis of chronic pancreatitis are incompletely understood. A major limiting factor is a lack of a reliable animal model to study this problem. Nevertheless, factors associated with chronic pancreatitis allow some speculation as to its etiology. Longstanding alcohol abuse is the most common factor associated with chronic pancreatitis. In fact, some investigators question whether this disease can occur without a history of alcoholism. The exact mechanism by which alcohol causes chronic pancreatitis is not known although a direct toxic effect of ethanol on the pancreas remains a popular theory.

Several investigators have reported an increase in the protein concentration and a decrease in the bicarbonate and pancreatic secretory trypsin inhibitor concentration in the pancreatic juice of patients consuming large amounts of alcohol (1–3). Multigner and coworkers (4) have reported a low molecular weight protein in pancreatic juice that inhibits precipitation of calcium salts. Named pancreatic stone protein, its level is lower in the pancreatic exocrine fluid of patients with chronic alcoholic pancreatitis (5). Increased dietary protein and alcohol may cause an increase in pancreatic protein secretion, but this theory is still speculative. Premature enzyme activation resulting from decreased concentrations of pancreatic secretory trypsin inhibitor and decreased protein solubility secondary to decreased pancreatic stone protein concentration can result in the intraductal formation of protein plugs in chronic pancreatitis. These protein plugs could cause duct obstruction and duct hypertension with resulting pain and secondary inflammatory changes. Although this hypothesis is attractive, further investigation is needed to prove its validity. It is uncertain whether diabetes has any influence on the factors affecting this hypothesis.

Pancreatic duct obstruction is also a central factor in other theories of the pathogenesis of chronic pancreatitis. Repeated passage of common bile duct stones with resulting pancreatic duct obstruction was once thought to be a cause of chronic pancreatitis. Although this is a widely accepted mechanism for acute pancreatitis, gallstone passage plays little or no role in the development of chronic pancreatitis. In patients with chronic pancreatitis and cholelithiasis, gallstones are usually a coincidental finding as these patients almost always have a history of excessive alcohol intake.

Pancreatic divisum, the failure of fusion of the dorsal and ventral pancreatic ducts, has been implicated as a cause of pancreatitis. Proponents claim that relative stenosis at the lesser papilla results in increased pancreatic duct pressure. Arguments against this theory are that pancreas divisum occurs in many patients who do not have pancreatitis, and sphincteroplasty has failed to relieve pain and prevent recurrent attacks of pancreatitis in many patients with pancreas divisum. Pancreatic divisum is best viewed as a normal anatomic variant that rarely causes acute or chronic pancreatitis (6). Although rare, pancreatic trauma whether due to surgery or blunt or penetrating injury may result in ductal strictures that cause complete or partial obstruction of the pancreatic duct with resulting chronic pancreatitis. This is most common with injuries to the head of the pancreas. Chronic pancreatitis is a frequent finding in the pancreas of patients with pancreatic carcinoma and it remains a topic of debate whether this is a cause or result of the tumor. There is evidence for both sides of this issue and further study is required to resolve whether chronic pancreatitis predisposes to the development of pancreatic cancer.

Once duct obstruction occurs, inflammatory changes develop in the pancreatic parenchyma that result in fibrosis, atrophy, and eventual endocrine and exocrine insufficiency. Animal studies show that pancreatic duct ligation can result in acinar atrophy and fibrosis in the pancreas. Yeo and associates (7), using a canine pancreatic duct ligation model, reported progressive deterioration in both intravenous and oral glucose tolerance. Glucose intolerance was detected one week after pancreatic duct ligation, which progressed for 4 months. Between 4 and 6 months after duct ligation, the deterioration of glucose tolerance stabilized. The associated histologic changes were parallel to the functional changes. Initially, there was edema, polymorphonuclear leukocyte infiltration, and zymogen granule depletion. By 4 to 6 months, the acute inflammation had resolved, and the islets of Langerhans were relatively well preserved. These authors, although recognizing the interplay of many factors, believe that the glucose intolerance documented in this model is the result of decreased islet cell responsiveness and consequent decreased insulin output.

Although endocrine and/or exocrine insufficiency develop in many patients with chronic pancreatitis, it is pain that prompts them to seek medical care. The pain of chronic pancreatitis is difficult to control medically and is a frequent indication for surgery. Nevertheless, the cause of pain in this disease remains uncertain. Most theories focus on ductal obstruction with duct distention and hypertension. Another theory is that the inflammatory process within the pancreas involves visceral pain fibers in the parenchyma of the gland itself or in adjacent tissue. The surgical treatment of chronic pancreatitis hinges upon these theories of pain. If the pain is due to ductal obstruction, drainage of the duct is reasonable. However, if the pain is due to inflammatory involvement of visceral pain nerves and no ductal hypertension is present, pancreatic drainage is inappropriate and pancreatic resection is necessary.

A classic finding in chronic pancreatitis is strictures alternating with multiple areas of pancreatic duct dilatation (Fig. 1). This is known as a chain of lakes appearance of the pancreatic duct. Although by no means universal, the majority of patients with pain from chronic pancreatitis have a dilated pancreatic duct. In these patients, ductal dilatation and pain are most likely the result of ductal hypertension. Bradley (8) reported increased pancreatic duct pressures in patients with chronic pancreatitis and dilated pancreatic ducts. Okazaki (9) demonstrated increased pancreatic duct pressures associated with chronic pancreatitis regardless of duct size using transampullary manometry. Ebbehoj (10) showed that pancreatic tissue pressure corresponded to pancreatic duct pressure and was increased in chronic pancreatitis.

Direct neuronal damage by the inflammatory process of chronic pancreatitis may also contribute to pain. Keith and coworkers (11) have shown perineuronal eosinophilic infiltration in patients with chronic pancreatitis undergoing pancreatic resection. Bockman and associates (12) have described changes in the nerve sheath of intrapancreatic and peripancreatic nerves in chronic pancreatitis.

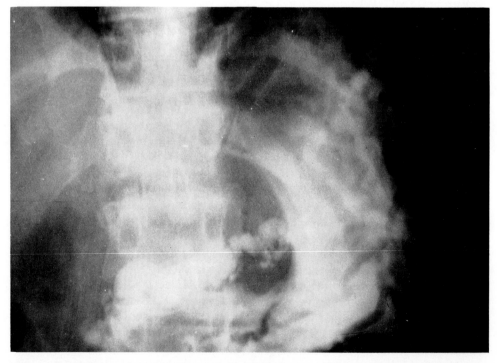

FIG. 1. Endoscopic retrograde cholangiopancreatography (ERCP) demonstrates dilation of the pancreatic duct with multiple strictures (chain of lakes). There is reflux of dye into the stomach.

Pancreatic duct obstruction and nerve inflammation may not constitute mutually exclusive hypotheses. Patients with chronic pancreatitis may have different causes for pain. This is supported by the fact that not all patients with chronic pancreatitis have a dilated pancreatic duct. Yet patients with a dilated duct receive substantial pain relief from pancreatic duct drainage. Pain most likely is due to varying combinations of ductal obstruction and nerve inflammation. The surgeon must be aware of these variations when choosing an operation to treat these patients.

The course of pain in this disease is variable and unpredictable. Some investigators have estimated that 30–50% of patients with chronic pancreatitis will have some lessening of their pain over time. This is believed to be the result of acinar atrophy with decreased ductal pressure as the inflammation in the pancreas "burns out." Ammann (13) and associates supported this concept with a report that maximum pain relief occurred at a mean of 4.5 years after the onset of symptoms. These data are controversial for several reasons. First, there is no way to predict which patients with chronic pancreatitis, if any, will experience spontaneous amelioration of their pain. Second, it is hard to explain why surgical results in all series of patients operated upon for the pain of chronic pancreatitis deteriorate with time, while the results of medical therapy improve with time. Finally, it seems unreasonable to relegate patients to years of pain, narcotic addiction, and all the subsequent medical and social sequelae of chronic pancreatitis when effective surgical modalities are available to treat their disease.

The endocrine and exocrine consequences of chronic pancreatitis have been extensively studied. Generally, deterioration of exocrine and endocrine function are parallel to each other, although histologically, some relative preservation of pancreatic islet cells may be seen. Clinically, endocrine and exocrine insufficiency is not noted until as much as 90% of the pancreas is destroyed. Therefore much damage can occur "silently."

The ongoing fibrosis and inflammation of chronic pancreatitis causes progressive loss of beta cell mass. As a result of these physiologic derangements, insulin-dependent diabetes mellitus develops in at least 35–50% of patients with chronic pancreatitis. As many as two thirds of the patients with chronic pancreatitis will have impaired glucose tolerance (14–16). The preoperative incidence of diabetes mellitus as evidenced by an elevated fasting blood glucose level in 100 patients with chronic pancreatitis undergoing lateral pancreaticojejunostomy reported by Prinz and coworkers was 34% (17). Of these, approximately one third were insulin dependent.

The microvascular complications of diabetes mellitus are less common in patients with diabetes secondary to chronic pancreatitis. Ketoacidosis and nephropathy are also uncommon (16). The incidence of retinopathy is the same as in idiopathic diabetes mellitus (18). Neuropathies may be somewhat more prevalent and are probably related to malnutrition and the direct toxic effects of alcohol (16). It is not known whether these effects are synergistic with diabetes.

Fasting insulin levels are normal or slightly decreased in patients with chronic pancreatitis (19). Insulin secretion in response to various stimulants is significantly decreased, however (19). In addition to this impaired insulin secretion, clinical and experimental evidence suggest that altered hepatic glucose metabolism contributes significantly to the glucose intolerance frequently associated with chronic pancreatitis (20–22). This alteration in hepatic glucose metabolism is the result of a primary hepatic resistance to insulin (22,23). Andersen and coworkers (23) have demonstrated in an *in vitro,* isolated, perfused rat liver model that administration of exogenous pancreatic polypeptide reverses hepatic insulin resistance. Pancreatic poly-peptide administration in dogs and humans has also been shown to reverse diminished hepatic response to insulin (20,21).

In patients with chronic pancreatitis, circulating levels of pancreatic polypeptide are normal or decreased (19,24). Secretion of pancreatic polypeptide in response to a meal is markedly diminished, however (19,24). It may be that in addition to decreased insulin secretion, glucose intolerance results from a decreased hepatic response to insulin, which in turn is a consequence of decreased pancreatic polypeptide secretion. If this is a significant factor in the development of diabetes, therapy with pancreatic polypeptide may have a role in the prevention and treatment of glucose intolerance secondary to chronic pancreatitis.

Secretion of other pancreatic peptides is also impaired by chronic pancreatitis. Fasting glucagon levels are generally, but not universally, decreased (19). There is a subgroup of patients with pancreatic diabetes who are prone to hypoglycemic episodes. This subgroup has been shown to have a consistently decreased glucagon response to hypoglycemia. Major pancreatic resections further decrease the already diminished alpha-cell mass and the result is decreased glucagon release in response to hypoglycemia. As one of the major regulatory functions of glucagon is the prevention of hypoglycemia via glycogenolysis and gluconeogenesis, the loss of glucagon activity in patients with chronic pancreatitis (especially after pancreatic resection) severely limits their ability to maintain glucose hemostasis.

Both basal levels of gastric inhibitory peptide (GIP) and the response of GIP to oral glucose or a test meal are consistently increased (19). As GIP is thought to be a major enteric factor involved in the release of insulin, this increase may represent appropriate up regulation of GIP in response to decreased levels of insulin. Fasting plasma levels of secretin and gastrin in patients with chronic pancreatitis have been found to be normal (19). Some evidence suggests, however, that the secretin response to intraduodenal acid may be impaired (19). Finally, although difficult to reliably measure, CCK-PZ levels are probably increased in CP (19). In spite of our increasing understanding of the hormonal consequences of chronic pancreatitis, the interplay of these various factors and their cumulative effect on gastrointestinal function must still be elucidated.

Exocrine insufficiency also occurs frequently in patients with chronic pancreatitis. Of the 100 patients undergoing pancreatic duct drainage reported by Prinz and co-workers (17), 17 had preoperative steatorrhea requiring oral enzyme supplements. The incidence of gross steatorrhea secondary to chronic pancreatitis reported in the literature is 7–17% with two thirds of the patients demonstrating fat malabsorption (25). Although not as life threatening as diabetes mellitus, exocrine insufficiency results in malnutrition and long-term disability. Patients can be easily treated with oral enzyme administration.

In discussing the natural history of chronic pancreatitis and in planning therapy, it must be remembered that the life expectancy of patients with chronic pancreatitis is substantially shortened by their disease. Of 87 patients who underwent pancreatic duct drainage for chronic pancreatitis, only 41 were alive on long-term follow-up ranging up to 21 years after surgery (17). Mean survival following operation was 6.1 years and the 5-year mortality rate was 40%. Continued alcoholism was the most important factor affecting survival of the patients in this study. In patients who stopped drinking after surgery, there was a 25% mortality rate with long-term follow-up. There was a 63% mortality rate among those who continued to drink. Other studies also emphasize the potentially malignant nature of this benign disease (26).

Optimal treatment of chronic pancreatitis is controversial. Ammann and coworkers (13) reported that 85% of a group of 145 patients with alcohol-induced chronic pancreatitis had spontaneous pain relief within 5 years of initiating supportive medical treatment. The results of surgery in 76 patients were compared with the results of medical treatment in 87 patients with chronic pancreatitis. No difference in pain relief was found between these two groups, but this study has been criticized because of major flaws in both patient selection for surgery and the types of operations performed. Operations not generally considered beneficial for pain relief were included in the surgical group. On the other hand, Nealon (27) and associates have recently suggested that earlier operative intervention for pain relief in chronic pancreatitis may actually decrease the rate of pancreatic endocrine and exocrine insufficiency. They evaluated 85 patients with chronic pancreatitis with endoscopic retrograde cholangiopancreatography (ERCP) and exocrine and endocrine function testing. Of these 85 patients, 41 underwent a pancreatic duct drainage procedure. Seventy-one percent of the patients who did not undergo surgery progressed to severe disease compared to only 16% in the group who did have surgery. Furthermore, 87% of the patients in the operative group gained weight after surgery (mean 4.2 kg); none in the nonoperative group gained weight. Although encouraging, this report must be viewed cautiously as the mean follow-up was only 14 months.

Chronic pancreatitis is not primarily a surgical disease and should be managed medically until a surgically correctable complication develops. Medical management of pancreatitis is primarily supportive and includes optimization of nutrition, control of diabetes mellitus, replacement of pancreatic enzymes and pain control. Diabetes mellitus is treated, as it is in the patient without chronic pancreatitis, by dietary management, oral hypoglycemic agents, and insulin. Because continued alcoholism complicates patient care and adversely affects pancreatic function and patient survival, an alcohol rehabilitation program is essential. Nutritional management of the patient with chronic pancreatitis should include regular administration of vitamin B_{12} because the pancreatic component of intrinsic factor may be diminished or absent.

Pain control in chronic pancreatitis requires the use of analgesics. Narcotics are often necessary, but should be used with extreme caution because of the high potential for addiction in these patients. Other avenues of treatment include pancreatic enzyme administration. Slaff and coworkers (28) have shown in patients with chronic pancreatitis, not due to alcoholism, substantial pain relief can be obtained by administration of pancreatic enzymes. Other nonoperative means of pain control have included the use of oral citrate to dissolve pancreatic duct stones (29) and extracorporeal shock wave lithotripsy to clear the pancreatic duct of stones (30). These techniques, although innovative, remain unproven.

Surgical treatment of chronic pancreatitis is reserved for those patients in whom a surgically correctable complication develops or who fail medical management. The indications for surgery in chronic pancreatitis are listed in Table 2. The need for surgery is clear in cases complicated by pseudocysts, pancreatic abscess, pancreatic fistula or ascites, fibrotic obstruction of the intrapancreatic portion of the common bile duct or the duodenum, or hemorrhage secondary to splenic vein obstruction. However, most patients are referred to the surgeon because of severe incapacitating

TABLE 2. *Surgical indications in chronic pancreatitis*

Incapacitating pain
Biliary obstruction
Gastrointestinal obstruction
Pseudocyst
Pancreatic fistula
Pancreatic ascites
Hemorrhage secondary to splenic vein obstruction
Differentiation from carcinoma

pain that has been refractory to medical therapy. Relief of pain in chronic pancreatitis is a difficult and challenging problem for the surgeon. Many procedures have been devised and tried to lessen the pain of chronic pancreatitis, but only pancreatic duct drainage and pancreatic resection have proven beneficial. In treating these patients, the surgeon must be aware that pain is the end product of a wide spectrum of pathologic changes in the pancreas and must consider the particular anatomy and level of pancreatic function in choosing the operation that best suits the individual patient.

The ideal operation for chronic pancreatitis should relieve pain and preserve endocrine and exocrine function. We have favored pancreatic duct drainage as the operation best suited to attain this goal in patients who have pain and a dilated pancreatic duct. Although there is some debate as to what actually constitutes a dilated duct, we employ this procedure in patients whose pancreatic duct measures more than 5.0 mm in diameter. Our experience with 100 patients treated over a 25-year period with pancreatic duct drainage supports the contention that satisfactory pain relief can be achieved without major sacrifice of pancreatic exocrine and endocrine function (17). These results have been confirmed in the 80 patients we have treated subsequent to this report. Preoperatively, diabetes mellitus was present in 34 of the 87 patients available for long-term follow-up (Fig. 2). Ten of these 34 had insulin-dependent diabetes mellitus. With long-term postoperative follow-up, diabetes developed in 11 of the 53 nondiabetic patients, and of these only eight were insulin

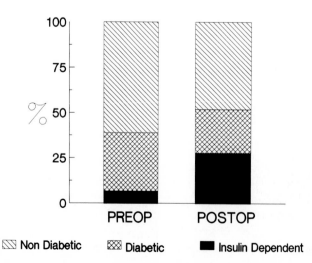

FIG. 2. Thirty-four of 87 patients available for follow-up were diabetic prior to pancreaticojejunostomy, but only ten of these patients required insulin. Diabetes developed in 11 of the 53 nondiabetic patients, and eight of these required insulin. Only 28% of patients are insulin-dependent diabetics.

dependent. Thus, almost one half of our 87 patients did not become diabetic after pancreaticojejunostomy and only 24 required insulin therapy. We believe these numbers are consistent with the natural history of chronic pancreatitis and illustrate that pancreatic duct drainage does not accelerate the development of endocrine insufficiency in chronic pancreatitis. The ability to preserve pancreatic endocrine function is a crucial advantage for pancreatic duct drainage.

Preoperative pancreatic exocrine insufficiency, defined by the need for oral enzyme replacement therapy, was present in 17 of the 87 patients available for long-term follow-up after pancreaticojejunostomy (17) (Fig. 3). Following surgery, an additional ten patients eventually required enzyme supplements. This may have resulted in part from improved nutrition with liberalized fat intake following relief of pain associated with eating. Pancreatic exocrine function remains sufficient for adequate digestion in most patients after pancreatic duct drainage.

Complete pain relief was obtained in 32 of the 87 patients undergoing pancreaticojejunostomy. An additional 39 experienced substantial pain relief. Overall, 82% of the patients undergoing pancreatic duct drainage benefitted in terms of pain relief. These results were obtained without a substantial increase in exocrine or endocrine dysfunction. Others report that 65 to 90% of patients have pain relief with lateral pancreaticojejunostomy. The operative mortality in our series was 4%, and has ranged from 0 to 5% in other reports of pancreatic duct drainage (27,31–33).

A lateral side-to-side pancreaticojejunostomy (17,34) is our preferred method of draining the pancreatic duct (Fig. 4). The abdomen is entered through an upper abdominal transverse or midline incision. The entire anterior surface of the pancreas is exposed by dividing the gastrocolic omentum and mobilizing the stomach superiorly and the colon inferiorly. A thorough Kocher maneuver is performed so that the entire head of the pancreas can be evaluated. The anterior surface of the pancreas is palpated and the pancreatic duct is located by feeling fluctuation of fluid under pressure. This is confirmed by needle aspiration of water clear exocrine fluid. If the pancreatic duct cannot be palpated, we have used intraoperative ultrasound as an aid to locate the duct. An oblique incision to the expected course of the main pancreatic duct is made in an area away from major vessels. Once the duct is entered, the overlying pancreas is incised so the duct of Wirsung and the duct of Santorini are unroofed throughout their entire course. The dissection is carried from as close as possible to the duodenum in both ducts to the distal

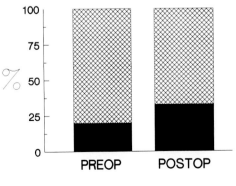

FIG. 3. Seventeen of 87 patients required pancreatic enzyme treatment before pancreatic duct drainage. After operation, 12 more patients required enzyme therapy.

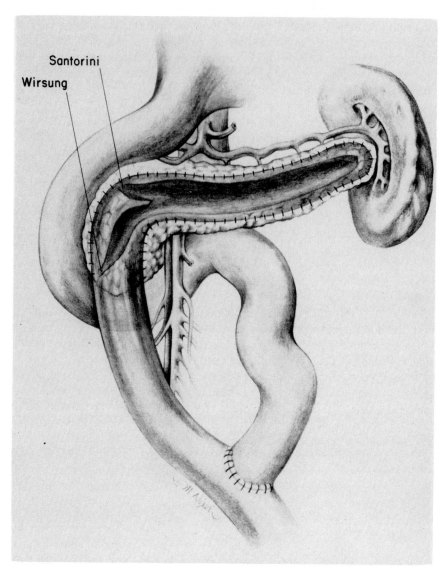

FIG. 4. Complete pancreatic duct drainage is achieved by unroofing the duct of Santorini and the duct of Wirsung from the tail to as close as possible to the duodenum in the head of the gland. (From Prinz RA, Aranha GV, and Greenlee HB. Redrainage of the pancreatic duct in chronic pancreatitis. *Am J Surg* 1986; 151:150–156.)

denum in both ducts to the distal portion of the major pancreatic duct in the tail of the gland. It is especially difficult to achieve complete ductal drainage in the head of the pancreas. In this portion of the gland, the duct courses posteriorly and the amount of pancreatic tissue is at its greatest, often resulting in a pseudotumor. Special efforts, including resection of overlying pancreas, must be used to ensure that all dilated segments of pancreatic duct in this area are drained. Any intraductal calculi encountered in the pancreatic duct system are removed, particularly those in the head of the gland beause they may cause persistent or recurrent obstruction.

After the duct is opened, the pancreas is palpated to be sure that all diseased areas are drained. A biopsy of any suspicious area is done to be certain that there is no underlying unsuspected malignancy. Even if no suspicious areas are encountered, we routinely perform a biopsy of the pancreas to confirm our diagnosis of chronic pancreatitis. A Roux-en-Y limb of jejunum is passed retrocolic to the anterior surface of the pancreas. A side-to-side one layer anastomosis is performed. Mesenteric defects are closed. External drainage of the pancreatic bed is usually not required after pancreaticojejunostomy for chronic pancreatitis. We have stressed complete opening of the pancreatic duct rather than achieving an anastomosis of any particular length and believe this is important if the best results are to be achieved.

In patients who have persistent or continued pain after pancreaticojejunostomy, a thorough evaluation is indicated. Other causes of pain must be ruled out including peptic ulcer disease, biliary tract disease, and intestinal ischemia. If no other cause is found, the adequacy of the initial drainage procedure must be evaluated. This is best done by ERCP. Failure to visualize the Roux loop or demonstration of strictures or undrained areas should prompt the consideration of reexploration and redrainage. We have reported our experience with 14 patients who initially underwent drainage procedures but had persistent or recurrent pain (34). Nine of these patients had an ERCP showing areas of undrained ducts or strictures in the head of the gland. Redrainage resulted in complete or substantial pain relief in 10 of these 14 patients. Three patients had no pain relief and there was one surgical mortality. These results are similar to those obtained in patients undergoing initial pancreatic duct drainage. We believe redrainage of the pancreatic duct should be attempted whenever possible because substantial pain relief is achieved without sacrificing pancreatic exocrine or endocrine function.

Continued alcohol abuse has been the most important factor associated with a poor surgical result. Of the 23 patients in our series who abstained from alcohol, 21 experienced substantial pain relief. On the other hand, of the 16 patients who had little or no pain relief following pancreatic duct drainage, 14 continued to drink heavily. Alcohol had a similar detrimental effect on patient survival. Of patients who quit drinking, 75% were alive as compared with only 37% of those who continued to drink.

Pancreatic resection is another operative approach to pain relief in chronic pancreatitis. The major drawback to pancreatic resection has been the inevitable development of insulin-dependent diabetes and pancreatic exocrine insufficiency as greater amounts of pancreas are removed. Insulin dependence in the setting of alcohol and narcotic dependence is a major problem. Rapid fluctuations in blood glucose levels can be seen, and ketoacidosis and hypoglycemia are not infrequent. Four of our patients undergoing pancreatic resection for chronic pancreatitis have died from complications related to diabetes. Although reported rates of morbidity and mortality from pancreatic resection are quite similar to those with pancreatic duct drainage (35), we believe that extended pancreatic resections are technically much more difficult than pancreatic duct drainage.

Our indications for pancreatic resection in patients with chronic pancreatitis are disabling pain in a patient with a small duct, which by definition is less than 5.0 mm in diameter, or the suspicion of an underlying pancreatic malignancy. The latter indication is somewhat subjective because it is frequently difficult, if not impossible, to confirm a diagnosis of malignancy prior to resection. Palpation of the enlarged fibrotic head of the pancreas is of little help. Biopsy is associated with a high false-negative rate in patients with chronic pancreatitis. In our series of pancreatic duct drainage now totaling 180 patients, four died of pancreatic cancer within one year of surgery. All of these patients had pancreatic biopsies at the time of their pancreatic duct drainage that showed only chronic pancreatitis. White and coworkers (36) emphasized the risk of occult carcinoma in patients with chronic pancreatitis, reporting that nine of 55 patients undergoing pancreatic drainage had unsuspected pancreatic cancer. Six of these nine died within six months of surgery.

Other authors have advocated pancreatic resection for patients with chronic pancreatitis and concomitant pseudocysts. Our approach to this problem has been to combine lateral pancreaticojejunostomy with internal pseudocyst drainage usually through the same Roux-Y loop (37). The overall incidence of pseudocyst in 87 consecutive patients undergoing lateral pancreaticojejunostomy was 39% (26 of 87 patients). There was no significant difference in morbidity or mortality between patients undergoing pseudocyst drainage in combination with lateral pancreaticojejunostomy or lateral pancreaticojejunostomy alone. Morbidity and mortality rates in patients with combined drainage was 19 and 8%, respectively; morbidity and mortality with lateral pancreaticojejunostomy alone was 18 and 2%, respectively. Substantial pain relief was achieved in 81% of patients who underwent combined drainage procedures and 84% of those undergoing lateral pancreaticojejunostomy. There were no recurrent cysts on follow-up in either group of patients. We believe this approach is superior to pancreatic resection in patients requiring surgery for a pseudocyst and chronic pancreatitis.

Another traditional indication for pancreatic resection has been the failure of an initial pancreatic duct drainage operation to relieve pain. As already discussed, patients who have persistent or continued pain after pancreaticojejunostomy require a thorough evaluation. If no other cause of pain is identified and the pancreatic duct is adequately drained, as evidenced by ERCP, pancreatic resection may be appropriate.

Some authors have suggested that patients with preexisting insulin-dependent diabetes mellitus who require surgery for control of the pain of chronic pancreatitis are best treated by resection. Although these patients already require insulin preoperatively, we believe that preservation of any remaining endocrine and exocrine function is extremely important. Resection decreases the beta-cell mass and diminishes insulin secretion. It also decreases the alpha-cell mass and glucagon secretion. Both of these factors increase the difficulty of diabetic management. Resection increases the number of patients who will require insulin as well as the amount of insulin required by each patient.

The risk of hypoglycemia is greatly enhanced by pancreatic resection while the patient's ability to respond to hypoglycemia by glucagon secretion is greatly diminished. In these poorly compliant patients, many of whom continue to drink, hypoglycemia is not infrequent due to the patient's inability to appropriately regulate diet and insulin dosage. Severe hypoglycemia can occur in this setting. In fact, three of five patients reported in our series of patients who underwent pancreatic resection after a failed lateral pancreaticojejunostomy died of uncontrolled diabetes mellitus. Two of these three had severe recurrent hypoglycemic episodes. This experience illustrates the extreme caution we believe is necessary when recommending pancreatic resection. The inevitable consequences of diabetes and steatorrhea must be considered and weighed carefully against the possible benefits of surgery.

Distal pancreatectomy is the simplest resection with the lowest morbidity. There is a large disparity in reported results with this procedure probably because of varying amounts of tissue removed. The amount of pancreas removed with a distal pancreatectomy varies from 40 to 90% of the gland, depending upon the aggressiveness of individual surgeons. As the extent of resection is increased, the results of pain relief are improved, but the frequency of insulin-dependent diabetes and pancreatic exocrine insufficiency is also increased. With the exception of true focal disease in the tail, which is usually traumatic in origin, it is hard to justify distal pancreatectomy of 75% or less.

Chronic pancreatitis of alcoholic origin is a diffuse disease and not confined to the head or tail of the pancreas. For alcoholic pancreatitis, near total or 80–95% resection of the gland may be appropriate. This removes the inferior portion of the head of the pancreas, but leaves the common bile duct in continuity. Diabetes mellitus and pancreatic exocrine insufficiency are almost always the result of these extended resections and temper our enthusiasm for this approach.

A pancreaticoduodenectomy or Whipple procedure is advocated by some surgeons because the cellular changes of chronic pancreatitis often begin and are most prominent in the head and uncinate process of the gland. This procedure usually preserves enough islet cells in the tail of the normal gland to prevent endocrine insufficiency. Unfortunately, diabetes following Whipple resection occurs much more frequently in patients with chronic pancreatitis. Preservation of the pylorus is usually possible with this form of pancreaticoduodenectomy. This leaves the motor, secretory, and reservoir functions of the stomach intact and diminishes the risk of dumping syndrome. Stone and coworkers (38) reported 15 patients undergoing Whipple procedures for chronic pancreatitis with small duct disease without operative mortality. Complete or substantial pain relief was obtained in 53% and 27% respectively, of his patients during a mean follow-up of 6.2 years. Postoperative exocrine and endocrine insufficiency developed in eight and six of the 15 patients, respectively. There were no late deaths related to diabetes mellitus. Sato and coworkers (39) reported satisfactory pain relief in 50% of 16 patients and Rossi and coworkers (40) reported a 79% satisfactory outcome following Whipple resection in 73 patients with chronic pancreatitis. Mean duration of follow-up for Rossi was five years. These results are comparable to those obtained by pancreatic duct drainage. Nonetheless, pancreaticoduodenectomy is a formidable operation in chronic pancreatitis where peripancreatic inflammation and fibrosis have obliterated normal tissue planes. We hesitate to recommend it as the initial procedure for chronic pancreatitis because of its increased operative mortality and increased long-term metabolic problems.

One innovative approach to prevent diabetes following near total or 95% pancreatectomy is pancreatic autotransplantation. Both islet and segmental pancreas autotransplantation have been performed. Najarian and coworkers (41) performed pancreatic islet cell autotransplantation in ten patients undergoing 95% pancreatectomy for disabling pain secondary to chronic pancreatitis. At the time of pancreatectomy, the resected pancreas was mechanically minced, dispersed by collagenase digestion, and transplanted into the liver by portal vein infusion. One patient died of an unrelated complication. Of the nine surviving patients, three were insulin independent at 1–38 months following the procedure. Cameron and colleagues (42) reported nine patients who underwent pancreatic islet autotransplantation. As with the Minnesota group, partially purified islet material was injected into the liver via the portal vein. Portal hypertension developed in all eight patients (14–60 cm H_2O) during islet infusion. One patient required emergent mesocaval shunting 24 hours after the inital procedure and subsequently died with renal failure and massive hepatic necrosis. Portal hypertension developed in a second patient and disseminated intravascular coagulopathy (DIC) with resultant massive hemorrhage requiring 39 units of blood. Although initially severe, the portal hypertension was transient in surviving patients. Hyperglycemia requiring insulin therapy immediately following surgery, developed in all eight surviving patients undergoing islet autotransplant in Cameron's series (41). Of the eight, only three did not require insulin on follow-up ranging from 9 to 22 months.

Only six of the 18 patients in these two series remained insulin independent during a short follow-up. This relatively poor outcome, combined with the risks of portal hypertension, DIC, and the difficulty of obtaining adequate numbers of islets from the fibrotic inflamed pancreas prompted Rossi and coworkers (43) to attempt segmental pancreas autotransplantation. They reported ten patients undergoing near total pancreatectomy for disabling pain who had the body and tail of the gland autotransplanted into the femoral area (43). The pancreatic duct was occluded and the graft was vascularized using the splenic and femoral vessels. Eight of the ten autografts were technically successful and seven of these eight patients remain insulin independent with a follow-up of 24–54 months. That the autotransplanted pancreas was capable of maintaining normoglycemia was demonstrated by two patients who underwent distal pancreatectomy and segmental autotransplantation followed by completion pancreatectomy for continued pain. Both of these patients remained normoglycemic with only the autotransplanted pancreatic segment. Although follow-up is relatively short and the number of patients is small, the results obtained by this group suggest that segmental pancreatic autotransplantation may provide a means of avoiding IDDM in highly selected patients with chronic pancreatitis who require pancreatic resection.

REFERENCES

1. Renner IG, Rinderknecht H, Douglas AP. Profiles of pure pancreatic secretions in patients with acute pancreatitis: The possible role of proteolytic enzymes in pathogenesis. *Gastroenterology* 1978;75:1090–1098.
2. Renner IG, Rinderknecht H, Valenzuela JE, et al. Studies of pure pancreatic secretions in chronic alcoholic subjects without pancreatic insufficiency. *Scand J Gastroenterol* 1980;15:241–244.
3. Sahel J, Sarles H. Modifications of pure human pancreatic juice induced by chronic alcohol consumption. *Dig Dis Sci* 1979;24:897–905.
4. Multigner L, Sarles H, Lombardo D., and DeCaro A. Pancreatic stone protein. I. Implications in stone formation during the course of chronic calcifying pancreatitis. *Gastroenterology* 1985;89:387–391.
5. Sarles H, DeCaro A, Multigner L, Martin E. Giant pancreatic stones in teetotal women due to the absence of the "stone protein"? *Lancet* 1982;2:714–715.
6. Sugawa C, Watt AJ, Nunez DC, Masuyama H. Pancreatic divisum: Is it a normal variant? *Am J Surg* 1987;153:62–67.
7. Yeo CJ, Bastidas JA, Schmieg RE, et al. Pancreatic structure and glucose tolerance in a longitudinal study of experimental pancreatitis induced diabetes. *Ann Surg* 1989;210(2):150–158.
8. Bradley EL III. Pancreatic duct pressure in chronic pancreatitis. *Am J Surg* 1982;144:313–316.
9. Okazaki K, Yamamoto Y, Ito K. Endoscopic measurement of papillary sphincter zone and pancreatic main ductal pressure in patients with chronic pancreatitis. *Gastroenterology* 1980;91:409–418.

10. Ebbehoj N, Borly L, Madsen P, et al. Pancreatic tissue pressure and pain in chronic pancreatitis. *Pancreas* 1986;1:556.
11. Keith RG, Keshavjee SH, Kerenyi NR. Neuropathology of chronic pancreatitis in humans. *Can J Surg* 1985;28:207–211.
12. Bockman DE, Buchler M, Malfertheiner P, et al. Analysis of nerves in chronic pancreatitis. *Gastroenterology* 1988;94:1459–1469.
13. Ammann RW, Akovbiantz A, Largiader F, Schueler G. Course and outcome of chronic pancreatitis. Longitudinal study of a mixed medical–surgical series of 245 patients. *Gastroenterology* 1984;86:820–828.
14. Linde J, Nilsson LH, Barany FR. Diabetes and hypoglycemia in chronic pancreatitis. *Scand J Gastroenterol* 1977;12:369–373.
15. Larsen S, Hilsted J, Tronier B, Worning H. Metabolic control and B cell function in patients with insulin-dependent diabetes mellitus secondary to chronic pancreatitis. *Metabolism* 1987;36:964–967.
16. Bank S, Marks IN, Vinik AI. Clinical and hormonal aspects of pancreatic diabetes. *Am J Gastroenterol* 1975;64:13–22.
17. Prinz RA, Greenlee HB. Pancreatic duct drainage in 100 patients with chronic pancreatitis. *Ann Surg* 1981;194:313–320.
18. Covet C, Genton P, Pointel JP, et al. The prevalence of retinopathy is similar in diabetes mellitus secondary to chronic pancreatitis with or without pancreatectomy and in idiopathic diabetes mellitus. *Diabetes Care* 1985;8:323–328.
19. Stasiewicz J, Adler M, and Delcourt A. Pancreatic and gastrointestinal hormones in chronic pancreatitis. *Hepatogastroenterology* 1980;27:152–160.
20. Tanaka Y, Druck P, Brunicardi FC, et al. Reversal of abnormal glucose production in chronic pancreatitis by administration of gastric inhibitory peptide (GIP) and pancreatic polypeptide (PP). *Surg Forum* 1987;38:149–151.
21. Bruncardi FC, Chaiken RL, Seymour NE, et al. Reversal of abnormal glucose metabolism in chronic pancreatitis by pancreatic polypeptide administration in man [Abstract]. *Diabetes* 1987;21(suppl 1)36:38A.
22. Seymour NE, Turk JB, Laster MK, et al. In vitro hepatic insulin resistance in chronic pancreatitis in the rat. *J Surg Res* 1989;46:450–456.
23. Goldstein JA, Kirwin JD, Seymour NE, et al. Reversal of in vitro hepatic insulin resistance in chronic pancreatitis by pancreatic polypeptide in the rat. *Surgery* 1989;106:1128–1133.
24. Valenzuela JE, Taylor IL, Walsh JH. Pancreatic polypeptide response in patients with chronic pancreatitis. *Dig Dis Sci* 1979;24:862–864.
25. Frey CF. Role of subtotal pancreatectomy and pancreaticojejunostomy in chronic pancreatitis. *J Surg Res* 1981;31:361–370.
26. Leger L, Lenriot JP, Lemaigre G. Five to twenty year follow-up after surgery for chronic pancreatitis in 148 patients. *Ann Surg* 1974;180:185–191.
27. Nealon WH, Townsend CM, Thompson JC. Operative drainage of the pancreatic duct delays functional impairment in patients with chronic pancreatitis: A prospective analysis. *Ann Surg* 1988;208:321–329.
28. Slaff J, Jacobson DJ, Tillman CR, Curington C, Toskes P. Protease-specific suppression of pancreatic exocrine secretion. *Gastroenterology* 1984;87:44–52.
29. Sahel J, Sarles H. Citrate therapy in chronic calcifying pancreatis. In: Mitchell CJ, Kelleher J, eds. *Pancreatic disease in clinical practice*. London: Pitman, 1981;346–353.
30. Cremer M, Van der Meeren A, Delhage M. Extracorporeal shock wave lithotripsy for pancreatic stones. *Gastroenterology* 1988;94:80.
31. Sato T, Saitoh Y, Noto N, Matsuno K. Appraisal of operative treatment for chronic pancreatitis with special reference to side to side pancreaticojejunostomy. *Am J Surg* 1975;129:621–628.
32. Warshaw AL, Popp JW, Schapiro RH. Long term patency, pancreatic function, and pain relief after lateral pancreaticojejunostomy for chronic pancreatitis. *Gastroenterology* 1980;79:289–293.
33. Bradley EL III. Long term results of pancreaticojejunostomy in patients with chronic pancreatitis. *Am J Surg* 1987;153:207–213.
34. Prinz RA, Aranha GV, Greenlee HB. Redrainage of the pancreatic duct in chronic pancreatitis. *Am J Surg* 1986;151:150–156.
35. Frey CF, Suzuki M, Jsaji S, Zhu Y. Pancreatic resection for chronic pancreatitis. *Surg Clin North Am* 1989;69:499–528.
36. White TT, Slavotinek AH. Result of surgical treatment of chronic pancreatitis. *Ann Surg* 1979;189:217–224.
37. Munn JS, Aranha GV, Greenlee HB, Prinz RA. Simultaneous treatment of chronic pancreatitis and pancreatic pseudocyst. *Arch Surg* 1987;122:662–667.
38. Stone WM, Sarr MG, Nagorney DM, McIlrath DC. Chronic pancreatitis: Results of Whipple's resection and total pancreatectomy. *Arch Surg* 1988;123:815–819.

39. Sato T, Miyashita E, Yamauchi H. The rule of surgical treatment for chronic pancreatitis. *Ann Surg* 1986;203:266–271.
40. Rossi RL, Rothschild J, Braasch JW, et al. Pancreaticoduodenectomy in the management of chronic pancreatitis. *Arch Surg* 1987;112:416–420.
41. Najarian JS, Sutherland DER, Baumgartner D, et al. Total or near total pancreatectomy and islet autotransplantation for the treatment of chronic pancreatitis. *Ann Surg* 1980;192:526–542.
42. Cameron JL, Mehigan DG, Broe PJ, Zuidema GD. Distal pancreatectomy and islet autotransplantation for chronic pancreatitis. *Ann Surg* 1981;193:312–317.
43. Rossi RL, Heiss FW, Watkins E, Jr., et al. Segmental pancreatic autotransplantation with pancreatic ductal occlusion after near total or total pancreatic resection for chronic pancreatitis: Results at 5 to 54 month follow-up evaluation. *Ann Surg* 1986;203:626–636.

Surgical Management of the Diabetic Patient,
edited by Michael Bergman and Gregorio A. Sicard.
Raven Press, Ltd., New York © 1991.

14

Diabetes Associated with Other Endocrine Disorders

Jeffrey J. Wang and Dean H. Lockwood

Endocrine-Metabolism Unit, University of Rochester, School of Medicine and Dentistry, Rochester, New York 14642

In 1979, the National Diabetes Data Group revised the nomenclatures and classifications of diabetes mellitus (1). One of the classifications is "Other Types of Diabetes Mellitus," which includes numerous categories including pancreatic disease, hormonal causes, drug or chemically induced, insulin-receptor abnormalities, genetic syndromes, and other special types of diabetes such as diabetes associated with the malnourished. This chapter discusses diabetes associated with other endocrine disorders. These conditions usually present with a noninsulin-dependent diabetes-like pattern and the pathophysiology is either due to relative insulin deficiency and/or insulin resistance. For example, primary hyperaldosteronism leads to hypokalemia and defects in insulin secretion. Glucocorticoid excess results in marked insulin resistance, and pheochromocytomas can cause inhibition of insulin secretion and insulin resistance. In most of the cases of diabetes associated with other endocrine disorders, there must also be a genetic predisposition. This is especially true of those endocrine disorders that induce insulin resistance, e.g., acromegaly, glucagonoma.

The focus of this chapter is endocrine disorders whose excessive or deficient hormone secretion can significantly affect glucose homeostasis. Insulin is the major anabolic hormone in man and its actions are generally opposed by the counterregulatory hormones, glucagon, epinephrine, growth hormone, and glucocorticoids. It is not unexpected that an adenoma or carcinoma producing large amounts of a counterregulatory hormone could provoke hyperglycemia and, conversely, deficiencies of these hormones could lead to significant hypoglycemia. Although most cases of diabetes associated with other endocrine disorders do not present a unique challenge to the surgeon regarding management of diabetes, it is important to identify concomitant disorders because they can influence surgical outcomes. For example, a state of glucocorticoid excess can markedly prolong wound healing, an unrecognized pheochromocytoma could result in a hypertensive crisis during surgery, and surgery in an untreated patient with Addison's disease could lead to profound hypoglycemia. Furthermore, recognition and treatment of these associated endocrine disorders should result in significant amelioration of the diabetic condition.

GROWTH HORMONE EXCESS

Growth hormone (GH; somatotropin) is a single-chain peptide hormone with 191 amino acids (MW 22,000). It is synthesized and secreted by somatotrophic cells in the anterior pituitary gland.

The hypothalamic regulators of pituitary GH release are the stimulator growth hormone-releasing hormone (GRH) and the inhibitor somatostatin. They are in turn regulated by a number of neural, metabolic, and hormonal factors in the human body.

Human GRH is similar in structure to the group of peptide hormones in the gastrointestinal tract, i.e., secretin, gastrin, vasoactive intestinal polypeptide (VIP), and gastric inhibitory peptide (GIP). Somatostatin is a cyclic peptide and is present in various tissues, including hypothalamus, D cells of the pancreas, and the gastrointestinal tract. It has multiple physiological functions. In addition to its potent inhibitory effects on pituitary GH release, somatostatin also inhibits secretion of thyroid-stimulating hormone (TSH), insulin, glucagon, secretin, gastrin, and VIP.

The basal secretion of GH follows an episodic pattern and is under the control of not yet fully understood neural factors. The peak levels occur during sleep stages 3 and 4.

The physiological effect of growth hormone is promotion of linear growth which is mediated through somatomedins, a family of peptides produced in the liver and probably in other tissues.

At least two types of somatomedins with 62% homology of amino acid sequences have been identified. Both are structurally homologous with proinsulin, and have effects simulating that of insulin. Because of these characteristics, somatomedins are abbreviated as IGF-1 and IGF-II (insulin-like growth factors).

The somatomedins are the only hormones known to be produced by the liver. After release, somatomedins are bound to specific carrier proteins that are also synthesized in the liver and other tissues.

The plasma levels of somatomedins are primarily regulated by GH. Secretion of IGF-I is stimulated by GH after birth, and it exerts negative feedback control on GH by stimulating hypothalamic somatostatin release and by inhibiting the action of GRH on somatotrophs. IGF-II is only weakly regulated by GH and probably is the somatomedin responsible for growth in fetal stage.

The principal effects of growth hormone regarding growth promotion are in protein metabolism. The anabolic action increases transport of amino acids into tissues and accelerates their incorporation into proteins resulting in net protein synthesis and hence positive nitrogen balance.

Growth hormone decreases glucose uptake and its utilization by cells. It is noteworthy that growth hormone exerts insulin resistance independent of somatomedins.

Growth hormone excess leads to the classic syndromes of acromegaly in adults and gigantism in children. The etiology of chronic growth hormone hypersecretion is almost invariably due to a pituitary adenoma. Ectopic GRH secretion from carcinoid tumors or islet cell tumors accounts for only a handful of cases of acromegaly/gigantism.

In children and adolescents, chronic growth hormone excess leads to the overgrowth of long bones with striking body heights. Many gigantic patients also have hypogonadism, which delays fusion of epiphysis of long bones and further promotes additional linear growth.

In adults, the clinical manifestations of acromegaly include acral enlargement, soft-tissue overgrowth, headache, visual field defects, weight gain, hyperhidrosis, acanthosis nigricans, hypertension, cardiomegaly, lethargy, peripheral neuropathy, menstrual disorders, impotence, galactorrhea, renal calculi, hyperinsulinemia, and glucose intolerance.

The characteristic appearances of acromegaly are usually obvious. The normal basal fasting plasma GH levels are between 1–5 ng/ml. In about 90% of acromegalic patients the levels are greater than 10 ng/ml and can be considerably higher. A single determination may fail to demonstrate elevated plasma GH levels, however, because GH secretion may be episodic in acromegaly. Oral glucose suppressibility is the most simple test for acromegaly. One hundred grams of glucose given orally suppresses GH levels to less than 5 ng/ml at 60 minutes in normal subjects. In acromegaly, GH levels may respond differently. They can increase or show no change.

Transsphenoidal adenomectomy remains the best initial treatment if there are no contraindications. Bromocriptine may be useful when surgery fails or the tumor recurs. The newly developed somatostatin analogue, octreotide, is even more effective than bromocriptine in reducing GH levels in acromegalic patients and the action is longer, although it has the disadvantage of requiring subcutaneous administration. Radiation therapy is employed when both surgical and medical therapy fail, but it has the disadvantage of being slowly effective and ultimately causing hypopituitarism (2).

Impairment of carbohydrate tolerance is a well recognized feature of acromegaly. Review of two large series indicate that approximately 20% of the patients fulfill the diagnostic criteria for diabetes (3). Even in those patients with normal glucose tolerance, evidence for insulin resistance is apparent (4). The mechanisms by which excessive growth hormone causes insulin resistance (hyperinsulinemia) and diabetes can be at least partially explained by GH stimulation of lipolysis, which results in increased gluconeogenesis. The hormone also antagonizes the effects of insulin by decreasing glucose uptake and utilization by cells. The phenomenon of insulin resistance seen in acromegaly appears to be the direct effect of GH instead of somatomedin excess.

It has been reported that the glycemic control improves if the underlying growth hormone excess is corrected by radiation therapy (5), hypophysectomy (5,6), bromocriptine (3,7), or a somatostatin analogue (8). Yet the time required before restoration of glucose tolerance varies (5). In addition, the improvement in carbohydrate abnormalities may not always correlate with the absolute levels of plasma GH, both before and after treatment. There are no definite factors to determine the susceptibility for diabetes in acromegalic patients. No correlations have been found among GH levels, duration of disease, family history, pancreatic islet cell antibodies, or HLA typing and glucose intolerance.

Patients with acromegaly who undergo surgery should have no special problems related to diabetes mellitus. The surgeon should be aware, however, that acromegalic patients frequently have hypertension, cardiomegaly, and, occasionally, cardiomyopathy.

PITUITARY INSUFFICIENCY

Pituitary insufficiency is either caused by destruction of the anterior pituitary gland or by a deficiency of hypothalamic hormones regulating it.

Cases of selective pituitary hormone insufficiency are well documented, but panhypopituitarism is still the most common disorder. Eighty-five percent of the pituitary function must be destroyed before signs and symptoms develop. The most vulnerable hormone deficiencies are, in descending order: gonadotropins [follicle-stimulating hormone (FSH) and luteinizing hormone (LH)], GH, TSH, adrenocorticotropic hormone (ACTH), and prolactin (PRL).

The etiology of hypopituitarism may be any one of the following: tumor compression, infarction, infiltrative disorders, trauma, surgery, radiation therapy, granulomatous infections, autoimmune disease, familial, and idiopathic etiologies.

A space-occupying lesion, such as craniopharyngioma (the most common tumor in the hypothalamic–pituitary region in children), a large pituitary adenoma, aneurysm, encephalocele, meningioma, or glioma, which either arises from the pituitary gland or lies in proximity to it, may result in hypopituitarism through local pressure or direct invasion.

Radiation therapy over the pituitary–hypothalamus region has been applied in patients in whom surgery for pituitary adenomas has been unsuccessful. Using either supravoltage x-ray or accelerated alpha particle (proton beam) irradiation, the incidence of delayed onset of hypopituitarism is high. The same complication occurs in irradiation of tumors in the head and neck regions. Transsphenoidal surgery for discrete adenomas is usually not complicated by hypopituitarism.

The clinical manifestations of hypopituitarism reflect the deficiency of individual or multiple pituitary hormones. Because gonadotropins are frequently the first hormones to diminish, amenorrhea in women and decreased libido and impotence in men may be the most common initial symptoms. For some patients, fasting hypoglycemia caused by GH deficiency and/or ACTH deficiency may be the first to occur. The clinical picture of secondary hypothyroidism resulting from pituitary TSH insufficiency is similar to the primary condition, except that goiters are usually absent. The lack of ACTH results in a clinical picture similar to that of Addison's disease. Failure of the cardiovascular system is usually absent, however, because of the intact renin-angiotensin system. Hyperpigmentation commonly observed in Addison's disease is usually lacking. In addition, the severity of secondary adrenal insufficiency is less and may go undetected except during periods of stress.

In addition to a thorough clinical history and physical examination, basal levels of thyroid hormones, testosterone, prolactin, as well as a rapid ACTH stimulation test (see below) evaluating glucocorticoid reserve help demonstrate the existence of target organ failure. If the functions of target organs are subnormal, measurement of basal levels of pituitary hormones can differentiate between primary and secondary hypofunction. TSH, FSH, LH, or ACTH are elevated if it is primary endocrine gland failure. Low or normal values of these pituitary hormones suggest dysfunction of the hypothalamus and/or pituitary gland. Provocative endocrine tests should be used to establish the diagnosis and determine the degree of anterior pituitary hypofunction (9).

The relationship between pituitary hormones, especially that of GH, and diabetes mellitus has provoked a lot of interest. Houssay first observed that pituitary ablation in diabetic dogs results in increased insulin sensitivity and decreased insulin requirements needed to control diabetes. This observation led to the speculation that GH is an etiological factor in diabetes (10). Furthermore, it was observed that the devastating complications of diabetic retinopathy are relatively rare in sexual ateliotic dwarfism (11). This condition is characterized by GH deficiency, glucose intolerance or diabetes, and lipid abnormalities. The striking lack of retinopathy in this form of dwarfism suggested that GH is the factor responsible for the development of angiopathy in diabetes. In fact, pituitary ablation by a variety of methods was tried in an attempt to halt the progression of diabetic retinopathy in the 1960s (12). It is now rarely performed for that purpose.

Hypopituitarism is characterized by enhanced insulin sensitivity with lower than average plasma insulin levels and spontaneous hypoglycemia. About 30% of hypopituitary children suffer from fasting hypoglycemia with blood glucose level below 50 mg/dl (13). Both symptomatic and asymptomatic hypoglycemia occur with equal frequency in children with isolated GH and multiple anterior pituitary deficiencies (14). Children and adults who have secondary adrenal failure are also prone to hypoglycemia.

Hypopituitarism may develop at a later date in patients with diabetes mellitus. In fact, postpartum pituitary necrosis (Sheehan's syndrome) occurs with a higher incidence in diabetic women. The compromised circulation in the pituitary stalk accelerated by diabetic angiopathy renders the gland more vulnerable to vascular incompetence and infarction.

Fasting hypoglycemia in children improves with cortisone plus GH therapy in panhypopituitarism. Cortisone replacement alone is not adequate to prevent hypoglycemia (15).

GLUCOCORTICOID EXCESS

Microscopically, the adrenal cortex is composed of three zones. The outer zona granulosa produces aldosterone, which is the major mineralocorticoid and is controlled by the renin–angiotensin system. The two inner zones—zona fasciculata and reticularis—are one functional unit producing cortisol, the major glucocorticoid, and a few adrenal androgens.

Glucocorticoids accelerate protein catabolism in most tissues, such as muscle, bone, connective tissue, and lymphatic tissue. They also increase lipolysis of adipose tissue resulting in release of glycerol and free fatty acids. These effects provide substrate for intermediary metabolism. In muscle and adipose tissue, glucocorticoids also inhibit glucose uptake and impede the action of insulin. This insulin antagonism can result in increased insulin secretion in chronic glucocorticoid excess.

The actions of glucocorticoids on the liver are quite different from the "peripheral" tissues. Glucocorticoids increase gluconeogenesis through these mechanisms:

1. Stimulation of certain gluconeogenic enzymes
2. Enhancement of the hepatic response to the gluconeogenic hormones, glucagon and catecholamines
3. An increase in the release of gluconeogenic substrates from peripheral tissues (amino acids, free fatty acid, and glycerol).

The etiology of chronic glucocorticoid excess (Cushing's syndrome) can be divided into iatrogenic and "spontaneous." Iatrogenic Cushing's syndrome resulting from chronic glucocorticoid therapy is by far the most common cause of this disease entity. The spontaneous causes can be classified with respect to whether it is ACTH dependent or independent. The former variety include Cushing's disease [ACTH-producing pituitary adenoma, and much less commonly, hypothalamic corticotrophin (ACTH)-releasing hormone (CRH) hypersecretion], and ectopic ACTH syndrome (ACTH-secreting nonpituitary tumors, such as oat-cell carcinoma of lung, thymoma, islet cell tumors of pancreas, carcinoid tumors). The ACTH-independent causes include autonomous cortisol-secreting adrenal adenomas and carcinomas.

The most characteristic clinical features of Cushing's syndrome is the centripetal obesity. "Moon facies" describes the deposition of fat on the face with facial plethora; "buffalo hump" the accumulation of fat in the dorsocervical fat pads; and central obesity that occurs in the trunk and abdomen with relative sparing of extremities.

The other clinical symptoms and signs include purple striae and easy bruisability of the skin, hirsutism, acne, hyperpigmentation, muscle weakness; menstrual dysfunctions; hypertension, edema, congestive heart failure; psychological symptoms; headache; nephrolithiasis, and diabetes mellitus.

In patients with suspected Cushing's syndrome, the overnight 1 mg dexamethasone suppression test with a morning plasma cortisol determination and measurement of 24 hour urinary-free cortisol remain the best screening procedures (16). If both are normal, hypercortisolism is excluded. Positive screening tests should prompt endocrine consultation to establish whether the patient has ACTH-dependent or independent Cushing's syndrome.

"Steroid diabetes" caused by prolonged glucocorticoid excess is a well-defined entity. In their series of 50 patients with Cushing's syndrome who ranged in age from 11 months to 68 years, Soffer et al. (17) reported an 84% prevalence of diabetes mellitus, 30% defined by fasting hyperglycemia and 54% by abnormal glucose tolerance curves. Hyperglycemia and glycosuria may well be the first manifestations of Cushing's syndrome before other symptoms and signs emerge. Following successful removal of an adrenal adenoma, the fasting hyperglycemia and abnormal glucose tolerance usually returns to normal. But in those patients with adrenal cortical carcinoma, recurrence of diabetes following initial improvement may be an indication of functional metastasis. Exogenous glucocorticoids are used to treat a wide variety of diseases. The incidence of steroid-induced diabetes may be as high as 50% (18). Exogenous glucocorticoids may extend impaired glucose intolerance to frank diabetes, or even nonketotic hyperosmolar coma (19). Ketoacidosis, however, is unusual as the patient maintains insulin reserves. Administration of pharmacological amounts of glucocorticoids leads to hyperinsulinemia, a reflection of insulin resistance (19). Approximately one-half of steroid-induced diabetic patients need chronic insulin therapy to adequately control their hyperglycemia (18). The diabetes may have a rapid onset within a few days or as late as a few months after the initiation of steroid therapy. The diabetes is usually temporary, sometimes becomes less severe after prolonged administration of glucocorticoids and disappears after discontinuing them (19).

ADRENOCORTICAL INSUFFICIENCY

The causes of deficiency in glucocorticoids and/or mineralocorticoids are classified as primary and secondary. Primary adrenocortical insufficiency is caused by destruction of the adrenal cortex with resultant uninhibited ACTH secretion. Secondary adrenocortical insufficiency results from deficient ACTH secretion, either by exogenous glucocorticoid therapy or by destructive lesions in the pituitary.

Primary adrenocortical insufficiency (Addison's disease) can be idiopathic (most common), or due to tuberculosis, hemorrhage and infarction, fungal infections, and metastatic malignancy. It is now recognized that many patients with acquired immunodeficiency syndrome (AIDS) have adrenal insufficiency. In these patients, cytomegalic virus (CMV) infection and/or ketoconazole treatment are the major etiologic factors.

The idiopathic etiology occurs in about 80% of affected patients and is often associated with adrenal autoantibodies in the plasma. It is also frequently associated with other autoimmune endocrine gland failure. The common components of this syndrome include ovarian or testicular failure, thyroid disorders, insulin-dependent diabetes mellitus, hypoparathyroidism, pernicious anemia, and atrophic gastritis.

The clinical manifestations of adrenal insufficiency depend upon the extent of insufficiency, whether the onset of disease course is acute or chronic, primary or secondary, and the presence or absence of concomitant mineralocorticoid deficiency. Fatigue, weakness, weight loss, hyperpigmentation, supine or postural hypotension, anorexia, nausea, and vomiting are the most common manifestations of Addison's disease. The onset of secondary adrenal insufficiency is usually insidious and the clinical picture similar to that of the primary disease, except that hyperpigmentation is absent and symptoms related to mineralocorticoid deficiency, such as dehydration, hypotension and hyperkalemia, are rare. A cushingoid appearance suggests exogenous glucocorticoid therapy.

Acute adrenal crisis occurs in patients with chronic adrenal insufficiency when exposed to greater physiological demands, such as infection, injury, surgical procedures or dehydration. Nausea, vomiting, vascular collapse, weakness, apathy, confusion, abdominal pain, fever, hyponatremia, hyperkalemia, and hypoglycemia are the principal features. Shock and coma can rapidly lead to death in untreated patients. Acute adrenal hemorrhage follows a course similar to that of acute adrenal crisis superimposed upon chronic insufficiency, plus abdominal, flank, or back pain and tenderness often misdiagnosed as other abdominal emergencies.

The diagnosis of impaired adrenal reserve can be achieved by the "rapid" ACTH stimulation test. A synthetic human ACTH fragment, cosyntropin, is administered and plasma cortisol levels are determined at basal, 30, and 60 minutes. Basal plasma cortisol level greater than 5 μg/dl, an increment greater than 7 μg/dl, and peak level greater than 18 μg/dl at either 30 or 60 minutes are considered normal responses. A subnormal cortisol response indicates the presence of either primary or secondary adrenal insufficiency. Plasma ACTH determinations can help differentiate between the two forms.

Coexisting Addison's disease and diabetes mellitus are not common, but the incidence has been increasing (20). In the majority of cases, adrenal insufficiency develops after the onset of diabetes (21). Increased episodes of hypoglycemia and decreased insulin requirement are the most significant findings in the early stages of adrenal insufficiency (22). With glucocorticoid replacement therapy, the insulin dose required usually resumes the original level (20). In those few patients whose diabetes developed after the onset of adrenal insufficiency, hyperglycemia is usually mild and discovered only by routine blood sugar examinations. Modest amounts of insulin may or may not be needed.

MINERALOCORTICOID EXCESS

Mineralocorticoids constitute a group of adrenal steroid hormones having electrolyte-regulating activity. Aldosterone is the principal mineralocorticoid hormone, which is produced exclusively in the zona glomerulosa. Other steroid hormones possessing mineralocorticoid activities are produced in the zona fasciculata.

The major effects of aldosterone are on the reabsorption of sodium and the excretion of potassium ions in the distal tubules of the kidney, as well as salivary glands, sweat glands, and the gastrointestinal tract. Ammonium and magnesium excretion are also increased by aldosterone.

The major regulator of aldosterone secretion in humans is the renin–angiotensin system. Intravascular volume reduction is the most important stimulus to renin secretion. The fall in blood pressure increases the renin output by stimulating baroreceptors in juxtaglomerular cells of the kidney. The decreased blood pressure also reduces the glomerular filtration rate and therefore the filtered sodium load, which also induces renin secretion. Renal sympathetic nerves also participate by enhancing renin output. The net effects of the renin–angiotensin–aldosterone system are that angiotensin II helps maintain blood pressure by its vasoconstricting actions and aldosterone retains sodium to maintain the volume. Serum electrolytes, ACTH, and catecholamines are less important regulators.

Mineralocorticoid excess can be primary or secondary. Primary hyperaldosteronism is caused by excessive production of aldosterone from an adenoma, carcinoma, or hyperplasia. It is characterized by sodium retention with normal or elevated serum sodium; increased extracellular fluid volume and reduced hematocrit; suppressed plasma renin activity; hypokalemia and alkalosis. The patient may complain of tiredness, weakness, and lassitude. Thirst and polyuria may occur with severe hypokalemia because of the associated resistance to antidiuretic hormone. The blood pressure may be borderline high or frankly elevated. Postural hypotension may occur if potassium is severely depleted because of the blunted baroreceptor reflex.

Impaired glucose tolerance has been reported to be as high as 52% in patients with primary aldosteronism subsequently proved to have aldosterone-producing adenomas by surgery (23). This high incidence is probably not related to the glucocorticoid activity of aldosterone, but instead the resultant hypokalemia. Repletion of potassium in those still harboring the adenoma improves the glucose tolerance curves, and removal of the tumor usually results in total recovery of the glucose impairment. Secretion of insulin from the pancreatic β-cells requires potassium ions.

PHEOCHROMOCYTOMA

The adrenal medulla is composed of chromaffin cells (pheochromocytes) containing catecholamines. Catecholamines include epinephrine, norepinephrine, and dopamine, which are derived from the amino acid, tyrosine. Epinephrine is mainly synthesized, stored, and secreted in the adrenal medulla, whereas norepinephrine is distributed in the adrenal medulla, central nervous system, and sympathetic system.

The physiological functions of adrenergic hormones are manyfold. It depends not only on the type of receptor(s) present on the cell surface, but also on the presence of a number of other factors. Generally, the sympathetic nervous system is mainly responsible for the minute-to-minute adjustment of internal body environment, whereas the adrenal medulla exerts its functions in the presence of stress.

The effects of epinephrine and norepinephrine on intermediary metabolism are mainly mediated through the β-adrenergic receptor, followed by adenyl cyclase activation, cyclic adenosine monophosphate (cAMP) production, and activation/suppression of associated enzymes. In the liver, adrenergic hormones activate glycogenolysis and enhance gluconeogenesis, resulting in increased glucose production. In adipose tissue, they activate hormone-sensitive lipase resulting in lipolysis. In muscle, adrenergic agents inhibit glucose uptake. Finally, catecholamines act as hyperglycemic agent by inhibiting insulin secretion.

Pheochromocytomas are the tumors derived from chromaffin cells. The adrenal medulla is the most common site but pheochromocytomas can arise in extraadrenal chromaffin tissues, such as near the kidney, in the organ of Zucherkandl, sympathetic ganglia, and nerve plexi.

Pheochromocytomas can also be a component of multiple endocrine neoplasia (MEN). MEN type I consists of tumors of the parathyroid, pituitary, and pancreas (gastrinomas and insulinomas). The components of MEN type IIa are medullary thyroid carcinoma, parathyroid hyperplasia or adenoma, and pheochromocytoma. MEN type IIb is composed of medullary thyroid carcinoma, pheochromocytoma, marfanoid habitus, and multiple mucosal neuroma. Pheochromocytoma is often the first clinical indication of MEN. Approximately 15% of the tumors are malignant (24).

The symptoms and signs of pheochromocytoma are headache, perspiration, palpitations, pallor, nausea/vomiting, tremor, trembling, weakness, exhaustion, anxiety, chest pain, dyspnea, flushing, warmth, and numbness. Because the catecholamines can be released from the tumor episodically, paroxysmal attacks are characteristic in affected patients. Postural change or strenuous work can precipitate attacks, but sometimes there is no identifiable cause. The duration of individual episodes varies from minutes to hours. The intervals between attack are also variable from a few times a day to once in several weeks or months.

Assays for plasma or urine catecholamines and their metabolites can be used to screen not only those patients with typical clinical manifestations of pheochromocytoma, but also those at high risk. The high-risk group consists of young hypertensive patients, as well as hypertensive patients with a family history of pheochromocytoma or medullary thyroid carcinoma, neurofibromatosis, and mucosal neuromas. In patients with pheochromocytoma who have continuous hypertension and other symptoms, levels of catecholamines and their metabolites are usually clearly elevated. In those patients with equivocal levels of catecholamines and their metabolites, such as infrequent paroxysms, diagnosis may be more difficult. Timed collection of blood and urine samples are necessary. The clonidine test, an α_2-agonist, can be used when it is not feasible to collect blood under resting conditions.

Diabetes mellitus may occur in about two-thirds of patients with pheochromocytoma (25,26), and the prevalence is even higher in those with sustained hypertension with or without paroxysms, which implies more or less continuous hypersecretion of catecholamines (26).

The glucose intolerance and diabetes mellitus associated with pheochromocytoma are usually mild and reversible after tumor removal. A patient with a pheochromocytoma can cause problems at surgery with a hypertensive crisis. The patient should be treated preoperatively with oral phenoxylbenzamine, an alpha-blocker. The dose is raised from 10 mg twice daily until hypertension is controlled or paroxysms are prevented. The patient should also be volume repleted and diuretics should be discontinued. During surgery the blood pressure is carefully monitored and if hypertension occurs acutely, iv phentolamine is indicated. Some people believe the patient should have partial beta-adrenergic blockade. This should occur only after alpha blockade has been accomplished. Concomitant beta blockade minimizes arrhythmias.

THYROID HORMONE EXCESS

Thyroid hormones (thyroxine, T_4; triiodothyronine, T_3) affect metabolic processes in most organs. They are also vital in the intrauterine and postnatal development of the fetus, especially the neural and skeletal systems. Intrauterine deficiency leads to cretinism (dwarfism and mental retardation).

Under physiological conditions, thyroid hormone maintains basal metabolic rate, body heat production, heart rate, and cardiac output. It exerts many of its effects by potentiating the action of catecholamines in the heart. It also increases the metabolism and clearance of various hormones and accelerates both bone formation and resorption.

Thyroid hormone also has a profound effect upon intermediary metabolism. The synthesis, mobilization and degradation of all lipids are increased. Because the degradative effects predominate, lipid levels, including triglycerides, phospholipids, and cholesterol, usually decline with thyroid hormone excess. The reverse effects are seen in hypothyroidism. Under physiological conditions, thyroid hormone enhances protein synthesis and also stimulates the normal growth of animals by indirectly increasing the synthesis and secretion of growth hormone. In the hyperthyroid state, however, the process of protein synthesis is retarded and growth is inhibited.

Thyroid hormone exerts its effects on carbohydrate metabolism in close collaboration with catecholamines and insulin. Under physiological conditions, thyroid hormone potentiates both the glycogenolytic actions of epinephrine and the effects of insulin on the glycogen synthesis. In the hyperthyroid state, however, both the glycogenolysis and gluconeogenesis are increased.

In diabetic patients, deterioration of metabolic control occurs when hyperthyroidism occurs. In addition, the incidence of glucose intolerance increases in hyperthyroidism (27). Factors attributed to these phenomena include enhanced gastric emptying time and intestinal absorption rate, and increased hepatic glucose output. Traditionally it was considered that thyroid hormones affect the insulin sensitivity of target tissue as well as the secretion of insulin. Recently the peripheral insulin sensitivity in hyperthyroidism has been shown to be unaltered (28). The findings regarding insulin secretion have been conflicting, but generally it is considered unaffected or augmented in hyperthyroidism (29). Increased glucose production from the liver in hyperthyroid patients has been demonstrated (28,30,31). Direct effects of thyroid hormones on gluconeogenesis, indirect action through enhanced β-adrenergic activity, and antagonism between the effect of insulin and thyroid hormones on hepatic glucose output probably play a concerted role (32). Clinically, the diabetes is generally mild.

GLUCAGONOMA

Glucagon is a single-chain polypeptide of 29 amino acids produced and secreted by the alpha cells of pancreatic islets. Its secretion is inhibited by glucose, fatty acids, insulin, and somatostatin, and is stimulated by some amino acids (e.g., arginine, alanine), catecholamines, gastrointestinal hormones, and the autonomic nervous system. The major function of glucagon is to channel stored fuels for tissue utilization during the fasting state. This catabolic hormone enhances glycogenolysis, gluconeogenesis, and ketogenesis in the liver. It stimulates hepatic uptake of certain amino acids. These functions probably prevent hypoglycemia that could occur when insulin secretion is excessive after a large meal of protein and carbohydrates. The sole human target organ for glucagon is the liver. No peripheral action of the hormone has been identified.

A glucagonoma is a pancreatic islet tumor producing an excessive amount of glucagon. The etiology is unknown. The most striking clinical manifestation of glucagonoma is a migratory necrolytic erythema. In fact, more often than not the patients seek help in the dermatology clinic (33). The characteristic skin lesions are polymorphous confluent erythematous eruptions with superficial vesiculation, which lead to erosion, necrosis, secondary infection, healing, and pigmentation (34). The most frequent sites are the perioral area (angular stomatitis), groin, perineum, and lower extremities. These characteristic lesions probably result from hyperglucagonemia or nutritional deficiency (e.g., amino acids or zinc) because surgical removal of the tumor or zinc supplement can improve the lesions.

Other manifestations of glucagonoma include painful glossitis, weight loss, intermittent diarrhea, abdominal mass, normocytic normochromic anemia, hypoaminoacidemia, venous thrombosis, pulmonary embolism, and mild diabetes mellitus.

Glucagonoma can be a component of MEN, but the incidence is quite small.

The combined occurrence of diabetes and migratory necrolytic erythema in an individual indicates the necessity to determine the fasting serum-glucagon level. Levels greater than 300 pmol/l are usually diagnostic. Dynamic tests such as glucose (suppressor) or arginine (stimulant) infusion have given no consistent results. Noninvasive diagnostic methods such as abdominal ultrasonography, computerized tomography, and a liver scan might help detect the tumor. Selective celiac axis arteriography and catheterization of various pancreatic venous tributaries might help to locate the tumor more precisely (35).

The majority of reported cases of glucagonoma demonstrated either fasting hyperglycemia or a diabetic glucose tolerance test (33,35–37). The diabetes is usually mild. Satisfactory blood glucose level control may be obtained by diet alone; rarely does it take insulin to attain normoglycemia (37). Sulphonylurea should be used with caution because tolbutamide markedly stimulated glucagon secretion in a patient affected with a glucagonoma (38). Ketoacidosis is rare even though glucagon is ketogenic. The paradox may be explained by the enhanced insulin release and the down regulation of hepatic glucagon receptors (36). The severity of diabetes is not correlated with plasma glucagon levels. There is no evidence of increased incidence of chronic diabetic complications.

SOMATOSTATINOMA

The first case of somatostatinoma was reported in 1977 (39). Somatostatinoma is an extremely rare tumor; fewer than 30 cases have been reported in the literature (40). The clinical features are characterized by cholelithiasis (bile stasis in gall bladder), hypochlorhydria (inhibition of gastric acid secretion), steatorrhea (reduced pancreatic exocrine functions), and diabetes (inhibition of both insulin and glucagon) (39,41). Because the symptoms are nonspecific, the diagnosis was previously made by radiological and/or surgical exploration. Since the somatostatin immunoassay has become available, the above-mentioned symptom complex warrants a preoperative assessment for the possibility of somatostatinoma.

The diabetes associated with a somatostatinoma usually demonstrates mild-fasting hyperglycemia or fits the diagnosis only by glucose tolerance testing. It is the result of insulin suppression. Ketoacidosis is typically rare because of the simultaneous inhibition of secretion of glucagon, a ketogenic agent. In a few cases of somatostatinoma, ketoacidosis has occurred. In these cases there has been an excess of the precursor of somatostatin, and it is postulated that this agent suppresses insulin secretion to a greater extent (40,42).

PARATHYROID HORMONE EXCESS

It has been observed that the incidence of diabetes mellitus is approximately 8% in patients with hyperparathyroidism (43). It has been shown that hypercalcemia and/or hypophosphatemia enhance insulin secretory response to a glucose challenge, but at the same time impair the insulin response at target tissue (44,45).

Several investigators have determined whether parathyroidectomy improves diabetic control or reduces the need for insulin in those patients with both diabetes and hyperparathyroidism (43,46–49). The larger studies have shown that normalization of serum calcium and phosphate levels by surgical management do not affect the diabetic control and the required dosage of insulin (43,49). Insulin levels were found to be inversely correlated with serum phosphate rather than calcium levels. Furthermore, it is the phosphate depletion that enhances the insulin secretory response and impairs the tissue insulin sensitivity (50).

SUMMARY

In this chapter we have indicated that there are numerous endocrine disorders that are associated with diabetes. With the exception of the autoimmune disorder of multiple end organ failure, diabetes usually occurs because the other endocrine disorder leads to alterations in glucose metabolism or insulin secretion that places a significant stress on the endocrine pancreas. In an individual who has a genetic susceptibility for diabetes, the stress is greater than the compensatory capacity of the pancreas, and overt diabetes becomes evident. However, most of these states of diabetes are relatively mild and are usually controlled by diet alone, or diet plus oral hypoglycemic agents, or modest doses of insulin. We have presented a brief discussion of the pathophysiology of the diabetes associated with these endocrine disorders, the clinical picture, the magnitude of the diabetic problem, screening tests for these disorders, and some comments about treatment of the associated endocrine disorders. We have not provided full details of the endocrine diagnostic workup because these are best handled by an endocrinologist. Where possible, in our discussions of associated endocrine disorders we have tried to identify potential serious medical problems that could occur during surgery and the perioperative period. This emphasizes the need for the surgeon to be aware that mild diabetes either known or discovered during a routine preoperative workup can signal a much greater problem of surgical interest.

REFERENCES

1. National diabetes data group. Classification and diagnosis of diabetes mellitus and other categories of glucose intolerance. *Diabetes* 1979;28:1039–57.
2. Melmed S. Medical progress: acromegaly. *N Engl J Med* 1990;322:966–77.
3. Wass JAH, Cudworth AG, Bottazzo GF, Woodrow JC, Besser GM. An assessment of glucose intolerance in acromegaly and its response to medical treatment. *Clin Endocrinol* 1980;12:53–9.
4. Karlander S, Vranic M, Efendic S. Increased glucose turnover and glucose cycling in acromegalic patients with normal glucose tolerance. *Diabetologia* 1986;29:778–83.
5. Gordon DA, Hill FM, Ezrin C. Acromegaly: a review of 100 cases. *Can Med Assoc J* 1962; 87:1106–9.
6. Sönksen PH, Greenwood FC, Ellis JP, Lowy C, Rutherford A, Nabarro JDN. Changes of carbohydrate tolerance in acromegaly with progress of the diabetes and in response to treatment. *J Clin Endocrinol Metab* 1967;27:1418–30.
7. Popovic V, Micic D, Nesovic M, Djordjevic P, Micic J, Djuric DS. Chronic bromocriptine treatment and glucose intolerance in acromegaly. *Exp Clin Endocrinol* 1985;85:351–7.
8. Cantalamessa L, Catania A, Baldini M, Orsatti A. Improvement of diabetes after treatment with somatostatin analogue SMS 201-995 in an acromegalic patient. *Horm Metab Res* 1986;18:790–1.
9. Lufkin EG, Kao PC, O'Fallon WM, Mangan MA. Combined testing of anterior pituitary gland with insulin, thyrotropin-releasing hormone, and luteinizing hormone-releasing hormone. *Am J Med* 1983;75:471–5.
10. Harvey JC, deKlerk J. The Houssay phenomenon in man. *Am J Med* 1955;19:327–36.
11. Merimee TJ, Fineberg SE, McKusick VA, Hall J. Diabetes mellitus and sexual ateliotic dwarfism: a comparative study. *J Clin Invest* 1970;49:1096–1102.
12. Wright AD, Kohner EM, Oakley NW, Hartog M, Joplin GF, Fraser TR. Serum growth hormone levels and the response of diabetic retinopathy to pituitary ablation. *Br Med J* 1969;2:346–8.
13. Brasel JA, Wright JC, Wilkins L, Blizzard RM. An evaluation of seventy-five patients with hypopituitarism beginning in childhood. *Am J Med* 1965;38:484–98.
14. Hopwood NJ, Forsman PJ, Kenny FM, Drash AL. Hypoglycemia in hypopituitary children. *Am J Dis Child* 1975;129:918–26.
15. Haymond MW, Karl I, Weldon VV, Pagliara AS. The role of growth hormone and cortisone on glucose and gluconeogenic substrate regulation in fasted hypopituitary children. *J Clin Endocrinol Metab* 1976;42:846–56.
16. Tyrrell JB, Forsham PH. Glucocorticoids and adrenal androgens. In: Greenspan FS, Forsham PH, eds. *Basic and clinical endocrinology*, 2nd ed. Los Altos, CA: Lange, 1986;272–309.
17. Soffer LJ, Iannaccone A, Gabrilove JL. Cushing's syndrome: a study of fifty patients. *Am J Med* 1961;30:129–46.
18. Arner P, Gunnarsson R, Blomdahl S, Groth C-G. Some characteristics of steroid diabetes: a study in renal-transplant recipients receiving high-dose corticosteroid therapy. *Diabetes Care* 1983;6:23–5.
19. Olefsky JM, Kimmerling G. Effects of glucocorticoids on carbohydrate metabolism. *Am J Med Sci* 1976;271:202–10.
20. Kenna AP. Addison's disease and diabetes mellitus. *Arch Dis Child* 1967;42:319–21.
21. Gharib H, Gastineau CF. Coexisting Addison's disease and diabetes mellitus: report of 24 cases with review of literature. *Mayo Clin Proc* 1969;44:217–27.

22. Matsaniotis N, Tzortzatou-Stathopoulou F, Thomaidis TH, Karakatsani-Kerasioti Z, Theodoridis CH, Dacou-Voutetakis C. Diabetes mellitus and Addison's disease in an adolescent female. *Acta Paediatr Scand* 1981;70:949–50.
23. Conn JW. Hypertension, the potassium ion and impaired carbohydrate tolerance. *N Engl J Med* 1965;273:1135–43.
24. Gifford RW, Kvale WF, Maher FT, Roth GM, Priestley JT. Clinical features, diagnosis and treatment of pheochromocytoma: a review of 76 cases. *Mayo Clin Proc* 1964;39:281–301.
25. Modlin IM, Farndon JR, Shepherd A, et al. Phaeochromocytomas in 72 patients: clinical and diagnostic features, treatment and long term results. *Br J Surg* 1979;66:456–65.
26. Stenström G, Sjöström L, Smith U. Diabetes mellitus in phaeochromocytoma. *Acta Endocrinol* 1984;106:511–5.
27. Mouradian M, Abourizk N. Diabetes mellitus and thyroid disease. *Diabetes Care* 1983;6:512–20.
28. Laville M, Riou JP, Bougneres PF, et al. Glucose metabolism in experimental hyperthyroidism: intact in vivo sensitivity to insulin with abnormal binding and increased glucose turnover. *J Clin Endocrinol Metab* 1984;58:960–5.
29. Ahren B. Hyperthyroidism and glucose intolerance. *Acta Med Scand* 1986;220:5–14.
30. McCulloch AJ, Nosadini R, Pernet A, et al. Glucose turnover and indices of recycling in thyrotoxicosis and primary thyroid failure. *Clin Sci* 1983;64:41–7.
31. Saunders J, Hall SEH, Sönksen P. Glucose and free fatty acid turnover in thyrotoxicosis and hypothyroidism before and after treatment. *Clin Endocrinol* 1980;13:33–44.
32. Bratusch-Marrain PR, Komjati M, Waldhäusl WK. Glucose metabolism in noninsulin-dependent diabetic patients with experimental hyperthyroidism. *J Clin Endocrinol Metab* 1985;60:1063–8.
33. Mallinson CN, Bloom SR, Warin AP, Salmon PR, Cox B. A glucagonoma syndrome. *Lancet* 1974;2:1–5.
34. Sibbald RG, Schachter RK. The skin and diabetes mellitus. *Int J Dermatol* 1984;23:567–84.
35. Higgins GA, Recant L, Fischman AB. The glucagonoma syndrome: surgically curable diabetes. *Am J Surg* 1979;137:142–8.
36. Stacpoole PW. The glucagonoma syndrome: clinical features, diagnosis, and treatment. *Endocr Rev* 1981;2:347–61.
37. Bloom SR, Polak JM. The glucagonoma syndrome. *Adv Exp Med Biol* 1978;106:183–94.
38. Soler NG, Oates GD, Malins JM, Cassar J, Bloom SR. Glucagonoma syndrome in a young man. *Proc Royal Soc Med* 1976;69:429–31.
39. Larsson L-I, Hirsch MA, Holst JJ, et al. Pancreatic somatostatinoma: clinical features and physiological implications. *Lancet* 1977;1:666–8.
40. Willcox PA, Immelman EJ, Barron JL, et al. Pancreatic somatostatinoma: presentation with recurrent episodes of severe hyperglycemia and ketoacidosis. *Q J Med* 1988;255:559–71.
41. Krejs GJ, Orci L, Conlon JM, et al. Somatostatinoma syndrome. Biochemical, morphologic and clinical features. *N Engl J Med* 1979;301:285–92.
42. Jackson JA, Raju BU, Fachnie JD. Malignant somatostatinoma presenting with diabetic ketoacidosis. *Clin Endocrinol* 1987;26:609–21.
43. Ljunghall S, Palmér M, Åkerström G, Wide L. Diabetes mellitus, glucose tolerance and insulin response to glucose in patients with primary hyperparathyroidism before and after parathyroidectomy. *Eur J Clin Invest* 1983;13:373–7.
44. Kim H, Kalkhoff RK, Costrini NV, Cerletty JM, Jacobson M. Plasma insulin disturbances in primary hyperparathyroidism. *J Clin Invest* 1971;50:2596–2605.
45. Yasuda K, Hurukawa Y, Okuyama M, Kikuchi M, Yoshinaga K. Glucose tolerance and insulin secretion in patients with parathyroid disorders. *N Engl J Med* 1975;292:501–4.
46. Cheung PSY, Thompson NW, Brothers TE, Vinik AI. Effect of hyperparathyroidism on the control of diabetes mellitus. *Surgery* 1986;100:1039–47.
47. Walsh CH, Soler NG, Malins JM. Diabetes mellitus and primary hyperparathyroidism. *Postgrad Med J* 1975;51:446–9.
48. Akgun S, Ertel NH. Hyperparathyroidism and coexisting diabetes mellitus: altered carbohydrate metabolism. *Arch Intern Med* 1978;138:1500–2.
49. Bannon MP, van Heerden JA, Palumbo PJ, Ilstrup DM. The relationship between primary hyperparathyroidism and diabetes mellitus. *Ann Surg* 1988;207:430–3.
50. DeFronzo RA, Lang R. Hypophosphatemia and glucose intolerance: evidence for tissue insensitivity to insulin. *N Engl J Med* 1980;303:1259–63.

Surgical Management of the Diabetic Patient,
edited by Michael Bergman and Gregorio A. Sicard.
Raven Press, Ltd., New York © 1991.

15

Surgical Management of Pediatric and Adolescent Patients with Type I Insulin-Dependent Diabetes Mellitus

Fredda Ginsberg-Fellner, Paula Liguori, and Signe Larson

Division of Pediatric Endocrinology and Metabolism, and the Carole and Michael Friedman and Family Young People's Diabetes Unit, Department of Pediatrics, Mount Sinai School of Medicine of the City University of New York, New York, New York 10029

Insulin, fluid, electrolyte, and antibiotic therapy in the management of the pediatric and adolescent patient with type I diabetes mellitus prior to, during, and after surgical procedures requires understanding of normal physiology, responses to stress, specific alterations in metabolic requirements imposed by insulin-dependent diabetes mellitus, and then careful preoperative assessment and intraoperative and postoperative follow-up of each patient individually. Thus, in the nondiabetic individual, insulin release is adjusted automatically consonant with the body's needs at all times; this is obviously not the case for diabetic patients. For example, surgical procedures are not equivalent in length, type of anesthesia required, or duration of recovery, which will effect what can be ingested orally and at what time postoperatively, and the degree of stress to the patient. Even short procedures have the potential to become unexpectedly more prolonged and complex, resulting in more difficult management problems. Rosenstock (1) has defined major surgery as any procedure requiring general anesthesia. All surgery, even that involving only local or regional anesthesia, is, however, serious. The metabolic derangements inherent in type I diabetes add to an already complex situation. Advance planning for potential problems can make management more predictable, prevent major avoidable complications, and thus smooth the course for the child or adolescent and his/her anxious parents. As type I insulin-dependent diabetes mellitus is the most common endocrine disorder in childhood and adolescence, currently affecting at least one in 350 such individuals (2), surgery in young diabetic patients occurs frequently and thus poses a challenge to both the surgeon and the diabetologist. Type II or noninsulin-dependent diabetes mellitus of significant degree is not usually diagnosed in young people and thus rarely is a major consideration during surgical procedures in this population.

PREOPERATIVE CONSIDERATIONS

Surgery, including the induction of anesthesia, initiates a stress response. Intubation and mechanical ventilation provoke a sympathetic response resulting in rapid elevation of hormones including catecholamines, glucagon, and cortisol (3), and perhaps growth hormone, all of which are known to antagonize the effects of insulin. The action of these glucose counter-regulatory hormones results in increased hepatic gluconeogenesis and reduced insulin-mediated glucose utilization. Surgery itself, analogous to a state of prolonged starvation, accelerates gluconeogenesis, glycogenolysis, lipolysis, and ketogenesis, and the result is significant catabolism affecting protein and lipid stores (4). The diabetic patient, particularly when hyperglycemia is present, is thus at risk for the development of osmotic diuresis, dehydration, and electrolyte imbalance due to decreased insulin availability. Ketosis can develop with prolonged stress via an increase in mobilization of free fatty acids from lipid stores. Concomitant hyperglycemia and fluid loss accelerate this picture. If these metabolic derangements are not appropriately and rapidly corrected, ketosis and later ketoacidosis may result. Increased concentrations of ketone bodies can often lead to nausea and then vomiting, compounding the metabolic derangements already present in the diabetic individual. Anesthetic agents, independently, are capable of causing an increase in ACTH, cortisol, and catecholamine secretion (4). Although effects of stress hormones on the immune system must still be thoroughly elucidated, receptors for them are found on lymphocytes (5,6). As red blood cell and immune system, particularly phagocytic, functions may already be compromised in diabetes (7,8), correction of blood glucose level elevations and insulin deficiency become of great importance to the healing processes. Insulin can reverse the adverse effects of stress and starvation but usually this will require administering an amount well above the usual basal needs.

The route of administration of insulin when stress is prominent is a debatable issue. Subcutaneously injected insulin has a variable absorption rate depending on the site of its administration, and hydration status and degree of adiposity of the patient (9,10). Its onset of action is also influenced by the brand and species of origin of the insulin used (11), the presence of insulin autoantibodies and immune complexes (12), and whether crystalline insulin is given alone, or in combination with, intermediate-acting insulin, either neutral protamine Hagedorn (NPH) or Lente (13). Crystalline insulin given intravenously has a rapid onset of action, i.e., 6–10 minutes, and a biological half-life of about 20 minutes (14). Thus, a bolus of regular insulin has a very brief effect and therefore bolus therapy cannot be used effectively for other than very short-term maintenance of normoglycemia in a diabetic individual; even then, boluses must be given every 10–15 minutes and therefore is not a practical mode of treatment. An intravenous infusion of insulin is most effective in maintaining close to normal blood glucose levels consistently over time, particularly if the blood glucose level is measured frequently and the insulin infusion rate is adjusted appropriately (15,16). Therefore, just as with temperature, blood pressure, and respiratory rates, blood glucose levels should be frequently monitored pre-, intra- and postoperatively. Under ideal circumstances, especially during surgery, an experienced diabetologist and/or diabetes nurse educator should perform these tests so that insulin doses can be appropriately and rapidly adjusted. Clearly, a diabetes care team would most appropriately undertake these responsibilities and in nonemergency situations in particular would be the ideal group to supervise the care of the diabetic child or adolescent. Alternatively, the child's diabetologist or pediatrician can assume this role. Most large hospitals, where young diabetic patients are normally treated, now require a pediatrician as well as a surgeon to provide care for all patients under 14–16 years of age undergoing surgery, thus providing support for the medical aspects of surgical care. In emergency situations, such expertise may not always be immediately available but the patient's diabetologist or pediatrician should speak with the anesthesiologist and surgeon prior to surgery, if at all possible. Capillary blood glucose level testing is quick and, when done correctly, using a calibrated meter, has been shown to be accurate (17). Visual reading of test strips is also accurate, if performed by a competent, well-trained individual. In our opinion, intravenous insulin via constant infusion, as will be more fully discussed, is the therapy of choice during surgical procedures, particularly in labile type I diabetic youngsters and teenagers and during long operations.

PREOPERATIVE EVALUATION

A comprehensive evaluation of the young person with insulin-dependent diabetes mellitus (IDDM) is of critical importance if a surgical admission is prearranged, as for an elective procedure, e.g., herniorrhaphy, adenoidectomy, etc. When a surgical emergency occurs, the evaluation may of necessity have to be considerably condensed but as much data as possible should be rapidly collected. A child or adolescent whose diabetes is less than adequately controlled can be expected to tolerate intraoperative hyperglycemia to a lesser degree than a similar patient with near-normoglycemia resulting in intraoperative ketonemia and, less frequently, acidosis. Thus, it must always be borne in mind that the following preoperative concerns are important:

1. The degree of previous glycemic control, including episodes of ketoacidosis, recurrent infections, compliance with diabetic regimen, duration of diabetes, stage of sexual development (which influences fluid and insulin needs), dietary habits, exercise patterns.
2. Previous medical care received; diabetes knowledge particularly concerning self-management techniques.
3. The presence of secondary complications associated with IDDM: gastropathy, thyroid disease, enteropathy, autonomic neuropathy, lipoatrophy and hypertrophy, retinopathy, nephropathy, hypertension, obesity, and anorexia.
4. The nature and extent of the surgery and the expected duration of the recovery period. If infection is present, special attention must be paid to its proper diagnosis and treatment. The need for antibiotics should be carefully considered even when obvious infection is not noted. It should also be noted that fever increases fluid needs and meticulous attention to this fact is most important in diabetic patients.
5. Coping abilities of the patient and family.
6. Allergies and immunizations; medications taken in addition to insulin.

BLOOD GLUCOSE LEVELS AND COMPLICATIONS IN DIABETES MELLITUS

The levels of glycosylated hemoglobin (hemoglobin A,C, glycohemoglobin) are usually reliable indicators of the degree of control of blood glucose levels if a sufficient number of values previously obtained every 3–4 months are available (18). An average level greater than 1½ times the upper limit for normal values in the laboratory employed requires attention. Such individuals are significantly hyperglycemic (i.e., majority of blood glucose levels >200–250 mg/dl) for most of the day. Assessment of the growth and development is also important; previous heights and weights should be obtained, and growth rates plotted on appropriate charts (e.g., as obtained from the Center for Disease Control). A child whose growth rate is below normal, has unusual fluctuations of weight, and/or a delay in sexual maturation can be suspected to have poor glycemic control (19).

THYROID DISEASE AND DIABETES

Hashimoto's thyroiditis associated with significant concentrations of antimicrosomal and antithyroglobulin autoantibodies is a common finding in IDDM associated with insidious development of hypothyroidism (20,21). As defective thyroid status can affect all stages of operative procedures, thyroid function should be normal prior to surgery. If this is not possible, appropriate precautions should be instituted to ensure that normal cardiovascular function and temperature control are maintained. No difficulties will be encountered if it is necessary to withhold oral thyroid hormone preparations from the patient for 1 to 2 days, as these hormones are bound to serum proteins and therefore have a long half-life. Thus, in most situations, parenteral administration will not be required. Hyperthyroidism is rare, but its presence dictates the need for appropriate therapy (e.g., beta adrenergic blockers prior to, during, and after surgery) (22,23).

ADRENAL DISEASE AND DIABETES

Addison's disease is a rare complication associated with IDDM through the adolescent period (24). Adrenal cortical autoantibodies (25) may contribute to its pathogenesis but are not routinely measured. Thus, physical signs to look for during the physical examination include skin hyperpigmentation, depressed pulse rate, and blood pressure. Measurement of serum electrolytes, including sodium, potassium, chloride, and bicarbonate, should be done and if abnormalities are identified, plasma cortisol levels should be measured at 8 AM and 4 PM, to ensure that they are normal and that the diurnal variation (i.e., higher values at 8 AM and lower values at 4 PM) are present (26). If there is any indication that adrenal hypofunction is present, the patient must be treated with daily cortisol preparations or the synthetic equivalents; the required stress dose—three to five times the daily required dose (27)—should then be administered orally, intramuscularly, or intravenously the day before, the day of, and the day after surgery, and for as long thereafter as is required until the patient is eating well, all vital signs are normal, and the surgical incision is healing well. Thereafter, if the treatment period is not greater than 1 week, the dose can be rapidly tapered to its preoperative level. If treatment with corticosteroids is required for more than 7 days in the non-Addisonian patient, the dose should be gradually tapered and then discontinued. Adrenal function should then be evaluated to ensure that the patient's adrenal glands have not been suppressed. Patients should also be instructed that they might be at risk for adrenal hypofunction during periods of stress for as long as 1 year, and appropriate arrangements for follow-up care should be made. If not done preoperatively, endogenous adrenal function should be evaluated in the postoperative period to determine if maintenance corticosteroids will be required. If there is a question of adrenal hypofunction, it is far safer to administer stress doses of corticosteroids and then rapidly taper them after surgery rather than to risk an adrenal crisis. In addition, serum sodium and potassium concentrations should be monitored carefully so that appropriate intravenous solutions are administered.

VASCULAR, NEUROPATHIC, RENAL AND OTHER COMPLICATIONS OF DIABETES

Micro- and macrovascular complications may be present in children with IDDM, although major complications of diabetes are rarely seen before puberty (28). Autonomic neuropathies may be present after a relatively short duration of diabetes but may be difficult to demonstrate (29). It now appears that autonomic dysfunction may be related not only to the degree of blood glucose level control, but also to the presence of autoantibodies against adrenal medullary and other nerve tissue (30). An electrocardiogram (EKG) with 5 seconds of breath holding and 5 seconds exhalation can elicit a loss of beat-to-beat variability in the R-R interval (31). Postural hypotension may occur, most often in the postoperative period. Autonomic dysfunction may also be suspected in the presence of symptoms suggestive of delayed gastric emptying, prolonged and/or marked postprandial fullness, or when erratic postprandial glucose excursions are noted (32). In this situation the stomach contents should be emptied via gastric suction prior to emergency surgery under general anesthesia (33). Autonomic dysfunction has been reported to cause cardiorespiratory arrest (4).

As diabetic nephropathy may also influence surgical management, a thorough evaluation of renal status should be obtained preoperatively. Renal impairment may be suspected with proteinuria greater than 500 mg/24 hours, significant microalbuminuria (if this test is available) and/or an elevated creatinine and blood urea nitrogen (BUN) (34,35). It should be noted that creatinine clearance may be increased early in the course of type I diabetes and begins to decrease later on in the course of the disease. An elevated blood pressure along with renal impairment increases the concern about the progression of renal disease (36). Significant hypertension (e.g., greater than 130/85 in adolescents) should be investigated and treated, usually with an angiotensin-converting enzyme inhibitor, e.g., enalapril (37). If renal failure appears to be incipient, fluid administration should be carefully adjusted and urine output checked frequently. It should also be noted that bladder tone may be diminished in the child with IDDM, resulting in increased volume capacity, urine retention, increased difficulty in voiding on command, and the tendency to an increased number and frequency of urinary tract infections (38). Teenage girls with this complication frequently have recurrent infections; urine cultures therefore should be done prior to surgery and postoperatively, particularly if bladder catheterization has been performed. However, we prefer not to catheterize our patients unless it is absolutely necessary. Adolescent girls often also have vaginal moniliasis, which can be significantly exacerbated with antibiotic therapy (39). Antifungal treatment should be instituted if moniliasis is present and should be considered in all young diabetic women receiving other than very short courses of antibiotics.

IMPROVING BLOOD GLUCOSE LEVEL CONTROL PRIOR TO ELECTIVE SURGERY

Preparing for Surgery

For elective surgical procedures, it is not unreasonable to attempt, if feasible, a 1–2-month period of intensified insulin therapy with blood glucose level monitoring in an effort to improve glycemic control; diet and exercise should also be included in the treatment plan. This period can also be used for evaluating psychologic factors and parent and child education. Elective surgery then should await optimum metabolic control when possible. The preoperative evaluation should include a retinal examination if this has not been performed within the last 12 months.

Extensive surgery, e.g., open-heart surgery, requires long-term planning. Nutritional status should be assessed if prolonged periods of "starvation" are expected. Nutritional support is available for long recovery periods and insulin can be added to intravenous hyperalimentation fluids to control hyperglycemia.

As with all children, diabetic youngsters should be prepared for surgery by talking about hospitals, visiting special care units and the recovery room, and reading stories about the hospital. This will help dispel myths and attenuate fears, which when diabetes is present is of even greater importance because blunting of the stress response, as discussed previously, can help prevent more major metabolic derangements. Many hospitals have Child Life Programs that prepare the pediatric patient for surgery by introducing intravenous procedures, operating room procedures, and recovery room management routines. Parents must be allowed to remain with small children, should be encouraged to stay with diabetic youngsters if at all feasible, and can often be integrated into their child's diabetes management. Such planning is most appropriately performed preoperatively via discussions with the "Diabetes Team" if the latter is available.

ADMISSION AND PREOPERATIVE MANAGEMENT

Emergency Admissions

Children and adolescents with diabetes are, of course, prone to having the same types of emergency surgical conditions develop as are nondiabetic individuals of comparative age; these include acute appendicitis, fractures requiring reduction under anesthesia, and traumatic injuries requiring immediate surgery. In such cases, the surgical emergency may override the best therapy for diabetes. However, significant degrees of ketoacidosis, which can accompany such situations, should be corrected with intravenous fluids and sodium bicarbonate, the latter only if the arterial pH is less than 7.0; in that case 1 mEq/kg body weight of sodium bicarbonate can be administered slowly by intravenous infusion. Blood glucose levels should be measured frequently, up to every half-hour, and intravenous crystalline insulin given, as described below, to maintain the blood glucose levels between 120 and 180 mg/dl, if at all possible. In such situations, an expert in diabetes management may not be immediately available but should be contacted as soon as possible for advice.

Nonemergent Admissions

Optimally, a child with IDDM should be admitted to the hospital early on the day before an elective procedure. This allows time for a thorough evaluation of the patient and preparation for surgery. In practice, even with new rules regarding admission to the hospital, a diabetic youngster usually receives approval for admission the day before surgery. As a complete blood count is a normal part of a preoperative evaluation, it should be noted that stress and ketosis can lead to both increased white blood cell counts and increased numbers of polymorphonuclear neutrophils, which may not be secondary to an infection.

INSULIN ADMINISTRATION

Morning and prelunch (if given) crystalline and intermediate-acting insulin doses will normally be administered the same as at home. If patients are receiving long-lasting insulin, such as Ultralente, we prefer to discontinue it the day before surgery and use just crystalline insulin four times per day, before each meal and at bedtime. In most children and adolescents who had diabetes for more than 1 year, approximate daily total insulin requirements are 1 unit/kg of body weight. Some adolescents, however, may require up to 1.5–2 units/kg. It should be remembered that while stress increases blood glucose levels, they may be decreased in the presence of anorexia, frequently associated with stress. Insulin dosages need to be adjusted accordingly. Before dinner, the normal crystalline insulin dose can be administered. If the surgical procedure requires that the patient not eat during the night, it is our experience that either no insulin or a reduced dose of the intermediate-acting form should be given to reduce the risk of hypoglycemia developing during sleeping hours. Nocturnal hypoglycemia can be missed resulting in rebound hyperglycemia in the morning (40) or it could necessitate the administration of oral liquids or glucagon, which can have an adverse effect on the planned surgery. If intermediate-acting insulin is used prior to dinner or at bedtime, we recommend that 50% of the usual dose be administered. In the presence of significant hyperglycemia, an insulin infusion can be started the night before the procedure, if necessary. In that case, the evening intermediate acting insulin (NPH, Lente) should be withheld. These regimens minimize the risks of overnight hypoglycemia, a problem in the diabetic child who is not allowed to take food or fluids by mouth. Although children in general do not eat after 10–11 PM, the situation before surgery is often such that the patient has been somewhat anorexic for several days, adding to the possibility that nocturnal hypoglycemia may occur, particularly if liver glycogen stores have been significantly depleted. In practice, if blood glucose levels are less than 200 mg/dl, an insulin infusion is not necessary until the morning of surgery and its absence may make the patient more comfortable and more able to sleep during that night. When insulin sensitivity is not known, an insulin infusion of 0.025–0.05 units/kg body weight/hr can be empirically initiated. Using hourly capillary blood glucose level measurements initially, the insulin infusion can be adjusted to maintain a serum glucose level in the desired range of 120 to 200 mg/dl. In emergencies, where the child's insulin dose is unknown, a starting infusion dose of 0.025 units/kg body weight/hr is always safe and can be increased if indicated. A child whose blood glucose levels are less than optimally controlled may initially feel hypoglycemic if the serum glucose is quickly brought to the normal range. A more gradual lowering may be necessary to keep the child comfortable. Frequent monitoring is essential because many children may not be able to voice or interpret their sensations of hypoglycemia. Blood glucose level testing at hourly to four hourly intervals, as indicated by the patient's status, will allay the family's anxiety regarding diabetes control and reassure them that their child's entire situation is being carefully observed and managed. Properly instructed nurses can perform this monitoring skill in 3–5 minutes and often the child need not be awakened during the night by the fingerstick if a lancet device is used. On the night before surgery, at least one blood glucose level should be checked between midnight and 7 AM to ensure that hypoglycemia or significant hyperglycemia has not occurred. If such conditions are found, intravenous glucose or increased insulin should be administered. If the child needs to be on an altered caloric diet preoperatively for more than a short time, intravenous insulin should be considered during this period along with hyperalimentation fluids. Insulin can be added to a soluset at a concentration that can be varied to adjust fluid infusion depending on the need to restrict fluid volume. The insulin infusion should be separate from the hydration infusion but can be "piggybacked" into the same line. Ten units of regular insulin per 100 ml of ½ normal saline (0.45%) or normal saline (0.9%) provides a concentration of 0.1 unit/ml. Likewise, 20 units/ 100 ml of diluent gives a concentration of 0.2 units/ml. After mixing 20–50 ml the solution should be flushed through the plastic tubing to allow saturation of the tubing with insulin; this prevents any significant change in the actual amount of insulin delivered secondary to its adherence to glass or plastic (41). Insulin doses usually need to be increased intraoperatively, starting immediately during induction of anesthesia. An algorithm can be used initially (Tables 1 and 2) but may not be suitable in every situation and frequent monitoring of blood glucose levels in the operating room determines how much insulin is needed, remembering that an increase in intravenous rate will lower the blood glucose level in about 10 minutes and a decrease in the insulin delivery rate will likewise increase blood glucose in about 10 minutes. The use of a delivery pump to accurately control infusion rate is advisable.

At times, it may be necessary to use less complicated, although less optimal,

---

TABLE 1. *Diabetes management during surgery for child or adolescent with type I IDDM*

Insulin-glucose infusion regimen when child or adolescent is NPO:
1. Mix 25 units crystalline insulin in 250 ml normal (0.9%) or ½ normal (0.45%) saline (insulin concentration = 0.1 unit/ml).
   Adjust rate of delivery to give 0.025–0.05 units of insulin/kg body weight/hr. (See example below.) The higher rate and perhaps a rate up to 0.1 units/kg body weight per hour may be required in the presence of significant ketonemia and/or infection.
2. Use an intravenous infusion pump for the insulin solution.
3. Add dextrose 5% in ¼ normal (0.225%) or ½ normal (0.45%) saline or dextrose 10% in ¼ or ½ normal saline plus 10–30 mEq KCl/l to infusion system by "piggybacking" into insulin infusion via second intravenous infusion pump. Fluid needs will vary from maintenance (50 ml/kg body weight/24 hr) to 1½–2 times maintenance depending on hydration status and presence of ketonemia. Dextrose is important as a supply of calories, thus decreasing ketone body formation that would impair insulin action. (See example below.)
4. Measure capillary blood glucose (BG) levels hourly using bedside glucose monitoring system.
5. Increase insulin scale (unit/hr) slowly if blood glucose level is persistently >240 mg/dl; decrease slowly if persistently <80 mg/dl.

TABLE 2. *Intraoperative fluid and insulin administration for child or adolescent who weighs at least 20 kg*

BG	Insulin		10% Glucose + ¼–½ NS + KCl	5% Glucose + ¼–½ NS + KCl
(mg/dl)	(Units/hr)	(ml/hr)	(ml/hr)	(ml/hr)
<80	0.5	5	63	125
80–120	1	10	63	125
121–180	1.5	15	63	125
181–240	2	20	50	100
241–400	2.5	25	50	100
>400	3	30	38	75

Sample calculations are for a 40 kg patient

If blood glucose level is <70 mg/dl, give bolus of 25% dextrose in water (15–20 ml) and measure BG level in 15 minutes

At times additional fluid may be required

modes of insulin administration during surgical procedures. In these instances, it may be appropriate to administer one-half the usual dose of intermediate acting insulin subcutaneously in the morning before surgery and then to supplement with crystalline insulin 2–10 units subcutaneously depending on the weight of the patient every 2–4 hours if blood glucose concentrations increase to levels greater than 200 mg/dl.

INTRAVENOUS HYDRATING SOLUTIONS

An intravenous line should be placed in all patients with diabetes undergoing surgery, who are to receive general anesthesia or significant amounts of analgesia, or who cannot eat for more than 8–12 hours. At the level of significant hyperglycemia, (i.e., greater than 300–500 mg/dl), glucose may not be needed in the intravenous fluids and is contraindicated when blood glucose levels exceed 500 mg/dl because hyperosmolality and osmotic diuresis can ensue. Glucose may be added later to the fluid regimen when the blood glucose level falls below 300 mg/dl and dehydration is corrected. If intravenous insulin is required, intravenous solutions containing 2.5–5% dextrose should also be used concomitantly to prevent starvation ketosis (which interferes with insulin action) and to help maintain serum glucose levels in the desired range. If the patient is not ketotic, the amount of fluid that is required is about 50 ml/kg body weight per day (maintenance); if oral liquids can be given and tolerated, this volume may be reduced by an equivalent amount. If ketonemia or vomiting are present, additional fluid may be required; normally 10–20% above maintenance is suggested. The insulin infusion rate should be adjusted at the same time; at least 10–20% additional insulin is required if ketosis is present.

ADDITIONAL PRECAUTIONS IN VERY YOUNG CHILDREN WITH IDDM

Although the prevalence of IDDM in patients under the age of two years is very low (i.e., less than 1:50,000 (42)), the administration of intravenous fluids and insulin during surgery is complicated and ideally should be performed by an experienced diabetologist. In emergency situations, when a consultant is not available, intravenous insulin should be cautiously administered. A small dose of 0.02 units/kg body weight/hr should be administered as young children are extremely sensitive to crystalline insulin. In addition, the risk of hypoglycemia to the developing brain may be significant. Thus, 5% dextrose should always be used in the hydrating solutions unless the initial blood glucose level is significantly greater than 500 mg/dl. Fluid needs may also be higher than in older children and amounts up to 75–100 ml/kg/day may be required. These children, should therefore be monitored extremely closely.

POTASSIUM ADMINISTRATION

Intravenous potassium is also necessary during long surgical procedures. In procedures lasting more than 4 hours, serum potassium levels should be measured and/or an electrocardiogram taken to ensure that hyper- or hypokalemia is not developing. We recommend 20–30 mEq of potassium chloride per liter of intravenous fluid if renal function is normal; at times as little as 10 mEq per liter or as much as 40 mEq may be required. It should be noted that insulin increases potassium entry into cells and that in the presence of insufficient insulin, intracellular potassium is low, while serum potassium levels may be elevated. Serum potassium should be measured periodically, until intravenous hydration is terminated.

ADMINISTRATION OF ANTIBIOTICS

The prophylactic use of antibiotics for surgical procedures in type I diabetics, is controversial. Carefully performed studies, particularly in children and adolescents have not been performed which provide guidelines. Nevertheless, appropriate antibiotics should be administered under the following circumstances:

1. When overt infection (e.g., peritonitis) is present: appropriate cultures should be taken before the start of the antibiotics and after the responsible organism has been identified and its sensitivities to drugs determined, the antibiotic can be changed, if indicated.
2. In the presence of temperature greater than 101° F: again, appropriate cultures should be taken, the most appropriate antibiotic given and then continued or discontinued based on culture results.
3. When pneumonia or other respiratory infections are detected on physical examination.
4. When a history of recurrent urinary tract infections is obtained and there is not sufficient time preoperatively to obtain the results of a urine culture. If the culture is found later to be sterile, antibiotics should be discontinued unless the bladder was catheterized during the surgical procedure, in which case they should be continued until postoperative cultures are also sterile. The urine should again be cultured 48 hours after antibiotics have been discontinued.
5. After major abdominal or neurosurgical procedures where a single large dose of antibiotics is routinely administered immediately after surgery.
6. When open wounds are present.

TABLE 3. *Sample postoperative insulin sliding scale for 40 kg child*

Subcutaneous injections for premeal and bedtime doses (QID)	
Blood glucose level	Insulin (crystalline)
(mg/dl)	(units)
>400	12
>240–400	11
>180–240	9
>120–180	8
>80–120	7
≤80	6

Add 3–4 units of NPH or Lente at bedtime and decrease crystalline insulin dose by 50% if small bedtime snack used

POSTOPERATIVE MANAGEMENT

Intravenous insulin therapy can be continued until solid food is well tolerated. This obviates problems with wide and unpredictable swings in blood glucose levels if vomiting or nausea make intake unpredictable. Blood glucose testing can usually be spaced at 2 to 4-hour intervals once the blood glucose values have been stable for 4 to 6 hours and insulin adjustments are not required as frequently. When subcutaneous insulin therapy is resumed, at least a 45-minute overlap is needed before discontinuing intravenous insulin to prevent rebound hyperglycemia. In some patients the transition may be made smoother by tapering the intravenous insulin as subcutaneous insulin saturates receptors and controls the blood glucose levels. Subcutaneous crystalline insulin can be given by variable dose based on body weight and blood glucose levels before meals. (Table 3) Adding a small amount of intermediate insulin with the bedtime snack prevents AM ketosis and hyperglycemia. Usually not more than 2–5 units of NPH or Lente are necessary depending on the weight of the child. In a very small child, insulin increments may be tolerated only if alterations are made in half-unit increments. The results of the postprandial blood glucose level after one meal can be used to adjust the insulin dose sliding scale. Obviously, the goal is to achieve the target glucose range smoothly without wide swings in glycemia. If the insulin dose scale is too low and hyperglycemia results, supplemental insulin can be given cautiously after 2–2½ hours as long as blood glucose testing confirms ongoing hyperglycemia. In the occasional case where oral feedings cannot be tolerated after 3–5 days, intravenous hyperalimentation should be considered because negative nitrogen balance develops rapidly along with protein catabolism, which is not advantageous to the metabolism of the growing child or adolescent with diabetes mellitus (15).

In summary, careful attention to the details of blood glucose levels, nutrition, and hydration decreases surgical risks and facilitates a faster and smoother recovery in children and adolescents with type I diabetes mellitus.

REFERENCES

1. Rosenstock J, Raskin P. Surgery! Practical guidelines for diabetes management. *Clin. Diabetes* 1987;5:49–61.

2. Kyllo KJ, Nuttall FQ. Prevalence of diabetes mellitus in school-age children in Minnesota. *Diabetes* 1978;27:57–60.
3. Clarke RSJ, Johnston H, Sheridan B. The influence of anaesthesia and surgery on plasma cortisol, insulin and free fatty acids. *Br J Anaesth* 1970;42:295–301.
4. Allison SP, Tomlin PJ, Chamberlain MJ. Some effects of anaesthesia and surgery on carbohydrate and fat metabolism. *Br J Anaesth* 1969;41:588–593.
5. Smith EMA, Morrill C, Meyer WJ, Blalock JE. Corticotropin releasing factor induction of leukocyte derived immunoreactive ACTH and endorphins. *Nature* 1986;32:881–887.
6. Kavelaars A, Ballieux RE, Heijnen CB. The role of IL-1 in the corticotropin-releasing factor and arginine vasopressin-induced secretion of immunoreactive B-endorphin by human peripheral blood mononuclear cells. *J Immunol* 1989;142:2338–2346.
7. Bagdade JD, Nielson KL, Bulger RJ. Reversible abnormalities in phagocytic function in poorly-controlled diabetic patients. *Am J Med Sci* 1972;263:451–456.
8. Wagner H, Junge-Hulsing G, Otto H, Adler J, Hauss WH. Animal experiments concerning the disturbed wound-healing in diabetes mellitus. *Diabetologia* 1970;6:412–413.
9. Pezzarossa A, et al. Perioperative management of diabetic subjects. *Diabetes Care* 1988;11:52–58.
10. Kemmer FW, Sonnenberg G, Cuppers HJ, Berger M. Absorption kinetics of semisynthetic human insulin and biosynthetic (recombinant DNA) human insulin. *Diabetes Care* 1982;5(Suppl 2):23–28.
11. Galloway JA. Insulin treatment for the 80s. Facts and questions about old and new insulins and their usage. *Diabetes Care* 1980;3:615–622.
12. Schernthaner G. Affinity of IgG-insulin antibodies to human (recombinant DNA) insulin and porcine insulin in insulin-treated diabetic individuals with and without insulin resistance. *Diabetes Care* 1982;5(Suppl 2):114–118.
13. Sailer D, Ludwig Th, Kolb S. Comparison of the activity profiles of two fixed combinations of regular/NPH human insulin (recombinant DNA) of different compositions with a fixed regular/NPH porcine insulin combination in insulin-dependent diabetic individuals. *Diabetes Care* 1982;5(Suppl 2):57–59.
14. Weinges K, Ehrhardt M, Nell G, Enzman F. Pharmacodynamics of human insulin (recombinant DNA)-regular, NPH and mixtures obtained by the Gerritzen method in healthy volunteers. *Diabetes Care* 1982;5(Suppl 2):67–70.
15. Alberti KG, Gill GV, Elliot MJ. Insulin delivery during surgery in the diabetic patient. *Diabetes Care* 1982;5(Suppl 1):65–77.
16. Husband DJ, Thai AC, Alberti KG. Management of diabetes during surgery with glucose-insulin-potassium infusion. *Diabetic Med* 1986;3:69–74.
17. Skyler J, ed. Symposium on home glucose self-monitoring. *Diabetes Care* 1981;4:392–426.
18. Koenig RJ, Peterson CM, Jones RL, Saudek C, Lehrman M, Cerami A. Correlation of glucose regulation and hemoglobin A1C in diabetes mellitus. *N Engl J Med* 1976;295:417–420.
19. Jackson RL, Holland E, Chatman ID, Guthrie D, Hewett JE. Growth and maturation of the child with insulin-dependent diabetes mellitus. *Diabetes Care* 1978;1:96–107.
20. Riley WJ, MacLaren NK, Lezotte DC, Spillar RP, Rosenbloom AR. Thyroid autoimmunity in insulin-dependent diabetes mellitus: the case for routine screening. *J Pediatr* 1981;98:350–354.
21. Riley WJ, Winer A, Goldstein D. Coincident presence of thyro-gastric autoimmunity at onset of Type I (insulin-dependent) diabetes. *Diabetologia* 1983;24:418–421.
22. Farid NR, Hawe BS, Walfish PG. Increased frequency of HLA DR3 and 5 in the syndrome of painless thyroiditis with transient thyrotoxicosis: Evidence for an autoimmune etiology. *Clin Endocrinol* 1983;19:699–704.
23. Biro J. Thyroid-stimulating antibodies in Graves' disease and the effect of thyrotrophin-binding globulins on their determination. *J Endocrinol* 1982;92:175–184.
24. Neufeld N, MacLaren N, Blizzard RM. Two types of autoimmune Addison's disease associated with different polyglandular autoimmune (PGA) syndromes. *Medicine* 1981;60:355–362.
25. Riley WJ, MacLaren NK, Neufeld M. Adrenal autoantibodies and Addison disease in insulin-dependent diabetes mellitus. *J Pediatr* 1980;97:191–195.
26. Migeon CJ. Physiology and pathology of adrenocortical function in infancy and childhood. In: Collu R, ed. *Pediatric endocrinology,* vol. 1. New York: Raven Press, 1981;465–522.
27. Migeon CJ, Lanes R. Adrenal cortex: Hypo- and hyperfunction. In: Lifshitz F, ed. *Pediatric endocrinology,* vol 3, Clinical Pediatrics. New York: Marcel Dekker, Inc. 1985;179–202.
28. Knowles H Jr, Guest G, Lampe J, Kessler M, Skillman T. The course of juvenile diabetes treated with unmeasured diet. *Diabetes* 1965;14:239–264.
29. Page MMcB, Watkins PJ. Cardiorespiratory arrest with diabetic autonomic neuropathy. *Lancet* 1978;1:14–16.
30. Rabinowe SL, Brown FM, Whatts M. Antisympathetic ganglia antibodies and postural blood pressure in IDDM subjects of varying duration and patients at high risk of developing IDDM. *Diabetes Care* 1989;12:1–16.
31. Bennett T, Hosking PJ, Hampton JR. Cardiovascular control in diabetes mellitus. *Br Med J* 1975;2:585–9.

32. Kassander P. Asymptomatic gastric retention in diabetics (Gastroparesis diabeticorum). *Ann Intern Med* 1958;48:797–800.
33. Root HF. Pre-operative care of the diabetic patient. *Postgrad Med* 1966;40:439–444.
34. Steffes MW. The predictive value of microalbuminuria. *Am J Kidney Dis* 1989;13:25–28.
35. Chavers BM. Glomerular lesions and urinary albumin excretion in type 1 diabetes without overt proteinuria. *N Engl J Med* 1989;320:966–970.
36. Hommel E. Acute reduction of arterial blood pressure reduces urinary albumin excretion in type I (insulin-dependent) diabetic patients with incipient nephropathy. *Diabetologia* 1986;29:211–215.
37. Passa P. Effects of enalapril in insulin-dependent diabetic subjects with mild to moderate uncomplicated hypertension. *Diabetes Care* 1987;10:200–204.
38. Guthrie RA. Special problems. In: Jackson RL, Guthrie RA, eds. *The physiological management of diabetes in children.* New York: Elsevier Science Publishing Co. Inc., 1986;236–257.
39. Kozak GP, Krall LP. Disorders of the skin in diabetes. In: Marble A, Krall L, Bradley R, Christlieb AR, Soeldner JS, eds. *Joslin's diabetes mellitus,* 12th ed. Philadelphia: Lea & Febiger, 1985;777–779.
40. Gale EAM, Tattersall RB. Unrecognized nocturnal hypoglycemia in insulin-treated diabetics. *Lancet* 1979;1:1049–51.
41. Peterson L, Caldwell J, Hoffman J. Insulin adsorbance to polyvinylchloride surfaces with implications for constant infusion therapy. *Diabetes* 1976;25:72–74.
42. La Porte RE, Fishbein HA, Drash AL, et al. Pittsburgh insulin-dependent diabetes mellitus (IDDM) registry—The incidence of insulin-dependent diabetes mellitus in Allegheny County, Pennsylvania (1965–1976). *Diabetes* 1981;30:279–283.

Surgical Management of the Diabetic Patient,
edited by Michael Bergman and Gregorio A. Sicard.
Raven Press, Ltd., New York © 1991.

16

Predischarge Planning

Daniel L. Lorber

Diabetes Control Foundation, Flushing, New York 11355

Discharge planning for the surgical patient with diabetes is unique for several reasons:

1. People with diabetes are more likely to require surgery than the general population. More than one-half of people with diabetes will require surgery at some time in their lives (1). This increase in surgery results from the long-term complications of diabetes and the impact on surgical disease. An increased rate of cataract and vitreo-retinal disorders leads to ophthalmic surgery; accelerated arteriosclerotic heart disease (ASHD) leads to increased coronary bypass surgery; peripheral vascular disease and peripheral neuropathy combine to increase the risk of lower extremity amputation or vascular reconstructive surgery; autonomic neuropathy can lead to surgery for impotence or for urinary retention.
2. Diabetes is often asymptomatic and undiagnosed until the patient comes to medical attention for an acute problem. As many as one-sixth of surgical patients (2) have undiagnosed diabetes.
3. Patients with diabetes are often admitted to the hospital for surgical procedures that would otherwise be performed in the ambulatory operating room. In addition to an increased hospitalization rate, people with diabetes often have a prolonged hospitalization. This is the result of the impact of diabetes on every stage of the hospital stay.
4. The standard recommendation that diabetic patients have surgery early in the morning makes surgical scheduling more difficult and can introduce delays.
5. Diabetes is often out of control in acutely ill patients, requiring a delay in surgery until the metabolism is stabilized.
6. Surgical complications, such as intraoperative myocardial infarction or postoperative infection are more common in diabetic patients (3,4).
7. The complications of diabetes will have an impact on many aspects of the postoperative course and on the patient's ability to perform self-care after discharge. Peripheral neuropathy and peripheral vascular disease (PVD) lead to an increased rate of heel decubiti; autonomic neuropathy and postural hypotension lead to delayed ambulation and an increased risk of urinary retention. Diabetic gastropathy delays a return to a normal diet and the resulting dysmetabolism is further complicated by the high carbohydrate content of most dietary supplements, tube feedings, and clear fluids.
8. Poorly controlled diabetes in the postoperative period will lead to a delay in discharge from the hospital until the diabetes is stabilized.

9. Diabetes is a chronic disease that depends upon daily self-care and self-management in the home.

Diabetic complications can cause decreased ability to provide self-care, due to decreased vision (retinopathy), decreased mobility, and decreased dexterity (neuropathy and PVD). As a result, discharge is delayed until either the patient is taught alternative self-care techniques or an alternate care-giver is identified.

Self-care requires that specific knowledge and skills be mastered before it is safe to discharge the patient from the hospital. If education is delayed to the period immediately prior to discharge, this mastery will be incomplete and inadequate. Hospital admission and surgery often result in changes in the patient's diabetes management, requiring further patient education. Discharge is, therefore, delayed to teach the patient insulin use or to arrange for its administration at home.

Diabetes thus has an impact on all phases of the surgical patient's hospital course. It increases hospitalization rates and may complicate or delay discharge at every step between admission and discharge from the acute care setting. Effective discharge planning for the diabetic surgical patient must, therefore, be implemented at every stage of the patient's surgical admission.

The last decade has seen dramatic changes in the financing of health care and, as a result, its practice. With the onset of prospective payment and Diagnosis Related Groups (DRGs) has come increased pressure to shorten length of stay for all hospitalized patients, including those with diabetes. Insurers, whose programs in the past encouraged hospitalization by refusing to pay for outpatient procedures, have changed these same programs to encourage ambulatory and same-day surgery for many procedures.

These changes have had an impact on the health-care system in many ways. One of the most important is a change in the function of discharge planning. In the past, discharge planning was carried out primarily by social workers whose function was primarily to expedite patient placement in long-term care facilities. Discharge planning as currently practiced is a comprehensive program to expedite discharge from the hospital to the community.

This chapter reviews discharge planning in a chronological sequence from preadmission planning to postdischarge follow-up.

It will not provide a comprehensive overview of discharge planning or of diabetes education, but rather an approach to specific aspects of discharge planning for the patient with diabetes who is undergoing surgery. For a comprehensive review of discharge planning and of diabetes education, the reader is referred to O'Hara and Terry (5), Zarle (6).

GOALS OF DISCHARGE PLANNING

The primary goal of discharge planning is to facilitate smooth transitions for the patient. This includes transition within the hospital (discharge from the recovery room or intensive-care unit to the floor) or from hospital to home or alternate-care facility. A discharge planning program ensures that patients who enter the acute-care institution have a planned program for continuing care needs and a follow-up plan when they leave the hospital. Discharge planning provides for all necessary arrangements for continuing care—be it to home or to an alternate-care setting.

Secondary goals of discharge planning for the person with diabetes include training in self-care skills necessary to avoid rehospitalization and provision for further diabetes care and education after discharge.

STRUCTURE OF DISCHARGE PLANNING

Discharge planning is "a centralized, coordinated program developed by a hospital to ensure that each patient has a planned program for needed continuing follow-up care." It requires "a program which coordinates assessment, planning, and follow-up procedures by providing a multidisciplinary team approach to patients with post-hospital needs." (5)

During the 1980s there have been a number of alternative structures for discharge planning. For many years, discharge planning was carried out by the social-work department with input from the patient's primary nurse. As discharge planning has grown in importance, most hospitals have developed departments of discharge planning. These departments have a multidisciplinary structure that includes nurse-specialists, social workers, and others.

Three levels of interdisciplinary team have an impact on any patient's discharge planning.

- The *primary care team* includes the patient, floor nurse, physician, rehabilitation specialists and dietitian—those who direct the patient's hospital stay.
- The *resource team* includes the continuing care nurse specialist, home health-care nurses, other nurse-specialists (diabetes educators, ostomy nurses, etc.) discharge planning specialists (usually a nurse or social worker), the utilization review team, pharmacists, and administration.
- The *community team* includes the primary physician, home health care agencies, physical and occupational therapists, dietitian, and diabetes educators.

The structure of these teams varies from community to community and from hospital to hospital. Whatever the specific structure may be, certain constants hold true. Proper discharge planning depends upon communication within the team and between teams; coordination is essential to avoid duplicate or incomplete efforts. Efficient discharge planning requires the varied skills of a multidisciplinary team; this must be recognized in the department structure.

THE PROCESS OF DISCHARGE PLANNING

It is essential that any discharge planning process provide for early identification of patients who will need more complex posthospital care.

Once patients are identified, the process of discharge planning follows a structured format similar to other areas of the nursing process. The four principal steps involved are: assessment, planning, implementation, and evaluation.

Assessment

Assessment of the patient's discharge needs should begin before hospitalization (if possible) and continue throughout the admission and discharge period.

The assessment process in discharge planning takes a holistic view of the patient's needs. It includes social, physical, and psychological aspects of the patient's function. In particular, it asks, "Does the patient need help? If so, what kind of help and has the help been effective in the past?" These data are usually available from the patient or family member, primary health care team, or other health agencies.

Discharge planning diagnoses commonly follow a series of Functional Health Patterns (6), including queries into health self-management, nutrition, elimination, activity, cognitive function, sleep patterns, self-concept, role and relationships, sexuality, stress and coping, and values and beliefs. The problems identified are described in diagnostic terms amenable to nursing therapy, e.g., rather than "diabetic neuropathy," a discharge planning diagnosis would be "impaired mobility secondary to diabetic neuropathy."

The needs assessment for any patient should include: functional capacity, nursing and other care requirements, and social and family resources available. For the person with diabetes, assessment must address additional specific aspects of diabetes care. These include: ability to prepare and tolerate diet, medication administration, self-monitoring of blood glucose level and urine ketones, activity/exercise, sick day management, and knowing when to contact the physician. A final point on the assessment process: full documentation of the assessment is essential as in all phases of discharge planning.

Planning

Once functional diagnoses have been established, programs to meet the needs identified are developed in the planning phase. The steps include: assigning priorities to diagnosed problems, identifying whom will resolve which problems, developing nursing-care plans to develop nursing orders, indicating specific nursing orders (including education), identifying short, intermediate, and long-term goals, identifying desired behavioral outcomes of the care, and documentating.

Each health care discipline develops individual outcome goals that contribute to overall goals for the patient. Coordination is essential to avoid conflict and to avoid sending mixed messages to an already stressed patient. The patient's and family's goals may differ markedly from those of the health professionals. It is essential, therefore, that the patient and family be integrated into the planning phase of any discharge plan.

Implementation

The implementation phase of discharge planning can begin with the patient's entry into the health care system. It involves coordination of nursing and medical care plans and requires explicit communication between physician and nurse.

Implementation of discharge planning programs for diabetes is *not* a process that begins on the day of discharge. The person with diabetes who needs instruction on insulin or other diabetes education should be started on this process well in advance of the planned discharge. If arrangements are needed for home health care or other community services, these must also be implemented in advance.

Documentation becomes especially important in the implementation phase of discharge planning. The patient is in flux between the acute care setting and home or extended care facility. He is changing health-care teams from the primary floor nurse to either self-care or a community health resource. Careful communication by use of referral forms or nursing discharge summaries is essential.

Evaluation

The evaluation phase of discharge planning takes place after patient discharge. It has a number of interlocking levels, including: evaluation of individual patient results, evaluation of individual programs, such as home health care, visiting nurse services (VNS), outpatient diabetes education, or skilled nursing facility (SNF) referrals; and evaluation of the institution's entire discharge planning program.

For the evaluation phase to be effective, individual follow-up with phone calls, home visits, and chart audit are necessary. Careful documentation is again essential to the process; documentation is needed for communication among professionals, for medico-legal reasons, and to document compliance with third-party requirements.

PREADMISSION PLANNING

Current fiscal regulations have dictated extremely brief preoperative hospital stays. As a result, there is a limited amount of time to initiate discharge planning and patient education before the patient goes to surgery. Of necessity, this brief period must be devoted to admission, orientation, and basic preoperative teaching. Careful assessment of discharge needs is delayed because preoperative teaching is a priority. Shortened stays mean that one cannot wait until two or three days after surgery, when the patient is feeling better, to begin planning for return to the home environment. With delayed planning, hospitalization becomes prolonged or discharge planning becomes incomplete.

Discharge planning need not wait until hospital admission. The patient scheduled for elective surgery provides a unique opportunity for early and effective discharge planning. The discharge plan process can identify BEFORE admission the posthospital needs of the patient.

The first questions to be asked are, "Why is this patient being admitted? Is this admission necessary because of diabetes? If so, can the procedure be performed in the ambulatory operating room if diabetes is otherwise controlled? If yes, is there time to initiate a program of better diabetes control?"

For the patient who will be able to eat shortly after surgery and does not require admission for parenteral medications, catheters, etc., ambulatory diabetes management and surgery is often preferable to hospital admission. A brief period of outpatient education in self-care skills, including self blood glucose monitoring, urine acetone testing, insulin adjustment for decreased appetite or activity, and sick-day management may be all that is needed to avert a hospital stay of several days. This educational program requires an available multidisciplinary diabetes care team, including internist/diabetologist, diabetes nurse-educator, and nutritionist. Patient self-monitoring of blood glucose levels, careful guidelines, and telephone availability of the diabetes care team can often obviate the need for hospitalization.

For the patient requiring hospitalization, preadmission assessment determines where the patient came from and whether a return to that environment is feasible. If it is, what additional supports will be needed? If not, what alternatives are available? A plan can be developed to meet these needs and implementation begun before admission. Patients and family members are made familiar with community resources and preoperative teaching is begun. The patient and family knowledge base can be assessed during the preadmission period.

Often the person with diabetes manages the diabetes the best. Patients should be encouraged to bring their capillary blood glucose monitoring equipment and to participate actively in their care (12). Preadmission assessment should include accuracy of the patient's capillary blood glucose level monitoring technique, particularly if testing will be performed in the hospital.

Preadmission education in postoperative self-care shortens hospitalization (8–10) and improves the performance of postoperative tasks by the patient (11). Postoperatively, the patient's attention span is shortened due to the effect of pain and medications. The preadmission time provides an excellent opportunity for teaching. This is also the time to decide on perioperative diabetes management:

- Who will be managing the patient's diabetes in the perioperative period? Will it be the internist, surgeon, or surgical housestaff?
- Should this patient be admitted to the medical service for diabetes stabilization or is direct surgical admission feasible?
- What will constitute the preoperative and postoperative diet?
- What perioperative diabetes treatment will be needed?
- What will the perioperative fluids be? What effects will the fluids chosen have on the patient and what changes in insulin or oral agents will be needed?
- What education will be needed for postsurgical self-care in the hospital? This includes appropriate activity and exercises.
- What education will be needed for diabetes self-care in the hospital?
- What education will be needed for postdischarge care?
- What postdischarge diabetic and postsurgical care will be needed?
- Who will carry out postdischarge care? Can they be educated now?
- What other arrangements are necessary for postdischarge support? These may include home health aides, nursing services, dressing supplies, and durable goods.

Who assesses the patient's needs before admission? Clearly, the primary physician is involved. In addition, assigning a Clinical Nurse Specialist (CNS) to the preadmission unit can be an effective solution to this problem (10). The CNS can identify elements of preoperative care that a surgical patient needs during the hospital stay and for discharge. The role of the CNS includes assessment, teaching, counselling, emotional support, and orientation to the hospital. Other tasks include coordination or referral and consultation for support services such as physical therapy, home health care, and social work.

Provision of nursing services in the preadmission unit facilitates early management of educational, psychosocial, and discharge planning needs. Further liaison between the admitting and discharge planning units can include assigning a social worker or discharge planning coordinator to the preadmission unit. With effective coordination, discharge planning can often be completed before the patient is admitted.

Same-day or ambulatory surgery present additional needs for a CNS in the preadmission phase (13). A telephone conference between the CNS and patient provides an opportunity to answer the patient's questions about the procedure, discuss the time and duration of surgery and aid in planning home support for a brief hospital stay or ambulatory procedure. Often, diabetes self-management may be impossible after an otherwise simple procedure. For example, a right-handed patient with insulin-dependent diabetes cannot easily administer insulin after carpal tunnel or hand surgery on the dominant hand. A brief preoperative referral to home health care or education for a family member can prevent a great deal of postoperative stress.

PREOPERATIVE INPATIENT ASSESSMENT

Preoperative inpatient assessment should include any areas not covered in the preadmission assessment. It is important to not assume accurate diabetes knowledge in even the most educated patient (14). Many patients have had no formal diabetes education; even those who have been taught may not remember or perform rudimentary tasks accurately.

Assessment at this time should include knowledge of diabetes survival skills and of basic postoperative behavior. To plan a logical knowledge and skill progression to discharge, the assessor must evaluate what the patient and family know and what they will need to know for posthospital self-care, including knowledge, skills, and attitudes about diabetes. What resources are now in use by the patient, including family members, physicians, diabetes educators, or others? What will be needed?

PREOPERATIVE DISCHARGE PLANNING TASKS

Preoperative tasks for the diabetic surgical patient can be divided into two groups: tasks that facilitate recovery, and tasks that facilitate discharge.

To facilitate postoperative recovery in patients with diabetes, the goal is to avoid the metabolic perturbations associated with severe hyperglycemia or hypoglycemia. The steps to this goal include:

• Planning preoperative meals and medication
• Planning perioperative medications and fluids
• Planning postoperative medications and diet progression from nothing by mouth (NPO) to normal eating
• Education in postoperative self-care, including coughing, movement, pain medication, and appropriate exercises.

Early structured teaching in self-care tasks shortens hospitalization and improves self-care activities both in the hospital and after discharge (8,11).

Tasks that facilitate discharge include:

• Tasks listed above that improve postoperative recovery
• Development of a discharge plan and review of this plan with the patient and family
• Answering patient and family questions about the discharge plan
• Initiation of education in diabetes mellitus survival skills if time is available.

Survival skills, including insulin and blood glucose monitoring, and basic diet understanding can be briefly introduced. Rather than overwhelm the patient with postoperative self-care and diabetes self-care at this time, it is advisable to delay most diabetes education until the interval between the immediate postoperative period and discharge. A preoperative "total immersion" program in both diabetes and surgical self-care is likely to result in confusion, with little learning. It is more effective to focus on postoperative self-care activities such as coughing, deep breathing, and exercises at this time and delay more detailed diabetes education.

IMMEDIATE POSTOPERATIVE PERIOD

The first 24 hours of the postoperative period are marked by metabolic instability and rapid changes in diet, fluids, and diabetes management. Discharge or transfer from one unit within the hospital to another requires a different form of discharge planning. The nursing process of "giving report" on patient transfer accomplishes part of this process. Another essential part is carried out by the physician writing postoperative orders. In addition to standard postoperative orders, diabetes requires planning for blood glucose level monitoring and reinstitution of diet and of insulin or oral hypoglycemic agents. All too often, these orders are written by the least experienced surgical house officer, who is likely to be experienced in standard postoperative orders but totally unsophisticated in adjusting diabetes management for the metastable postoperative period.

The progression of the patient from the operating room to eventual hospital discharge depends upon smooth diabetes control and the rapid reinstitution of the diabetic diet and medications. The internist or diabetes specialist expedites this process by guiding the patient's metabolic management from arrival in the recovery room, rather than waiting for the next day's rounds. In many cases, the preoperative medical consultation includes guidelines for postoperative fluids, diet and insulin, or sulfonylureas. The patient is on the road to metabolic balance with little delay.

Many patients are treated with insulin/dextrose infusions through the surgical period. We have found the following approach easiest for the transfer to food in the patient treated with insulin:

1. Total the patient's preoperative insulin doses for an average 24-hour period.
2. Multiply the patient's weight in kg by 0.4.
3. Take the lesser of 1 and 2 and divide by 4.
4. The resulting number is the premeal regular insulin dose. Institute with the first postoperative meal and adjust based on the resulting blood glucose level before the next meal.
5. The resulting number is also the neutral protamine Hagedorn (NPH) or Lénte insulin dose taken at bedtime (hs). Institute at bedtime after the first postoperative meal and adjust based on the next day's fasting blood sugar (FBS).

For example, if an 80 kg man has been treated with 30 units of NPH insulin in the morning and 14 units at hs, the calculations are as follows:

1. Total insulin: $30 + 14 = 44$
2. Weight $\times 0.4 = 32$
3. The lesser number (32) divided by $4 = 8$
4. The insulin orders are: regular insulin 8 units subcutaneous (sc) before meals; NPH 8 units sc at hs.

Continue the intravenous insulin/dextrose infusion until the first postoperative meal is consumed. With the first meal, institute sc regular insulin following the above regimen. This approach provides the flexibility necessary for patients to eat lunch or supper as their first postoperative meal. If the first meal is breakfast, this regimen can be used as well. As an alternative, however, many diabetologists prefer to resume the patient's prior insulin regimen.

The patient treated with oral hypoglycemic agents presents a different problem. If the diabetes was well controlled with an oral agent, it is easiest to resume its use with preoperative feedings. If the first meal is breakfast or lunch, the usual day's dose can be given. If supper is the first meal, one-half of the prior dose can be given before supper. The usual medication regimen can be resumed on the first full postoperative day. As an alternative, insulin can be used in the same fashion as for the patient who requires insulin (above).

DIABETES MANAGEMENT FOR THE INTERVAL BETWEEN THE IMMEDIATE POSTOPERATIVE AND IMMEDIATE PREDISCHARGE PERIOD

The goals of the recovery period between surgery and discharge are both metabolic and educational.

The metabolic goal during this interval is to avoid excessive nitrogen and calorie loss. The patient should be returned to a stable diet and stable metabolism as quickly as possible and should be ambulated as soon as is feasible. In addition to the improved respiratory and other advantages to early ambulation, normal activity is essential to diabetes management. Achieving diabetes control in a patient who spends most of the time in bed bears little relationship to what will be needed in the more active home situation. Early ambulation should include postprandial walking in order to more closely mimic the patient's usual home activity pattern.

The next step in the progression from surgery to discharge is achieving a medical regimen that can be implemented by the patient at home. The usual hospital regimen of multiple regular insulin injections based on capillary blood glucose results is not easy for most patients. Now is the time to reassess the patient's preadmission diabetes regimen. Is insulin necessary? If so, what regimen? How many shots a day? Can the patient be managed with sulfonylureas plus diet or with diet alone?

Developing and implementing a regimen of diabetes management early in the postoperative period expedites metabolic stability and provides more time for directed patient education in application of this regimen. With the advent of self blood glucose monitoring and patient education in advanced diabetes self-management, the best approach is often to allow the patient to achieve diabetes control by him or herself. We prefer to allow educated patients to determine and administer their own insulin doses as soon as possible. The well-educated patient can provide essential guidance to the professional and often knows his body's response to different foods and insulin doses better than the physician.

DIABETES EDUCATION FOR THE INTERVAL BETWEEN THE IMMEDIATE POSTOPERATIVE AND IMMEDIATE PRE-DISCHARGE PERIOD

This period represents the most important phase of discharge planning for the diabetic patient. If he or she is to be discharged home, diabetes management will be, of necessity, carried out primarily by the patient or immediate family.

The stresses of hospitalization make comprehensive diabetes education impossible. Ideally, therefore, teaching begins in the hospital and is expanded and reinforced in the community. Education in the hospital focuses on survival skills. These skills include a basic understanding of diet, technical facility in capillary blood glucose and urine ketone monitoring, and technical facility in measuring and administering insulin, if needed. For most hospitalized patients, these tasks are all that is needed and all that can be achieved prior to discharge. The diabetes educator should have a plan and, ideally, a checklist of what is to be taught.

Education in self-care is begun as soon as possible in the postoperative period. All too often, the diabetes nurse educator is called the day before discharge and asked to teach how to administer insulin so that the patient will be able to go home. As for all of discharge planning, the process of education must include both the patient and family members.

The Patient with Preexisting Diabetes

For the person with preexisting diabetes, the education process begins with a directed knowledge assessment. It should never be assumed that even the most experienced patient thoroughly understands diabetes self-management. Assess the patient's and family's knowledge of diet and of the past medication regimen. Have the patient demonstrate technical skills such as insulin measurement and administration and capillary blood glucose monitoring. A thorough nursing assessment is needed to determine not only the patient's knowledge and home situation but also the impact diabetes may have on the individual's home life and vice versa.

Hospitalization and surgery often lead to significant changes in the patient's psychological and medical response to diabetes. Surgery exacerbates the sense of loss and social isolation common in people with diabetes. It may lead to changes in the medication regimen (such as the need for insulin), which can be perceived as a worsening of the diabetes. Changes in the patient's diabetes management must be introduced with the psychological effects in mind. Planning and implementing diabetes education should begin simultaneously with the knowledge assessment. The education plan includes a review of prior knowledge with correction of misconceptions and errors of technique. New techniques should be instituted as soon as possible to allow for repeated reinforcement prior to discharge.

The Patient with Newly Diagnosed Diabetes

One-sixth of the patients admitted for surgery may have undiagnosed diabetes (1). The education process for these patients differs from that needed for the person with known preexisting diabetes, but the goals are much the same. The person with newly diagnosed diabetes requires knowledge of diet basics and facility with the technical skills necessary for self-management.

Assessment of the newly diagnosed diabetic patient should include:

• Lifestyle and habits
• Coping mechanisms
• Family support
• Dietary needs and preferences
• Medication needs
• Medical sophistication

The planning of an education program for the postoperative patient with newly diagnosed diabetes includes a basic introduction to diabetes—what is it, how is it treated. This is followed by the survival skills—diet basics, capillary blood glucose and urine ketone testing, and use of insulin or oral agents. The education program begins as soon as the patient or family member is able to listen and learn.

The hospital is not the place for a comprehensive education in all of diabetes management for the newly diagnosed patient. Education begins in the hospital; it is reinforced and complemented by education in the outpatient setting, either the clinic or a diabetes education program. Procedures that cause the most anxiety must be taught as early as possible. If insulin injection or obtaining capillary blood glucose samples are delayed, the patient's apprehension about these potentially painful procedures will interfere with learning any other necessary information. We recommend that self-injection with a saline-containing insulin syringe be done at the same time as the patient is first told of the need for insulin self-treatment. The usual process of teaching the patient about insulin measurement and mixing followed by practicing injections on an orange delays the learning process unnecessarily.

If it is apparent that the patient and family will not master needed skills prior to discharge, now is the time to consider alternate possibilities. Home health agencies, including the Visiting Nurse Services, will continue the education process, administer insulin, pre-fill insulin syringes for patient use, and perform blood glucose monitoring.

What of the patient who will be discharged to an alternate-care facility? Education plays a small role in care at this time. Discharge planning must concentrate instead on achieving a medical regimen that can be carried out at the receiving facility. The use of adjusted insulin doses or capillary blood glucose level monitoring is more difficult in a skilled nursing facility (SNF) than in the hospital, and may not be practical. The Discharge Planning department can provide information about alternative care settings and which diabetes regimens are feasible.

THE PREDISCHARGE PERIOD—PLANNING FOR POSTHOSPITAL CARE

This phase of hospitalization overlaps with the previous one. As the time of discharge approaches, many of the questions raised earlier gain a new immediacy.

1. Where will the patient be going?
   SNF, HRF, home, other (6)
2. What tasks will be necessary?
   food preparation
   medication administration
   follow-up education
   skilled nursing needs
   other nondiabetes-related needs
3. Who will be delivering care?
   patient
   family
   skilled nurses
   community resources

With proper discharge planning, many of these questions will have been answered before admission or early in the patient's hospital course. The immediate predischarge phase will be a period of consolidation rather than introduction. It provides an opportunity to address specific patient concerns, such as diet, medications (15), pain management, and self-care tasks.

Funding for home health care is in a state of flux at the time of this writing. In particular, the definition of skilled nursing needs is more restricted than in the past. For the person with diabetes, specific skilled nursing needs can include measurement and administration of insulin (usually only once a day) and further patient education in diabetes self-management. Home health nurses should not be viewed as a permanent part of the patient's care, but rather as an educational resource and aid in transition to family or patient self-care.

It is during the immediate predischarge period that arrangements for community resources are made. Referral to home health agencies are instituted at this time.

TRANSITION TO HOME

Discharge represents a transition from hospital care to community care. It requires implementation of the plan of self-care that had been instituted in the hospital.

With proper patient education, the survival skills necessary for basic self-management have been learned in the hospital and discharge merely requires being sure that necessary supplies are in place. A few days before discharge the family should be given a list of necessary supplies and appropriate prescriptions. These supplies can include dressings and other surgical needs as well as medications, syringes, and blood glucose and urine acetone monitoring equipment needed for diabetes care. Food shopping should precede discharge to facilitate resumption of the diabetic diet.

Now is the time to complete final referral paperwork. Coordination of care with involved community resources, including the primary physician, home health agencies, outpatient diabetes education centers, and others requires detailed, written communication. Follow-up arrangements are made as needed with the physician, nurse-educators, and dietitians. The entire carefully implemented discharge plan that began prior to admission will be useless if not carefully carried through to the home situation.

Any medical program requires evaluation of its results. Diabetes discharge planning is evaluated on an individual and programmatic level. Individual patient follow-up may include telephone contact, home visits, or questionnaires. Programmatic evaluation is more complex and has been described elsewhere (5,6).

TRANSITION TO THE ALTERNATE-CARE FACILITY

The elderly hospital patient is 30 times more likely to require posthospital care in an SNF than the younger counterpart (16), and is also far more likely to have diabetes (17). Transition to an SNF requires special care for the person with diabetes. Referral forms must include detailed information about diet and medication. In most cases, the patient's primary physician relinquishes direct care to the SNF physician. Careful communication of medical information is necessary among physicians, nurses, and dietitians to ensure a smooth transfer and avert readmission for decompensated diabetes.

DISCHARGE PLANNING FOR AMBULATORY SURGERY

Ambulatory surgery depends upon the ability of the patient and family to provide for the patient's postoperative medical needs. For the person with diabetes, these needs include the basic survival skills and other, more sophisticated care, such as continuous sc insulin infusion pumps.

Preadmission planning for ambulatory surgery includes predischarge planning as well. The same questions are asked as for inpatient discharge planning. What diet, medications, and monitoring will be necessary? Who will be meeting these needs? Will the patient be able to carry out self-management or will assistance be needed? A nurse-clinician assigned to the ambulatory unit can call the patient before surgery to discuss necessary arrangements. The diabetologist should include preoperative and postoperative insulin treatment and dietary modifications in the preoperative medical clearance. These recommendations are transmitted in writing to the patient and to the ambulatory unit.

If the planned surgical procedure is likely to interfere with dexterity or vision, discharge planning includes arrangements for a family member or other caregiver to carry out blood glucose level monitoring and insulin treatment, if needed. Common ambulatory procedures, such as cataract extraction and hand surgery fall into this category. In most cases, surgery results in a transient change in eating and activity patterns. Diet and medication planning in advance decreases the metabolic disruption caused by these changes.

SUMMARY

1. Discharge planning for the surgical patient with diabetes is a process that begins prior to admission and continues throughout all phases of the hospitalization and discharge process. Its goal is the safe return of the patient to diabetes self-management.

2. Discharge planning for all diabetic patients begins with an assessment of diabetes-related knowledge, skills, and attitudes. This assessment includes the major aspects of diabetes survival skills: diet, blood glucose and urine ketone level monitoring, and proper use of insulin or oral hypoglycemic agents.

3. In-hospital diabetes education primarily addresses the basic diabetes survival skills. Comprehensive diabetes education is continued after discharge. Discharge planning for the patient with diabetes includes identification and referral to an appropriate community diabetes program for continued education.

4. Discharge planning and patient education must begin early in the hospitalization. Delaying diabetes education to the immediate predischarge period results in unnecessarily prolonged hospitalization or incomplete learning of diabetes survival skills.

5. The discharge planning process is a multidisciplinary process, including nurses, physicians, social workers, and, most important, the patient and family.

Each phase of hospitalization represents a period of specific need that can be met by the discharge planning process. With early assessment, planning, and implementation of a diabetes care and education program, and early involvement of the patient and family, there need be no delay in discharge for the postoperative patient with diabetes.

ACKNOWLEDGMENTS

The author thanks Maria Nazario, RN, and Alice Curley, RN, Department of Discharge Planning, Booth Memorial Medical Center, for their invaluable advice in preparation of this chapter.

REFERENCES

1. Alberti KG, Thomas DJ. The management of diabetes during surgery. *Br J Anasth* 1979;51:693–710.
2. Galloway J, Shuman C. Diabetes and surgery: A study of 667 cases. *Am J Med* 1963;34:177.
3. Lilienfeld DE, Vlahov D, Tenney J, and McLaughlin JS. Obesity and diabetes as risk factors for postoperative wound infections after cardiac surgery. *Am J Infect Control* 1988;16:3–6.
4. Nagachinta T, Stephens M, Reitz B, Polk BF. Risk factors for surgical-wound infection following cardiac surgery. *J Infect Dis* 1987;156:967–973.
5. O'Hare PA, Terry MA. *Discharge planning: strategies for assuring continuity of care.* Rockville: Aspen Publishers, 1988.
6. Zarle NC. *Continuing care: the process and practice of discharge planning.* Rockville: Aspen Publishers, 1987.
7. American Diabetes Association. Quality recognition for diabetes patient education programs. *Diabetes Care* 1986;9:XXXVI–XL.
8. Reiner IJ. Early discharge after vaginal hysterectomy. *Obstet Gynecol* 1988;71:416–418.
9. Devine EC, Cook TD. A meta-analytic analysis of psychoeducational interventions on length of postsurgical hospital stay. *Nurs Res* 1983;32:267–274.
10. Phipps CG. Effectiveness of the clinical nurse specialist in preadmission testing. *Health Matrix* 1987–8;5:23–27.
11. Williams PD. Valderrama DM, Gloria MD, et al. Effects of preparation for mastectomy/hysterectomy on women's postoperative self-care behaviors. *Int J Nurs Stud* 1988;25:191–206.
12. Molitch M. What to tell the hospital. *Diabetes Forecast* 1989;May:69–73.
13. Craig D. Discharge planning checklist boosts facility's effectiveness. *Same-day Surgery* 1980; February-March:21–23.
14. Miller LV, Goldstein J, Nicolaisen G. Evaluation of patients' knowledge of diabetes self-care. *Diabetes Care* 1978;1:275–280.
15. Leyder BL, Pieper B. Identifying discharge concerns. *AORN J* 1986;43:1298–1304.
16. Podolsky R, Mason JH. Geriatric discharge planning and follow-up. *Illinois Medical Journal* 1980;May:291–292.
17. Harris MI, Hadden WC, Knowler WC, et al. Prevalence of diabetes and impaired glucose tolerance and plasma glucose levels in U.S. population aged 20–74 yr. *Diabetes* 1987;36:523–534.

Surgical Management of the Diabetic Patient,
edited by Michael Bergman and Gregorio A. Sicard.
Raven Press, Ltd., New York © 1991.

17

Diabetic Foot Care

*Vilray P. Blair, III, *Dolores A. Drury, and †Marvin E. Levin

*Division of Orthopedic Surgery, Washington University School of Medicine, St.
Louis, Missouri 63110, and †Department of Internal Medicine, Washington University
School of Medicine, Chesterfield, Missouri 63017

This and the subsequent chapter (see chapter 18) review state-of-the-art considerations for providing comprehensive foot care management of the diabetic patient.

Limb loss is perhaps the most feared complication of diabetes. The statistics associated with amputation create a very real concern. Fifty percent of all nontraumatic amputations occur in the diabetic patient (1). Each year, six of every 1,000 diabetic individuals undergo surgery for an amputation (2). Education of the diabetic patient and frequent foot examinations have been shown by Davidson et al. (2) to decrease the amputation rate by 50%. In spite of these hopeful statistics, Cohen et al. (4) found that 40% of patients entering the examination room wearing shoes did not receive specific foot examinations. Bailey et al. (5) found that patients who presented to the examining physician without shoes were three times more likely to have their feet examined. Thus, the first step to good diabetic foot care is the proper examination of patients barefoot (3).

PATHOGENESIS OF AMPUTATION

Diabetic patients are arbitrarily categorized into two groups: those with angiopathy and those with neuropathy. This is somewhat of a false division because most patients with diabetes have elements of both neuropathy and vascular disease. Many patients have predominant findings, however, and their pathology can be assigned into one of these two groups (Fig. 1). Angiopathy can be divided into two major groups: macrovascular disease (large vessel), and microvascular disease (small vessel). Small-vessel disease is distinct from those changes seen in the capillaries, including the thickened capillary basement membranes; it refers to disease of the smaller arteries of the foot and toes (4a).

Neuropathy, on the other hand, affects the foot in three different ways: involvement of the autonomic nervous system; loss of sensation; and involvement of motor nerves with subsequent foot deformity. Aberrant autonomic nervous system function decreases perspiration, which leads to dry, cracking, scaling, skin that may serve as a portal of entry for infection. In addition, involvement of the autonomic nervous system prevents the typical flare reaction that normally occurs with noxious stimuli. A normal flare reaction indicates an increased delivery of blood flow to the affected area, an effect that may be absent in the diabetic patient. Destruction of the sympathetic nerves in the foot may mimic an autosympathectomy with resultant

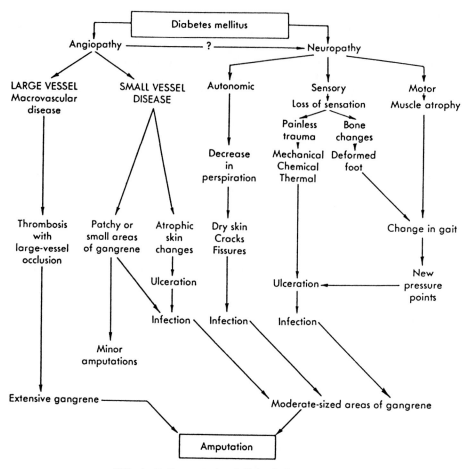

FIG. 1. Pathogenesis of diabetic foot lesions.

increase in blood flow. This increased flow can contribute to bone absorption and the development of the Charcot foot (6).

Insensitivity causes diabetic foot ulcers, which ultimately can lead to amputation. Ulcers resulting from insensitivity require hospitalization three times more often than those caused by vascular disease. The development of insensitivity has an insidious course. Patients may complain of pain as neuropathy develops, but they frequently will not complain of insensitivity. With the loss of protective sensation, relatively minor mechanical disturbances, such as bony prominences, small foreign objects within the shoe, areas of prominence in the lining of the shoe, wrinkles in the socks, or undue shear forces can cause local skin injury that is due to local ischemia (7). If this ischemia is prolonged, full thickness ulcers can be the result. Although these normal mechanical disturbances can occur in the normally sensate foot, they produce pain at least at a subconscious level, which causes the individual to correct the abnormality. Once an ulcer has formed, it continues to be painless and may persist for months and often longer. Infection is frequently the presenting complaint in a diabetic patient with a neuropathic foot ulcer.

These neuropathic ulcers are seen in other pathologic conditions that cause insensitivity, such as Tabes dorsalis, Hansen's disease, and myelomeningocele. Diabetic foot ulcers respond to medical treatment in an identical fashion to those ulcers caused by other forms of neuropathy.

Finally, the deformity that is the result of motor neuropathy causes a change in gait and produces new pressure points, which ultimately cause ulceration. Once infection develops in these ulcers, the final catalyst of events of major foot deformity, gangrene and amputation, is predictable (8). When peripheral vascular disease complicates neuropathy, the impaired delivery of antibiotics, oxygen, and nutrients may prevent healing. Loss of sensation may also lead to the changes consistent with Charcot foot. It is believed that this process is secondary to the repeated stress applied to an insensate foot (7). The most common focus of the Charcot changes is at the midtarsal joints where the metatarsals meet the tarsal bones on the medial side of the foot (3). Stress fractures at the navicular cuneiform and first metatarsal joint cause swelling and inflammation. Collapse of the weight-bearing support structures on the medial side lead to increased stress and eventual failure of the load-bearing bones in the middle and lateral parts of the foot. These changes occur in those diseases that produce insensitivity as well as in diabetes. The typical deformity that results in the Charcot foot is a loss of the longitudinal arch with a flattening of the foot and even a reserve arch or rocker bottom deformity (3). Other changes include dislocation of tarsal bones, which may cause ischemic pressure on the skin of the foot. The natural history of the Charcot foot in a weight-bearing individual leads to progressive foot deformity with ulceration over the predictable bony prominences.

OFFICE EXAMINATION

As has been previously noted, an adequate physical examination always begins with inspection. This inspection requires that the patient remove shoes and socks, a procedure that should be performed at every office visit. In patients with a history of peripheral vascular disease or neuropathy, these examinations should occur every 3–4 months. Signs of significant ischemia in the foot include the loss of hair on the dorsum of the foot and toes. Atrophic skin changes include a shiny appearance, and the patient often appears drawn because of the loss of subcutaneous fat.

Dependent rubor is indicative of severe peripheral vascular disease. This is also reflected by delayed capillary filling and is assessed by having the patient lay supine with the legs elevated at a 45° angle until the feet blanch (3). Then the patient sits in an upright position with the feet dangling. The time required for capillary filling is estimated in Table 1.

Muscular contractures in the diabetic foot are suggestive of neuropathic change. Neuropathic changes can frequently be suspected by the muscular contractures with which they are often associated. The foot may have a prominent heel or calcaneous

TABLE 1. *The estimated time required for capillary filling*

Capillary filling time on dependency
Normal: 10–15 sec
Moderate ischemia: 15–25 sec
Severe ischemia: 25–40 sec
Very severe ischemia: 40 + sec

pattern with an increased longitudinal arch and clawing of the toes. Presence of a plantar ulcer should certainly add to the suspicion of an insensate foot. In addition to inspection for large and obvious ulcers, care should be taken to examine between the toes. One must check for calluses on the weight-bearing areas and corns interdigitally or on the dorsum of the toes. Bruising or bleeding into or around the callus or corn can indicate impending ulceration. Attention should be paid to how the patient takes care of his or her feet. Specifically, the cleanliness of the shoes and socks and any "bathroom" surgery performed by the patient should be discouraged. The shoes should also be inspected for their adequacy in relieving areas of bony prominence and supporting the plantar surface of an insensate foot.

Inspection should include noting the condition of the skin. Dry skin can lead to cracking and possible fungal or bacterial infection. The nails should also be inspected noting any ingrowth, overgrowth, loose nails, exudative, or abnormal nails. Overgrown nails frequently indicate the inability of the patient to provide self-care due to a decreased range of motion in the joints, obesity, or poor vision.

PALPATION

Changes in the temperature of the skin are frequently the most sensitive and earliest alteration suggesting a pathologic condition (7). Simple palpation by the palm or back of the hand is sufficient to detect temperature changes of less than 1° C. In patients who have had previous deformity secondary to Charcot foot, the change in temperature alone is the most sensitive indicator of the course of the process. Those patients with persistent deformity and swelling with a cool extremity are managed conservatively; those with warmth frequently require emergent treatment.

Palpation of the pulses is critical and includes the femoral, popliteal, dorsalis pedis, and posterior tibial. Auscultation for bruits can also indicate the presence of atheromatous plaques and narrowing of the arterial lumen.

Gross swelling should be carefully palpated to rule out fluctuance and possible abscess formation versus pedal edema secondary to venous insufficiency or soft-tissue swelling secondary to injury, which would be accompanied by warmth and rubor. Crepitance may also be palpated in the presence of an occult fracture or ongoing Charcot change.

Sensory testing is best performed with a Simms-Weinstein monofilament[1] (9). Testing for sensation with an uncalibrated light touch, either with a finger, a brush, or even a needle, is insufficient in diagnosing the level of neuropathy in the diabetic foot. The Simms-Weinstein monofilaments have been calibrated and documented to show whether the patient has protective sensation. This level of sensation is critical in decision-making as to the patient's need for a protective shoe and prognosis for future foot problems. These monofilaments come in three different thicknesses, 4.17, 5.07, and 6.10. It is simply placed against the skin and applied until the filament buckles. The patient should be able to detect the presence of the monofilament before it buckles. The thickness of 5.07 is equal to 10 g of linear pressure and is the

---

[1]These monofilaments may be obtained from the Gillis W. Long Hansen's Disease Center, Nylon Monofilament Project, Carville, LA 70721.

limit used to determine protective sensation (9). According to Mueller et al. (10) if the patient can feel 80% of the trials with the 5.07 monofilament, protective sensation is intact.

Although a variety of sophisticated techniques is available for measurement of vibratory sense, a simple tuning fork with a 256 cycle is sufficient. This examination should include vibratory sense not only at the ankle, but at the tibia and the tip of the toes.

To determine the patients' ability to perceive temperature, testing small nerve fiber thermal sensitivity can also be carried out. Guy et al. (11) found that the lateral aspect of the foot was the most sensitive location for the measurement of thermal sensation. These authors noted loss of thermal sensation in all feet with neuropathic ulcerations and in those with Charcot changes. When thermal sensitivity was compared with vibratory perception threshold, thermal sensitivity was sometimes selectively affected, especially in those patients with painful neuropathy; this suggests that the small fibers are more vulnerable in the diabetic individual. Measurement of thermal sensation was made using a Mars Stock Stimulator (Somedic, Stockholm, Sweden), which consists of a metal plate through which a current of three amps is delivered. The patient presses a switch as soon as the plate is felt to be warm or cool. The current is then reversed to change the temperature. This device gives an objective and quantitative measure of temperature sensation (12). Using test tubes of cold and warm water, however, gives a simple quantitative and reasonable means of detecting thermal sensation.

LABORATORY TESTING

A simple hand-held Doppler is a relatively inexpensive and easy way to evaluate peripheral vascular status and can be performed in the office. Although absolute pressures are useful, the ratio of the ankle pressure compared with the brachial pressure is considered the standard. The ratio of the ankle pressure and brachial pressure should equal 1. An ankle/arm index below 0.9 indicates the presence of peripheral vascular disease, indices below 0.45 are indicative of severe peripheral vascular disease (13,14). These patients should be referred to a vascular surgeon. Because of the severe degree of calcification of the vessels frequently seen in diabetic patients, erroneously high ankle pressures may be noted in about 15% of cases (15,16). These patients should demonstrate nonelastic waveforms on their vascular study and the suspicion of vascular disease in these patients should be high despite an ankle/arm index of 1 or greater.

Loss of range of motion is a common physical finding in neuropathic feet (17). This loss of range of motion should be carefully documented as it can lead to bony prominences that may cause ulcer formation in the insensitive foot. Recognition of these bony prominences and this loss of motion allows the proper insoles, footwear, and prosthetic alterations to be fabricated (18).

Examination using x-rays is recommended for diabetic patients with a foot deformity as well as those patients with a history of ulcer formation, warmth, or swelling. The latter should be reviewed for deformities, Charcot changes, fractures, and osteomyelitis. The radiographic diagnosis of osteomyelitis can be somewhat troublesome as diabetic patients can also show periosteal changes secondary to neuropathy and stress reactions, which can often be confused with osteomyelitis. Nuclear medicine scans, such as bone scans, Technesium, and differential scans with Gallium can be helpful, as can Indium-labeled leukocyte scans.

Culturing open ulcers may be useful but can also be deceptive. Patients who have had ulcers for significant periods of time have colonization of an inordinate number of different bacterial species that may or may not be pathogens. The culturing of wounds is more critical in those patients who are exhibiting physical signs of overt infection, such as redness, warmth, swelling, or copious or foul-smelling exudate (19). These cultures may show a predominance of a pathologic organism and, therefore, are informative. Aerobic and anaerobic cultures must be taken. Bone biopsies may also be helpful, although their yield of an organism in a known case of osteomyelitis may be no greater than 50%. Biopsies can be obtained by percutaneous needle aspiration under sterile conditions or by open biopsy in the operating room through uncontaminated tissues.

TREATMENT

The treatment of patients with diabetic foot problems that are primarily the result of vascular insufficiency should be managed by the vascular surgeon. Recalcitrant ulcers frequently heal rapidly after revascularization if they are caused by lack of blood flow.

Diabetic patients who have foot problems due to neuropathy should be treated for their deformities, protected against further injury, and, in the future, screened for the potential causes of injury (20). An example of the history and physical examination performed in a screening clinic for neuropathic feet is shown in Fig. 2 (21).

SKIN CARE

Thickened callus and corns should be pared with a scalpel by a professional. Any bruising or bleeding into or around the callus or corn can indicate impending ulceration and requires immediate débridement. Patients can remove some of their corns and calluses by using an emery board (21), but should, however, be discouraged from using over-the-counter callus preparations as they can destroy normal tissue along with the hyperkeratotic areas. A real risk for the diabetic foot is home "bathroom" surgery or picking at nails and calluses. Substituting an emery board to smooth rough spots and reduce the calluses helps to modify this behavior (21). Shoes or orthotics should be adjusted to unweight the area of persistent callus formation combined with paring of the thickened callus (20).

Dry skin can be a source of cracking and potential skin infection (22). Patients should use an emollient daily or more often if necessary. Patients need to be instructed regarding the importance of checking their feet every day for cracks, sores, and foreign bodies as well as for temperature changes. Toenails are a frequent source of problems in the diabetic patient. Loose nails should be removed as they can cause damage to the nailbed and cause possible infection. Onychomycosis is also common in the diabetic patient. Overgrown nails should be trimmed frequently. A Dremmel sander can be used to reduce their size. Nails should be trimmed straight across and the sharp edges should be sanded with an emery board (Fig. 3A). The nails should not be rounded at the corners (Fig. 3B). The entire nail needs to be cut and nail

BARNES HOSPITAL
DIABETIC FOOT CENTER

Date:_____
Referring physician_____
Blood glucose_____
Presenting complaint_____
_____
_____

HISTORY

1. Diabetes: Onset_____ Control_____ Insulin_____ Oral agents_____
   Diet control_____
2. Significant medical complications_____
3. History of vascular disease: Claudication_____ Rest pain_____ Smoking_____
   Vascular studies_____ Surgery_____
4. Foot problems: Ulcers_____ When_____ Where_____
   Previous foot surgery_____
5. Footwear_____
6. Are shoes and socks clean?_____
7. Ambulation: Community_____ Household_____ Bed_____ Wheelchair_____
   Walker or crutches_____ (May be more than one)

PHYSICAL

Inspection

Condition of nails: Ingrown_____ Overgrown_____ Diseased_____ Missing_____

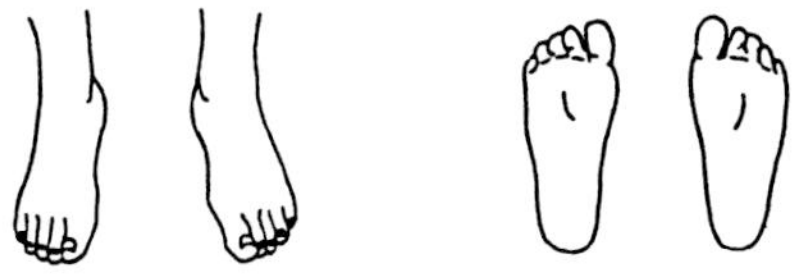

Label:
C = Calluses or corns
E = Erythema
T = Temperature (radiometer reading)
U = Ulceration
L = Skin lesions

DEFORMITY	R	L
Hammertoe/Clawtoe		
Bony prominences		
Rigid hallux		
Equinus		
Foot drop		
Partial foot resection		
Complete amputation		
Overlapping digits		

MUSCLE STRENGTH	R	L
Dorso flexion		
Plantar flexion		
Great toe extension		
Great toe flexion		
Inversion		
Eversion		

Vascular

Pulses: Right: POP_____ PT_____ DP_____ Left: POP_____ PT_____ DP_____
Atrophic skin changes_____ Rubor_____ Pallor_____
Capillary filling_____

FIG. 2. Example of history and physical examination performed in a screening clinic for neuropathetic feet. (*Figure continues.*)

Neurological

A.J._____ Joint position _____

K.J._____ Vibrations _____

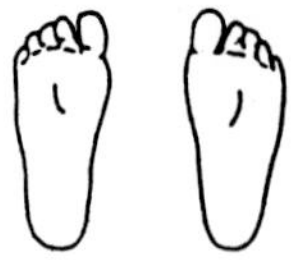

SENSORY LEVEL/MONOFILAMENT TEST	
1	4.17 (Mean + 5 for normal)
2	5.07 (Protective sensation)
3	6.10 (Loss of protective sensation)
4	> 6.10

Chart results on picture.

Gait: Limp_____ Antalgic_____ Broad based_____

ASSESSMENT

Plantar ulcer_____ Total contact casting_____ Dorsal ulcer_____

Protective shoes:_____ Other Rx_____

No ulcer risk category:

LEVEL	PROTECTIVE SENSATIONS	HISTORY OF ULCERS	FOOT DEFORMITY	CATEGORY	FOOTWEAR
0	Yes	No	Yes/No	0	Properly fitting shoes
1	No	No	Yes/No	1	Nonmolded insoles, extra-depth shoe
2	No	Yes	No	2	Molded insoles, extra-depth rocker shoes
3	No	Yes	Yes	3	Molded insoles, extra-depth rockers/custom shoes
4	No	No/Yes	Charcot's foot	4	Molded insoles, extra-depth rocker, or fabricated walker

CATEGORY	RETURN VISIT
1	1 year
2	6 months
3	3 months
4	1 month

PLAN

Follow-up diabetic foot center_____

Referral to: Medicine_____

              Metabolism_____

              Foot care_____

              Vascular_____

              Education_____ Films_____ Classes_____

              Private physician_____

Casting_____

Footwear_____

X-rays_____

NOTES:

_____
Assessor/Title

FIG. 2. *Continued*

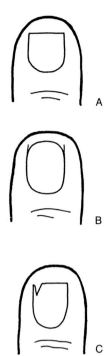

FIG. 3. Examples of proper toenail trimming (A) and improper trimming (B,C).

spicules left in the nail fold should be avoided as they can grow into the soft tissue as the nail grows out (Fig. 3C).

MALPERFORANS ULCER

Ulcers secondary to insensitivity with little or no vascular component are best treated by unweighting the affected area (18). Complete bedrest is essential because if the patient is allowed to assume a standing weight-bearing position even once daily, the ulcer will rarely heal. Many attempts at other forms of modified weight-bearing have been attempted including healing sandals and orthotics for shoes. These methods have had limited success but are generally unreliable. Total contact casting has been perhaps the most successful ambulatory method of healing neuropathic nonvascular ulcer formation (6,10,23).

A total contact cast is a rigid bandage that completely encompasses the foot from the knee to the toe. It is applied with very little padding so that weight-bearing forces are hydraulically shared under the majority of the surface area of the cast. This allows very little pressure to be placed on the area of the ulcer, which allows healing. Total contact casting has the advantage of predictable and rapid wound healing while allowing the patient to be ambulatory and generally functional. [Contrary to Mueller et al.'s findings (10), the disadvantage of a total contact cast is the potential for an infection to spread beneath the cast without being observed by the patient or the examiner.] Because the cast is applied with very little padding, bony prominences can cause new ulceration to occur in the insensitive foot. Even the removal of the cast can be somewhat difficult because the small amount of padding can cause frequent cast saw abrasions upon removal. The potential for infection means that care must be taken before casting to be sure the ulcer is stable and unlikely to become infected during the casting. Therefore, care must be taken in applying the total contact cast to protect bony prominences and caution must also be exercised when the cast is removed to protect the skin from cast saw abrasions (10).

Custom-molded braces may replace casts in the future for the treatment of neuropathic ulcers. These custom-molded braces can be quite expensive and poorly accommodate the changes in size of the extremity which is frequently seen during total contact casting. The first cast is usually changed within 5 days to 1 week of its application to be sure there is no further skin breakdown or undiagnosed infection. The ulcer is débrided of hyperkeratotic material about its edges and redressed prior to recasting. Second and third casts may be kept on for a longer period, up to 2 weeks if the patient tolerates the cast well. Most ulcers heal within a 6–8-week period. Contraindications to casting include skin problems, such as cracking and peeling of the skin, fungal infections, or vascular lesions (24). Overtly infected ulcers are also a contraindication to casting (10). Patients with ulcers may need to be hospitalized for complete total bedrest and antibiotic therapy. The ulcers are observed until it is certain that they are free of infection. Ulcers that are deeper than they are wide are also a relative contraindication to casting as they tend to seal over superficially, causing the potential for abscess formation. When casting patients for neuropathic ulcers it is a good idea to have the molds made for their custom-molded insole before the casting process is finished. There is frequently a lag of 1 or 2 weeks after the molds are made before the finished insole and extra-depth shoes are available. In that way, when the patient comes out of the final cast, shoes with custom-molded insoles will be ready.

PROPER FOOTWEAR

History and physical examination allow the patient to be categorized in prognostic groups (Table 2). Level 0 patients have normal protective sensation using Simms-Weinstein monofilaments and have had no history of ulcer formation on their feet. They have good pulses and a normal vascular examination otherwise. These patients are treated with properly fitting shoes and are discouraged from wearing high heels or shoes with restrictive, pointy toes.

Level 2 patients are those who have lost protective sensation, but have not yet

TABLE 2. *Prognostic groups for diabetic patients*

Level	Protective sensations	History of ulcers	Foot deformity	Category	Footwear	Return visit (months)
0	Yes	No	Yes/No	0	Properly fitting shoes	—
1	No	No	Yes/No	1	Nonmolded insoles, extra-depth shoe	12
2	No	Yes	No	2	Molded insoles, extra-depth rocker shoes	6
3	No	Yes	Yes	3	Molded insoles, extra-depth rockers/custom shoes	3
4	No	No/Yes	Charcot's foot	4	Molded insoles, extra-depth rocker, or fabricated walker	1

experienced skin breakdown or ulcer formation. Because of their loss of protective sensation, these patients need to have extra-depth shoes made to protect their forefoot as well as to provide enough room for a nonmolded foam orthotic. Custom-molded orthotics are preferable, but they tend to be more expensive.

Level 3 patients have loss of protective sensation and a history of ulcer formation. They do not, however, have a significant foot deformity that requires a custom-molded shoe. Once adequate ulcer healing has been achieved, these patients are placed in extra-depth shoes with custom-molded insoles. Because many of these ulcers are in the forefoot, it has been helpful to add rigid rocker bottom soles, which alleviate forefoot pressures. Patients with a history of an ulcer who also have foot deformity are categorized in Level 3 and usually require custom-molded shoes to protect the bony prominences that are the result of their foot deformity.

Finally, patients in Level 4 have Charcot changes in their foot that not only require a custom-molded shoe with custom-molded insoles, but require orthotic support of either the foot or ankle (21). Our custom-molded insoles are currently fabricated with semi-rigid foam products, such as Plastizote and Alizote, and are frequently backed with a close cell foam, such as PPT (18). These are heat molded from a positive mold allowing exact fit and adequate support. These insoles can collapse over a period of time and should be evaluated at least every 3 months to inspect for "bottoming out." Varus and valgus deformities at the heel and ankle can be accommodated with heel flares and posting of the orthotic. However, severe varus or valgus deformities usually require an ankle/foot orthosis incorporated in the shoe.

Diabetic patients who do not have insensitivity need information about proper footwear. A list of shoe stores in your city that have functional footwear and trained shoe fitters should be made available to assist patients in their search.

A functional shoe has a low heel and the toe box of the shoe completely covers the forefoot without cramping the toes (Fig. 4). The uppers should be made from leather or fabric. Man-made materials do not stretch or mold to the shape of the

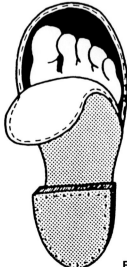

FIG. 4. Sample of functional shoe for diabetic foot.

foot. The soles of the shoes should be a soft material such as Vibram. Running or walking shoes (25) are excellent choices. Shoes should be purchased in the evening when the feet are larger, and should be comfortable when new so they do not have to be broken in. Patients should insist on having their feet measured each time they buy new shoes.

Shoes should be kept in good repair, as rundown heels or broken shoe contours change the weight-bearing forces in the foot, causing new pressure points. Torn lining or stitching can cause abrasions to the insensitive foot.

INJURY PREVENTION

Preventive care is the key to reducing the risk of major diabetic foot problems (4). Some factors to discuss with diabetic patients include not walking barefoot or in stocking feet because foreign bodies can puncture the foot, leading to infection. Hot water bottles, heating pads, or soaking the foot in hot water can quickly burn an insensitive foot without the patient being aware. Patients should be warned to test the temperatures of the bathwater first with their hand before immersing their feet. Avoiding exposure to the sun or using a high-factor sunscreen should be addressed. Caution patients to keep their feet warm and dry in cold weather to avoid frostbite. Patients should avoid warming their feet in front of the fire or with a space heater because of the potential for burns.

PROPHYLACTIC SURGERY

Prophylactic surgery on bony prominences and other disorders of the feet is usually contraindicated in the diabetic patient. Because these individuals have a propensity for infection and vascular complications, surgery should be reserved for those lesions that cannot be accommodated by custom shoe wear.

The demands of care for the diabetic foot are high. These patients require not only screening by vascular and orthopedic surgeons but constant examination and care by foot-care nurses, diabetes nurse practitioners, and educators. Most diabetic foot problems require the involvement of an orthotist. The use of total contact casting requires a physical therapist or specifically trained cast technician. We have found that the multispecialty approach in a diabetic foot center provides the patient with the most comprehensive foot care (21).

REFERENCES

1. Palumbo PJ, Melton LJ. Peripheral vascular disease and diabetes. In: *Diabetes in America*: Diabetes data compiled 1984. NIH pub. no. 85-1468. Washington, DC: U.S. Govt. Printing Office, 1985;1–21.
2. Bild DE, Selby JV, Sinnock P, Prowner WS, Braverman P, Showstack JA. Lower extremity amputation in people with diabetes. Epidemiology and prevention. *Diabetes Care* 1989;12:24–31.
3. Davidson JK, Alogna M, Goldsmith M, Borden J. Assessment of program effectiveness at Grady Memorial Hospital, Atlanta. In: Steiner G, Lawrence PA, eds. *Educating diabetic patients*. New York: Springer, 1981;329.
4. Cohen SJ. Potential barriers to diabetes care. *Diabetes Care* 1983;6:499–500.
4a. Levin ME. The diabetic foot: Pathophysiology, evaluation and treatment. In: Levin ME, O'Neal LW, eds. *The diabetic foot,* 4th ed. St. Louis: C.V. Mosby, 1988;1–50.
5. Bailey TS, Yu HM, Rayfield EJ. Patterns of foot examination in a diabetic clinic. *Am J Med* 1985;78:371–374.

6. Boulton AJM, Scarpello JHB, Ward JD. Venous oxygenation in the diabetic neuropathic foot: Evidence of arterial venous shunting. *Diabetologia* 1982;22:6–8.
7. Brand PW. Repetitive stress in the development of diabetic foot ulcer. In: Levin ME, O'Neal LW, eds. *The diabetic foot,* 4th ed. St. Louis: C.V. Mosby, 1988;83–90.
8. Taylor LM, Jr, Porter JM. The clinical course of diabetics who require emergent foot surgery because of infection or ischemia. *J Vasc Surg* 1987;6:454–459.
9. Birke JA, Sims DA. Plantar sensory threshold in the ulcerative foot. *Lepr Rev* 1986;57:261–267.
10. Mueller M, Diamond J, Sinacore D, et al. Total contact casting in treatment of diabetic plantar ulcers. *Diabetes Care* 1989;12:384–388.
11. Guy RJC, Clark CA, Malcolm PN, Watkins PJ. Evaluation of thermal and vibration sensation in diabetic neuropathy. *Diabetologia* 1985;28:131–137.
12. Fruhstorfer H, Lindblom U, Schmidt WG. Method for quantitive estimation of thermal thresholds in patients. *J Neurol Neurosurg Psychiatry* 1976;39:1071–1075.
13. Levin ME, Sicard GA. Evaluating and treating diabetic peripheral vascular disease, part I. *Clin Diabetes* 1987;62–70.
14. Levin ME, Sicard GA. Evaluating and treating diabetic peripheral vascular disease, part II. *Clin Diabetes* 1987;5:80–93.
15. Taylor LM, Jr, Porter JM. The clinical course of diabetics who require emergent foot surgery because of infection or ischemia. *J Vasc Surg* 1987;6:454–459.
16. LoGerfo FW, Gibbons GW. Ischemia in the diabetic foot: Modern concepts and management. *Clin Diabetes* 1989;7:72–74.
17. Mueller MJ, Diamond JE, Delitto A. Limited joint mobility, insensitivity and plantar ulcers in patients with diabetes. *Phys Ther* 1989;69:453–462.
18. Boulton AJM, Franks CI, Betts RP, Duckworth T, Ward JD. Reduction of abnormal foot pressures in diabetic neuropathy using a new polymer insole material. *Diabetes Care* 1984;7:42–46.
19. Little JR, Kobayashi GS. Infection of the diabetic foot. In: Levin ME, O'Neal LW, eds. *The diabetic foot* 4th ed. St. Louis: C.V. Mosby, 1988;104–118.
20. Edmonds ME, Blundell MP, Morris HE, et al. Improved survival of the diabetic foot: The role of a specialized foot clinic. *Q J Med* 1986;60:763–771.
21. Blair VP, Drury DA. Starting the diabetic foot center: In: Levin ME, O'Neal LW, eds. *The diabetic foot,* 4th ed. St. Louis: C.V. Mosby, 1988;342–350.
22. Jelinke JE, ed. *Diabetes and the skin.* Philadelphia: Lea and Febiger, 1985.
23. Boulton AJM, Bowker JH, Gadia M, et al. Use of plaster casts in the management of diabetic neuropathy foot ulcers. *Diabetes Care* 1986;9:149–152.
24. Sinacore DR. Total contact casting in the treatment of diabetic neuropathic ulcers. In: Levin ME, O'Neal LW, eds. *The diabetic foot,* 4th ed. St. Louis: C.V. Mosby, 1988;273–292.
25. Soulier SM. The prevention of plantar ulceration in the diabetic foot through the use of running shoes. *J Am Podiatr Med Assn* 1986;76(7):395–400.

Surgical Management of the Diabetic Patient,
edited by Michael Bergman and Gregorio A. Sicard.
Raven Press, Ltd., New York © 1991.

18

Diabetic Foot Management

*Brian Butler, †Kevin T. Jules, and †Michael J. Trepal

*Department of Medicine, New York Medical College, Valhalla, New York; and
Departments of *Community Medicine and †Surgical Sciences, New York College of
Podiatric Medicine, New York, New York 10035

Foot problems pose potential major complications for persons with diabetes. They are a major cause of diabetes-related morbidity and mortality (1). Diabetic persons are five times more susceptible to gangrene than the general population and approximately 15% of these cases eventually require amputation (1). Ablation of a limb has devastating implications for the diabetic individual. After amputation of a leg, two-thirds of diabetic patients will not be alive in 5 years (2). It is well established that diabetic neuropathy and diabetes-associated vascular disease predispose to injury and infection. Twenty percent of hospitalizations for diabetic patients are for foot-related conditions and these conditions require more in-hospital time than any other complication of diabetes (2). Fortunately, however, foot complications are not inevitable and are generally far more amenable to prevention through proper care than are other diabetes-related problems. Recent retrospective studies of foot-care programs at medical centers in London, England; Atlanta, Georgia; and Geneva, Switzerland, persuasively demonstrate that provision of foot-care services for vascularly compromised patients can significantly reduce utilization of labor-intensive health-care services. Lower extremity amputation (LEA) rates at Atlanta's Grady Memorial Hospital dropped by 50% annually when comprehensive podiatric services were provided for diabetic patients. The LEA rate at London's King's College Hospital dropped by 44% over a 2-year period when comprehensive podiatric services were provided for diabetic patients, and at the University of Geneva the LEA rate dropped by 85% over a 4-year period after "patient education and training in foot care was instituted for those with diabetes." (3).

The prevalence of foot problems is high. A British study noted that in an acute-care facility, 94 of 100 patients examined had three or four foot problems ranging from dystrophic toenails to ulcers, five patients had toe deformities only, and one patient had no foot problems (4). Macroscopic surveys indicate that more than ten million Americans suffer from soft-tissue complaints and static foot deformities (5). Rothenberg has estimated the prevalence of foot problems over a person's lifetime at 100% (5). Today, the need for diabetic foot care is appreciated and a "strong consensus exists for the critical role of the podiatrist in caring for diabetics." (5) Although there may be some overlap in the care provided by podiatrists and other specialists, the volume and focus of foot treatment that is provided differ markedly. "In comparing aggregate visits to podiatrists with visits to (other physicians) for soft tissue disease and static foot deformities, the ratio is 6:1." (5) Only 1 to 2% of outpatient visits to other physicians are for foot problems (5). "Furthermore, in the specific case of orthopedic physicians, foot problems per se were not identifiable as one of the ten most common principal diagnoses rendered" (5).

The human foot is both a complex anatomical structure and a biomechanical wonder. Fifty-two of the 208 bones in the human body are in the feet and with each step gravity-induced pressure of three to six times total body weight must be carried by the feet (6). As the foot contacts the ground, it adapts to a variety of surfaces by pronating. The foot then supinates into a rigid lever in order to be ready to propel itself off the ground. Because of its complicated structure and function, the foot is vulnerable to a variety of medical conditions. Inadequate treatment of a foot problem in a diabetic person can result in ruinous consequences for the patient. A simple hyperkeratotic lesion over a bony prominence can ulcerate, become infected, and lead to cellulitis before the patient is aware that there is a problem. Studies of diabetic patients undergoing amputation of the leg report a hospital mortality rate of 23%, with only 61% of these patients surviving 3 years after the first amputation (7).

Although treatment of an ischemic foot differs from that of the neurotrophic foot, the diabetic foot does not occur as an isolated neurologic or vascular complication. Both ischemic and neurologic complications are associated in the diabetic foot and the incidence of all complications, including retinopathy, nephropathy, and coronary artery disease, increases with the duration of the diabetes. (2). A multiplicity of clinical factors places the diabetic foot at risk. Vascular, neurotrophic, skeletal, cutaneous, and biomechanical factors expose the diabetic foot to ischemic, thermal, mechanical, and frictional trauma. Because of the dimunition of tissue oxygenation and proprioceptive sensation secondary to large-vessel disease, small-vessel disease, and neuropathy (2), the diabetic foot is particularly vulnerable to the concomitant hazards of ulceration. Infected ulcers can extend and lead to cellulitis, osteomyelitis, and sepsis. Apparently trivial conditions if not evaluated and treated can precipitate a fulminant infection. Prompt, safe, and definitive podiatric therapy is, therefore, an essential component of total management of the diabetic patient.

Wagner's diabetic foot grading system Grade 0 to Grade 5 is helpful in organizing a therapeutic approach to diabetes-related foot problems (8). The Grade 0 diabetic foot has intact skin. There are no open lesions but the appearance of the foot can vary from a supple, well-hydrated healthy foot, to a dyshydrotic foot with multiple osseous deformities and nonpalpable pulses, to a partially amputated foot with no evidence of ulceration. The feet of an early diabetic person have normal sensation and circulation and generally respond to infection and injury like those of a nondiabetic individual. As the disease progresses, the patient's vascular and neurologic status begins to deteriorate. It is unusual to find patients with long-term diabetes who do not have evidence of neuropathy (2). Neuropathy involving the small, intrinsic muscles of the feet ultimately causes contracture and deviation of the toes. Vascular lesions are two to three times more common in patients with neuropathy (2). The primary therapeutic aim for the Grade 0 foot consists of conservative management. Regularly scheduled podiatric evaluations are indicated for the diabetic patient. Palliative débridement and padding of hyperkeratotic lesions, which can ultimately ulcerate, and skillful onychodébridement of dystrophic and onychocryptotic toenails is a service not to be underestimated. In addition, the patient's gait biomechanics should be evaluated and attention should be directed to balancing the feet and redistributing body weight to ensure tissue viability at points of osseous pressure. Orthotic prosthetic therapy is of fundamental importance in rectifying problematic gait patterns. As proprioception deteriorates, Charcot-type joint changes begin. For this less dynamic foot type, molded shoes should be utilized. Because of hereditary predisposition and diabetes-related intrinsic foot musculature imbalance, the diabetic patient frequently evidences ingrown toe nails, hammer toes, plantarflexed metatarsals, tailor's bunions, hallux valgus, and exostoses at various sites on the feet. Because these abnormalities can lead to a break in the skin, prophylactic surgical intervention should be considered. All too often these deformities are ignored as they are well tolerated. With the passage of time, these foot abnormalities generally become more symptomatic. Later, the patient's condition may have deteriorated and the patient may then be a poor surgical risk. Although the type and extent of surgical treatment in the foot may be modified by complications in other organs, definitive podiatric surgical intervention for nail, toe, and foot abnormalities should be attempted when the patient is best able to tolerate surgery (9). If the foot is ischemic, podiatric surgery should not be considered until after successful revascularization. Doppler "toe-arm" indices of 0.70 or higher can predict healing with a high degree of success with local foot surgery (7). The aim of all diabetic foot care is to sustain the diabetic foot at Grade 0.

The Grade 1 diabetic foot is characterized by a superficial ulceration that does not penetrate completely through the dermis and is not infected. There are two types of ulcers: ischemic and neurotrophic. The presentation and management of ischemic and neurotrophic ulcers differ. Ischemic ulcers can be found anywhere on the foot. Eschars may be evident with surrounding hyperemia. There is usually no significant hyperkeratosis. These lesions are painful and will become quickly infected if not treated early. Although good wound care is essential in the management of any ulcer, a high index of suspicion must be maintained in dealing with dysvascular lesions. Débridement of the ischemic lesion reveals deeper fibrotic ischemic tissue. Ischemic ulcers are highly resistant to treatment. A vascular consult is indicated, as there may be no improvement until the foot is revascularized. Total contact casts are contraindicated in the treatment of ischemic ulcers (7). The neurotrophic ulcer is associated with chronic pressure patterns. These lesions are painless and generally hyperkeratotic. Débridement of these keratotic lesions is indicated to allow granulation and epithelization. The neurotrophic lesion invariably bleeds with aggressive débridement. Weight dispersal is of paramount importance. In treating deeper neurotrophic ulcers, total contact casting is recommended. Unless an uncontrolled infection is present, neurotrophic lesions have a good prognosis for healing (7).

The Grade 2 diabetic foot indicates a deep infected ulcer with the possible exposure of tendon and bone. Débridement and drainage of all abscesses should be performed as early as possible. Appropriate cultures should be taken and antibiotic coverage should be initiated. The only contraindication to débridement and drainage of an infected ulcer is gangrene or an infection so extensive that the initial therapy should be amputation (2). If the lesion is ischemic, a vascular consult should be requested to determine whether revascularization is required. If vascularity is adequate, therapy consists of antibiosis, débridement, padding, dressing changes, and contact-cast therapy. Throughout the management of this condition, an acute awareness must be maintained of the volatile nature of a diabetic infection; within an amazingly brief period of time, a clinically controlled diabetic infection can become a fulminant infection (11).

Although anatomical structures in and near the superficial transverse ligament form natural barriers to infection, a furtively infective diabetic microangiopathy can destroy these anatomic barriers and permit the spread of infection along structures that would normally retard the spread of infection (2). In addition to narrowing of the blood vessels, two specific microcirculatory abnormalities are also associated with diabetes: decreased red-cell flexibility and increased blood viscosity (12). Thrombotic occlusion in the blood vessels immediately adjoining an infection site is common. In normal blood vessels this process only occurs at the margin of the infection. After control of the infection, these tissues recanalize and form granulation tissue. In the diabetic, a vascular predisposition can exaggerate this occlusive process so that the infection can expand to ever-enlarging areas of necrosis. This can be further exaggerated by multiple segmental arteriosclerotic blockades causing an end-artery situation to develop in the diabetic foot (2). When the end-artery is occluded, there is no way to compensate for its function and the tissue supplied by the artery dies. Ideal glucose control can correct these abnormalities; however, glucose levels do fluctuate and diabetic patients remain constantly at risk. Radiographs of the Grade 2 foot may evidence osteolysis. This condition can be caused by physiologic resorption of bone or by osteomyelitis.

Charcot osteoarthropathy is a progressive, painless, destructive disorder that primarily involves the foot and ankle. The onset of Charcot osteoarthropathy is the result of a combination of neurotraumatic and neurovascular events that subject bone to fracture and joint damage. A major study conducted at the Joslin Diabetes Center noted that the most frequent location of Charcot foot involvement was at the level of the tarsal-metatarsal joints followed by the metatarsalphalangeal joints (14). Bone cultures should be taken to differentiate the Charcot-type condition from osteomyelitis. If osteomyelitis is diagnosed, this condition should be treated vigorously. If a Charcot-type condition is diagnosed, the possibility of ostectomies or joint fusions should be entertained once the infection is controlled and the foot is in a latent stage. With conservative care Grade 2 ulcers can close (14). Should conservative care prove ineffectual, however, bone excision and grafting procedures can be utilized to achieve wound closure.

The Grade 3 diabetic foot differs from Grade 2 by the presence of localized cellulitis, edema, and warmth. The infectious process of the Grade 3 diabetic foot may include a midfoot fascial plane infection as well as deep abscess formation and septic tracts to the level of bone resulting in necrotizing fasciitis, osteomyelitis, gas gangrene, and synergistic necrotizing cellulitis. Hospital admission with initiation of parenteral antibiotics is indicated. Baseline radiographs should be ordered to rule out osseous involvement as well as the presence of gas in soft tissues. Nuclear medicine scans using Technetium (^{99m}Tc) and Gallium-67 Citrate (Ga-67) permit better assessment of the vascular status of the foot, osteoblastic function, and degree of inflammatory activity (15). The use of Indium-111 white blood cell scans (In-111 WBC) is being evaluated for use in differentiating osteomyelitis from Charcot osteoarthropathy, and Magnetic Resonance Imaging is being used to differentiate soft-tissue and osseous pathology in the diabetic foot.

Siegel, investigating the objective prognosis in the healing of foot ulcers, utilized ^{99m}Tc Macroaggregated Albumin (^{99m}Tc MAA), to contrast healthy tissue patterns of blood flow with pathologic states and found that ulcers that healed without amputation demonstrated hyperemia in the vicinity of the ulcer bed. Ninety percent of ulcers that healed with conservative therapy had 3.5 times the blood delivery as compared with the uninvolved tissues of the same foot. Ulcers that did not demonstrate this level of hyperemia required amputations 90% of the time (15). This prognosticator of healing prevents unnecessary amputations. It also helps to delineate which patients require hyperbaric oxygen therapy or chemoneurolysis of sympathetic ganglia to promote oxygenation and blood flow to an affected extremity (15). Thallium-201 (Tl-201) intravenous technique can be used to obtain the same information as the ^{99m}Tc MAA arterial injection technique. With Tl-201, the ratio of ulcer bed to uninvolved soft-tissue activity is less than or equal to 1.5.

Nuclear medicine techniques are highly sensitive but their specificity is less than optimum. To effectively use these techniques, a close correlation of clinical and radiographic findings is necessary (16). Drainage and débridement of dysvascular tissue should be accomplished as quickly as possible. Appropriate deep bacterial cultures should be taken and vigilance maintained for the possibility of extending sinus tracts and dissecting tissue planes. Sinus tracts must be irrigated and left open. Sequestrae and devitalized tissue must be surgically excised. Parenteral antibiotics are continued until microbiologic studies are negative and laboratory parameters have returned to normal. Closure is usually accomplished by secondary intention although primary closure of a clean wound may be possible. Should this not be possible, split thickness skin grafts can be used when the bacterial count falls below 10 × 5 organisms/g of tissue (17). In managing a Grade 3 diabetic foot, the patient's best interest is served by a coordinated health-care team effort to attempt to restore the foot to Grade 0.

The Grade 4 diabetic foot involves frank forefoot gangrene. Gangrene mandates amputation of the compromised body part at an appropriate level. Every effort should be made to preserve as much of the foot as is functional. However, the chances of salvaging a Grade 4 foot are markedly reduced in the presence of vascular insufficiency. There is a greater potential for failure and higher level amputation is usually indicated. Revascularization before amputation can limit the extent of surgery. Toe amputation, ray resection, and transmetatarsal amputation are more conservative procedures and should be considered before a more radical amputation is performed. Those patients who do tolerate localized amputations of the foot need to be followed postoperatively with shoe gear that compensates for the amputated body part and allows for both static and propulsive activity. Gait training should start as soon as possible and attention should also be directed to preserving intact the non-involved foot.

The Grade 5 diabetic foot is a gangrenous foot and requires amputation at the ankle or higher. Patients with adequate vascular status and gangrene only in the forefoot are possible candidates for a Syme's amputation or ankle disarticulation. Other patients require above-knee or below-knee amputation. Because of the high mortality rate subsequent to amputation, aggressive postoperative follow-up by the diabetes health-care team is indicated. Rehabilitation and prosthetic gait training should be initiated expeditiously (18). The remaining extremity frequently becomes compromised and undergoes a similar fate shortly following the initial amputation (18).

The importance of diabetic foot management is underscored by the fact that the total number of diabetic persons in the United States is increasing as medical advances continue to expand their overall life span. Unfortunately, with age, the susceptibility to foot pathology increases. Despite significant improvement in the medical management of the diabetic patient, their neurotrophic and vascular problems persist (16).

Proper treatment of the diabetic foot, therefore, has important implications both for saving limbs and returning ambulation and independence to the patient.

REFERENCES

1. Olsen CL, et al. Delivery of podiatric care to persons with diabetes in New York State. *NY State J Med* 1982;1041.
2. Levin ME, O'Neal LW. *The diabetic foot*. St Louis: C.V. Mosby, 1977;196.
3. Bild DE, Selby JV, Sinnock D, et al. Lower-extremity amputation in people with diabetes, epidemiology and prevention. *Diabetes Care* 1989;12:24–31.
4. Ebrahim SB, et al. Foot problems of the elderly. *Br Med J.* 1981;283:949–950.
5. Rothenberg R. Podiatry's role in health care, it's time to examine the shibboleths. *Postgrad Med* 1983;73:201.
6. Graham JL. A Mayo Clinic podiatrist reviews the most commonly diagnosed—and most commonly misdiagnosed—diabetic foot problems. *Transition* 1984;39.
7. Sage R, Doyle, D. Surgical treatment of diabetic ulcers: A review of forty-eight cases. *J Foot Surg* 1984;23:102.
8. Wagner FW. Orthopedic rehabilitation of the dysvascular limb. *Ortho Clin North Am* 1978;9:325–349.
9. Greteman B. Digital amputations in neurotrophic feet. *J Am Podiatr Med Assoc* 1990;80:120–126.
10. Sanders L. Amputations in the diabetic foot. *Clin Podiatr Med Surg* 1984;4:481–502.
11. LoGero FW. Coffman JD. Vascular and microvascular disease of the foot in diabetes. *N Engl J Med* 311, No 25, 1984;311:1615–1618.
12. Chren S. Determinants of blood viscosity and red cell deformability. Abstracts, 6, International Symposium on Filterability and Red Blood Cell Deformability, Goteberg, Sweden, Sept 11–13, 1980.
13. Lowe, GDO, et al. Blood and plasma viscosity in prediction of venous thombosis. International Symposium on Filterability and Red Blood Cell Deformability, Goteberg, Sweden, Sept 11–13, 1980;77.
14. Frykberg RG. Osteoarthropathy. *Clin Podiatr Med Surg* 1987;4:351.
15. Hartshorne MF Peters V. Nuclear medicine applications for the diabetic foot. *Clin Podiatr Med Surg* 1987;4:361–372.
16. Shenaq SM. Diabetic foot ulcers. *Postgrad Med* 1989;85:328.
17. Calhoun JH, et al. Treatment of diabetic foot infections, Wagner Classification, Therapy, and outcome. *Foot Ankle* 1988;9:104.
18. Helfand AE. Preventing diabetic foot problems, rehabilitation of the foot. *Clin Podiatr Med Surg* August, 1984;1:343–351.

Surgical Management of the Diabetic Patient,
edited by Michael Bergman and Gregorio A. Sicard.
Raven Press, Ltd., New York © 1991.

19

Vascular Surgery

Peter B. Alden and Gregorio A. Sicard

Department of Surgery, Washington University School of Medicine,
St. Louis, Missouri 63110

There is a strong tendency towards accelerated atherosclerosis in diabetic patients. The vascular surgeon is thus frequently called upon to evaluate and treat the diabetic patient with peripheral vascular disease. Some degree of occlusive arterial disease is seen in all diabetic patients, but it becomes more prevalent with increasing age (1,2). The incidence has been estimated to be 15% at 10 years and 45%, after 20 years from the initial diagnosis. Progressive vascular disease is a major factor in the increased mortality and morbidity of diabetic patients.

So-called "microvascular" disease is often described in diabetes and is implicated in the pathogenesis of foot ulcers, even in the presence of palpable pedal pulses. This concept was advanced by Goldenberg in 1959 (3), who described lesions of intimal hyperplasia that stained periodic acid-Schiff (PAS) positive but negative for colloidal iron in the arterioles of amputated lower extremities of diabetic patients. This was then touted as a specific variant of atherosclerosis, which is unique to diabetic patients. Similar lesions in the glomeruli and retinae of diabetic patients had been described earlier (4,5). Subsequent investigators, however, were unable to confirm or duplicate Goldenberg's findings in the peripheral arteries of the feet. Strandness et al. (6) studied 42 diabetic and 35 nondiabetic patients with basic clinical assessment and noninvasive vascular testing. Approximately one-half of each group underwent lower extremity amputation and histologic study of the specimen. No evidence of physiologic or histologic abnormalities implicating a diabetic arteriolar lesion was found, thus casting further doubt on Goldenberg's findings. Likewise, a study by Conrad (7), in which casts of the vessels of amputated extremities were made by injection of acrylic plastic, showed no propensity for small-vessel occlusive disease in diabetic patients. Goldenberg also described thickening of capillary basement membranes in skin and muscle. Subsequent studies confirmed basement membrane thickening in muscle (8), but not in skin (9). There may be functional abnormalities in capillaries of diabetic patients. For instance, the movement of albumin through the capillary into the interstitium is increased (10). Despite conflicting data, there is no solid evidence to support the concept of *arteriolar occlusive* disease in the extremities of diabetic patients.

Sensory and motor neuropathy, as well as depressed host resistance to infection, appear to be the main factors that promote soft-tissue destruction and gangrenous changes in the diabetic foot (11). The sensory neuropathy allows repeated excessive mechanical stresses in the insensate foot. The motor neuropathy affecting the intrin-

sic muscles of the foot creates a "claw foot" deformity where weight is borne principally upon the metatarsal heads. This promotes localized pressure and callous formation, which in turn leads to trophic ulcers. Once an ulcer forms, adequate blood
flow is necessary for healing to occur. Usually, good foot care allows healing without
the need for invasive vascular treatment (see Chapter 17, Diabetic Foot Care). In
those situations in which a critical proximal arterial occlusion exists, pedal blood
flow must be increased by surgical bypass or percutaneous transluminal angioplasty
if ulcer healing is to occur.

   Although the concept of diabetic arteriolar obstructive disease is questioned, there
are aspects of diabetic large-vessel disease that are unique. The pattern of disease
affecting diabetic patients is different from that of the general population of atherosclerotic patients. Generally, only very elderly nondiabetic individuals (8th or 9th
decade) manifest a pattern of distal disease similar to that seen in patients with diabetes. Diabetic patients have a propensity for disease in the infrapopliteal vessels of
the legs (6). In a large study of the results of arterial reconstruction, 20% of the total
patients were diabetic, but they were disproportionally represented in the group with
distal disease (12). Only 10% of all aortoiliac occlusive patients had diabetes, and
35% of all of the patients with tibial artery disease were diabetic (Fig. 1). Disease of

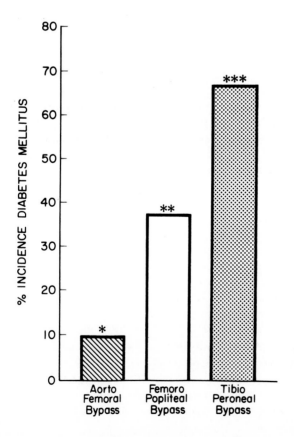

FIG. 1. Incidence of diabetes in
selected reports of peripheral arterial bypass procedures. *references 13–17; **references 18–
22; ***references 23–29. From
Levin ME, O'Neal LW. *The diabetic foot.* St. Louis, CV Mosby,
1977;165 with permission.

the small digital arteries of the hand and foot is a problem seen more commonly in insulin-dependent diabetes with other complications, including renal failure (30). These patients may require amputations in spite of normal peripheral pulses and in the absence of repetitive trauma. The incidence of aneurysmal disease does not increase in diabetic patients. In a large series, only 3% of 441 patients with an abdominal aortic aneurysm had diabetes (31). These data confirm the fact that peripheral vascular disease that requires revascularization surgery is mainly infrainguinal and most commonly infrapopliteal.

DIAGNOSIS

The clinical evaluation of the diabetic patient with peripheral vascular disease is made simpler by knowledge of the most common anatomic disease patterns, as well as the consideration of concomitant problems of sensory and motor neuropathy. Thus, the surgeon learns to expect infragenicular occlusive disease in the diabetic patient with a mal perforans ulcer and no pulses palpable below the femoral artery. Nonetheless, it is important to screen for the presence of aortoiliac occlusive disease in each patient, as this might influence the approach to arteriography (in cases with significant renal impairment) as well as therapeutic options.

In general, patients with peripheral vascular disease present with ischemic ulceration or gangrene, rest pain, or claudication. In diabetic patients, the symptoms of rest pain or claudication may be altered or erased by neuropathy. In the noninsulin-dependent diabetic patient with minimal neuropathy, however, these symptoms still remain a reliable marker of peripheral vascular occlusive disease.

Intermittent claudication is usually described by the patient as a muscular cramping pain induced by exercise and promptly relieved by rest. It is not necessary to lie or sit to obtain this relief, and relief usually occurs in 2 to 3 minutes. Other causes of leg pain with ambulation that my be confused with intermittent claudication include degenerative arthritis of the spine, hips, and knees, neuritis, and venous claudication. These are collectively referred to as pseudoclaudication symptoms. The symptoms of spinal stenosis with lumbosacral plexopathy mimic the symptoms of claudication due to aortoiliac disease more closely than other pseudoclaudication symptoms. Noninvasive vascular testing and spinal computerized tomography (CT) or magnetic resonance imaging (MRI) can help clarify the diagnosis. Diabetic patients with marked neuropathy may experience their claudication as leg weakness ("my leg goes out on me") rather than pain and this may, at times, make diagnosis confusing.

The symptoms of claudication may give a reasonable indication of the level of arterial blockage. Thus, cramping and tiredness in the buttocks is associated with aortic occlusion or aortoiliac occlusive disease. In men, this may be associated with impotence due to decreased internal iliac blood flow; in diabetic patients, however, impotence may result from other causes. Calf claudication suggests superficial femoral artery blockage. Foot cramping with ambulation is uncommon, usually because of the frequently associated neuropathy. When present, however, it can be a manifestation of infrapopliteal arterial occlusive disease.

As the severity of claudication increases and the patient's ability to walk distances becomes shorter and shorter, other symptoms may become manifest. The patient may begin to complain of foot numbness, night pain, and later, rest pain, ischemic ulcers, or gangrene. Nighttime numbness and foot pain (frequently stocking-like in nature) are common complaints. As the blood pressure drops during sleep, collateral blood flow to the foot decreases. This severe burning pain in the toes and forefoot often wakes the patient. The patient gets relief not from further rest, as in intermittent claudication, but by walking a few steps or dangling the foot in a dependent position. This presumably elevates the blood pressure, thus adequately supplying enough blood through collateral vessels to the feet. The patient may demonstrate unilateral leg edema, which is secondary not to venous thrombosis, but instead due to prolonged dependency in an effort to relieve rest pain. The symptoms of rest pain, persistent numbness, painful ulcers, and gangrene are all indicative of severe involvement of the large- and intermediate-size vessels and should be promptly investigated. A thorough and complete physical examination is important in the assessment of the degree of vascular involvement in the diabetic patient. Examination of the extracranial carotid artery may detect a thrill or a bruit, either of which would indicate the need for further evaluation of the cerebral circulation. The presence of hypertension, cardiomegaly, or heart failure indicates severe cardiovascular involvement.

Palpation and auscultation of the abdomen may detect an asymptomatic abdominal aortic aneurysm or bruits associated with visceral renal or iliac occlusive disease. Careful evaluation of the extremities can often pinpoint the site of most vascular occlusive involvement. The absence of femoral pulses indicates aortoiliac occlusive disease, which, though less common than distal disease in diabetic patients, should always be sought because it is often easily treated. Palpation of popliteal, posterior tibial, and dorsalis pedis pulses determines the extent of the peripheral occlusive disease. Although uncommon, but occasionally a weak pedal pulse may be palpated even in the presence of an occluded superficial femoral artery, which indicates well-developed collateral blood flow. In diabetic patients, careful inspection of the feet is important. Sensory changes should be noted. The presence of erythematous pressure points, ischemic ulcers, neuropathic ulcers (mal perforans ulcers), gangrenous toes, callouses, and hypertrophic nails can provide important information regarding the degree of vascular or neuropathic involvement of the extremity. Cyanosis and rubor of the feet may indicate arterial insufficiency. It is not specific for patients with arterial disease as these features may also be seen in patients with venous disease. Cyanosis and rubor are more indicative of arterial insufficiency when unilateral. Dependent rubor is the result of arteriolar vasodilation secondary to chronic ischemia.

In the diabetic patient with a mal perforans ulcer, any hint of arterial insufficiency should be investigated. Although neuropathy does contribute to the development of ulcers and gangrenous changes in diabetic feet, the combination of small- and large-vessel disease is probably responsible for the increased frequency of limb loss. Before débriding ulcers or performing small amputations in diabetic patients, further objective assessment of the pedal circulation is recommended. The first step is to obtain noninvasive segmental lower extremity pressures and waveforms. These lower extremity pressures and waveforms usually include the femoral, popliteal, posterior tibial, and dorsalis pedis arteries. Toe pressures and waveforms are important, specifically in the diabetic patient with toe ulcerations. If significant arterial occlusive disease is demonstrated in the femoral, popliteal, or tibial vessels, arteriography is indicated to better assess the possible need for revascularization prior or concomitant to surgery on the foot.

Noninvasive Diagnostic Techniques

Once peripheral vascular disease is suspected on the basis of history and physical examination, the next step is usually noninvasive vascular testing. The most widely used modality is the measurement of segmental lower extremity blood pressures and analysis of arterial Doppler waveforms. The use of treadmill testing can help differentiate those patients with claudication from those with arthritis or spinal stenosis. Systolic blood pressures measured at various levels at the lower extremities correlate well with plethysmographic measurements of blood flow. The use of a strain-gauge manometer, which measures pulse volume displacement, or standard auscultation with the Doppler probe below a cuff are both acceptable. Use of the Doppler is less cumbersome and is more widely used. Correlation between the two methods is good (32).

Pressures are measured in both arms, high thigh, above the knee, below the knee, and at the ankle. Arterial obstruction results in a fall in pressures measured by cuffs placed below the level of the obstruction. Ankle pressure is measured in both the dorsalis pedis (anterior tibial) and posterior tibial arteries. The higher ankle pressure compared with the higher arm pressure in a ratio known as the ankle/arm index (AAI) or ankle brachial index (ABI). A normal AAI equals 1.0. Rest pain and/or gangrene are frequently seen with AAIs less than 0.4. Obstruction at the iliofemoral level may be detected by a fall in the high-thigh pressure, but often this may be falsely elevated in limbs of large diameter. Analysis of the analogue tracing of the femoral Doppler waveforms can identify iliofemoral occlusive disease. The normal arterial waveform is triphasic with a brisk forward flow in systole, a brief flow reversal early in diastole, and smaller forward flow in late diastole. This triphasic wave is blunted in the presence of upstream occlusive disease.

Extensive medial calcification develops in the arteries of some diabetic patients. Although discussed in another chapter, it is nonetheless worthwhile indicating that when a cuff is inflated on such a vessel, it will not collapse. This leads to a false elevation of the segmental pressures, even in the face of arterial occlusive disease (33). Pressures measured in severely calcified, rigid vessels are in excess of 300 mm Hg. In general, diabetic patients tend to have increased foot pressures compared with nondiabetic individuals, and this is particularly true of those who have had the disease for more than 10 years (34). Qualitative analysis of Doppler waveforms can be helpful in the diabetic patient with falsely elevated segmental pressures (Fig. 2). Some of the most difficult problems in noninvasive assessment of diabetic patients arise not when vessels are completely incompressible, but when vessels are marginally less compressible. The meaning of segmental pressures may be very difficult to assess under such circumstances. In this case, evaluation of the waveform is very useful (Fig. 3).

Another technique that is useful for noninvasive assessment of the peripheral vascular system in the presence of incompressible arteries is the measurement of toe pressures. Small cuffs have been designed for measurement of toe pressures and the quantitative assessment can be performed (32) by photoplethysmography or strain-gauge plethysmography. A toe brachial index (TBI) is calculated in a manner analogous to calculation of the AAI. Toe pressures are not falsely elevated in the presence of arterial calcification unless the digital arteries themselves are calcified. The TBI correlates well with clinical assessment (claudication versus threatened limb) even in the presence of incompressible arteries. The degree of small-vessel disease

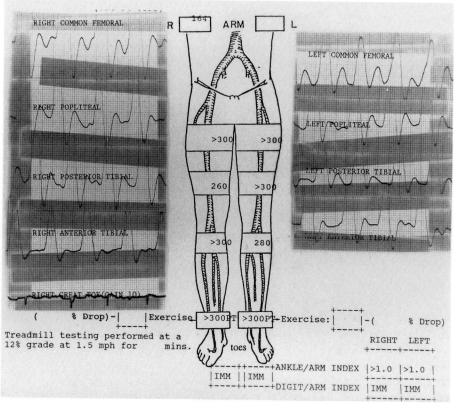

FIG. 2. Lower extremity segmental arterial pressures and Doppler waveforms in diabetic patient with incompressible vessels and small-vessel disease. Note normal Doppler waveforms down through the anterior and posterior tibial vessels. The right great toe waveforms are flat and toe pressure is not detectable (patient had a previous left transmetatarsal amputation). Compare with toe pressure waveforms in Fig. 3.

can be quantitated by comparing ankle and toe pressures and expressing this as a toe/ankle index. A normal range for the toe/ankle index is 0.55 or greater (35).

Several studies have correlated amputation healing with toe pressures. Data from these studies may be extrapolated to predict healing of foot ulcers and the need for arteriography and revascularization. Although there is some variability in the data, it appears that toe pressures in the range of 25 to 45 mm Hg are associated with successful primary healing of toe amputations. Therefore, in patients with ischemic ulcerations and toe pressures below this range, surgical correction of proximal obstructive lesions should be considered (see Chapter 22 on Amputation).

Other techniques have been described in the assessment of the degree of ischemia, but are not as widely utilized as the segmental pressure and Doppler waveform analyses. Intradermal xenon-111 washout was highly touted as a predictor of critical ischemia and primary amputation healing (36,37). The techinque is cumbersome, however, and initial enthusiasm has substantially diminished in subsequent reports (38). The transcutaneous measurement of PO_2 has shown great promise in multiple studies as a predictor of primary amputation healing (38–41). Because oxygen delivery to tissues is a primary metabolic determinant to healing, $TcPO_2$ is a logical parameter to measure. The transcutaneous oxygen electrode is fixed to the skin with

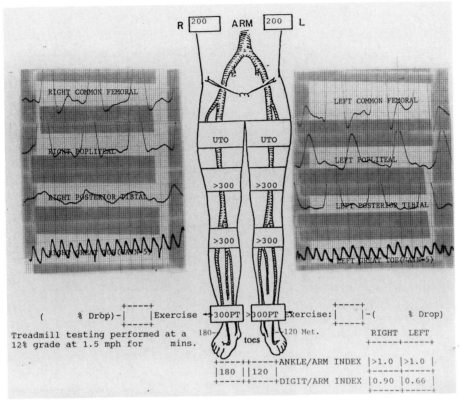

FIG. 3. Lower extremity segmental arterial pressures and Doppler waveforms in diabetic patient with imcompressible vessels. Note that pressures at all levels are in excess of 300 mm Hg. The right posterior tibial Doppler waveform is damped, indicating occlusive disease in this vessel.

an adhesive ring. A thermistor raises the skin temperature to approximately 45°C, causing capillary dilatation, increased blood flow, and diffusion of oxygen to the skin surface where it is electrochemically reduced to allow quantification of PO_2. A sensor is placed on the chest or upper arm as a reference; additional sensors are placed on the dorsum of the foot, or below the knee, depending on the level of amputation planned. The sensors can be placed adjacent to ulcers to predict the success of healing without surgical revascularization. Measurements can be taken supine or with the foot elevated to determine the contribution of large-vessel arterial disease to $TcPO_2$ abnormalities. There is a reasonable consensus from several studies that amputations or ulcers with adjacent $TcPO_2$s of less than 20–30 mm Hg have a poor prognosis for healing; however, above this level the prognosis is good (39–41). The test appears to be a more accurate predictor of healing when results are expressed as an index of the $TcPO_2$ below the knee divided by the $TcPO_2$ measured over the biceps brachialis (40). In Kram et al.'s study (23), six of six patients with a PO_2 index ≤ 0.20 failed to heal below knee amputations. Thirty-three of 34 patients with PO_2 indices > 0.20 healed primarily. $TcPO_2$ measurements may be particularly helpful in diabetic patients with incompressible vessels and unreliable segmental lower extremity pressures. Hauser and associates (42) reported on the use of this technique in the limbs of 64 diabetic patients. They showed that $TcPO_2$ measurements had a higher accuracy than ankle/brachial pressures indices, pulse volume recordings, and toe pulse reappearance time. These investigators recommended TcPO$_2$ as the initial noninvasive diagnostic procedure of choice in patients with severe lower extremity ischemia.

One other finding regarding diabetic patients is that the TcPO$_2$ in feet with ulcers or gangrene tends to be higher than in nondiabetics. Presumably this reflects the other factors promoting gangrene in diabetic patients, such as neuropathy, trauma, and poor host resistance to infection (43). Again, the technique may help define the subgroup of diabetic patients with ulcers who need angiography and vascular reconstruction to achieve ulcer healing, or before they undergo extensive débridement or amputation.

Angiography

With a combination of clinical skills and noninvasive testing, a subgroup of diabetic patients emerges in whom lower extremity angiography is appropriate. In addition to the risks of local complications, (e.g., hematoma, thrombosis, pseudoaneurysm, and arteriovenous fistula) there are the potential systemic problems of allergic contrast reaction and renal failure (44). This last complication is of particular significance in the diabetic patient.

In a survey of 83,000 procedures performed in 5,114 hospitals, the incidence of local puncture site complications was 0.47% for angiography using the femoral approach (44). Local complications are more frequent with the transaxillary approach. Allergic contrast reactions are classified on the basis of severity as minor, intermediate, or major. Minor non-life-threatening reactions include headache, chills, vomiting, hives, and edema. Major, life-threatening reactions include bronchospasm, laryngeal edema, convulsions, and severe hypotension. It is estimated that major reactions occur with a frequency of about one in 1,000 infusions of intravenous contrast (45,46). In Hessel's survey, the incidence of laryngeal edema was 0.04% (44). Nonionic contrast media have been introduced relatively recently and it is hoped that such dyes will decrease the incidence of allergic reactions. Kinnison et al. (47) reviewed 45 randomized trials of nonionic versus ionic contrast agents and found no significant difference in life-threatening reactions. Other nonrandomized trials, however, have shown a decrease in adverse reactions with nonionic agents (48). The high cost of these agents mandates selective usage (49). In a patient with a history of a contrast reaction, pretreatment with prednisone and antihistamines is recommended (50,51). We generally use 50 mg of prednisone by mouth (po) every 8 hours for 3 doses, plus 50 mg of diphenhydramine intramuscularly, 1 hour before angiography.

The incidence of renal dysfunction after administration of iodinated contrast medium is increased in diabetic patients and those with underlying renal insufficiency; the combination of the two is worse than either condition alone (52,53). Parfrey et al. (54) reported an incidence of renal dysfunction associated with *intravenous* (iv) contrast administration of 8.8% in diabetics with preexisting renal dysfunction and 2.4% in diabetic patients without renal insufficiency. The frequency of renal dysfunction is obviously affected by how renal insufficiency is defined in these studies. Nonetheless, recent studies indicate a lower risk of renal insufficiency than previously reported. The incidence of renal failure after arteriography appears higher than that associated with iv contrast. In unselected patients, a rate of 7–12% has been reported (55–57). In all of these series, diabetes and/or preexisting renal failure insufficiency substantially increased the risks of renal failure. Preangiography hydration (58–60) as well as limiting the contrast dose administered (60)[1] are both important measures that decrease the risk of contrast-induced nephropathy. Thus, virtually all of our diabetic patients receive intravenous fluids before angiography. We also administer 12.5–25.0 g mannitol iv just before giving contrast in most diabetics. This osmotic agent induces brisk diuresis, which facilitates urinary dye excretion. In addition, its free radical scavenger properties (6) may limit renal injury. Finally, nonionic contrast is preferentially used in diabetic patients. Even though evidence of a decreased incidence of contrast-induced neuropathy with nonionic dyes is lacking (62), there are many theoretical reasons it should be less nephrotoxic (63). Saline hydration and/or mannitol must be used cautiously, especially in patients with diminished cardiac reserve or history of congestive heart failure.

If the creatinine level rises after angiography, we try to maintain a good urinary output with fluids and diuretics as necessary. The response to diuretics may separate patients with mild from those with severe renal injury. Even though there is no evidence of an actual therapeutic benefit from diuretics in this situation, management is simplified by maintenance, if good urine flow is maintained. Fortunately, the vast majority of cases of contrast-related nephropathy do correct spontaneously, with the incidence of permanent renal failure requiring dialysis ranging from 0–0.8% (52,54). Another way to reduce dye load in high-risk patients undergoing angiography is to use digital subtraction techniques. Intravenous digital studies involve a large volume of contrast injection and yield relatively low-quality images. The intraarterial digital subtraction method, however, uses smaller contrast volumes and currently is the preferred method for imaging vessels below the knee.

MEDICAL MANAGEMENT

Once the diagnosis of significant peripheral vascular disease is made, one must decide whether it is appropriate to obtain an angiogram. This decision hinges on whether or not one believes the symptoms warrant any intervention. The indications for intervention are variable. No one debates the appropriateness of revascularization or angioplasty for rest pain or ischemic gangrene. The appropriate treatment for a claudicator however, is more problematic. The point at which claudication becomes truly disabling is subject to debate. Furthermore, one can reasonably question whether more mild claudication should be followed conservatively or be treated with semi-invasive techniques such as balloon angioplasty. The decision of whether or not to proceed to angiography can only be made by thorough and frank discussion of the situation with the patient. In the patient with simple, intermittent claudication of mild degree, angiography should not be obtained simply because of the fear that the disease could progress to gangrene. In nondiabetic patients it has been shown often that stable, intermittent claudication, in general, does not portend gangrene or amputation (64–66). Boyd (64) followed 1,440 patients with intermittent claudication

---

[1]A practical formula for limiting the dye dose has been suggested by Cigarroa. The formula is:

$$\text{contrast material limit} = \frac{5 \text{ ml contrast/kg/bw}}{\text{serum creatinine/mg/dl}}$$

Maximum 300 ml of contrast. This formula is for Renografin-76, which contains 66% meglumine diatrizoate, 10% sodium diatrizoate, and 370 mg/ml iodine.

and found an amputation rate of 7.2% and 12.2% at 5 and 10 years, respectively. McAllister (67) followed 100 patients with intermittent claudication for an average of 6 years and found an amputation rate of 7%. Interestingly, six of the seven patients (86%) who required amputation were diabetic (67). Furthermore, in 82% of the patients, the claudicatory symptoms either improved or remained stable during the follow-up period. Similarly, in the study by Imparato and collaborators (65), 79% of the patients with claudication improved or remained stable with an exercise program. Thus, in most patients with mild to moderate claudication, conservative management seems the most prudent course of action. On the other hand, in diabetic patients with moderate to severe claudication who demonstrate marked peripheral vascular disease progression over a short period of time or those who have significant neuropathy, prompt and aggressive evaluation is the correct course. The physician should obtain noninvasive lower extremity vascular studies to document the extent of disease and should strongly advise that the patient quit smoking. Patients often have the impression that exercise to the point of pain further damages their circulation, which, of course, is completely counter to the truth. Exercise to the point of tolerance enhances the development of collaterals. Control of glucose, cholesterol, and triglyceride levels may slow progression of the disease. Meticulous foot care with daily inspections, bathing, and application of moisturizing lotion to prevent drying and cracking of the skin, is crucial for diabetic individuals. Furthermore, the patient should understand that continued follow-up is necessary and, should their condition deteriorate, intervention may be necessary. The patient must clearly understand that any lesion on the foot, regardless of how trivial, should be evaluated by a physician. The physician, likewise, must understand that any abrasion, blister, or crack can lead to a loss of limb because of the combined problems of neuropathy, poor wound healing, and poor resistance to infection in the presence of impaired tissue perfusion. Although it is reasonable to treat mild claudication conservatively, any sign of progressive symptoms should probably be investigated in the diabetic individual because of the strong propensity for accelerated atherosclerosis (68). Investigators have noted that it is frequently possible to intervene and correct a stenosis prior to complete occlusion using angiographic techniques, and thereby avoid or at least postpone bypass operations in this high-risk subset of patients (67).

Although vasodilators have never been demonstrated to be effective in claudication, new agents that improve the deformability of red blood cells have been shown to be effective in some patients with mild to moderate claudication (69). Pentoxifylline is the only agent currently available in the United States. It acts to increase red blood cell membrane fluidity and thereby improve the flow of blood through small collaterals by enhancing the deformability of the red cell. It is not the appropriate therapy for limb-threatening ischemia.

SURGICAL MANAGEMENT

Once angiogram information is available, decisions need to be made regarding intervention, assuming that the reasons for obtaining an angiogram were valid. In this section, surgical options are considered, as well as invasive radiologic options [e.g., percutaneous transluminal angioplasty (PTA)]. More often than not, these two modalities are complementary rather than competitive. The discussion of surgical treatment is divided into three main anatomic regions: aortoiliac, femoropopliteal, and infrapopliteal. As previously mentioned, the patterns of atherosclerotic disease in diabetic patients are different from those without diabetes. Aortoiliac occlusive disease is less common in diabetic than in nondiabetic patients with peripheral vascular disease. Conversely, infrapopliteal or combined superficial femoral artery disease with infrapopliteal obstruction is more common in diabetic than in nondiabetic patients.

Aortoiliac Disease

Although isolated aortoiliac occlusive disease occurs less frequently in diabetic patients than in nondiabetic patients with arteriosclerosis obliterans, it is important to identify such disease because it radically effects treatment. Classically, thigh and buttock claudication, impotence, and diminished femoral pulses with bruits characterize the patient with Leriche's syndrome that is due to aortoiliac occlusive disease. Some patients, however, will only experience calf claudication. Limb-threatening ischemia is not typically seen with isolated aortoiliac disease because of the effective and usually extensive collateral blood supply that is seen in these patients. If severe ischemia is seen, tandem distal lesions are usually present. Segmental arterial pressures as well as exercise (treadmill) and femoral Doppler waveform analysis help identify aortoiliac occlusive disease. Noncontrast "scout" films can be useful in assessing the degree of vascular calcification that may affect the therapeutic options (Fig. 4). Multiplanar arteriography and measurement of pressure gradients across

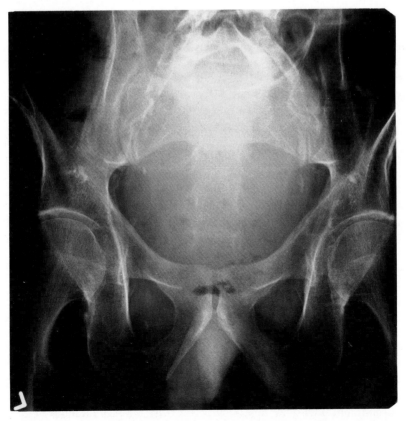

FIG. 4. Extensive iliac and femoral arterial calcification in diabetic patient.

stenotic lesions at the time of angiogram are helpful in assessing the hemodynamic significance of the lesion(s).

A variety of options is available for the treatment of aortoiliac occlusive disease. The appropriate approach in any given patient depends upon age, general health, cardiac status, and the nature of the lesions on angiography.

Nonsurgical Invasive Options

Of the options available, percutaneous transluminal balloon angioplasty (PTA) is the easiest on the patient in terms of morbidity, length of hospital stay, disability, and cost (70). The mechanism of successful PTA depends upon cracking of the diseased intima with separation from the media so that, in effect, the result is a localized dissection. The media then distends under the pressure of flowing blood and carries the broken intima with it outward (71). The best results of this modality are seen in the iliac arteries, as compared with more distal sites (72). Short segment stenoses are best suited to PTA and good, long-term patency can be achieved (73). Occlusions that can be crossed with a guidewire are also suitable for PTA (74). Long-segment stenoses or occlusions (i.e., > 4cm) and multiple stenoses in series, are better managed by surgical reconstruction, when this is possible (73). Concentric narrowings respond better to PTA than eccentric plaques (74). Atherectomy devices, such as the Simpson catheter, intuitively seem better suited than balloon angioplasty for these eccentric plaques, but more data are necessary to assess the efficacy of this modality (75,76). Lasers are popular subjects in the lay press, and are heavily advertised. For the most part, however, it has not been demonstrated that these devices offer a significant advantage over conventional balloon angioplasty and/or atherectomy (77).

Overall, the durability of iliac PTA is probably inferior to direct surgical reconstruction (78). The series that judges success by the absence of symptoms tends to overestimate success (79); on the other hand, those whose criteria for success are hemodynamic measurements (i.e., AAI), give lower patency rates (80). Multiple studies have shown higher patency rates when the indication for PTA is claudication as opposed to limb salvage (73,81). This discrepancy is also seen with surgical reconstruction. A larger review of multiple reports of iliac PTA (2,697 procedures) showed an average 2-year patency rate of 81% and a 5-year patency rate of 72% (74). Several studies have documented a negative effect of diabetes on long-term patency (72,73), but this has not been the most important factor in overall patency.

The complications of PTA have been reviewed by Weibull et al. (82). In their series, the 30-day periprocedural mortality was 2.2%, with septic complications accounting for a surprising 5.5%. Other potential problems include renal dysfunction and vessel perforation or thrombosis, which requires urgent surgery.

Use of PTA should be limited to patients with suitable lesions. If diffuse disease is present, direct surgical reconstruction is preferable, if, from a medical standpoint, the patient is a suitable candidate for surgery. There is a tendency among some clinicians, in an effort to avoid surgery, to use PTA even when a lesion is not angiographically suitable. This often simply subjects the patient to the combined risk of angioplasty and the inevitable direct surgical reconstruction. Furthermore, progression of disease after failed angioplasty can limit surgical options or make reconstruction more difficult. Thus, the best results are most often obtained by close consultation between the radiologist and the vascular surgeon working in collaboration rather than in competition.

Surgical Options

Direct surgical options for aortoiliac disease include aortoiliac or aortobifemoral grafting procedures and a variety of endarterectomy procedures. As mentioned above, these procedures are applicable to a wider variety of lesions and are generally more durable than PTA. As expected, morbidity and mortality rates are greater with direct aortic reconstruction. Operations that require aortic cross-clamping can induce marked and sudden shifts in cardiac dynamics with changes in myocardial blood flow, particularly with coexistent coronary artery disease. Reports from several large centers have shown an approximate 6% risk of perioperative myocardial infarction, with 20–50% of those being fatal (84–86). Nonetheless, with modern anesthetic management in properly selected patients, aortic procedures can be performed safely. Aortobifemoral bypass graft is the most commonly used surgical approach to aortoiliac occlusive disease. The 5- and 10-year patency rates for aortofemoral grafting procedures from selected series are summarized in Table 1. On average, an 80–90% patency rate at 5 years and a 70% rate at 10 years can be expected (16,86–90). Progression of the disease in the vessels distal to the bypass accounts for most of the late failures. In addition to the cardiac risk, there is other potential morbidity associated with grafting, including wound complications and graft infection. The infection of a vascular prosthesis in the aortic position is a devastating event; fortunately this occurs in only about 1% of all procedures (90).

An alternative to prosthetic bypass grafting is aortoiliac endarterectomy. This is infrequently used in many centers, probably because of the increased technical complexity to endarterectomy as compared with bypass grafting. Aortoiliac endarterectomy has the advantage of avoiding the use of prosthetics, and patency rates are comparable to those achieved with aortofemoral grafting, as evidenced by the Barnes Hospital series reported by Butcher and Jaffe (91). These authors reported a 5-year patency rate of 84% for nondiabetic patients and 70% for diabetic patients. Operations on the aorta and iliac can be performed either by the transperitoneal (i.e., midline incision) route or the retroperitoneal approach. There is some controversy as to which approach is better. A recent prospective study of these two approaches from the Massachusetts General Hospital showed no difference in morbidity rates

TABLE 1. *Aortoiliofemoral graft patency rates*

Authors	Year reported	Number of patients	Operative mortality (%)	Functional success	
				5 years (%)	10 years (%)
Malone, et al. (87)	1975	180	2.5	82	66
Brewster, et al. (88)	1978	406	1.1	88	74
Nevelsteen, et al. (16)	1980	352	5.1	80	62
Crawford, et al. (86)	1981	949	3.8	87	79
King, et al. (89)	1983	79	4.8	79	—
Szilagyi, et al. (90)	1986	1,647	5.0	85	80
Total		3,613	4.1	85	77

between the two (92); in a retrospective study from Barnes Hospital, however, operative time was similar and postoperative ileus and hospital stay were reduced with the retroperitoneal approach (93). Nevelsteen and coworkers (94), in a randomized trial comparing both of these surgical approaches to aortic surgery, found reduced pulmonary complications with the retroperitoneal approach. We tend to favor this approach for the more debilitated patient, believing that fluid shifts, ileus, and discomfort are reduced by staying out of the peritoneum. The retroperitoneal approach is also favored any time a suprarenal clamp is anticipated, because excellent exposure of the suprarenal aorta can be achieved with this approach.

The final alternative to PTA, or direct correction of aortoiliac disease, is extraanatomic bypass grafting. For unilateral iliac occlusive disease with a normal contralateral iliac and femoral artery, femorofemoral bypass can be used. With bilateral aortoiliac disease, the axillary artery can be used for inflow in construction of an axillobifemoral bypass graft. The advantage of these grafts is that aortic cross-clamping is avoided and body cavities are not entered. They are therefore appropriate in patients with prohibitive medical risks for general anesthesia. Although patency rates approaching those of direct aortobifemoral bypass grafting have been reported (95), the experience has not been as favorable for Rutherford and associates (96), who seem to agree that these grafts tend to thrombose, but are frequently salvageable with secondary procedures. Poor patency rates of unilateral axillofemoral grafts can be markedly improved by adding a femorofemoral bypass, thereby increasing the run-off (97). The quality of the native run-off vessels also seems important. With a patent recipient superficial femoral artery, 5-year patency rates of approximately 70% are achieved, compared with 35% when run-off is via the profunda femoris alone (96). Because of inferior long-term patency of extraanatomical bypass, we limit this surgical option to the high-risk patient who cannot tolerate aortic cross-clamping.

As mentioned above, isolated aortoiliac occlusion is relatively infrequent in diabetic patients, although calcification of the aortoiliac vessels is not infrequent (Fig. 4). When aortoiliac stenotic lesions are seen, they are usually in conjunction with infrainguinal disease, most often superficial femoral artery occlusion or stenosis. Occasionally it is difficult to determine whether the iliac or the infrainguinal disease, or both, should be reconstructed. A time-honored dictum in vascular surgery is "fix the inflow first" (i.e., correct the upstream lesions first). If the inflow disease is suitable for PTA, this should be done before considering distal reconstruction. Analysis of femoral Doppler waveforms before and after exercise can give qualitative information on the hemodynamics of an iliac occlusion as well (98). When there is mild aortic bifurcation disease angiographically, it may be difficult to judge the hemodynamic significance. Measurement of pressure gradients at the time of angiogram may be helpful. A significant (i.e., 30 mm Hg) increase in pressure gradient across the lesion with injection of a vasodilator such as Papaverine, indicates that it is hemodynamically significant (98,99). In the majority (60–80%) of patients with combined aortoiliac and femoropopliteal occlusive disease, correction of the inflow obstruction can relieve most symptoms (100). During the recovery period, the hemodynamic and functional results can be assessed noninvasively and the patients followed symptomatically. In cases of critical ischemia (i.e., gangrene) with a unilateral iliac occlusion, we often perform an iliac endarterectomy through a low, limited retroperitoneal exposure in combination with a femoropopliteal or femoral distal saphenous vein bypass. The retroperitoneal incision seems to have limited morbidity and the patients recover much as they would from a simple femoropopliteal bypass.

Femoropopliteal Disease

Femoropopliteal disease is, unfortunately, often seen in conjunction with trifurcation occlusions in the diabetic patient. The most common symptom of isolated femoropopliteal occlusive disease is calf claudication. As discussed above, this condition is certainly not limb threatening and therefore most cases can be followed medically with an excercise program and cessation of smoking. The decision to perform arteriography in this group of patients must be made on the basis of how a given patient's symptoms affect their lifestyle. The advent of PTA has changed the indications for angiography in patients with superficial femoral artery obstruction determined by noninvasive Doppler studies. Patients with incapacitating claudication should undergo arteriography and if a lesion amendable to PTA is found, this should be considered as the initial therapy (101). The characteristics of the lesion, such as length, eccentricity, and focal or diffuse nature of the disease, influence PTA's success in the superficial femoral artery (81). Lesions less than 4–6 cm in length can be dilated with high initial success rates and 4-year patency of 60–70% (102,103). Segments longer than 7 cm can be dilated, but at 6 months, the patency is only 23% (104). A prospective randomized VA cooperative study compared the results of PTA and surgery for iliac and superficial femoral artery lesions deemed suitable for therapy by both radiologists and vascular surgeons. The durability of superficial femoral PTA was equivalent to that of surgical reconstruction, 59 versus 70% at 4 years, respectively (101). Thus, if a patient has a suitable lesion, PTA should be attempted first.

The presence of diabetes has a negative impact on femoral PTA results. Gallino et al. (80), reported long-term success rates of 42% in diabetic patients and 68% in nondiabetic patients. Presumably, this difference is related to the presence of infratrifurcation disease in diabetic patients, as well as accelerated disease progression.

For longer segment superficial femoral artery occlusions, femoropopliteal bypass grafting is the procedure of choice. The distal anastomosis of the graft is placed above or below the knee, depending on the angiographic appearance of the popliteal artery, as well as the surgeon's assessment of the popliteal artery in the operating room.

The "gold standard" is the use of autogenous saphenous vein graft. This may be reversed or left *in situ* with the valves rendered incompetent. If the vein is unsuitable or unavailable, a prosthetic graft such as polytetrafluoroethylene (PTFE, Goretex) can be used. When the distal anastomosis is above the knee, PTFE performs very well. The multicenter prospective randomized trial of PTFE versus saphenous vein for femoropopliteal bypass reported in 1986 (105) showed no significant difference in patency after 4 years, when the distal anastomosis was above the knee. However, the curves began to diverge after two years. The patency rates for reverse saphenous vein femoropopliteal bypasses are not affected by the location of the distal anastomosis (above knee versus below knee) (106–108). Two-year patency rates for reverse saphenous vein femoropopliteal bypasses range from 61–86% with the 5-year patency rates ranging from 57–72%. Short- and long-term patency results from several large series of reverse saphenous vein femoropopliteal bypass grafts are summarized in Table 2.

In contradistinction to vein, PTFE does not perform well when anastomosed to the below the knee popliteal level and beyond. In the same multicenter trial, PTFE and vein patency rates for femoral below-knee popliteal bypass were statistically equivalent at 2 years, but not at 4 years. Thus, PTFE is a reasonable choice when the saphenous vein is absent, unusable, or when life expectancy is short in a patient with significant ischemia of the lower extremities. It is also a reasonable choice when one wishes to save the vein for anticipated subsequent operations, such as coronary artery bypass or more distal reconstruction (107).

Arm veins can be used for infragenicular reconstructions, with some groups reporting results comparable to those achieved with saphenous vein (111). Human umbilical vein grafts perform as well as or better than PTFE (112,113), but they are prone to aneurysm formation and are technically difficult to work with. Thus, they have not achieved the popularity of PTFE.

When operating on a patient with severe lower extremity claudication due to femoropopliteal disease, one should consider the consequences of graft failure. There are data that support (22,114) and refute (115) the concept that the amputation level will be higher if a femoropopliteal graft fails as compared with the level where no graft is performed. We believe that as long as the operation does not in any way damage the profunda femoris artery, which is the most important source of collateral to the popliteal and infrapopliteal arterial tree, a failed graft should not alter the level of amputation. We recommend an aggressive approach to the diabetic patient with significant lower extremity vascular insufficiency, with less than one block calf claudication and with an ankle/arm index of 0.3 or less, especially if there has been a rapid progression of symptoms over a 6-month follow-up. Our philosophy is based on the well-known aggressive nature of diabetic atherosclerosis, especially in the neuropathic patient who may not manifest rest pain. It is extremely important to avoid cutaneous ulcers and the morbidity associated with them. Thus, in patients whose symptoms and noninvasive studies suggest advanced disease, early intervention to maintain satisfactory blood flow should be considered.

The durability of femoropopliteal bypass grafts in diabetic and nondiabetic patients is similar (22,105,110) so that diabetes is in no way detrimental to reconstruction results when compared with nondiabetic patients. The overall life expectancy

TABLE 2. *Patency rates of reversed saphenous vein femoropopliteal bypass grafts*

Authors	Year reported	Number of patients	Patency 2 years (%)	Patency 5 years (%)	Patency 10 years (%)
Darling & Linton (19)	1972	345	82	72	54
DeWeese and Rob (109)	1977	103	61	58	45
Szilagyi, et al. (22)	1979	364	66	56	45
Reichle, et al. (21)	1979	310	67	60	54
Codd, et al. (18)	1979	308	67	57	55
Taylor, et al. (108)	1986	239	86	—	—
Veith, et al. (105)	1986	147	81	68	—
Rafferty, et al. (110)	1987	227	84	65	—
Total		2,043	74	62	51

of these patients is limited. For example, overall survival of a group of patients undergoing arterial constructions was 50% at 5 years in a large Australian series (12). In that same series, diabetic patients with clinical myocardial ischemia had a 5-year survival rate of less than 40%. These factors enter into the decision as to what type of graft to utilize and at what stage in the patient's disease one should intervene.

Infrapopliteal Disease

Disease in the tibial and peroneal arteries accounts for much limb loss in diabetic patients (Figs. 5,6,7). The reintroduction by Leather and coworkers (116) of the *in situ* saphenous vein grafting technique has revolutionized the treatment of infragenicular atherosclerosis. The saphenous vein is left in its bed, the valves are incised intraluminally to render them incompetent, and side branches are ligated. There is controversy as to whether the *in situ* technique is truly superior to conventional reverse saphenous vein bypass (117,118). Nonetheless, the *in situ* technique is in

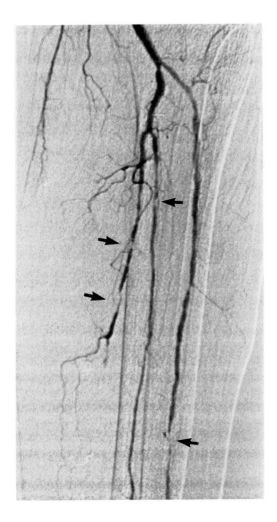

FIG. 5. Severe atherosclerotic change in the infrapopliteal vessels of a diabetic (digital subtraction arteriogram). Note multiple levels of stenosis and obstruction (arrows).

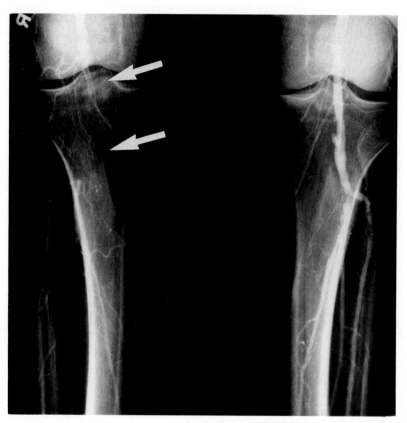

FIG. 6. Arteriogram from a patient with nonhealing mal perforans ulcer, right foot. Note occlusion of distal popliteal and proximal trifurcation vessels in the right leg (arrows).

wider use than reverse vein for tibial bypass. Putative advantages of the *in situ* technique are greater vein utilization, better size match of vein and artery at the distal anastomosis, and decreased endothelial ischemia. Meticulous technique is of paramount importance, with magnifying loupes and microvascular instruments used routinely.

Bypass to the distal vessels should be reserved for patients with ischemia that is truly limb threatening, rather than those with claudication (Figs. 8,9). The anterior and posterior tibial vessels are more easily exposed and in some series have more favorable patency rates as an outflow tract than the peroneal artery (25,27). If there is satisfactory collateralization between the peroneal and an intact pedal arch, good results can then be expected (25,119).

The patency rates of *in situ* infragenicular bypasses are excellent, with 2-year and 5-year patency rates of 80–90% and 70–80% reported (24,117–120). Table 3 summarizes results from several series. The length of the bypass does not appear to influence patency (121). Diabetes by itself has no deleterious effects on the patency of the bypass (120). In diabetic patients with disease limited to segments below the knee, the popliteal artery can be used for the inflow with excellent results (28,29). The introduction of digital subtraction arteriography allows for exact visualization

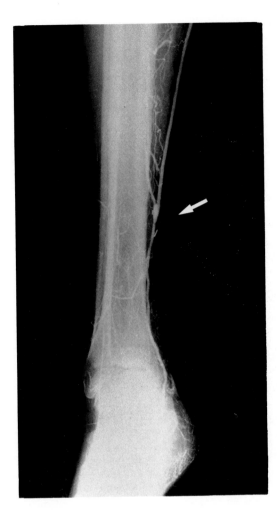

FIG. 7. Intraoperative (completion) arteriogram of a femoroposterior tibial *in situ* saphenous vein bypass (arrow).

of pedal arteries, which in selected cases may be used for plantar bypasses (Figs. 8,9). Andros and coworkers reported a patency rate of 73% at three years in 20 patients undergoing bypass grafts to the lateral plantar artery (122).

The patterns of failure in femoropopliteal and femoral distal bypass are illuminating. In general, there are three steps on the patency curves. Some grafts are lost in the first 30 postoperative days. Generally, thrombosis at such time is due to a technical error. Another subset of grafts thrombose in the first 6 to 12 months with neointimal hyperplasia at the anastomosis usually responsible for the failure. After 1 year, the patency curves become flatter with a steady attrition rate from progression of atherosclerosis, mainly in the distal native vessel(s). A routine follow-up program of noninvasive testing, including bypass graft velocity determination, can be useful in identifying lesions that may lead to graft thrombosis. Identification and correction of lesions before thrombosis occurs can help prolong graft patency (117,123).

A second lesson learned from examination of the patterns of graft failure is that limb salvage rates are usually 15–20% higher than graft patency rates. A healing

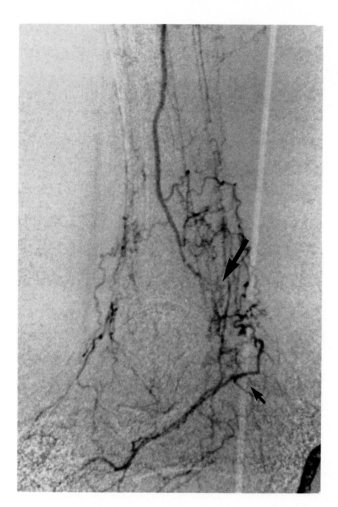

FIG. 8. Digital subtraction arteriogram of 70-year-old type II diabetic patient with gangrenous toes and nonhealing great toe amputation site. Note severe distal disease of peroneal artery (large arrow) as only distal run-off, but with severe occlusive disease of the posterior communicating branch. The only pedal run-off is the lateral plantar artery (small arrow).

cutaneous ulcer is metabolically more active than intact skin and thus requires increased blood flow for wound healing. A graft may remain patent long enough to allow healing of an ulcer and even if it thromboses, if the skin envelope remains intact, the limb should not be at risk.

There are recent reports of successful PTA of the infrapopliteal vessels (124). The technique is inherently riskier than PTA in larger diameter vessels because of risk of thrombosis and vessel rupture. However, many of the same catheters and techniques applicable to coronary angioplasty can be used in the infrapopliteal vessels. Preliminary reports of this technique in the infrapopliteal vessels describe initial technical success rates of 75% with 22-month clinical success rates of 67% in those which were successful (50% overall success) (124). Because infrapopliteal disease is often diffuse, patient selection is critical for good long-term results. However, if a PTA at this level remains patent long enough to allow ulcer healing, limb salvage may be achieved, even if the subsequent restenosis or occlusion occurs (126). Thus, PTA may prove useful in only a very select group of patients who are high risk for anesthesia and without suitable veins for vascular reconstruction.

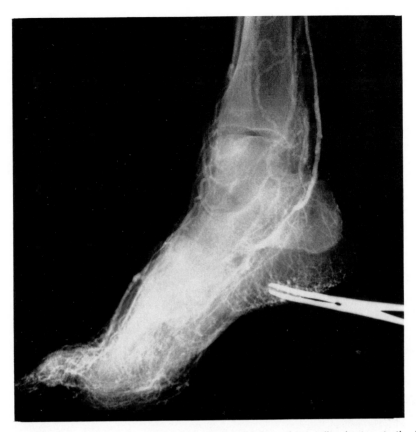

FIG. 9. Intraoperative arteriogram of *in situ* bypass graft from the popliteal artery to the lateral plantar artery in patient in Fig. 7. Note excellent filling of plantar vessels. Patient healed a transmetatarsal amputation performed postarteriogram.

TABLE 3. *Patency rates of bypasses to infrapopliteal vessels*

Authors	Year	Number of patients	Technique	Cumulative patency rate (%)				
				1 year	2 year	3 year	4 year	5 year
Karmody, et al. (119)	1984	391	*In situ*	89	28	67	67	—
Carney, et al. (24)	1985	21	*In situ*	85	72	72	—	—
Levine, et al. (120)	1985	55	*In situ*	83	72	72	—	—
Taylor, et al. (118)	1987	110	RSVG*	90	90	85	85	85
Berkowitz and Greenstein (117)	1987	102	RSVG*	78	74	74	70	70†
Total		679		87	78	72	71	78

*RSVG, reversed saphenous vein graft
†Secondary patency rate

Conclusion

The diabetic patient is often afflicted with aggressive atherosclerosis, which shows predilection for more distal vessels. Appropriate use of bedside clinical skills and noninvasive testing can help select appropriate patients for angiography and revascularization. A host of surgical and radiologic approaches is available for management of the ischemic limb. With a sound understanding of the natural history and relevant pathophysiology, as well as meticulous technique, lower extremities can be salvaged for many grateful patients.

Finally, the risks of peripheral arterial disease transcend the strict involvement of lower extremities. Because the presence of peripheral arterial disease enhances the risk of an acute cardiovascular event (127), patients presenting with manifestations of occlusive disease should also be assessed for the presence of atherosclerosis in the coronary arteries even in asymptomatic individuals.

REFERENCES

1. Kramer DW, Perilstein PK. Peripheral vascular complications in diabetes mellitus: A survery of 3,600 cases. *Diabetes* 1958;7:384–87.
2. Melton LJ, Macken KM, Palumbo PJ, Elveback LR. Evidence and prevalence of clinical peripheral vascular disease in a population-based cohort of diabetic patients. *Diabetes Care* 1980;3:650–54.
3. Goldenberg S. Non-atheromatous peripheral vascular disease of the lower extremity in diabetes mellitus. *Diabetes* 1959;8:261–73.
4. Koss LG. Hyaline material with staining reaction of fibrinoid in renal lesions in diabetes mellitus. *AMA Arch Pathol* 1952;54:528–47.
5. Friedenwald JS. Diabetic retinopathy. Fourth Francis I. proctor lecture. *Am J Ophthalmol* 1950;33:1187–99.
6. Strandness DE Jr, Priest RE, Gibbons GE. Combined clinical and pathologic study of diabetic and nondiabetic peripheral arterial disease. *Diabetes* 1964;13:366–77.
7. Conrad MC. Large and small artery occlusion in diabetics and nondiabetics with severe vascular disease. *Circulation* 1967;36:83–91.
8. Siperstein MD, Unger RH, Madison LL. Studies of muscle capillary basement membranes in normal subjects, diabetic and prediabetic patients. *J Clin Invest* 1968;47:1973–99.
9. Frederici HHR, Tucker WR, Schwartz TB. Observations on small blood vessels of skin in the normal and in diabetic patients. *Diabetes* 1960;15:233–50.
10. Parving HH, Rasmussen SM. Transcapillary escape rate of albumin and plasma volume in short- and long-term juvenile diabetics. *Scand J Clin Lab Invest* 1973;32:81–7.
11. LoGerfo FW, Coffman JD. Vascular and microvascular disease of the foot in diabetics: Implications for foot care. *N Engl J Med* 1984;311:1615–19.
12. Myers KA, King RB, Scott DF, Johnson N, et al. Surgical treatment of the severely ischemic leg: Survival rates. *Br J Surg* 1978;65:460–64.
13. Brewster DC, Perler BA, Robinson JG, Darling C. Aortofemoral graft for multilevel occlusive disease, predictors of success and need for distal bypass. *Arch Surg* 1982;117:1593–1600.
14. Duncan WC, Linton RR, Darling RC. Aortoilio-femoral atherosclerotic occlusive disease: Comparative results of endarterectomy and Dacron bypass grafts. *Surgery* 1971;70:974–84.
15. Minken SL, DeWeese JA, Southgate WA, Mahoney EB, et al. Aortoiliac reconstruction for atherosclerotic occlusive disease. *Surg Gynecol Obstet* 1968;126:1056–60.
16. Nevelsteen A, Suy R, Daenen W, Boel A, et al. Aortofemoral grafting: Factors influencing late results. *Surgery* 1980;88:642–53.
17. Pierce GE, Turrentine M, Stringfield S, Iliopoulos J, et al. Evaluation of end-to-side versus end-to-end proximal anastomosis in aortobifemoral bypass. *Arch Surg* 1982;117:1580–88.
18. Codd JE, Barner HB, Kaminski DL, Ramey A, et al. Extremity revascularization: A decade of experience. *Am J Surg* 1979;138:770–76.
19. Darling RC, Linton RR. Durability of femoropopliteal reconstructions. *Am J Surg* 1972;123: 472–79.
20. Kouchoukos NT, Levy JF, Balfour JF, Butcher HR. Operative therapy for femoral-popliteal

arterial occlusive disease: A comparison of therapeutic methods. *Circulation* 1967; 24(suppl):174–82.

21. Reichle FA, Rauken KP, Tyson R, Firestone AJ, et al. Long-term results of 474 arterial reconstructions for severely ischemic limbs: A fourteen-year follow-up. *Surgery* 1979;85:93–100.

22. Szilagyi DE, Hajeman JH, Smith RF, Elliot JP, et al. Autogenous vein grafting in femoropopliteal atherosclerosis: The limits of its effectiveness. *Surgery* 1979;86:836–51.

23. Auer AJ, Hurley JJ, Binnington HB, Nunelee JD, et al. Distal tibial vein grafts for limb salvage. *Arch Surg* 1983;118:597–602.

24. Carney WI, Balko A, Barrett MS. In situ femoropopliteal and infrapopliteal bypass: Two year experience. *Arch Surg* 1985;120:812–16.

25. Dardik H, Ibrahim IM, Dardik II. The role of the peroneal artery for limb salvage. *Ann Surg* 1979;189:189–98.

26. Hallin RW: In situ saphenous vein bypass grafting: Experience in 34 extremities over a two year period. *Am J Surg* 1983;145:626–29.

27. Reichle FA, Martinson MW, Rankin KP. Infrapopliteal arterial reconstruction in the severely ischemic lower extremity. *Ann Surg* 1980;191:59–65.

28. Samson RH, Gupta SK, Scher LA, Veith FJ. Treatment of limb-threatening ischemia despite a palpable popliteal pulse. *J Surg Res* 1982;32:535–39.

29. Schuler JJ, Flanigan P, Williams LR, Ryan TT, et al. Early experience with popliteal to infrapopliteal bypass for limb salvage. *Arch Surg* 1983;118:472–76.

30. Mitchell JC. End-stage renal failure in juvenile diabetes mellitus. *Mayo Clin Proc* 1977;52: 281–88.

31. Amundsen S, Trippestad A, Viste A, Spreide O. Abdominal aortic aneurysms: A national multicenter study. *Eur J Vasc Surg* 1987;1:239–43.

32. Gundersen J. Segmental measurements of systolic blood pressure in the extremities including the thumb and the great toe. *Acta Chir Scand* 1972;426(suppl 1):1–83.

33. Nielsen PE, Rasmussen SM. Indirect measurement of systolic blood pressure by strain gauge technique at finger, ankle and toe in diabetic patients without symptoms of occlusive arterial disease. *Diabetologia* 1973;9:25–9.

34. Tenembaum MM, Rayfield E, Junior J, Jacobson JH II, et al. Altered pressure and flow relationship in the diabetic foot. *J Surg Res* 1981;31:307–13.

35. Vincent D, Salles-Cunha S, Bernhard V, Towne J. Noninvasive assessment of toe systolic pressures with special reference to diabetes mellitus. *J Cardiovasc Surg* 1983;24:22–8.

36. Malone JM, Leal JM, Moore WS, Henry RE, et al. The "gold standard" for amputation level selection: Xenon-133 clearance. *J Surg Res* 1981;30:449–55.

37. Malone JM, Moore W, Leal JM, Childers SJ. Therapeutic and economic impact of a modern amputation program. *Ann Surg* 1979;189(6):798–802.

38. Malone JM, Anderson GG, Lalka SG, Hagaman RM, et al. Prospective comparison of noninvasive techniques for amputation level selection. *Am J Surg* 1987;154:179–184.

39. Burgess EM, Matsen FA, Wyss GR, Simmons W. Segmental transcutaneous measurements of PO_2 in patients requiring below-the-knee amputation for peripheral vascular insufficiency. *J Bone Joint Surg* 1982;64A(3):378–83.

40. Kram HB, Appel PL, Shoemaker NC. Multisensor transcutaneous oximetric mapping to predict below-knee amputation wound healing: Use of a critical PO_2 index. *J Vasc Surg* 1989;9(6): 796–800.

41. Rafliff DA, Klyne CAC, Chant ADB, Webster JHH. Prediction of amputation wound healing: The role of transcutaneous PO_2 assessment. *Br J Surg* 1984;71:219–22.

42. Hauser CJ, Clein SR, Mehringer CM, Appel P, et al. Superiority of transcutaneous oximetry in noninvasive vascular diagnosis in patients with diabetes. *Arch Surg* 1984;119:690–94.

43. Wyss CR, Matsen FA III, Simmons CW, Burgess EM. Transcutaneous oxygen tension measurements on limbs of diabetic and nondiabetic patients with peripheral vascular disease. *Surgery* 1984;95:339–45.

44. Hessel S, Adams D, Abrams H. Complications of angiography. *Radiology* 1981;138:273–81.

45. Greenberger PA. Contrast media reactions. *J Allergy Clin Immunol* 1984;74:600–05.

46. Lasser EC, Berry CC, Talner LB, Santini LC, et al. Pretreatment with corticosteroids to alleviate reactions to intravenous contrast material. *N Engl J Med* 1987;317:845–9.

47. Kinnison ML, Poew NR, Steinberg EP. Results of randomized controlled trials of low- versus high-osmolarity contrast media. *Radiology* 1989;170:381–89.

48. Wolf GL, Areson RL, Cross AP. A prospective trial of ionic versus nonionic contrast agents in routine clinical practice: Comparison of adverse effects. *AJR* 1989;152:939–44.

49. Lasser EC, Berry CC. Nonionic versus ionic contrast media: What do the data tell us? *AJR* 1989;152:945–46.

50. Kelly J, Patterson R, Liebermann P, et al. Radiographic contrast reactions in high-risk patients. *J Allergy Clin Immunol* 1978;62:181–84.

51. Greenberger PA, Patterson R, Raddin RC. Two pretreatment regiments for high-risk patients receiving radiographic contrast media. *J Allergy Clin Immunol* 1984;74:540–3.
52. Van Zee BE, Hoy WE, Talley TE, Jaenike JR. Renal injury associated with intravenous pyelography in nondiabetic and diabetic patients. *Ann Int Med* 1978;89:51–4.
53. Lang EK, Foreman J, Schlegel JU, Leslie C, et al. The incidence of contrast medium induced acute tubular necrosis following arteriography. *Radiology* 1981;138:203–6.
54. Parfrey PS, Griffiths SM, Barrett BJ, Paul MD, et al. Contrast material-induced renal failure in patients with diabetes mellitus, renal insufficiency or both: A prospective controlled study. *N Engl J Med* 1989;320:143–9.
55. Gomes AS, Baker JD, Martin-Paredero V, Dixon SM, et al. Acute renal dysfunction after major arteriography. *AJR* 1985;145:1249–52.
56. Martin-Paredero V, Dixon SM, Baker JD, Takiff H, et al. Risk of renal failure after major angiography. *Arch Surg* 1983;118:1417–20.
57. Swartz RD, Rubin JE, Leeming BW, Silva P. Renal failure following major angiography. *Am J Med* 1978;65:31–7.
58. Eisenberg R, Bank W, Hedgkolk M. Renal failure after major angiography can be avoided with hydration. *AJR* 1981;136:859–61.
59. Kerstein MD, Puyan FA. Value of preangiography hydration. *Surgery* 1984;96:919–22.
60. Cigarroa RG, Lange RA, Williams RH, Hillis LD. Dosing of contrast material to prevent contrast nephropathy in patients with renal disease. *Am J Med* 1989;86:649–52.
61. Morrison AR, Winokur TS, Brown WA. Inhibition of soybean lipoxygenase by Mannitol. *Biochem Biophys Res Comm* 1982;108:1757–62.
62. Schwab SJ, Hlatky MA, Pieper KS, Davidson CJ, et al. Contrast nephrotoxicity: A randomized controlled trial of a nonionic and ionic radiographic contrast agent. *N Engl J Med* 1989;320:149–53.
63. Golman K, Almen T. Contrast media-induced nephrotoxicity: Survey and present state: *Invest Radiol* 1985;20:593–97.
64. Boyd AM. The natural course of arteriosclerosis of the lower extremities. *Proc R Soc Med* 1962;55:591–93.
65. Imparato AM, Kim GE, Davidson T, Crowley JG. Intermittent claudication: Its natural course. *Surgery* 1975;78:795–99.
66. Cronenwett JL, Warner KG, Zelenock GB, et al. Intermittent claudication: Current results of nonoperative treatment. *Arch Surg* 1984;119:430–36.
67. McAllister FF. The fate of patients with intermittent claudication managed nonoperatively. *Am J Surg* 1976;132:593–95.
68. Bendick PJ, Glover JL, Kuebler TW, Dilley RS. Progression of atherosclerosis in diabetics. *Surgery* 1983;93:834.
69. DiPerri T, Guerrini M. Placebo-controlled double-blind study with pentoxifylline of walking performance in patients with intermittent claudication. *Angiology* 1983;34:40–45.
70. Jeans WD, Dauton RM, Baird RN, Horrocks M. A comparison of the costs of vascular surgery and balloon dilatation in lower limb ischemic disease. *Br J Radiol* 1986;59:453–56.
71. Castaneda-Zuniga WR, Formanek A, Tadavarthy M, Vladover Z, et al. The mechanism of balloon angioplasty. *Radiology* 1980;135(3):565–71.
72. Morin JF, Johnston KW, Wasserman L, Andrews D. Factors that determine the long-term results of percutaneous transluminal dilatation for peripheral arterial occlusive disease. *J Vasc Surg* 1986;4:68–72.
73. Cambria RP, Faust G, Gusberg G, Tilson MD, Zucker KA, Modlin IM. Percutaneous angioplasty for peripheral arterial occlusive disease: correlates of clinical success. *Arch Surg* 1987;122:283–87.
74. Becker GJ, Katzen BT, Dake MD. Noncoronary angioplasty. *Radiology* 1989;170:921–40.
75. Von Pölmitz A, Backa D, Remberger K, Höfling B. Restenosis after atherectomy shows increased intimal hyperplasia as compared to primary lesions. *J Vasc Med Biol* 1989;1:283–87.
76. Newman GE, Miner DG, Sussman SK, Phillips HR, Mikat EM, et al. Peripheral artery atherectomy: Description of techniques and report of initial results. *Radiology* 1988;169:677–80.
77. Wright JG, Belkin M, Greenfield AJ, Guben JK, Sanborn TA, et al. Laser angioplasty for limb salvage: Observations on early results. *J Vasc Surg* 1989;10:29–38.
78. Kwasnik EM, Siouffi SY, Jay ME, Khuri SF. Comparative results of angioplasty and aortofemoral bypass in patients with symptomatic iliac disease. *Arch Surg* 1987;122:288–91.
79. Van Andel GJ, Van Erp WFM, Krepel VM, Breslan PJ. Percutaneous transluminal dilatation of the iliac artery: Long-term results. *Radiology* 1985;156:321–23.
80. Gallino A, Mahler F, Probst P, Nachbur B. Percutaneous transluminal angioplasty of the arteries of the lower limbs: A 5 year follow-up. *Circulation* 1984;70(4):619–23.
81. Johnston KW, Ral M, Hogg-Johnston SA, Colapinto RF, et al. Five-year results of a prospective study of percutaneous transluminal angioplasty. *Ann Surg* 1987;206:403–12.

82. Weibull H, Bergqvist D, Jonsson K, Karlsson S, et al. Complications after percutaneous trans-luminal angioplasty in the iliac, femoral and popliteal arteries. *J Vasc Surg* 1987;5:681–86.

83. Jeffrey CC, Kunsman J, Cullen DJ, Brewster DC. A prospective evaluation of cardiac risk index. *Anesthesiology* 1983;58:462–64.

84. Brown OW, Hollier LH, Paerolero PC, et al. Abdominal aortic aneurysm and coronary artery disease: A reassessment. *Arch Surg* 1981;116:1484–88.

85. Hertzer NR. Fatal myocardial infarction following abdominal aortic aneurysm resection. Three hundred forty-three patients followed six to eleven years postoperatively. *Ann Surg* 1980; 192:667–73.

86. Crawford ES, Bomberger RA, Glaeser DH. Aortoiliac occlusive disease: Factors influencing survival and function following reconstructive operation over a twenty-five year period. *Surgery* 1981;90:1055–67.

87. Malone JM, Moore WS, Goldstone J. The natural history of bilateral aortofemoral bypass grafts for ischemia of the lower extremities. *Arch Surg* 1975;110:1300–06.

88. Brewster DC, Darling CR. Optimal methods of aortoiliac reconstruction. *Surgery* 1978;84: 739–48.

89. King RB, Myers KA, Scott DF, Denne TJ. The choice of operation in aortoiliac reconstructions for intermittent claudication. *World J Surg* 1983;7:334–39.

90. Szilagyi DE, Elliot JP, Smith RF: A thirty-year survey of the reconstructive surgical treatment of aortoiliac occlusive disease. *J Vasc Surg* 1986;3:421–36.

91. Butcher HR, Jaffe BM. Treatment of aortoiliac occlusive disease by endarterectomy. *Ann Surg* 1971;173:925–32.

92. Cambria RP, Brewster DC, Abbott WM, Freeham M, et al. Transperitoneal versus retroperito-neal approach for aortic reconstruction: A randomized prospective study. *J Vasc Surg* 1990; 11:314–25.

93. Sicard GA, Freeman MB, VanderWoude JC, Anderson CB: Comparison between the transab-dominal and retroperitoneal approach for reconstruction of the infrarenal abdominal aorta. *J Vasc Surg* 1987;5:19–27.

94. Nevelsteen A, Smet G, Weyman S, Depre H, et al. Transabdominal or retroperitoneal approach to the aortoiliac track: Pulmonary function studies. *Eur J Vasc Surg* 1988;2:229–32.

95. Johnson WC, LoGerfo FW, Vollmann RW, Corson JD, et al. Is axillo-bilateral femoral graft an effective substitute for aortic bilateral iliac-femoral graft? An analysis of ten years' experience. *Ann Surg* 1977;186:123–29.

96. Rutherford RB, Patt A, Pearce WH. Extra-anatomic bypass: A closer view. *J Vasc Surg* 1987; 6:437–46.

97. LoGerfo FW, Johnson WC, Corson JD, et al. A comparison of the late patency rates of axillo-bilateral femoral and axillounilateral femoral grafts. *Surgery* 1977;81:33–40.

98. Thiele BL, Bandyk DF, Zierler RE, Strandness DE. A systematic approach to the assessment of aortoiliac disease. *Arch Surg* 1983;118:477–81.

99. Archie JP. Some determinants of papaverine-induced femoral artery pressure gradients. *J Surg Res* 1990;48:211–16.

100. Brewster DC, Perler BA, Robinson JG, Darling RC. Aortofemoral graft for multilevel occlusive disease. *Arch Surg* 1982;117:1593–1600.

101. Wilson SE, Wolk GL, Cross AP. Percutaneous transluminal angioplasty versus operation for peripheral atherosclerosis. *J Vasc Surg* 1989;9:1–9.

102. Martin EC, Fankuchen EI, Karlson KB, Dolgin C, et al. Angioplasty for femoral artery occlu-sion: Comparison with surgery. *AJR* 1981;137:915–19.

103. Hewes RC, White RI, Murray RR, Kaufman SL, et al. Long-term results of superficial femoral artery angioplasty. *AJR* 1986;146:1025–29.

104. Murray RR, Hewes RC, White RI, Mitchell SE, et al. Long-segment femoropopliteal stenosis: Is angioplasty a boon or a bust? *Radiology* 1987;162:473–76.

105. Veith FJ, Gupta SK, Ascer E, White-Flores S, et al. Six-year prospective multicenter random-ized comparison of autologous saphenous vein and expanded polytetrafluoroethylene grafts in infrainguinal arterial reconstructions. *J Vasc Surg* 1986;3:104–14.

106. Michaels JA. Choice of material for above-knee femoropopliteal bypass graft. *Br J Surg* 1989;76:7–14.

107. Rosenthal D, Levine K, Stanton PE, Lamis PA. Femoropopliteal bypass: The preferred site for distal anastomosis. *Surgery* 1983;93:1–4.

108. Taylor LM, Phinney ES, Porter JM. Present status of reversed vein bypass for lower extremity revascularization. *J Vasc Surg* 1986;3:288–97.

109. DeWeese JA, Rob CG. Autogenous venous grafts ten years later. *Surgery* 1977;82(6):775–84.

110. Rafferty TD, Avellone JC, Farrell CJ, Hertzer NR, et al. A metropolitan experience with infrain-guinal revascularization: Operative risk and late results in northeastern Ohio. *J Vasc Surg* 1987;6:365–71.

111. Andros G, Harris RW, Salles-Cunha S, et al. Arm veins for arterial revascularization of the leg: Arteriographic and clinical observations. *J Vasc Surg* 1986;4:416–27.
112. Hirsch SA, Jarrett F. The use of stabilized human umbilical vein for femoropopliteal bypass. *Ann Surg* 1984;200:147–52.
113. Eickhoff JH, Broome A, Ericsson BF, Hansen HJB, et al. Four years' results of a prospective, randomized clinical trial comparing polytetrafluoroethylene and modified human umbilical vein for below-knee femoropopliteal bypass. *J Vasc Surg* 1987;6:506–11.
114. Kazmers M, Satiani B, Evans WE. Amputation level following unsuccessful distal limb salvage operations. *Surgery* 1980;87(6):683–87.
115. Samson RH, Gupta SK, Scher LA, Veith FJ. Level of amputation after failure of limb salvage procedures. *Surg Gynecol Obstet* 1982;154:56–58.
116. Leather RP, Power SR, Karmody AM. A reappraisal of the in situ saphenous vein arterial bypass: Its use in limb salvage. *Surgery* 1979;86:453–61.
117. Berkowitz HD, Greenstein SM. Improved patency in reversed femoral-infrapopliteal autogenous vein grafts by early detection and treatment of the failing graft. *J Vasc Surg* 1987;5:755–61.
118. Taylor LM Jr, Edwards JM, Phinney ES, et al. Reversed vein bypass to infrapopliteal arteries: Modern results are superior to or equivalent to in situ bypass for patency and vein utilization. *Ann Surg* 1987;205:90–97.
119. Karmody AM, Leather RP, Shah DM, Corson JD, et al. Peroneal artery bypass: A reappraisal of its value in limb salvage. *J Vasc Surg* 1984;1:809–16.
120. Levine AW, Bandyk DF, Bonier PH, Towne JB. Lessons learned in adopting the in situ saphenous vein bypass. *J Vasc Surg* 1985;2:145–53.
121. Corson JD, Karmody A, Shah DM, et al. In situ vein bypass to distal tibial and limited outflow tracts for limb salvage. *Surgery* 1984;96:756–63.
122. Andros G, Harris RW, Salles-Cunha SX, Dulawa LB, et al. Lateral plantar artery bypass grafting: Defining the limits of foot revascularization. *J Vasc Surg* 1989;10:511–21.
123. Bandyk DF, Cato RF, Towne JB. A low flow velocity predicts failure of femoropopliteal and femorotibial bypass grafts. *Surgery* 1985;98:799–809.
124. Brown KT, Schoenberg NY, Moore ED, Saddekni S. Percutaneous transluminal angioplasty of infrapopliteal vessels: Preliminary results and technical considerations. *Radiology* 1988;169:75–78.
125. Casarella WJ. Percutaneous tarnsluminal angioplasty below the knee: New techniques, excellent results. *Radiology* 1988;169:271–72.
126. Rush DS, Gewertz BL, Lu C, Ball DG, et al. Limb salvage in poor-risk patients using transluminal angioplasty. *Arch Surg* 1983;118:1209–12.
127. Abbott RD, Brand FN, Kannel WB. Epidemiology of some peripheral arterial findings in diabetic men and women: experiences from the Framingham study. *Am J Med* 1990;88:376–81.

Surgical Management of the Diabetic Patient,
edited by Michael Bergman and Gregorio A. Sicard.
Raven Press, Ltd., New York © 1991.

20

Carotid Artery Disease in the Diabetic Patient

Brian G. Rubin and Gregorio A. Sicard

*Department of Surgery, Washington University School of Medicine,
St. Louis, Missouri 63110*

Stroke is the fourth leading cause of death in America and accounts for approximately 8% of American deaths (1). Annual estimates of the care costs for stroke victims are staggering, reaching 9.5 billion dollars in disability care (2); it has been reported that the overall indirect cost was up to 20 billion dollars in 1985 alone (1). The majority of strokes are attributed to atherosclerosis of the extracranial circulation, usually from thromboembolic disease originating in the area of the carotid bifurcation. Surgical removal of plaque and debris from this region, termed carotid endarterectomy, is performed in an attempt to reduce the incidence of subsequent stroke and death. It has been estimated that in 1985, 80,000 to 110,000 carotid endarterectomies were performed in nonfederal hospitals at a cost of 1.25 billion dollars.

As with cerebrovascular disease, diabetes mellitus is quite common, with an estimated 8 million Americans afflicted with frank diabetes mellitus or glucose intolerance. Diabetes is a recognized risk factor for atherosclerosis. Optimal management of the diabetic patient includes recognition of the fact that atherosclerosis is a systemic disease, affecting all arterial beds, any one of which may be the most symptomatic at a given point in time. Twenty-year follow-up data from the Framingham study reveal that diabetic individuals are at approximately two-fold increased risk of cardiovascular events, including atherothrombotic brain infarction, congestive heart failure, symptomatic coronary heart disease, cardiovascular death, and intermittent claudication (3). Even after adjusting for age, systolic blood pressure, cigarettes per day, cholesterol levels, and left ventricular hypertrophy, the stroke rate in diabetic patients is increased 2.18-fold in men and 2.17-fold in women, compared with their nondiabetic counterparts. The attributable fraction of stroke due to diabetes has been estimated to be 10% in men and 14% in women. Not only do strokes occur with greater frequency in diabetic persons, but when they do occur they are associated with a 368% increase in mortality. This increase is most marked in the female insulin-dependent subgroup who suffer a 727% increased death risk (3). Moreover, when a cerebral ischemic event occurs in a diabetic person, it is twice as likely to result in a permanent neurologic deficit (stroke) rather than a transient deficit (TIA or RIND) when compared with a comparable group of nondiabetic persons with neurologic events (4). Alex and associates (5) found evidence of cerebrovascular accidents 10%

more often among diabetic individuals than in nondiabetic individuals. In a similar vein, Bell (6) reported an autopsy series in which the degree of encephalomalacia was 25% greater in diabetic patients older than 40 years of age, when compared with a similar nondiabetic group. This high rate of irreversible tissue damage in the diabetic population has been attributed to microvascular disease (4) and diminished ability to form collaterals.

Although atherosclerosis occurs at an accelerated rate in diabetic patients, this increase cannot be solely attributed to the effects of hyperglycemia (7). It is unclear whether hyperglycemia, hyperinsulinemia, or some other agent is responsible for the atherogenic effects of diabetes (8).

Several other significant risk factors for atherosclerosis occur in diabetic patients. Important determinants include whether the patient is type I or type II diabetic, and in the type I diabetic category, whether renal function is normal or abnormal. Type I diabetic individuals with impaired renal function and type II diabetic individuals frequently have associated hypertension, hypercholesterolemia, hypertriglyceridemia and decreased level of high-density lipoprotein (HDL) cholesterol. Type I diabetic persons with normal renal function have essentially normal parameters in these categories (9). Despite the frequent occurrence of comorbid disease, particularly hypertension and hyperlipidemia, there remains a residual effect due to diabetes alone that is manifested by increased cardiovascular morbidity and mortality (10).

In an attempt to reduce cerebrovascular mortality in patients with extracranial cerebrovascular disease, surgeons have popularized the use of carotid endarterectomy. When performed on symptomatic patients, and if associated with low perioperative stroke and death rates, this procedure improves short- and long-term survival rates (11–15). Suggestions regarding preoperative evaluation of carotid artery disease, and perioperative and long-term management of the patient undergoing carotid endarterectomy follow.

PREOPERATIVE WORKUP OF CAROTID ARTERY DISEASE

One of the more difficult problems that a clinician faces is which patients should undergo carotid artery evaluation. Certainly, all symptomatic patients with a history of amaurosis fugax, transient ischemic attacks, or RINDs should undergo noninvasive carotid artery evaluation. Management of the asymptomatic diabetic patient with or without a carotid bruit is more controversial. Early noninvasive studies using oculopneumoplethysmography (OPG) and carotid phonoangiography (CPA), revealed that 20% of diabetic patients had hemodynamically significant carotid artery stenosis (>50%). In a study by Kuebler et al. (16), the type of diabetes, its duration, and the degree of glucose control did not correlate with carotid disease.

Currently, noninvasive evaluation is best accomplished by duplex scanning technology. This method combines a pulsed Doppler unit with real-time spectral analysis and B-mode imaging. It allows direct visualization and determination of the appearance and echogenicity of the common, internal, and external carotid arteries, as well as interrogation of regions of stenosis by detecting areas of turbulence and increased flow (Fig. 1). When compared with standard carotid angiography, duplex scanning has been shown to be more than 90% sensitive and specific. Significant abnormalities

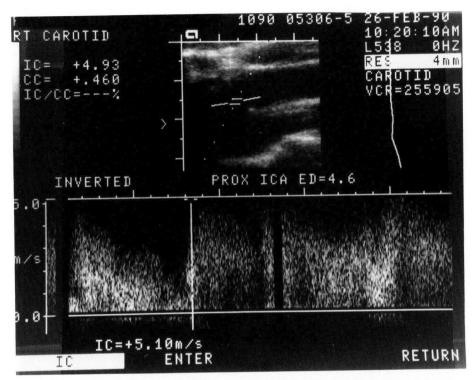

FIG. 1. Carotid duplex scan in patient with recent stroke and crescendo transient ischemic attacks. The upper panel shows the cursor in the stenotic area in the proximal internal carotid artery. Velocity waveforms determination in lower panel is consistent with very high-grade stenosis (80–99%).

determined by the duplex study include the presence of significant stenosis (>80%), occlusion of the internal carotid artery, or areas of ulceration with or without associated significant stenosis. In addition to the hemodynamic effect of a stenosis, the duplex scan allows for assessment of plaque morphology, which could be of significant prognostic importance by itself (17).

Using the duplex scanner, Chan and coworkers (18) have demonstrated that the percentage of diabetic patients with severe carotid disease (>80% stenosis) is 8.2% of noninsulin-dependent diabetics versus 0.7% of matched controls. Recognizing this accelerated occurrence of significant cerebrovascular disease in the diabetic population, clinicians can decide whether or not to screen the asymptomatic diabetic subgroup, especially those with a cervical bruit. Natural history studies of carotid artery disease show that the onset of neurologic symptoms is associated with progression of disease to greater than 80% stenosis or with occlusion of a carotid artery (19–22).

Major risk factors associated with disease progression include diabetes mellitus, cigarette smoking, and age—especially individuals under 65 years (23). Fifty-eight percent of diabetic patients demonstrate progression of disease by duplex scanning, compared with the nondiabetic population with a 35% incidence of disease progression over a study period of up to 36 months. Other authors, however, do not support this finding (19–21,24). Bogousslavsky et al. (25) have demonstrated that elevated blood glucose level is a risk factor for occlusion of the carotid artery in patients studied by angiography (25).

Drielsma et al. (26), using duplex ultrasound imaging of the carotid bifurcation, have found that diabetic and nondiabetic patients have similar ultrasound plaque types in symptomatic patients. They note, however, that in the subgroup treated with insulin, there is little evidence of echolucency (intraplaque hemorrhage or ulceration) and an increased percentage of dominantly echogenic or uniformly echogenic lesions.

Patients with significant duplex scanning abnormalities should undergo cerebral angiography (Fig. 2), as well as computerized tomography (Fig. 3), with and without

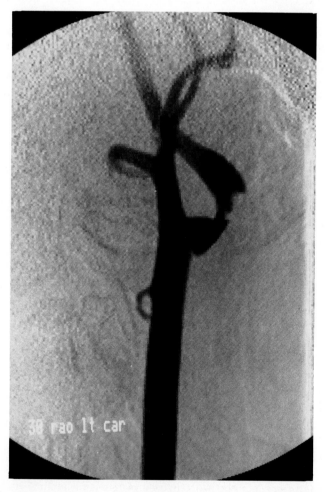

FIG. 2. Selective digital arteriogram of left carotid system in patient described in Fig. 1. Note high-grade lesion and irregularity in proximal internal carotid artery. Patient was successfully treated with emergent endarterectomy.

intravenous contrast. Cross-sectional imaging of the brain is suggested, as silent stroke is a frequent event, occurring in 10% of the stroke population in the Framingham series. Occasionally, patients with stroke in evolution or crescendo transient ischemic attacks show severe stenosis or "string sign" in the internal carotid artery requiring emergent endarterectomy (Fig. 4). Diabetic patients in particular should undergo computer tomography (CT) imaging as glucose intolerance is the sole risk factor that occurs more often in the group with silent lesions than in the group with evidence of acute stroke (27). If arteriography confirms significant unilateral or bilateral disease and CT scanning does not demonstrate evidence of a recent cerebrovascular accident, the patient should be considered for carotid endarterectomy. Patients with lesser degrees of pathology should be followed with duplex scanning on a 6-month basis (23).

PREOPERATIVE EVALUATION OF CORONARY ARTERY DISEASE

Of critical importance is the consideration of concomitant coronary artery disease. Diabetic populations have been demonstrated to have a three- to four-fold increase in the incidence of coronary artery disease, with an elevated percentage of this population with silent myocardial ischemia. Hertzer and colleagues (28) at the Cleveland Clinic Foundation performed coronary angiography in 1,000 patients referred for

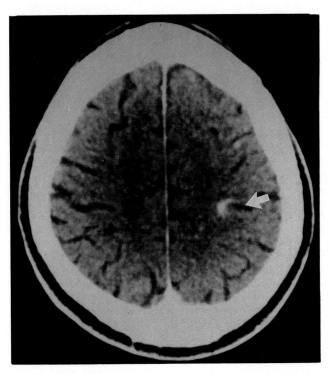

FIG. 3. Postarteriogram, CT scan showing enhanced lesion in left temporoparietal region in patient described in Figs. 1 and 2.

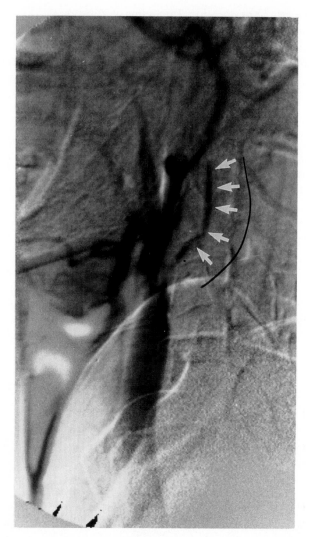

FIG. 4. Delayed view of selective carotid arteriogram in a 56-year-old diabetic patient admitted with acute stroke and recurrent transient ischemic attacks. Patient was treated with emergent carotid endarterectomy and symptoms improved.

noncardiac vascular disease. Results of cardiac catheterization were divided into patient groups with: normal coronary arteries; mild to moderate coronary artery disease (<70% stenosis); advanced but compensated coronary artery disease (>70% stenosis of one or more coronary artery with adequate intercoronary collateral circulation); severe correctable coronary artery disease (>70% stenosis of one or more coronary arteries serving unimpaired myocardium and thought to represent a risk for subsequent myocardial infarction); and severe inoperable coronary artery disease. Two hundred and ninety-five of these 1,000 patients were referred for cerebrovascular surgical procedures. In this group, 26–28% of the patients were identified as having severe correctable coronary artery disease (15,29). Severe, surgically correctable coronary artery disease was documented in 33% of the patients suspected to have coronary artery disease by clinical criteria. Surprisingly, it was also uncovered in 17% of patients with no clinical indications of coronary artery disease. In the group of patients with significant combined cardiac and carotid disease, those patients undergoing coronary artery bypass grafting and carotid endarterectomy had a 5-year survival rate of 83%, compared with those undergoing carotid endarterectomy without the indicated coronary artery bypass grafting who had a survival rate at 5 years of only 62% (15). Five-year survival rates in an equivalent patient group without carotid disease who were undergoing carotid artery bypass grafting was 90%. Since 1, the leading cause of death after carotid endarterectomy is myocardial infarction, 2, the rate of silent severe correctable coronary artery disease in patients with cerebrovascular disease is 17%; and 3, long-term survival after carotid endarterectomy appears improved in patients who had coronary artery bypass grafting when appropriate, these authors recommend that all patients with cerebrovascular disease undergo cardiac evaluation.

These points bear particular emphasis on preoperative evaluation of the diabetic, known to have an increased cardiac morbidity and mortality and a higher rate of silent myocardial ischemia. Long-term results reported by these same authors (30) demonstrated that in the subgroup with diabetes ($n = 170$) or glucose intolerance ($n = 107$), diabetic patients had a high mortality rate after coronary artery bypass (12%) and an increased 5-year mortality rate (57%—an increase of 2.5-fold) compared with nondiabetic patients who have undergone coronary artery bypass grafting.

Once the diabetic patient has had complete evaluation of extracranial circulation using invasive and noninvasive techniques, and evaluation of cardiac status and general medical condition, a decision can be made as to whether or not to proceed with carotid endarterectomy.

OPERATIVE TECHNIQUE

The procedure can be performed under general or regional anesthesia. The advantage of regional anesthesia is that in the awake patient, the neurologic consequences of carotid clamping are easily detected. General anesthesia allows increased patient comfort, but requires either routine shunting during the period of carotid clamping or monitoring for evidence of cerebral ischemia with selective shunting when ischemia becomes manifest. Our institutional preference is for general anesthesia with electroencephalogram (EEG) monitoring. We also routinely measure internal carotid artery stump pressures and suggest selective shunting for patients with contralateral occlusion or high-grade stenosis, previous cerebrovascular accidents, anticipated long periods of carotid cross-clamping, stump pressures of less than 40 mm Hg (mean blood pressure) or EEG changes after carotid artery clamping. After carefully dissecting the surrounding tissues away from the common, distal internal and external carotid arteries, occluding vascular clamps are applied and stump pressure is measured. Being mindful of the indications for placement of a shunt, a longitudinal arteriotomy is made over the common carotid artery through the bulb and extended into the origin of the internal carotid artery. Plaque removal is performed with careful determination of the cranial extent of the endarterectomy. Carotid artery patching is not routinely employed unless the internal carotid artery seems unusually small, or in patients with recurrent carotid artery stenosis following previous carotid artery endarterectomy. The longitudinal arteriotomy is closed and the patient awakened from anesthesia.

RESULTS OF CAROTID ENDARTERECTOMY

Although surgical techniques are standardized, indications for carotid endarterectomy and perioperative morbidity and mortality show wide variance. Carotid endarterectomy in the asymptomatic patient should not be performed by surgeons with combined stroke and death rates exceeding 3%. For symptomatic patients, benefit can be demonstrated after 2 years if the stroke plus death rate is less than 5%. Ideally, stroke rates should be less than 2% and perioperative mortality less than 1% in all patients undergoing cerebrovascular surgery. The institutional experience at Barnes Hospital/Washington University Medical Center, from July 1980 through December 1989, involved isolated carotid endarterectomy in 542 patients (Table 1). Indications for surgery in two-thirds of these patients were transient ischemic attacks, amaurosis fugax, or completed stroke; one-third of the patients were asymptomatic. Transient neurological deficits were seen in eight patients (1.5%), permanent neurological deficits in five patients (0.9%), and three patients (0.6%) died in the perioperative period. There was only one permanent neurologic deficit and no mortality among the asymptomatic subgroup.

With a large diabetic population base referred from the Joslin Clinic, Campbell et al. (31) at the New England Deaconess Hospital compared operative complication rates in diabetic and nondiabetic populations. Although the majority of their patients underwent surgery prior to 1980, they demonstrated a permanent neurologic deficit in 2.6%, myocardial infarction in 2.9%, and a death rate of 0.5% in all patients. There was no statistically significant difference in any of these complication rates between patients in the diabetic and nondiabetic subgroups. Long-term follow-up indicated an effective decrease in stroke rate in the diabetic population after carotid endarterectomy, with the expected significant increase in long-term mortality due to cardiac death.

Since introduction of a computerized Vascular Registry at the Barnes Hospital/ Washington University Medical Center Vascular Service in July of 1987, 65 carotid

TABLE 1. *Carotid endarterectomy results*

Indications	Number of patients (%)	Transient neurological deficit (%)	Permanent neurological deficit (%)	Mortality (%)
Transient ischemic attack and amaurosis fugax or stroke	366 (67.5)	7 (1.9)	4 (1.1)	3 (0.8)
Rind	4 (0.7)	0	0	0
Stroke in evolution	1 (0.2)	0	0	0
Asymptomatic	171 (31.6)	8 (1.5)	1 (0.5)	0
Total	542 (100%)	8 (1.5%)	5 (0.9%)	3 (0.5%)

Barnes Hospital: WUMC Vascular Service, July 1980–December 1989

TABLE 2. *Diabetic patients—carotid endarterectomy*

61 patients—65 carotid endarterectomies

Type of diabetes:	
Insulin dependent	20
Oral agent	25
Diet controlled	16
	61 patients
Indications for endarterectomy	
TIA	29
Amaurosis	10
Stroke	2
Asymptomatic	24
	65
Complications	
Temporary deficit –	2 (3%)
Permanent deficit –	0
Mortality –	0

Barnes Hospital—WUMC Vascular Service, July 1987 through October 1989

TABLE 3. *Carotid endarterectomy results*

188 patients—198 procedures
Permanent deficits—2.0%
Temporary—1.0%
Mortality—1.0%

Barnes Hospital—WUMC Vascular Service,
July 1987 through October 1989

endarterectomies were performed in 61 diabetic patients (Table 2). Twenty of these patients had insulin-dependent diabetes, 25 had disease controlled by oral agents, and 16 were controlled by diet alone. The indications for surgery were transient ischemic attacks in 29 patients, amaurosis fugax in 10 patients, previous stroke in two patients, and asymptomatic significant disease in 24 of the patients. In 65 procedures, two temporary deficits (3%) occurred with no permanent neurologic deficits or mortality observed. In this same time period, 198 procedures performed in 188 nondiabetic patients; a 2% permanent stroke rate was noted (1% transient neurologic deficits postoperatively and a 1% mortality rate) (Table 3). These data demonstrate that with appropriate preoperative screening and perioperative care, carotid endarterectomy can be performed safely in diabetic patients with morbidity and mortality rates comparable to their nondiabetic counterparts.

SURGICAL MANAGEMENT OF CONCOMITANT CORONARY AND CAROTID ARTERY DISEASE

The high incidence of concomitant cerebrovascular and coronary artery disease, especially in the diabetic patient, has been reviewed above. If preoperative evaluation reveals concomitant disease, optimal management of these patients requires careful planning. It has been suggested that in patients with significant carotid and coronary artery disease, both requiring surgery, that staged procedures be performed whenever possible. In general, the patient with severe symptomatic cerebrovascular disease without significant myocardial ischemia or with stable angina, should have the carotid endarterectomy performed first. In contrast, those patients with severe symptomatic cardiac disease and asymptomatic but significant cerebrovascular disease, may have coronary artery bypass grafting done as their primary procedure without simultaneous carotid endarterectomy. The incidence of perioperative stroke using the staged approach is approximately 1.5% and compares favorably with those undergoing elective carotid endarterectomy (15). The expected incidence of postoperative neurologic disturbances after cardiac operations alone is between 1.3 and 2.4% in large series, but frequently can be higher (32). A combined carotid endarterectomy and coronary artery bypass grafting can be performed simultaneously, but this is suggested only for those patients with severe coronary artery disease, or in those with unstable angina and high-grade symptomatic or bilateral carotid disease. Using this combined approach, neurologic complications occurred in approximately 9% in a recent large series (15). Of these, half were permanent and half were temporary neurologic deficits. Careful analysis of the published literature in a recent review supports the view that "Patient management is best determined by careful assessment of the symptomatology and severity of disease in each subsystem, with a combined procedure when conditions dictate, but staging whenever possible" (33).

In a recent report, 275 patients scheduled for coronary artery bypass surgery with previous neurologic events (29%), or asymptomatic severe (>70% diameter) stenosis (71%), were managed by one of three protocols (34). Those patients with stable cardiac disease had carotid endarterectomy before undergoing cardiac surgery ($n = 24$). Patients with symptomatic or bilateral carotid stenoses were managed on a selective basis ($n = 122$ patients) according to clinician preference. Prospective randomization was performed in those patients with unilateral asymptomatic carotid lesions to either combined procedures ($n = 71$) or coronary artery bypass grafting followed by carotid endarterectomy in a delayed operation ($n = 58$). In the subgroup of patients with unilateral asymptomatic carotid lesions who underwent combined procedures, the stroke rate was 2.8% (2/71) with a death rate of 4.2% (3/71). For those patients undergoing staged procedures, the stroke rate was 7.2% (eight of 111 operations) with a death rate of 2.7% (3/111) (34). All of these data reflect surgical series where combined procedures were performed by induction of general anesthesia, performance of carotid endarterectomy, subsequent performance of coronary artery bypass grafting with cardiopulmonary bypass support, and finally, closure of the sternal and neck incisions. In a smaller group of 47 patients undergoing combined procedures, there were improved stroke and death rates (1/47 = 2.1%), with slight modification of the technical aspects of the procedure. Carotid endarterectomy was not performed until cardiopulmonary bypass had been instituted with elevated pressures (70 to 90 mm Hg) and stabilized cardiac outputs of 2.5 to 3 l/min. As well, cardiopulmonary bypass was used to support the beating heart and provide pulsatile flow in a setting of hypothermia, hemodilution, and heparinization with ongoing EEG monitoring.

There is no surgical series of combined procedures with a large enough subset of diabetic patients to allow for meaningful analysis. Given the increased incidence of cerebrovascular disease and coronary artery disease in diabetic patients, however, severe concomitant disease is not unusual. Until further data are available, these patients should be managed in a manner similar to their nondiabetic counterparts.

CONCLUSIONS

Cerebrovascular disease is manifest in diabetic patients by an increased incidence of stroke and death from stroke. After careful preoperative evaluation of both the cerebral and coronary circulation, diabetic patients can undergo carotid endarterectomy with low perioperative morbidity and mortality, when compared with non-diabetic individuals, resulting in short- and long-term neurologic benefit.

REFERENCES

1. Callow AD. Cerebrovascular insufficiency. In: Haimovici H ed. *Vascular surgery: Principles and Techniques*. Connecticut, Appleton & Lange: 1989;719.
2. Wiebers DO, Whisnant JP, Sandok BA, et al. Effectiveness of carotid endarterectomy for asymptomatic carotid stenosis: Design of a clinical trial. *Mayo Clin Proc* 1989;64:897–904.
3. Garcia MJ, McNamara PM, Gordon T, Kannell WB. Morbidity and mortality in diabetics in the Framingham population. *Diabetes* 1974;23(2):105–111.
4. Asplund K, Hägg E, Helmers C, Lithner F, Strand T, Wester PO. The natural history of stroke in diabetic patients. *Acta Med Scand* 1980;207:417–424.
5. Alex M, Baron EK, Goldenberg S, Blumenthal HT. An autopsy study of cerebrovascular accident in diabetes mellitus. *Circulation* 1972;25:663–673.
6. Bell ET. A postmortem study of cerebrovascular disease in diabetics. *Arch Pathol* 1962;53:444–455.
7. Weinberger J, Biscarra V, Weisberg MK, Jacobson JH. Factors contributing to stroke in patients with atherosclerotic disease of the great vessels: The role of diabetes. *Stroke* 1983;14(5):709–712.
8. Giordano JM. Epidemiology and risk factors. In: Giordano JM, Trout HH, DePalma RG, eds. *The basic science of Vascular Surgery*. New York: Futura Publishing Company. 1988;351–357.
9. Ruderman NB, Haudenschild C. Diabetes as an atherogenic factor. *Prog Cardiovasc Dis* 1984;(5):373–412.
10. Kannel WB, McGee DL. Diabetes and cardiovascular disease: The Framingham study. *JAMA* 1979;241(19):2035–2038.
11. Thompson JE, Dale JA, Patman RD. Carotid endarterectomy for cerebrovascular insufficiency: Long-term results in 592 patients followed up to 13 years. *Ann Surg* 1970;184:663–679.
12. Callow AD, Mackey WC. Long-term follow up of surgically managed carotid bifurcation atherosclerosis: Justification for an aggressive approach. *Ann Surg* 1989;210:308–316.
13. Hertzer NR, Aronson R. Cumulative stroke and survival 10 years after carotid endarterectomy. *J Vasc Surg* 1985;2:661–668.
14. Stewart G, Ross-Russell RW, Browse NL. The long-term results of carotid endarterectomy for transient ischemic attacks. *J Vasc Surg* 1986;4:600–605.
15. O'Hara PJ, Hertzer NR. Concomitant carotid and coronary arterial occlusive disease. In: Ernst CB, Stanley JC eds. *Current therapy in vascular surgery*. Toronto: Brian C Decker, 1987;66–70.
16. Kuebler TW, Bendick PJ, Fineberg SE, et al. Diabetes mellitus and cerebrovascular disease: Prevalence of carotid artery occlusive disease and associated risk factors in 482 adult diabetic patients. *Diabetes Care* 1983;6(3):274–278.
17. Gomez CR. Carotid plaque morphology and risk for stroke. *Stroke* 1990;21:148–151.
18. Chan A, Beach KW, Martin DC, Strandness DE. Carotid artery disease in NIDDM diabetes. *Diabetes Care* 1983;6(6):562–569.
19. Chambers BR, Norris JW. Outcome in patients with asymptomatic neck bruits. *N Engl J Med* 1986;315:860–865.
20. Hemeric M, et al. Natural history of asymptomatic carotid artery occlusive lesions. *JAMA* 1987;258:2704–2707.
21. Bogousslavsky J, Despland PA, Regli F. Asymptomatic tight stenosis of the intimal carotid artery: Long-term progress. *Neurology* 1986;36:861–863.
22. Moneta GL, Taylor DC, Nicholls SC, et al. Operative versus nonoperative management of asymptomatic high-grade internal carotid artery stenosis: Improved results with endarterectomy. *Stroke* 1987;18:1005–10.
23. Roederer GO, Langlois YE, Jager KA, Primozich BS, et al. The natural history of carotid arterial disease in asymptomatic patients with cervical bruits. *Stroke* 1984;15(4):605–613.
24. Moneta GL, et al. Asymptomatic high grade internal carotid artery stenosis: Is stratification according to risk factors or duplex spectral analysis possible? *J Vasc Surg* 1989;10(5):475–483.

25. Bogousslavsky J, Regli F, Van Melle G. Risk factors and concomitants of internal carotid artery occlusion or stenosis. *Arch Neurol* 1985;42:864–867.
26. Drielsma RF, Burnett JR, Gray-Weale AC, et al. Carotid artery disease: The influence of diabetes mellitus. *J Cardiovasc Surg* 1988;29:692–696.
27. Kase CS, et al. Prevalence of silent stroke in patients presenting with initial stroke: The Framingham study. *Stroke* 1989;20(7):850–852.
28. Hertzer NR, Beven EG, Young JR, et al. Coronary artery disease in peripheral vascular patients: A classification of 1000 coronary angiograms and results of surgical management. *Ann Surg* 1984;199:223–233.
29. Graor RA, Hertzer NR. Management of coexistent carotid artery and coronary artery disease. *Stroke* 1988;19(11):1441–1444.
30. Hertzer NR, Young JR, Beven EG, et al. Late results of coronary bypass in patients with peripheral vascular disease: Five year survival according to sex, hypertension, and diabetes. *Cleve Clin J Med* 1987;54:15–23.
31. Campbell DR, Hoar CS, Wheelock FC. Carotid artery surgery in diabetic patients. *Arch Surg* 1984;119:1405–1407.
32. Minami K, Sagoo KS, Breymann T, et al. Operative strategy in combined coronary and carotid artery disease. *J Thorac Cardiovasc Surg* 1988;95:303–309.
33. Newman DC, Hicks RG. Combined carotid and coronary artery surgery: A review of the literature. *Ann Thorac Surg* 1988;45:574–581.
34. Hertzer NR, Loop FD, Beven EG, et al. Surgical staging for simultaneous coronary and carotid disease: A study including prospective randomization. *J Vasc Surg* 1989;9:455–463.

Surgical Management of the Diabetic Patient,
edited by Michael Bergman and Gregorio A. Sicard.
Raven Press, Ltd., New York © 1991.

21

Cutaneous Foot Ulcers

Charles B. Anderson and John S. Munn

Department of Surgery, Washington University School of Medicine,
St. Louis, Missouri 63110

Clinicians who treat diabetic patients frequently encounter cutaneous foot ulcers in these patients. Foot ulceration with secondary infection represents the number one septic cause for hospital admission in patients with diabetes (1) and disables approximately 25% of these patients (2). An epidemiological study suggests that the interrelated process of ulceration, infection, and gangrene may carry a prevalence of 10% in diabetic patients (3).

Diabetic foot ulcers have been divided into two main categories: ischemic ulcers and neurotrophic ulcers (4,5). Ischemic ulcers generally are superficial, painful lesions that have a rim of vascularized tissue and a necrotic center. They tend to occur in the friction areas between toes, or where they may overlie bony prominences such as the interphalangeal joints and metatarsal heads. Neurotrophic ulcers, also known as mal perforans ulcers, are painless. They have a deep, punched-out appearance with a surrounding, heaped-up callus. These lesions are most commonly found in contact areas such as under the first and second metatarsal heads, but they can occur anywhere on the plantar surface. These categories are not exclusive, however, and most diabetic foot ulcers have features of both ischemia and neuropathy with respect to cause and appearance.

Atherosclerosis runs an accelerated course in diabetes, and it is the most important cause of morbidity and mortality in these patients (6). The hallmark of peripheral vascular atherosclerosis in diabetes is severe trifurcation disease often with sparing of the femoral and popliteal segments (7). This phenomenon is demonstrated clinically by the fact that diabetic patients are more likely to have a palpable popliteal pulse with absent distal pulses when compared with atherosclerotic nondiabetic individuals. A predisposition for small-vessel disease of the foot in diabetes probably does not exist (7–9). In fact, intraoperative angiograms typically show an extensive vascular network in the diabetic foot. Nonetheless, diabetic patients tend to have increased resistance to flow in the vascular tree. It has been shown that for a given ankle pressure, flow in the diabetic foot is significantly less than that in atherosclerotic patients without diabetes (10). In addition, there is evidence of capillary basement membrane thickening in diabetic patients. This in turn may lead to a functional abnormality in the microcirculation, which could predispose these patients to ulceration or poor wound healing (8,9).

Ischemic ulceration develops when the diabetic foot, with compromised vascular supply, is subjected to trauma. Trauma is incurred during typical daily activities such as a pedicure, or walking barefoot; thermal injury may occur during bathing. Persistent pressure in an immobilized patient frequently leads to a heel ulcer. The presence of edema from congestive heart failure or venous insufficiency also increases the risk of ischemic ulceration. Once an ischemic ulcer is present, secondary infection can occur.

Neuropathy renders the foot more susceptible to trauma by affecting light touch, proprioception, and most importantly, pain sensation (11,12). Consequently, the diabetic patient may not be aware of trauma involving his foot. The inability to sense pain blocks the natural reflexes that would prevent further injury. Thus, constant friction or pressure from ill-fitting shoes causes tissue breakdown beneath the skin. Subsequent skin loss results in an ulcer. More advanced neuropathy may lead to Charcot joints, which usually involve the articulations of the tarsal and metatarsal bones. This resultant deformity leads to an abnormal contact surface on the sole of the foot, thus predisposing to ulceration. A more subtle consequence of neuropathy is its effect on the motor nerves of the foot that innervate the intrinsic muscles. Diminished function of these muscles can lead to extension of the metatarsophalangeal joint and flexion of the proximal interphalangeal joint, resulting in more pressure on the metatarsal heads (the so called "intrinsic-minus foot"). This configuration also leads to a distal migration of the metatarsal fat pads that would normally protect against friction during ambulation. Neuropathy may also involve the sympathetic fibers that regulate cutaneous blood flow and this alteration in circulation may retard ulcer healing (11–14).

An infected ulcer can predispose to further tissue loss and gangrene by one of two mechanisms. In the diabetic foot with vascular compromise, increased metabolism that is associated with local infection can exceed the blood supply and lead to gangrene. In addition, inflammatory cells and some bacteria may elaborate substances that act as procoagulants that cause small-vessel thrombosis and tissue necrosis. Patients with diabetes can also have a relatively compromised immune system, and this may further promote infection. Multiple mechanisms have been proposed for this immune defect including impaired leucocyte transformation, chemotaxis, and phagocytosis (2,15). Proper metabolic control of diabetes may partially reverse this immune deficiency (16).

Historically, diabetic foot ulcers have a bad prognosis. Because of the compromised immune state, established foot infections can rapidly progress to fulminant sepsis, resulting in risk to both the limb and the patient's life. In two studies of diabetic foot infections and ischemia, it was found that approximately 25% of affected limbs required amputation, and half of the patients with ulceration on one limb had an ulcer develop on the contralateral limb as well (17,18).

ULCER EVALUATION AND TREATMENT

Basic medical treatment of the diabetic foot ulcer requires assessment of the degree of infection, débridement, immobilization, metabolic control, antibiotics, and evaluation of the vascular status of the foot. Adequate treatment almost always requires hospitalization, at least for the initial period, until satisfactory progress has been identified.

The clinical presentation of a diabetic foot ulcer can range from a small, asymptomatic toe erosion to a deep excavation with extensive tissue loss and fulminant systemic sepsis (19). A cutaneous ulcer may be only the tip of the iceberg. It is not unusual for the infectious process to involve bones or joints. Ulcers on the plantar surface can also erode into the adjacent plantar space; diabetic patients may harbor severe plantar space abscesses while remaining relatively asymptomatic (20). Points of clinical interest during examination include the anatomic location of the ulcer, the nature of drainage, the presence of surrounding erythema or cellulitis, adjacent tissue necrosis, and involvement of bony structures. Consideration must be given also to the deep structures of the foot. Fluctuance or tenderness along the arch of the foot suggests a plantar space abscess. Systemic manifestations must also be checked including fever, white blood cell count, and toxic appearance. Roentgenograph studies may be helpful. The presence of gas does not necessarily indicate Clostridium gas gangrene; more likely it represents a severe, mixed infection of obligate anaerobes such as *Bacteroides fragilis* and *Peptostreptococcus,* combined with facultative enteric anaerobes such as *Proteus, Escherichia coli,* and *Klebsiella* (21). Careful ulcer evaluation also requires unroofing the overlying eschar, obtaining suitable tissue for culture, and careful probing for extension into the plantar space or into joints. The presence of bone at the base of an ulcer is always suspicious for osteomyelitis.

ANTIBIOTICS

The consensus among clinicians is that intravenous antibiotics are necessary for virtually all diabetic foot infections. However, definitive controlled studies are lacking with respect to: which ulcers should be treated, which antibiotics should be used, and how long treatment should be carried out (22). Antibiotic selection should be directed by culture results; several studies have looked at the microbial flora of diabetic foot ulcers (19,21–23). The most accurate cultures appear to come from carefully processed deep wound tissue specimens or curettings. Simple tissue swabs have a much poorer correlation. One fact that has emerged from several studies is that the flora of these ulcers is polymicrobial, with up to five organisms per patient. Commonly encountered organisms include the enteric bacteria such as *Proteus, E. coli,* and *Enterobacter.* Anaerobes are numerous and they include *Peptococcus, Clostridium* and several species of *Bacteroides. Enterococcus,* streptococci, and staphylococci are also frequently encountered. Thus, broad spectrum antibiotic coverage generally is required. A satisfactory regimen would include an aminoglycoside and a drug effective against anaerobes such as clindamycin or metronidazol. Ampicillin coverage may be required for *Enterococcus.* Patients with impaired renal function may be given either a third generation cephalosporin, a synthetic penicillin, or a ticarcillin-clavulanic acid combination. Patients with lesser degrees of foot sepsis may be satisfactorily covered with oral antibiotics with a suitable spectrum of activity. Antibiotic treatment alone, however, is not adequate in treating these ulcers, and débridement and careful wound management play a vital role.

DRAINAGE, DÉBRIDEMENT, AND AMPUTATION

Standard surgical techniques should be used for débridement. All necrotic, infected tissue must be removed. Débridement is facilitated by neuropathy, which typically renders the foot anesthetic. Occasionally a neglected ulcer rapidly evolves into a septic foot with severe, systemic toxicity. This is a surgical emergency and requires immediate wide incision and drainage of all infected areas. Consideration for subsequent reconstruction should be secondary to the goal of obtaining complete surgical drainage (2). After the initial incision and drainage, second and often multiple procedures may be required in order to insure adequate débridement (20). If the hindfoot is not salvageable or the patient has severe diffuse vascular disease, it may be prudent to proceed with guillotine amputation above the ankle (22). Wound dressings consist of fine-mesh gauze moistened with saline or dilute antiseptic solution. They are changed two to three times daily. The use of foot soaks or whirlpool treatments occasionally can be helpful; however, this may also cause tissue maceration.

Osteomyelitis should be suspected when there is erythema and drainage from a punctate ulcer over a bony prominence or if there is exposed bone at the base of an ulcer. Magnified roentgenograph views of the bony structures may be helpful in identifying osteomyelitis. The pertinent roentgenograph differential diagnosis for osteomyelitis includes Charcot joints and diabetic osteopathy. The latter is a resorptive process related to autonomic neuropathy that radiographically resembles osteomyelitis and does not require intervention (24). The differentiation is clinical. Diabetic osteopathy should be suspected, however, when there is multifocal involvement, bilaterality, and a peripheral distribution of bony lesions on roentgenograph. Evidence of osteomyelitis may also be obtained from a nuclear medicine bone scan or a sinogram performed in the ulcer bed. The presence of osteomyelitis is troublesome, because extensive medical treatment, including prolonged antibiotics or hyperbaric oxygen treatment, generally does not result in cure. All else being equal, the most cost-effective method of treating diabetic osteomyelitis in the foot is surgical: digital amputation for osteomyelitis of the toe, or resection of the involved metatarsal head (25). The technique for toe amputation as described by Sizer and Wheelock (26) has had excellent results with up to 98% of the wounds healing primarily. Highlights of their technique include division of skin, subcutaneous tissue, and tendons with the knife; ligation of bleeding points with fine suture; and delicate precision in creating flaps. Forceps and retractors are never used on the skin. The amputation wound may be closed primarily if it is a toe or a transmetatarsal amputation; there is no active infection at the site of amputation; all necrotic and infected material is removed; and the circulation is adequate. Sizer and Wheelock also recommend 7 to 10 days of antibiotics, a prolonged period of bedrest, and protection of the amputation site.

VASCULAR EVALUATION

Regardless of whether or not the diabetic ulcer is neurotrophic or ischemic, diminished blood flow is likely to be present, particularly in elderly patients. It is important to decide whether perfusion is adequate in order to allow for healing with local wound measures. The presence of a palpable pedal pulse and a warm, pink foot is a fairly reliable indicator of satisfactory perfusion, particularly if the pulses remain strong after exercise. Conversely, a chronically ischemic diabetic foot can be identified by lack of palpable pulses, by ruborous changes, and by characteristic cracked, dry skin. Other clinical observations (Table 1) can assist in determining whether local measures alone may suffice.

TABLE 1. *Clinical criteria predictive of foot ulcer healing*

Palpable pedal pulses
Absence of rest pain
Absence of dependent rubor
Pink color and warm foot
Lack of atrophy
Venous filling time less than 20 sec
Absence of infection

VASCULAR LABORATORY TESTS

Noninvasive laboratory techniques are detailed in Chapters 19 and 22. The following is meant to provide a brief overview of the procedures most commonly utilized in the assessment of foot ulcers.

Several vascular laboratory noninvasive tests provide further information regarding the circulatory status of the foot (27,28). The tests are relatively inexpensive and reliable and may be repeated without discomfort or risk. They may be used to measure the response to therapeutic maneuvers. We routinely perform Doppler studies of the lower extremities with segmental pressures and wave forms. Not only do these studies give information as to the nature of pedal circulation, but they can also anatomically localize the site of obstruction. Also important is that the ankle pressure may be used as a predictor of wound healing. Minor foot amputations in nondiabetic patients will not heal if the ankle pressure is less than 55 mm Hg (29). Most diabetic patients require a higher ankle pressure of at least 80–90 mm Hg to heal amputations such as digit or metatarsal resections (28,30). Other authors, however, have found that the correlation between ankle pressure and healing is not strong (31). There are two pitfalls to the Doppler ankle pressure study. First, the leg vessels in diabetic patients may be incompressible due to severe arterial medial calcification. This leads to a falsely elevated ankle pressure which on the average is 20 mm Hg higher than in the nondiabetic atherosclerotic patient. Secondly, diabetic patients can have additional disease beyond the ankle pressure cuff and this defect will not be recognized with standard ankle/arm index testing (28).

Better indicators of foot perfusion are the digital blood pressures and waveforms (32). The toe blood pressure may be measured using either the ultrasonic Doppler, the pulse volume recorder, or plethysmography. Several studies have indicated that diabetic patients require a minimum toe pressure ranging from 25–30 mm Hg (29,32) to higher pressures such as 45–50 mm Hg (31,33).

Additional techniques are available in some labs for the assessment of pedal perfusion (Table 2). Transcutaneous oxygen measurements may give important infor-

TABLE 2. *Laboratory determination of pedal circulation*

Pressures and waveforms
Digital blood pressure by
  Doppler
  Pulse volume recorder
  Photoplethysmography
Transcutaneous PO_2
Xenon 133 uptake
Angiography

mation on foot healing. The critical range for transcutaneous PO_2 for wound healing is between 25 and 40 mm Hg (34,35). Transcutaneous oxygen measurement is dependent on the patient's arterial PO_2, cardiac output, pulmonary function, hemoglobin concentration, skin thickness, and circulatory status. The uptake of subcutaneously injected radioactive Xenon 133 also gives an indication of foot perfusion. A Xenon 133 uptake greater than 2.2 ml/100g of tissue per minute has been associated with wound healing in 95% of patients tested (36).

ARTERIOGRAPHY

When noninvasive studies indicate that pedal perfusion is inadequate, an arteriogram is indicated. Arteriography does carry the risk of nephrotoxicity and this is especially increased in diabetic patients (37,38). The management of patients undergoing angiography is discussed in Chapter 19 (Vascular Surgery). Patients with significant renal dysfunction can have just the affected limb imaged. Computerized digital arteriographic techniques allow a further decrease in the amount of dye used. Arteriography should identify the level of obstruction and indicate the nature of the outflow vessels and a potential communication with the pedal arch. Not infrequently, the vascular disease is so severe and diffuse that satisfactory views of the pedal vessels cannot be obtained using standard angiographic techniques. One solution is to perform intraoperative prebypass arteriography. This is rarely necessary due to the development of high resolution digital subtraction angiographic techniques.

REVASCULARIZATION

The need for revascularization is based on clinical judgement and the results of vascular lab studies. The timing of revascularization depends on the clinical presentation. In cases of severe pedal sepsis with abcesses and cellulitis, control of the foot infection should be obtained before doing a bypass. On the other hand, minor wound débridements and amputations can be performed either in conjunction with or following revascularization. Angiography will typically disclose that the outflow vessel for bypass will be a distal tibial or peroneal artery. Not infrequently, the bypass may need to be performed in the foot. On occasion we have explored vessels that have not been demonstrated arteriographically but have had a satisfactory Doppler signal. Frequently we can use the popliteal artery as inflow. Many authors now suggest that shorter bypasses, when possible, are preferable to those originating from the femoral region (39,40). The conduit of choice for these distal bypasses clearly is saphenous vein. We prefer the *in situ* technique whenever possible (41).

   In most series, the results for distal bypass in diabetic patients are equal to and perhaps even better than nondiabetic patients (42). Long-term results indicate patency rates ranging from 50–95% (40–44). In our experience, roughly two-thirds of patients who require an operation for diabetic foot ulcer are candidates for an arterial bypass procedure. In those undergoing arterial bypass, early limb salvage is 91%.

   Other adjuncts are available to assist in healing diabetic foot ulcers. For patients with stable mal perforans or ischemic ulcers, extra-depth shoes or shoes with arch bars or specially preformed insoles can be designed that will relieve the weight from the affected areas. More extensive neurotrophic ulcers may benefit from total contact casting (45). This technique was developed in the 1930s, and allows ambulation

TABLE 3. *Prevention of diabetic foot infection*

Education
Good hygiene
Daily foot inspection
Avoid going barefoot
Adequately fitted footwear
Careful pedicure
Stop cigarette smoking
Periodic vascular exam
Control of blood pressure, weight, and glucose
Early intervention
Added protection for immobilized patients

while protecting the ulcer by diverting pressure and decreasing shear on the ulcer. Patient compliance with this modality is good. Contraindications to contact-casting include infection, deep ulcers, significant edema, or fragile skin. Contact-casting does carry the risk of joint stiffness and atrophy and it may also cause additional ulcers by abrasion.

The key to management of the diabetic foot is prevention (4,9). Preventive measures are summarized in Table 3. Prevention begins with patient education. It has been shown that diabetic patients with ulcers lack an understanding of the relationship between diabetes and the foot (46). Diabetic patients should be instructed not to go barefoot. Foot inspection should be performed regularly. Good hygiene requires that the feet be kept clean, warm, and dry at all times. Shoes that fit adequately are important and must allow room for the toes, metatarsal heads, and heel. Stiff, new shoes should be worn initially for short intervals until they are broken in. Foot care, including pedicure, should be performed by professionals, particularly in patients with diminished visual acuity. Cigarette smokers should quit. Additional consideration might include prophylactic podiatric surgery to resolve bony deformities before ulceration occurs (4).

A satisfactory outcome for diabetics with foot ulcers depends on careful clinical management. The surgeon can play an important role in the treatment of diabetic foot ulcers and restoration of limb function. In addition to ulcer evaluation, the surgeon must be able to provide adequate wound débridement and wound care. Equally important is the careful clinical assessment of the pedal circulation and the judgement of when arterial reconstruction is necessary.

REFERENCES

1. Whitehouse FW. Infections that hospitalize the diabetic. *Geriatrics* 1973;28:97–99.
2. Gibbons GW. The diabetic foot: amputations and drainage of infection. *J Vasc Surg* 1987;5:791–793.
3. Rosenqvist U. An epidemiological survey of diabetic foot problems in the Stockholm County, 1982. *Acta Med Scand (Supp.)* 1984;687:55–60.
4. Harkless LB, Dennis KJ. The role of the podiatrist. In: Levin ME, O'Neal LW, eds. *The diabetic foot.* St. Louis: C. V. Mosby Co., 1988;249–272.
5. Lee BY, Brancato RF. Perforating ulcers of the foot. In: Lee BY, ed. *Chronic ulcers of the skin.* New York: McGraw Hill Publishing Co., 1985;111–131.
6. Ruderman NB, Haudenschild CC. Diabetes as an atherogenic factor. *Prog Cardiovasc Dis* 1984;26:373–412.
7. Conrad MC. Large and small artery occlusion in diabetics and nondiabetics with severe vascular disease. *Circulation* 1967;36:83–91.

8. LoGerfo FW. Vascular disease, matrix abnormalities, and neuropathy: indications for limb salvage in diabetes mellitus. *J Vasc Surg* 1987;5:793–795.
9. LoGerfo FW, Coffmann JD. Vascular and microvascular disease of the foot in diabetics. *N Engl J Med* 1984;311:1615–1619.
10. Tenembaum MM, Rayfield E, Junior J, Jacobson JH, Giron F. Altered pressure flow relationships in the diabetic foot. *J Surg Res* 1981;31:307–313.
11. Brown MJ, Asbury AK. Diabetic neuropathy. *Ann Neurol* 1984;15:2–12.
12. Delbridge L, Ctercteko G, Fowler C, Reeve TS, Lequesne LP. The aetiology of diabetic neuropathic ulceration of the foot. *Br J Surg* 1985;72:1–6.
13. Wieman TJ, Huang KC, Tsueda K, Thomas MH, Lucas LF, Simpson F. Peripheral somatic sensory neuropathy and skin galvanic response in the feet of patients with diabetes. *Surg Gynecol Obstet* 1989;168:501–506.
14. Sundkvist G, Almer LO, Lilja B. Influence of autonomic neuropathy on leg circulation and toe temperature in diabetes mellitus. *Acta Med Scand (Suppl)* 1984;687:9–17.
15. Bagdade JD, Root RK, Bulger RJ. Impaired leukocyte function in patients with poorly controlled diabetes. *Diabetes* 1974;23:9–15.
16. Goodson WH III, Hunt TK. Wound healing in experimental diabetes mellitus: importance of early insulin therapy. *Surg Forum* 1978;29:95–98.
17. Klamer TW, Towne JB, Bandyk DF, Bonner MJ. The influence of sepsis and ischemia on the natural history of the diabetic foot. *Am Surg* 1987;53:490–494.
18. Kucan JD, Robson MC. Diabetic foot infections: fate of the contralateral foot. *Plast Reconstr Surg* 1986;77:439–441.
19. Axler DA. Microbiology of diabetic foot infections. *J Foot Surg* 1987;26:53–56.
20. Livingston R, Jacobs RL. Plantar abscess of the diabetic patient. *Foot Ankle* 1985;5:205–213.
21. Fierer J, Daniel D, Davis C. The fetid foot: lower extremity infections in patients with diabetes mellitus. *Rev Infect Dis* 1979;1:210–217.
22. McIntyre KE. Control of infection in the diabetic foot: the role of microbiology, immunopathology, antibiotics and guillotine amputation. *J Vasc Surg* 1987;5:787–790.
23. Sapico FL, Witte JL, Canawati HN, Montgomerie JZ, Bessman AN. The infected foot of the diabetic patient: quantitative microbiology and analysis of clinical features. *Rev Infect Dis* 1984 (Supp);6:S171–S176.
24. Friedman SA, Rakow RB. Osseous lesions of the foot in diabetic neuropathy. *Diabetes* 1971;20:302–307.
25. Benton GS, Kerstein MD. Cost effectiveness of early digital amputation in the patient with diabetes. *Surg Gynecol Obstet* 1985;161:523–524.
26. Sizer JS, Wheelock FC Jr. Digital amputations in diabetic patients. *Surgery* 1972;72:980–989.
27. Carter SA, Hamel ER. Role of pressure measurements in vascular disease. In: Bernstein EF, ed. *Noninvasive diagnostic techniques in vascular disease.* St. Louis: C. V. Mosby Co., 1982; 317–343.
28. Raines JK, Darling RC, Buth J, Brewster DC, Austen WG. Vascular laboratory criteria for the management of peripheral vascular disease of the lower extremities. *Surgery* 1976;79:21–29.
29. Barnes RW, Thornhill B, Nix L, Rittgers SE, Turley G. Prediction of amputation wound healing roles of doppler ultrasound and digit photoplethysmography. *Arch Surg* 1981;116:80–83.
30. Baker WH, Barnes RW. Minor forefoot amputation in patients with low ankle pressure. *Am J Surg* 1977;133:331–332.
31. Bone GE, Pomajzl MJ. Toe blood pressure by photoplethysmography: an index of healing in forefoot amputation. *Surgery* 1981;89:569–574.
32. Ramsey DE, Manke DA, Sumner DS. Toe blood pressure: a valuable adjunct to ankle pressure measurement for assessing peripheral arterial disease. *J Cardiovasc Dis* 1983;24:43–48.
33. Holstein P, Lassen NA. Healing of ulcers on the feet correlated with distal blood pressure measurements in occlusive arterial disease. *Acta Orthoped Scand* 1980;51:995–1006.
34. Cina C, Katsamouris A, Megerman J, et al. Utility of transcutaneous oxygen tension measurements in peripheral arterial occlusive disease. *J Vasc Surg* 1984;1:362–371.
35. Wyss CR, Robertson C, Love SJ, Harrington RM, Matsen FA. Relationship between transcutaneous oxygen tension, ankle blood pressure, and clinical outcome of vascular surgery in diabetic and nondiabetic patients. *Surgery* 1987;101:56–62.
36. Malone JM, Leal JM, Moore WS, et al. The "Gold Standard" for amputation level selection: xenon 133 clearance. *J Surg Res* 1981;30:449–455.
37. Parfrey PS, Griffiths SM, Barrett BJ, et al. Contrast material-induced renal failure in patients with diabetes mellitus, renal insufficiency, or both. *N Engl J Med* 1989;320:143–149.
38. Cruz C, Hricak H, Samhouri F, Smith RF, Eyler WR, Levin NW. Contrast media for angiography: effect on renal function. *Radiology* 1986;158:109–112.
39. Ascer E, Veith FJ, Gupta Sk, White SA, Bakal CW, Wengerter K, Sprayregen S. Short vein grafts: a superior option for arterial reconsructions to poor or compromised outflow tracts. *J Vasc Surg* 1988;7:370–378.

40. Rhodes GR, Rollins D, Sidawy AN, Skudder P, Buchbinder D. Popliteal to tibial in situ saphenous vein bypass for limb salvage in diabetic patients. *Am J Surg* 1987;154:245–247.
41. Leather RP, Shah DM, Chang BB, Kaufman JL. Resurrection of the in situ saphenous vein bypass 1000 cases later. *Ann Surg* 1988;208:435–442.
42. Hurley JJ, Aver AI, Hershey HB, et al. Distal arterial resconstructions: patency and limb salvage in diabetics. *J Vasc Surg* 1987;5:796–802.
43. Veterans Administrative Cooperative Study Group 141. Comparative evaluation of prosthetic, reversed, and in situ vein bypass grafts in distal popliteal and tibial-peroneal revascularization. *Arch Surg* 1988;123:434–438.
44. Buchbinder D, Pasch AR, Rollins DL, et al. Results of arterial reconstruction of the foot. *Arch Surg* 1986;121:673–677.
45. Sinacore DR. Total contact casting in the treatment of diabetic neuropathic ulcers. In: Levin ME, O'Neal LW, eds. *The diabetic foot.* St. Louis: C. V. Mosby Co., 1988;273–292.
46. Delbridge L, Appleberg M, Reeve TS. Factors associated with development of foot lesions in the diabetic. *Surgery* 1983;93:78–82.

Surgical Management of the Diabetic Patient,
edited by Michael Bergman and Gregorio A. Sicard.
Raven Press, Ltd., New York © 1991.

22

Lower Extremity Amputation in the Diabetic Patient

Daniel J. McGraw and Brent T. Allen

*Department of Surgery, Washington University School of Medicine,
St. Louis, Missouri 63110*

The management of lower extremity ischemia in the diabetic patient is a problem of enormous impact in the United States. There are approximately 10,000,000 diabetics in the United States, 25% of whom will consult a physician for diabetes-related foot or leg problems resulting from the triad of accelerated atherosclerosis, neuropathy, and infection. In particular, diabetic foot infections account for more in-hospital days than any other complication of diabetes. The severity of these problems is underscored by the observation that, in comparison to nondiabetic patients, gangrene occurs 53 times more frequently in diabetic men and 71 times more frequently in diabetic women (1). This propensity toward gangrene puts diabetic patients at particularly high risk for amputation. Indeed, the mean interval from the diagnosis of diabetes to amputation was only 13 years in one study (2). Most and Sinnock (3) have estimated the risk of amputation among diabetic patients discharged from short-term United States hospitals to be approximately 5.9 per 1,000 patients per year; other estimates range as high as eight per 1,000 patients per year (4). Thus, two-thirds of major amputations in the United States are performed on diabetic patients, at an age-adjusted risk approximately 15 times that of the nondiabetic population (3).

The tremendous commitment of health care resources to this problem is reflected in the estimated 500 million to 1.2 billion dollars spent on the approximately 50,000 amputations performed *annually* in the diabetic population (5,6). The frequency of this problem and its devastating impact on the patient mandate careful preoperative evaluation, operative technique, and postoperative follow-up if the best possible result is to be achieved.

CHOOSING AN AMPUTATION LEVEL IN THE DIABETIC PATIENT

Amputation in the diabetic patient is directed at removing all painful, infected, or gangrenous tissue. The level of amputation is determined by identifying the lowest possible level that will heal without complication and allow rehabilitation with or without a prosthetic device. Because as many as 50% of patients may undergo *con-*

tralateral amputation within 24 months, preservation of function in the amputated limb is of paramount importance (7). To achieve this goal, the surgeon has traditionally relied on the physical examination in selecting the amputation level. The past two decades have witnessed the establishment of the vascular laboratory and the refinement of angiographic techniques that are helpful in assessing the vascular status of the limb. However, these diagnostic modalities complement, but do not supplant, a careful physical examination by an experienced surgeon.

PHYSICAL EXAMINATION

Color, capillary refill, temperature, and the status of pulses all contribute to the clinical impression of tissue perfusion and the likelihood of primary healing of the amputation. Although a palpable pulse is often a good prognostic sign, the significance of its absence with respect to wound healing is more problematic. At the above knee (AK) level, it is commonly believed that 90% of amputations will heal regardless of the status of the femoral pulse (8). Squires et al., (9) however, achieved successful healing in only 45% of the patients lacking a palpable pulse while 82% of those with a pulse healed; these authors stressed the importance of superficial and profunda femoral artery patency in the success of primary healing. At more distal levels, Sizer and Wheelock (10) have shown that the presence of palpable pedal pulses is associated with healing in 98% of toe amputations; however, 89% of those performed in the absence of pulses also healed. The failures in the latter group were attributed to the greater extent of infection, which necessitated an open amputation. Finally, Andros et al. (11) described five diabetic patients with palpable foot pulses and gangrene who failed foot amputations; these authors stressed the need for arteriography in this setting. Pulse determinations alone, therefore, are less than discriminating indicators of healing.

THE VASCULAR LABORATORY EVALUATION

While several of these techniques have been discussed earlier (see Chapters 19 and 22), the following reviews these procedures as they pertain to amputation.

The most common adjunct to clinical judgement is the noninvasive vascular laboratory. Although few vascular laboratories perform all the noninvasive tests listed in Table 1, all perform at least several of the more common of these examinations, especially segmental limb pressures.

Segmental limb pressure measurement is the most basic of vascular laboratory examinations. It is predicated upon occluding the vessel of interest with an external pneumatic cuff. As the external pressure is released, the opening pressure of the vessel, as manifested by restoration of Doppler signals distally, is recorded. Although segmental limb pressures are highly accurate in predicting healing at the above and below knee level (12), the severity of diabetic peripheral vascular disease is often greatest in the calf. The calcific nature of medium-sized tibial arteries in diabetic patients renders these vessels incompressible and confounds the measurement of occlusion ankle pressures. Therefore, ankle pressures are not predictive of

TABLE 1. *Classification of diagnostic tests*

Noninvasive
    Careful physical examination
    Segmental arterial pressures
    Photoplethysmography
    Pulse volume recording
    Transcutaneous PO_2
    Laser Doppler velocimetry
    Photoelectric skin perfusion
    Skin temperature
Minimally invasive
    Isotopic clearance
    Fluorometry
Invasive
    Angiography

healing in diabetic forefoot amputations. Bone and Pomajzl (13) found 30% of amputations in diabetic patients with ankle pressures greater than 80 mm Hg failed to heal. Nicholas et al. (14) found ankle pressures in all patients (diabetic and nondiabetic) to have a sensitivity of 80% and a specificity of 97% when a pressure of greater than 70 mm Hg was chosen as a predictor of healing. Similarly, Welch et al. (15) found a pressure of 60 mm Hg to be essentially nonpredictive, and also noted no difference between diabetic and nondiabetic patients in this regard. Gibbons et al. (16) noted a 19% failure rate of forefoot amputations in those with ankle pressures greater than 70 mm Hg. Thus, ankle pressures are of limited usefulness in the nondiabetic patient and appear to be even more problematic in the diabetic patient.

The ankle/brachial index is derived from segmental limb pressures at these two locations and is the ratio of the ankle pressure to the arm pressure. In the normal population, this number is one or greater; in the presence of arterial occlusive disease, it is markedly reduced. Pinzur and colleagues (17) suggest a ratio of greater than 0.5 is predictive of foot amputations that will heal in the diabetic population. This seems, however, no more reliable than the values from which it is derived; although arm pressures are rarely affected by diabetes, the occlusion ankle pressure obtained in noncompliant diabetic arteries can remain falsely high, even in the presence of severely compromised pedal circulation (see chapter 19, Vascular Surgery).

Plethysmography (pulse volume recording) is less affected by the rigidity of the tibial vessels, as it is based on changes in limb volume as a function of arterial inflow. It may have more prognostic significance regarding the healing of minor amputations than ankle and toe pressure determinations. Raines et al. (18) noted a pulsatile pulse volume recording to be predictive of healing in 90% of patients. However, plethysmographic techniques have been demonstrated by Gibbons and colleagues in their series (16) to be of dubious predictive value, in that forefoot pulse volume recordings predicted failure in 50% of forefoot amputations that subsequently healed.

To overcome this prognostic dilemma, other more specialized tests can be used. Strain gauge digital plethysmography correlates volume change and blood pressure and is useful for predicting the healing of an adjacent toe amputation as the arterial medial calcification, which confounds this measurement more proximally, is often absent in the toe. Pressures of greater than 30 mm Hg predict healing of adjacent toe amputations in 78% of cases and foot and forefoot amputations in 80% of cases (19).

Digital photoplethysmography is commonly used in modern vascular laboratories to assess arterial perfusion at the toe level. Light near the infrared portion of the spectrum is emitted from a diode and reflected by the skin. Changes in the reflected light are a function of blood content of the skin. A digital blood pressure can, therefore, be measured as the digital occlusion cuff is relaxed. This technique has been reported to be 100% predictive of healing in toe amputation by some authors when pressures exceed 20 mm Hg (20) and forefoot amputations at pressures greater than 55 mm Hg (13).

Measurement of transcutaneous oxygen tension represents yet another technique to predict levels of successful amputation healing. Transcutaneous oxygen tension is a function of blood flow, oxygen extraction, oxyhemoglobin dissociation, and free oxygen diffusion through tissues. Because this parameter reflects several different processes, a transcutaneous oxygen tension of zero may exist in the presence of cutaneous blood flow detectable by other methods. For example, marginally perfused tissue extracts all available oxygen, yielding a transcutaneous oxygen tension of zero even though minimal blood flow is present. In contrast, in well perfused tissues, the transcutaneous oxygen tension is elevated because the oxygen supply far exceeds tissue demands. Thus, transcutaneous oxygen tension can reliably predict levels that will heal, but is not as reliable in predicting those levels that will not heal. Ratliff and colleagues (21) showed that all below knee (BK) amputations with a transcutaneous oxygen tension greater than 35 mm Hg healed and all those that failed had values less than 35 mm Hg. Some amputation levels however, with values less than 35 mm Hg also healed (21). Nevertheless, this technique provides a physiologic correlate to enhance the accuracy of other measurements and is not compromised by underlying calcific arterial disease as are most hemodynamic measurements.

Laser Doppler velocimetry measures blood flow velocity as a function of the frequency shift of light scattered by moving red blood cells near the skin surface. Although normal patients and those with vascular disease may have similar cutaneous blood flow under baseline conditions, the latter demonstrates a decreased hyperemic response in comparison to the former following local skin warming. Compared with transcutaneous oxygen tension measurements, laser Doppler velocimetry correctly predicted healing in 87% versus 95% (22).

Golbranson (23) has championed the technique of skin temperature measurement as a method of amputation level selection. In his series, all patients with skin temperature greater than 32°C at the level of amputation healed, and those with temperatures less than 30.5°C failed. Variable results were seen from 30.5°C to 32°C. In a prospective comparison of this technique to transcutaneous oxygen tension measurements, the former accurately predicted healing in 85% of cases versus 76% for the latter (23).

One of the more technically demanding and rarely available techniques to assess the suitability of amputation levels in the diabetic patient is the xenon-133 radioisotopic clearance technique as originally described by Nilsen (24) and Holstein (25). Flow rates greater than 2.4 ml/min per 100 g of tissue accurately predicted amputation healing in over 90% of reported cases (26). Other isotopes used have included [125]Iodo-antipyrine. These techniques require intradermal or epicutaneous injection of the isotope at the region of proposed skin incision for amputation and gamma camera imaging to quantitate washout of the injected isotope over time. Holstein

TABLE 2. *Preoperative level selection: The best commonly available tests*

Level of amputation	Selection criteria	Total successful primary and secondary healing (%)	Ref.
Toe	Palpable pedal pulses	98	10
	Photoplethysmographic pressure > 20 mm Hg	100	20
Transmetatarsal	Photoplethysmographic toe pressure > 55	100	13
Below knee	Transcutaneous PO_2 > 20	96	39
	> 35	100	
	Doppler calf pressure > 50 mm Hg	100	35
	Doppler thigh pressure > 80 mm Hg	92	35
Above knee	Clinical appearance	91	8
Transcutaneous	PO_2 > 20	100	39

(25) measured the external pressure required to prevent isotope washout; other techniques correlate washout and blood flow. The major disadvantages of isotope clearance techniques are the necessity for invasive injection of the isotope and requirement for operator expertise and imaging facilities. Another technique for evaluating amputation level is the use of fluorescein dye administered intravenously. A fluorometer can measure fluorescence at the proposed amputation site as a function of perfusion, allowing sensitive quantification of perfusion at the proposed amputation site (27). The commonly reported tests and their ability to help select the appropriate amputation levels are listed in Table 2.

THE RADIOLOGIC EVALUATION

Although the skin and soft tissues may appear viable, underlying osteomyelitis precludes successful amputation site healing. Plain radiologic films are useful in identifying occult osteomyelitis in the area of the amputation. Osteomyelitis suggested by cortical destruction seen on plain bone radiographs can be confirmed by increased radioisotope uptake on bone scan.

Ultimately, patients with threatened limb loss usually have angiography as part of their evaluation. If revascularization appears feasible, its performance as the initial procedure may lower the amputation level and optimize healing.

AMPUTATION: GENERAL PRINCIPLES

The objectives of amputation in diabetic patients are to control sepsis and to restore function. These goals often require more than one surgical procedure. Infection in the diabetic foot can rapidly lead to systemic sepsis and death. It should be approached aggressively as a potentially life-threatening problem, sometimes requiring emergency amputation. Amputation of noninfected appendages, on the other hand, can usually be approached electively as a definitive reconstructive procedure that removes useless tissue and promotes rehabilitation.

Amputation to Control Sepsis

The most disastrous complication in the diabetic patient is the development of a septic extremity with systemic manifestations of diabetic ketoacidosis and, on occasion, septic shock. The septic focus in the lower limb arises either as a superinfection of an inappropriately treated ulcer (Fig. 1A); a superficial abrasion or foreign body puncture that becomes secondarily infected (Fig. 1B); or bacterial invasion of gangrenous tissue. The susceptibility of the foot to infection is due not only to ischemia, but also to neuropathy. Although compromise of sensory function can lead to inadvertent impairment, motor dysfunction can result in derangements of the foot's weight-bearing capacity. Hammer toe, plantar prominence of the metatarsal heads, and proximal migration of the metatarsal fat pads leads to skin ulceration and erosion of the underlying soft tissues, exposing deep plantar spaces to bacterial invasion. Because of the patient's vascular insufficiency and peripheral neuropathy, these infections are often rapidly progressive in the absence of significant pain.

A septic foot represents a true surgical emergency. The polymicrobial nature of diabetic foot sepsis requires the administration of broad spectrum antibiotics. Because of the infection, diabetes is often uncontrolled and ketoacidosis, if present, requires emergent treatment. These stabilizing measures are in preparation for an expeditious débridement or amputation of all infected, nonviable tissue. Removal of infected tissue should be the primary goal with reconstruction of the limb being secondary in importance, often performed as a later procedure when the infection has been eradicated. If the infection has spread throughout the deep plantar spaces to involve the proximal portions of the foot, a guillotine amputation through viable noninfected tissue at the supramalleolar level may be necessary. Antibiotics, frequent dressing changes, and close observation are then followed by a reconstructive amputation at the appropriately selected level. If sepsis involves only the toes or forefoot, a more conservative amputation with sparing of the hind foot may be adequate. Any procedure is predicated on controlling the infection by removing all devitalized and infected debris back to bleeding viable tissue. Following débridement, wounds are left open and dressings changed frequently over the next few days. If there is any evidence of progression of infection or gangrene, further débridement is promptly carried out. While the wounds are being managed, the circulation of the limb is assessed in the vascular laboratory or with angiography. Plans for vascular reconstruction, if necessary, and secondary wound closure or definitive amputation are formulated when the wounds are clean.

Amputation to Restore Function

Amputation to restore function should be thought of as a reconstructive procedure. The most distal amputation that will allow complete healing is performed. In most situations, the more distal the amputation site, the better the chances for ambulation. The potential for rehabilitation in the elderly and often debilitated patient in large part is dependent on the energy requirements of prosthetic ambulation. A unilateral BK amputation requires a 10–40% energy expenditure increase compared with an AK amputation in which a 50–70% energy expenditure increase is required

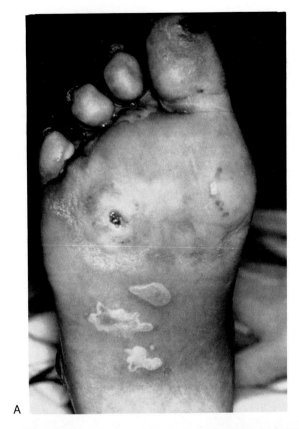

A

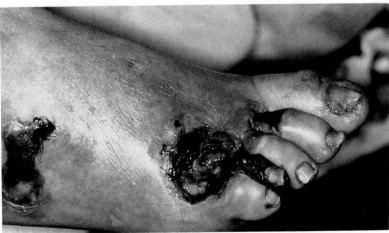

B

FIG. 1.A. Neglected mal perforans ulcer resulting in extensive infection of the foot. **B.** Neglected mal perforans ulcer resulting in extensive infection of the fourth toe.

in order to ambulate with a prosthesis (28). Length of the residual limb in a BK amputation has a relatively minor impact on energy consumption when compared to loss of the knee joint at the AK level. Inversely proportional to this increase in energy expenditure is the number of patients successfully rehabilitated. Multiple series show that although approximately 66% of those with BK amputations will be successfully rehabilitated, only 30–40% of those patients with AK amputations will be rehabilitated (29–31). It should be kept in mind that up to 50% of patients may undergo contralateral amputation in the ensuing 2 years that will further compromise the quality of life (7).

Even under elective conditions, an amputation should not be considered a "minor" operation. The manifestations of diabetes may not be confined to the threatened limb and in conjunction with other operative risk factors, e.g., cardiac, pulmonary, and renal dysfunction, can lead to significant surgical morbidity and mortality. Indeed, Plecha (32) compared the operative mortality rates of amputations from the transmetatarsal (TM) and more proximal level to those of major revascularization procedures and found the mortality from amputation to be higher than every type of major revascularization considered. Others, however, have reported substantially lower operative mortalities; Bunt et al. (33) demonstrated an operative mortality of 0.9% and 2.8% for BK and AK amputations, respectively.

Technical Considerations

Applicable to any level of amputation are several surgical principles, foremost of which is gentle handling of tissues. Bony structures should be precisely transsected. Angulated remnants and sharp edges should be beveled to create smooth contours and thereby avoid pressure points that may ulcerate. The periosteum should not be excessively removed. Small nerves should be sharply divided with some traction to allow retraction above the level of the amputation, but large nerves should be suture ligated to prevent bleeding from the vasa nervosum. Division of the muscles must be done with meticulous hemostasis. A proximal tourniquet that could obscure bleeding during amputation of an ischemic limb is contraindicated. It is necessary that hemostasis be absolute, as a hematoma may elevate an already tenuous skin flap causing necrosis or become a focus of subsequent infection. If complete hemostasis cannot be achieved, judicious use of closed suction drains to prevent hematoma formation, although controversial, may be helpful and in some cases indicated. In their analysis of wound complications, Squires et al. (9) found the use of drains to have no significant impact on subsequent complications. If close suction drains are placed, they should be removed within the first 24–48 hours following surgery. Penrose drains are to be avoided as they may allow for contamination of the wound with skin organisms. Finally, closure of the amputation stump must be performed gently and atraumatically. Exacting coaptation of skin edges leads to successful primary healing. If skin flaps are marginal or hemostasis inexact, secondary primary closure may be achieved by loosely placing monofilament sutures, which then may subsequently be tied down to more closely approximate skin edges. Surgical technique is as important as level selection in achieving wound healing; indeed, it may account for differences in results reported by different authors using the same method of selecting amputation levels. Various amputation sites are shown in Fig. 2.

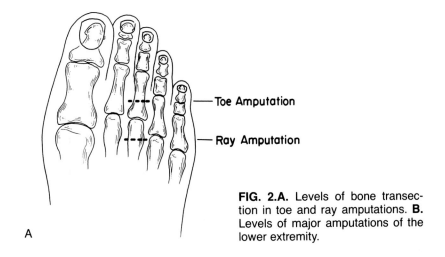

Toe Amputation

Ray Amputation

FIG. 2.A. Levels of bone transection in toe and ray amputations. **B.**
Levels of major amputations of the
lower extremity.

A

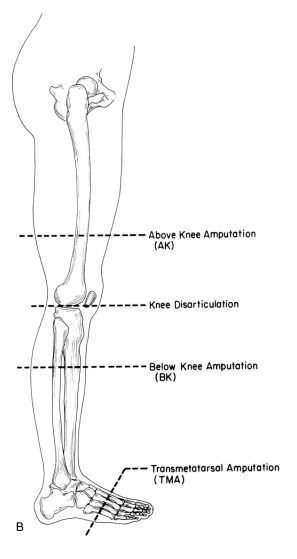

Above Knee Amputation
(AK)

Knee Disarticulation

Below Knee Amputation
(BK)

Transmetatarsal Amputation
(TMA)

B

AMPUTATION: OPERATIVE TECHNIQUE

Toe Amputation

Amputation of the toe is the most commonly performed amputation of the lower limb. Although the presence of dry gangrene may allow the patient to be expectantly treated to allow the process of autoamputation, this approach is rarely used as it prolongs the risk of converting dry gangrene to the wet, infected form and subsequent foot sepsis. Amputation of a dry mummified digit can safely be closed primarily; amputation and primary closure of a wet, infected digit is prone to failure. A single toe amputation is never performed by disarticulation through a phalangeal joint, but rather by transsection of the proximal phalanx leaving a small remnant of bone to protect the metatarsal head. Contraindications to the performance of amputation limited to the toe level include any infection or cellulitis proximal to the toes and dependent rubor of the toes. Prediction of healing at the level of the toe is most accurately done by the presence of palpable pedal pulses. This single finding has been reported to be predictive of healing in 98% of cases (10). In the absence of pedal pulses, digital systolic blood pressure measurements by photoplethysmography are the best available predictors of healing (17,20). An advantage of this level of amputation is that it has a minimal impact upon rehabilitation of the patient and no prosthesis is required to achieve ambulation. It is necessary to closely follow all patients who have undergone a toe amputation because there is a risk of progressive ischemia or intervening infection, and 75% of these patients may require additional ipsilateral amputation in subsequent years (34).

Ray Amputation

Ray amputation is carried out when gangrene or infection extends to the metatarsal phalangeal joint or involves the metatarsal head. In this situation, extension of the toe amputation to excise the metatarsal head effects removal of all infectious and gangrenous tissue. As with the toe amputation, the presence of any proximal cellulitis, infection, or gangrene is a contraindication to the performance of a ray amputation. A relative contraindication is involvement of three or more toes, in which case a transmetatarsal amputation may be more appropriate and allow for easier ambulation. Factors in healing at this level are no different from those used for a simple toe amputation. The common surgical technique is based upon a racket-shaped incision started with its most proximal component on the dorsum of the foot to expose the metatarsal head. All tendon remnants should be excised sharply and as far proximally as possible. The primary complication of this amputation is the possibility of chronic osteomyelitis in the metatarsal shaft remnant. In addition, ray amputation of the great toe may cause instability during ambulation. There are no requirements for a prosthetic device following this amputation.

Transmetatarsal Amputation

Transmetatarsal amputation is indicated for gangrene and infection of several toes. This amputation is also useful for disease that extends only a short distance past the metatarsal phalangeal crease. For a TM amputation to be successful, the plantar skin must be uninvolved with disease and well perfused. Therefore, contraindications to an amputation at this level include ostemyelitis of the proximal metatarsals, infection of the midfoot or plantar space, and gangrene or ischemic changes of the plantar skin. Prediction of healing at the transmetatarsal level is most accurately achieved with sophisticated techniques of fluorometry, xenon-133 skin blood flow assays, or transcutaneous oxygen measurements. In the absence of these, photoplethysmographic toe pressures of greater than 55 mm offer a reliable index of successful transmetatarsal amputation healing (13). It is notable that Doppler ankle systolic blood pressure measurements, as mentioned above, suffer from a lack of sensitivity and at absolute ankle pressures of 60–70 mm Hg healing cannot reliably be expected (15). In the diabetic patient, the Doppler ankle brachial index reported to predict healing is >0.5 (11); the shortcoming of the index in this setting has been discussed. The surgical technique utilizes a plantar skin flap developed proximal to the level of the metatarsal heads. A dorsal skin incision is made in the midmetatarsal region and carried down through the metatarsal bones, proximal to the metatarsal heads. Following excision of the bones and tissue of the forefoot, the plantar flap is brought over the transsected metatarsals and sutured to the dorsal skin of the midfoot.

Syme's Amputation

A Syme's amputation is generally contraindicated in the setting of diabetes. The possibility of neuropathy promotes late stump ulceration even after wound healing.

Below Knee Amputation

Below knee amputation is indicated in patients who have gangrene, infection, nonhealing ulcerations, or severe rest pain of the foot that cannot be corrected by revascularization or a more distal amputation. As mentioned above, in the diabetic patient, the BK amputation is usually preferable to the Syme's amputation. Often a BK amputation is the definitive procedure following an initial open guillotine amputation for a septic foot. Contraindications to performance of a BK amputation include flexion contracture at the knee and gangrene or infection that extends within 5–6 cm of the tibial tuberosity. Selection of a BK amputation level using clinical judgement alone leads to successful healing in about 80% of patients. Because preservation of the knee is an important factor in successful prosthetic ambulation, a BK amputation should be performed if there is a reasonable chance of healing. Although various sophisticated objective parameters such as fluorometry, laser Doppler, radioisotope clearance, and transcutaneous oxygen assays accurately predict healing in over 90% of the patients, these tests are not always available in all institutions. In their absence, Doppler segmental pressures in the thigh of >80 mm Hg and in the calf of >50 mm Hg, usually predict healing at the BK level (35).

The surgical technique of the BK amputation is based upon a choice of three basic skin flaps:

1. Equal-length anterior-posterior flaps, the so-called "fish mouth" technique
2. Creation of a long posterior flap based on the gastrocnemius and soleus muscles
3. Creation of equal-length medial and lateral flaps by sagittal incisions.

Although it was initially thought that the long posterior flap based on the gastroc-nemius and soleus circulation was superior because of a theoretical contention that the blood supply to these muscles was superior to that of the anterior compartment, this has not always held true. Most surgeons, however, prefer and have had excellent results with the long posterior flap technique.

Independent prosthetic ambulation can be achieved in 70% of all BK amputees, regardless of age, provided that they were ambulatory prior to amputation. Indeed, even the bilateral BK amputee has a good rehabilitation potential for successful am-bulation. The energy expenditure for ambulation with a BK prosthesis, however, is 40% greater than an amputation at the foot level.

Knee Disarticulation

A BK amputation is preferable to a knee disarticulation in any previously ambu-latory patient. The latter may be indicated in the occasional patient who presents with gangrene, cellulitis, or infection that precludes the creation of flaps necessary for closure of the BK amputation. The main disadvantage of amputation at this level is that the long skin flaps needed to close the wound are prone to poor healing. The probability of healing is similar to BK amputation. Advantages of knee disarticula-tion include a durable weight-bearing surface with the retention of a long powerful muscle-stabilized lever arm. Furthermore, there is improved stump proprioception and good potential for prosthetic control. The surgical technique involves disarticu-lation at the knee joint and remodeling of the femoral condyles. The latter allows an easier and safer skin flap closure. The three basic skin flaps used for closure of a knee disarticulation are a long anterior flap, equal anterior and posterior fish mouth flaps, and equal-length medial and lateral flaps via sagittal incisions. Of these three, the long anterior flap is probably the least reliable.

Above Knee Amputation

Above knee amputation is most commonly performed because of infection, gan-grene, or unreconstructible ischemia that precludes amputation at a more distal level. Approximately 90% of AK amputations heal when clinical judgement alone is used to select this level. Special consideration should be given to patients without a pal-pable femoral pulse. Vascular laboratory examination or angiography can be very helpful in these patients in defining the vascularity of the thigh. Those patients with occlusion of the superficial femoral artery and high-grade stenosis or occlusion of the profunda femoral artery and poor collateralization are at risk for ischemic break-down of the wound and may benefit from revascularization prior to amputation. Use of skin xenon-133 clearance or transcutaneous PO_2 levels, if available, may allow for better selection of levels.

The surgical technique of AK amputation is based upon three general levels. These are the supracondylar, midthigh, and high-thigh levels. A circular incision is placed distal to the proposed level of bone transection and the undermined skin flaps transversely closed. The choice of these levels is dependent upon the absence of gangrene or infection and the knowledge that the longer the femoral shaft the less energy is required for prosthetic ambulation and the more likely the patient will be able to successfully ambulate with a prosthesis. Indeed, compared with normal ambulation, relative energy costs for an AK ambulation is increased 50–70% (28). Although BK amputees may modify walking speed to maintain normal energy costs, AK amputees are not able to do this, which results in increased oxygen consumption, increased heart rate, and increased respiratory quotient (28). A successful rehabilitation following AK amputations is much less likely than in below the knee amputations and occurs in the range of 30–40% (29–31). Patients who undergo bilateral amputations above the knee are only rarely successfully rehabilitated.

ADJUNCT PROCEDURES

Although vascular bypass procedures are rarely planned solely to improve healing in major amputations (AK or BK), they commonly are used to allow more distal foot or toe amputations, and the augmentation of blood flow in the limb at risk is clearly advantageous. In patients with occlusion of the superficial femoral artery, the profunda femoral provides a collateral pathway of blood flow to the distal vascular tree. The efficacy of the profunda femoral collateral pathway is often limited by occlusive disease; therefore, in patients in whom a BK amputation is planned, a concomitant profundaplasty may improve results at the cost of minimal additional operating. Towne et al. (36) demonstrated the importance of profunda patency in healing of BK amputations. In their series, 17 of 19 (89%) AK amputations were in the setting of failed profundaplasty and all 24 successful BK amputations had patent profunda repairs.

A lack of ample soft-tissue coverage at a distal amputation site no longer dictates proceeding with a more proximal procedure. Revascularization combined with tissue transfer techniques done in collaboration with plastic surgeons permits the use of vascularized free-tissue flaps to cover large defects with considerable success. Shenaq et al. (37) achieved successful coverage in 13 of 15 flaps (87%); the majority of these was based upon the latissimus dorsi (37). Similar results have been reported by other researchers (38).

CONCLUSION

Amputation in the diabetic patient remains a significant problem. At Barnes Hospital, 326 amputations were performed between January 1987 and December 1989, 224 (89%) of which were in diabetic patients. Seventy-eight (56%) of 139 major amputations (AK or BK) and 142 (76%) of 187 minor (foot or toe) amputations were performed in diabetic patients. Utilizing lower extremity segmental arterial Doppler pressures and digital photoplethysmography to complement clinical judgement, only 10% of our patients with amputations of the foot and lower leg required revision to a more proximal level.

Amputation in the diabetic patient requires careful preoperative preparation, meticulous operative technique, and regular follow-up for the life of the patient. A multidisciplinary approach involving the internist, prosthetist and surgeon is of paramount importance in providing the best quality of life for the diabetic amputee.

REFERENCES

1. Bell, ET. Atherosclerotic gangrene of the lower extremities in diabetic and nondiabetic persons. *Am J Clin Pathol* 1957;28:27.
2. Liedberg E, Persson BM. Age, diabetes and smoking in lower limb amputation for arterial occlusive disease. *Acta Orthop Scand* 1983;54:383.
3. Most RS, Sinnock P. The epidemiology of lower extremity amputations in diabetic patients. *Diabetes Care* 1983;6:87.
4. Personal Communication, American Diabetes Foundation.
5. Bild DE, Selby JV, Sinnock P, et al. Lower extremity amputation in people with diabetes. *Diabetes Care* 1989;12:24.
6. Levin ME, Sicard GA. Evaluating and treating diabetic peripheral vascular disease. *Clin Diabetes* 1987;5:62.
7. Bodily KC, Burgess EM. Contralateral limb and patient survival after leg amputation. *Am J Surg* 1983;146:280.
8. Keagy BA, Schwartz JA, Kotb M, et al. Lower extremity amputations: The control series. *J Vasc Surg* 1986;4:321.
9. Squires JV, Johnson WC, Widrich WC, Nabseth DC. Cause of wound complications in elderly patients with above-knee amputation. *Am J Surg* 1982;143:523.
10. Sizer JS, Wheelock FC. Digital amputations in diabetic patients. *Surgery* 1972;72:980.
11. Andres G, Harris RW, Dulawa LB, et al. The need for arteriography in diabetic patients with gangrene and palpable foot pulses. *Arch Surg* 1984;119:1260.
12. Pollack SB, Ernst CB. Use of Doppler pressure measurements in predicting success in amputation of the leg. *Am J Surg* 1980;139:303.
13. Bone GE, Pomajzl MJ. Toe blood pressure by photoplethysmography: An index of healing in forefoot amputations. *Surgery* 1981;89:569.
14. Nicholas GG, Myers JL, Demuth WE. The role of vascular laboratory criteria in the selection of patients for lower extremity amputation. *Ann Surg* 1982;195:469.
15. Welch H, Lieberman DP, Pollock JG, Angerson W. Failure of Doppler ankle pressure to predict healing of conservative forefoot amputations. *Br J Surg* 1985;72:888.
16. Gibbons GW, Wheelock FC, Siembieda C, et al. Noninvasive prediction of amputation levels in diabetic patients. *Arch Surg* 1979;114:1253.
17. Pinzur M, Kaminsky M, Sage R, et al. Amputations at the middle level of the foot. *J Bone Joint Surg* 1986;68A:1061.
18. Raines JK, Darling RC, Buth J, et al. Vascular laboratory criteria for the management of peripheral vascular disease of the lower extremities. *Surgery* 1976;76:21.
19. Holstein P. The distal blood pressure predicts healing of amputations in the feet. *Acta Orthop Scand* 1984;55:227.
20. Schwartz JA, Schuler JJ, O'Connor RJA, Flanigan DP. Predictive value of distal perfusion pressure in the healing of amputation of the digits and the forefoot. *Surg Gynecol Obstet* 1982;154:865.
21. Ratliff DA, Clyne CAC, Chant ADB, Webster JHH. Prediction of amputation wound healing: The role of transcutaneous PO$_2$ assessment. *Br J Surg* 1984;71:219.
22. Karanfilian RG, Lynch TG, Zirul VT, et al. The value of laser doppler velocimetry and transcutaneous oxygen tension determination in predicting healing of ischemic forefoot ulcerations and amputations in diabetic and nondiabetic patients. *J Vasc Surg* 1986;4:511.
23. Golbranson FL. Amputation level selection by skin temperature measurement. In: Moore WS, Malone JM, eds. *Lower extremity amputation*. Philadelphia: W.B. Saunders, 1989;69.
24. Nilsen R, Dahn I, Lassen NA, Westling GA. On the estimation of local effective perfusion pressure in patients with obliterative arterial disease by means of external compression over a xenon-133 depot. *Scand J Clin Lab Invest* (Suppl) 1967;93:29.
25. Holstein P. Distal blood pressure as guidance in choice of amputation level. *Scand J Clin Lab Invest* 1973;31:245.
26. Moore WS, Henry RE, Malone JM, et al. Prospective use of xenon-133 clearance for amputation level selection. *Arch Surg* 1981;116:86.
27. Silverman DG, Rubin SW, Reilly GA, et al. Fluorometric prediction of successful amputation level in the ischemic limb. *J Rehab Res Dev* 1985;22:29.
28. Waters RL, Perry J, Antonelli D, Hislop H. Energy cost of walking amputees: The influence of level of amputation. *J Bone Joint Surg* 1976;58A:42.

29. Warren R, Kihn RB. Lower extremity amputations for ischemia. *Bull Soc Int Chir* 1969;28,394.
30. Kihn RB, Warren R, Beebe GW. The geriatric amputee. *Ann Surg* 1972;176:305.
31. Couch NP, David JK, Tilney NL, Crane C. Natural history of the leg amputee. *Am J Surg* 1977;133:469.
32. Plecha FR, Bertin VJ, Plecha EJ, et al. The early results of vascular surgery in patients 75 years of age or older: An analysis of 3259 cases. *J Vasc Surg* 1985;2:769.
33. Bunt TJ, Manship LL, Bynoe RPH, Haynes JL. Lower extremity amputation for peripheral vascular disease. *Am Surg* 1984;50:581.
34. Little JM, Stephen MS, Zylstra PL. Amputation of the toes for vascular disease: Fate of the affected leg. *Lancet* 1976;18:1318.
35. Yao JST, Bergan JJ. Application of ultrasound to arterial and venous diagnosis. *Surg Clin North Am* 1974;54:23.
36. Towne JB, Bernhard VM, Rollins DL, Baum PL. Profundaplasty in perspective: Limitations in the long-term management of limb ischemia. *Surgery* 1981;90:1037.
37. Shenaq SM, Krouskop T, Stal S, Spira M. Salvage of amputation stumps by secondary reconstruction utilizing microsurgical free tissue transfer. *Plast Reconstr Surg* 1987;79:861.
38. Gallico GA, Ehrlichman RJ, Jupiter J, May JW. Free flaps to preserve below knee amputation stumps: Long term evaluation. *Plast Reconstr Surg* 1987;79:871.
39. Christensen KS, Klarke M. Transcutaneous oxygen measurements in peripheral occlusive disease: An indicator of wound healing in leg amputation. *J Bone Joint Surg* 1986;68B:423.

Surgical Management of the Diabetic Patient,
edited by Michael Bergman and Gregorio A. Sicard.
Raven Press, Ltd., New York © 1991.

23

Gastrointestinal Surgery in Diabetics

*Nathaniel J. Soper, and †James M. Becker

*Department of Surgery, Washington University School of Medicine, St. Louis,
Missouri 63110, and †Department of Gastrointestinal Surgery, Harvard Medical
School, Brigham and Women's Hospital, Boston, Massachusetts 02115

Gastrointestinal surgery in patients with diabetes mellitus presents all of the problems of similar operations in nondiabetic patients, but with additional difficulties peculiar to diabetes and its complications. Other chapters in this text deal with general considerations of the diabetic medical condition before, during, and after surgery. The diabetic patient is susceptible to the same spectrum of gastrointestinal disease as the general population but there are several features of diabetes that are associated with distinctive disturbances of gut function. A number of processes can be involved in these derangements, including autonomic neuropathy and microangiopathy, metabolic changes, altered gut hormone release, and increased susceptibility to infections. This chapter reviews mechanisms causing alimentary disease in diabetic patients with specific reference to their operative management.

DIABETIC AUTONOMIC NEUROPATHY

The pathogenesis of diabetic autonomic neuropathy is unexplained, but a number of theories have been advanced. These include impaired neural protein synthesis, altered axoplasmic transport, and abnormal myoinositol metabolism (1,2). Anatomic evidence suggests that the number and densities of myelinated fibers within the enteric nervous system are diminished (3), but there may also be degeneration of the adrenergic nerves (4) and relative changes of various enteric neurotransmitters (5,6). Alternatively, imbalances in blood glucose and electrolyte levels may cause changes in gut motility independent of direct neural degeneration (7). There is as yet no good correlation of these abnormalities with the dysfunction of the gastrointestinal tract. It is clear, however, that other evidence of diabetic neuropathy (such as postural hypotension) often precedes gastrointestinal symptoms (8).

Esophageal Dysfunction

Most patients with diabetic neuropathy have abnormal esophageal motility, which is usually asymptomatic (9). The motor disorders that have been demonstrated range from mild impairment of peristalsis to total absence of coordinated peristaltic activity. The symptoms of patients with esophageal dysfunction are usually mild and consist of heartburn and occasional dysphagia. Investigation of these complaints often reveals manometric abnormalities such as diminished peristaltic activity, increased spastic contractions, and reduced lower esophageal sphincter pressure (10). Delayed esophageal emptying may be demonstrated by radionuclide transit studies (11). The prokinetic agent metoclopramide (Reglan) may be helpful in restoring normal resting pressure to the lower esophageal sphincter and thereby improve the rate of esophageal and gastric emptying in symptomatic patients. Metoclopramide, a benzamide derivative, exerts dual actions on gastrointestinal smooth muscle: inhibition of the neurotransmitter dopamine, and augmentation of acetylcholine release from postganglionic nerve terminals. Metoclopramide increases the amplitude of muscle contraction and appears to coordinate aborally-directed peristaltic activity (12). Antireflux operations are indicated only when symptomatic gastroesophageal reflux cannot be controlled by standard medical measures, and manometric studies demonstrate a hypotonic lower esophageal sphincter with preserved peristalsis of the more proximal esophagus.

Because of their esophageal dysmotility and increased susceptibility to infections, infections caused by *Candida albicans* are apt to develop in patients with diabetes. Because of this, candidiasis of the oral cavity and esophagus is more common in diabetic patients than in control populations. Esophagoscopy may reveal characteristic abnormalities, particularly when the typical whitish plaques are brushed and examined microscopically (13). Oral antifungal therapy is generally successful in eradicating the *Candida* infection.

Gastric Dysfunction

It is also common for patients with diabetic neuropathy to manifest impaired motor activity of the stomach, termed gastroparesis diabeticorum. Clinically, gastroparesis may cause vague postprandial abdominal discomfort or intractable nausea and vomiting. In severe cases, gastric stasis can lead to weight loss, poor diabetic control, and the formation of gastric bezoars (14). Classically, upper gastrointestinal contrast study reveals gastric dilatation, diminished peristalsis, and prolonged retention of barium. More sophisticated quantitative tests of gastric emptying, such as radionuclide studies, may show profoundly delayed emptying of scintigraphic markers (15). Manometric measurements have shown a variety of abnormalities, including absence of the antral component of Phase III of the interdigestive motor complex, which normally clears the stomach of indigestible solids (16) (Fig. 1), postprandial antral hypomotility, and nonpropagated powerful antral contractions (17). No single mechanism has been elucidated to explain the spectrum of abnormalities seen in gastroparesis diabeticorum. Defects in vagal nerve function and intrinsic neurons, altered release of gastrointestinal hormones, and even intrinsic myenteric smooth muscle dysfunction may all be involved (15,18,19).

Diagnosis of diabetic gastroparesis is suggested by the symptoms in a patient with other evidence of diabetic neuropathy and orthostatic hypotension. Physician examination may reveal a succussion splash. A barium upper gastrointestinal examination should be performed to rule out structural causes of obstruction, such as bezoars, and if present, the bezoar needs to be removed endoscopically. Perfor-

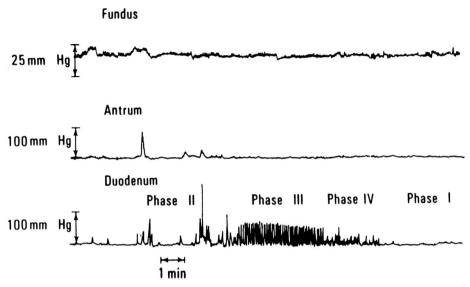

FIG. 1. Fundic, antral, and duodenal motor activity in a patient with diabetic gastroparesis. Typical high amplitude Phase III activity is observed in the duodenum without corresponding phasic changes in the fundus or antrum. (Reproduced with permission from Malagelada et al., ref. 16.)

mance of radiolabeled scintigraphy is the most reliable way to confirm and quantify the presence of a gastric emptying disorder and to follow the response to therapy.

Treatment of patients with gastroparesis diabeticorum is initiated with metoclopramide, 10 mg orally every 6 hours, which increases the amplitude of gastric contractions (16, Fig. 2), accelerates gastric emptying (20, Fig. 3) and decreases

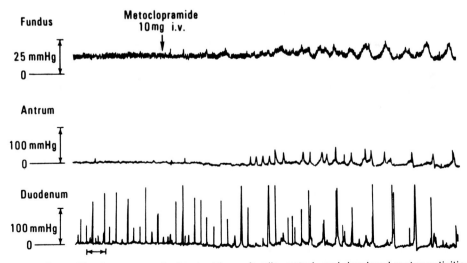

FIG. 2. Effect of intravenous metoclopramide on fundic, antral, and duodenal motor activities in a patient with diabetic gastroparesis. Metoclopramide causes onset of fundic and antral pressure waves. (Reproduced with permission from Malagelada et al., ref. 16.)

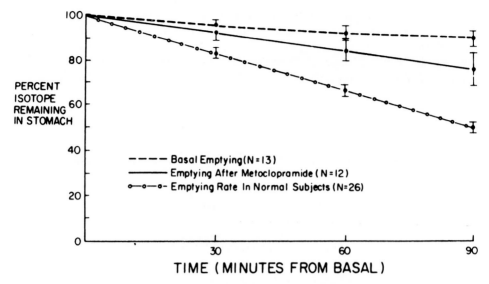

FIG. 3. Effect of metoclopramide (10 mg im) on gastric emptying in patients with diabetic gastroparesis. Metoclopramide accelerated the rate of emptying of the meal, but did not normalize gastric emptying. (Reproduced with permission from Ricci et al., ref. 20.)

postprandial gastric volumes. Metoclopramide may be augmented by using the cholinergic agent bethanechol. Newer prokinetic agents, such as domperidone (a dopamine antagonist that does not cross the blood-brain barrier readily) and cisapride (which enhances release of acetylcholine) are under investigation and may be commercially available soon. These newer drugs would be especially useful in those patients in whom extra-pyramidal side effects develop with metoclopramide.

Attempts at surgical correction of gastroparesis diabeticorum should be withheld until all of these pharmacologic therapies have proven fruitless. Results of gastric drainage procedures, such as gastroenterostomy or pyloroplasty, have been variable (21). In long-standing cases that are refractory to all other modes of therapy, near-total gastrectomy with Roux-en-Y gastrojejunostomy may be the only recourse (22).

Gastritis and Gastric Atrophy

Acute erosive gastritis is commonly seen during episodes of diabetic ketoacidosis and may cause upper gastrointestinal hemorrhage. This is usually amenable to treatment with histamine-2 blockers. Chronic gastritis and gastric atrophy frequently occur in diabetic patients. Because of this, the incidence of duodenal ulcer in diabetics is lower than in nondiabetic individuals (23). When peptic disease occurs in the diabetic patient it is managed in a fashion similar to that in the nondiabetic patient.

Small Bowel Abnormalities and Diabetic Diarrhea

Diabetes-induced small bowel disorders are more commonly symptomatic than are those of the esophagus or stomach. Diarrhea with or without steatorrhea may be present in up to 10% of patients (24). Diabetic diarrhea is most common in patients with poorly controlled diabetes complicated by neuropathy, and is characteristically intermittent, watery, profuse, and most bothersome in the nocturnal hours (25). In most patients, the cause of diarrhea is not clear. The presence of bacterial overgrowth of the small bowel, exocrine pancreatic insufficiency, and adult celiac disease must be investigated, however.

There is no characteristic abnormality of intestinal motility or transit (26). It is likely, however, that there is a motor disturbance of the small bowel (27). Conversely, diabetic patients may suffer from a syndrome indistinguishable from idiopathic intestinal pseudo-obstruction. In such cases plain abdominal radiographs reveal an obstructed pattern and perfused intestinal manometric catheters show abnormal small bowel motility.

The investigation of diabetic diarrhea includes tests of exocrine pancreatic function, celiac sprue, and bacterial overgrowth, and a trial of broad-spectrum antibiotics should be instituted. If no other abnormality is present, strict control of the blood glucose levels may help (28). Symptomatic control of the diarrhea can then be at-

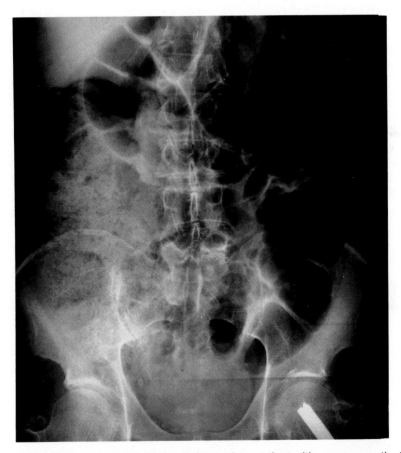

FIG. 4. Anteroposterior radiograph of the abdomen in a patient with severe constipation associated with diabetes. Note the dilated colon and large amount of stool in the right side of the colon. The patient's symptoms of abdominal pain and distention were relieved only after several days of therapy with enemas and cathartics.

tempted with loperamide (a synthetic, peripherally-active opioid) and psyllium; the use of clonidine, an alpha-adrenergic agonist, has also been shown to be beneficial recently (29). Similarly, the long-acting somatostatin analog, SMS 201-995, may ameliorate the symptoms of diabetic diarrhea (30).

Colorectal Motility Disorders

Chronic constipation is frequently seen in diabetic patients and may be related to diabetic autonomic neuropathy. This can become so severe as to cause colonic pseudo-obstruction similar to Ogilvie's syndrome (31; Fig. 4). Therapy for the constipation is initiated with enemas, laxatives, and prokinetic agents. Incontinence develops in a small percentage of diabetic patients, and occasionally coincides with the onset of diabetic diarrhea. Incontinence can be due to derangement of the internal anal sphincter mechanism (32); management is empiric and includes antidiarrheal therapy as well as biofeedback training.

THE ACUTE ABDOMEN IN THE DIABETIC

Just as in the nondiabetic person, an acute surgical abdomen can develop in individuals with diabetes. Because of diabetic neuropathy, however, the severity of the intraabdominal process can be masked by a relative lack of pain. As a result of this diminished pain sensation, the diabetic person may well present to the hospital at a later stage in the course of the abdominal catastrophe. It is generally believed that persons who are diabetic present more frequently with perforations of the gallbladder or appendix than do nondiabetic persons. Also, as a consequence of their known proclivity to infections, septic complications of abdominal disease may be more difficult to treat effectively. The differential diagnosis of the acute abdomen in diabetic persons is similar to nondiabetic individuals, and the appropriate cascade of diagnostic tests should be initiated immediately. Prior to operative intervention, meticulous attention must be given to rapid correction of fluid and electrolyte imbalances and hyperglycemia or hypoglycemia. When the operation is undertaken, aggressive surgery is necessary to treat the primary process and to avoid subsequent septic complications.

The surgeon must be aware of the gastrointestinal manifestations of diabetic ketoacidosis (DKA). Diffuse, often severe abdominal pain, nausea, and vomiting may all be seen during an episode of DKA with loss of metabolic control in patients with insulin-dependent diabetes. When recognized, the rapid administration of intravenous fluid, electrolytes, and insulin is usually associated with disappearance of the symptoms.

The situation may not be obvious, however, and the differential diagnosis may be made difficult when the DKA has resulted from an underlying intraabdominal process and is not the primary cause of the pain. Appropriately selected radiographic or radionuclide scanning procedures must be performed to rule out acute appendicitis or cholecystitis, perforation of a hollow viscus, acute pancreatitis, or mesenteric ischemia. Clinical acumen is crucial because death secondary to DKA may result from an underlying correctable surgical condition that is assumed to be due to DKA, and because DKA may suppress both mental function as well as abdominal signs and symptoms (33). The situation may be made more complex due to the well-known association between DKA and both gastritis and hyperamylasemia mimicking pancreatitis (34). The patient's history is helpful; patients with a surgical abdomen usually refer initial symptoms to the abdomen, and those with pain secondary to DKA generally experience abdominal distress only after they have had hours or days of other symptoms such as gastroenteritis, polydipsia/polyuria, and increasing weakness.

The "pancreatitis" of DKA is generally characterized by elevations of salivary-type amylase rather than the characteristic elevation of pancreatic isoamylase and lipase that is seen in true acute pancreatitis (35) (see also Chapter 13). When in doubt, imaging studies of the pancreas and biliary tract are indicated. If acute cholecystitis is suspected, ultrasound and/or scintigraphic biliary scans should be obtained.

Because atherosclerosis tends to develop in persons who are diabetic, they are prone to experience acute mesenteric arterial ischemia. Generally, pain out of proportion to the physical findings heralds the initiation of the process. When mesenteric ischemia is suspected, prompt arteriography and surgery are necessary to prevent intestinal gangrene.

BILIARY SURGERY IN THE DIABETIC PATIENT

It is thought that gallstones occur more frequently in diabetic than in non-diabetic individuals (36,37). There is no prospective study, however, of the incidence of cholelithiasis in diabetes controlled for the presence or absence of obesity. Two factors can account for an increase in the incidence of gallstones in diabetic persons. In adult-onset diabetics (type II), the bile is supersaturated with cholesterol with a concomitant reduced concentration of bile acids (38). Also, gallbladder emptying and peak ejection rate in response to cholecystokinin have been shown to be decreased in diabetic persons, particularly in those with diabetic autonomic neuropathy, thereby allowing stasis of bile in the gallbladder (39).

In the past, many surgeons have recommended prophylactic cholecystectomy for diabetic patients with asymptomatic gallstones (40,41). These recommendations were based on older retrospective data that suggested a much higher morbidity and mortality rate in diabetic patients than in nondiabetic patients undergoing surgery operated for gallbladder disease. More recent reports, however, suggest that diabetes has little effect on the overall mortality and morbidity of either elective or emergency biliary tract procedures (42–44). This issue remains controversial. The natural history of cholelithiasis in diabetic patients may not be parallel to that of nondiabetic patients, because acute cholecystitis and perforation may occur more commonly in those with diabetes and therefore require emergency surgery in a higher percentage of patients (45). Furthermore, a recent age- and sex-matched review of operations for acute cholecystitis revealed an increase in overall morbidity and, particularly, infection-related complications in diabetic patients (46). These data also suggested that diabetic patients more frequently had infected bile than their nondiabetic counterparts.

Largely due to the conflicting reports cited above, the role of prophylactic cholecystectomy in asymptomatic diabetic patients remains a matter of debate. The solution to the problem ultimately will depend on an accurate depiction of the natural course of asymptomatic gallstones in this group of patients. Support for expectant management of asymptomatic gallstones in diabetes has been afforded by decision-analysis techniques that revealed no advantage for prophylactic surgery in increasing life expectancy in any diabetic patient with asymptomatic gallstones (47). More fuel will be added to the fire by the recent implementation of nonoperative therapy of gallstones using lithotripsy, oral bile salts, or percutaneously instilled cholesterol solvents. The low morbidity and mortality rates of these procedures will once again raise the issue of prophylactic treatment of gallstones (48). At this time it seems prudent to advise against any prophylactic therapy of asymptomatic gallstones in diabetic patients, but rather to perform cholecystectomy or treat the stones by nonoperative means soon after the development of biliary symptoms.

DIABETES AND THE PANCREAS

As the seat of insulin-producing islet cells, the pancreas is key to the presence or absence of diabetes mellitus. (The topics of pancreatitis and pancreatic transplantation are covered in Chapters 13 and 26.) There are a number of other conditions, however, both natural and iatrogenic, that are associated with diabetes.

The incidence of pancreatic cancer in diabetic persons may be twice that of the general population. No other malignancy has been shown to be associated with diabetes. The abrupt onset of diabetes mellitus after age 40 has been said to be suggestive of the diagnosis of pancreatic cancer. Presumably the pancreatic cancer and diabetes coexist but no cause and effect relationship has been established.

Operative attempts at curing pancreatic cancer likewise may lead to diabetes. Pancreatoduodenectomy is usually not associated with the new onset of diabetes. Total pancreatectomy however, is necessarily followed by hypoinsulinemia. The severity of diabetes following total pancreatectomy varies from mild to severe, and may result in death. Indeed, in the Mayo Clinic series, there were more deaths from hypoglycemia (4%) than 5-year survivors after total pancreatectomy for ductal adenocarcinoma (2%) (49).

When performing total pancreatectomy, intraoperative blood glucose levels should be measured frequently and corrected with the appropriate dose of intravenous insulin. If wide swings in blood glucose levels are encountered, a blood glucose "clamp" technique with continuous monitoring of glucose levels and frequent small doses of insulin administered intravenously may be necessary. In the first 3 or 4 postoperative days, the patient's blood glucose level should be checked every 3–4 hrs and a continuous iv infusion of insulin can be given. It is desirable to maintain the blood glucose levels between 100–250 mg/dl at all times. During this time period, fluid shifts may be dramatic and systemic absorption is unpredictable; therefore, subcutaneous or intramuscular administration of insulin should be discouraged.

Once the patient's condition has been stabilized, a 5% dextrose solution should be maintained for 7–10 days with frequent glucose level monitoring. When oral feeding is initiated, the combination of neutral protamine Hagedorn (NPH) and regular insulin is given on a bid basis, with the usual dose being one-half to two-thirds of the daily requirement of the previous 3 days. The patient and his or her relatives should then be instructed in the appropriate management and precautions of the diabetic condition.

Two tumors of the nonbeta islet cells of the pancreas can also lead to diabetes mellitus. The glucagonoma syndrome is characterized by migratory necrolytic dermatitis, stomatitis, edema, weight loss, and diabetes mellitus. The presence of a prominent rash in a patient with diabetes should be enough to raise suspicions. Computed tomography (CT) scan with or without arteriography may help to localize the tumor, and confirmation of the diagnosis depends on demonstrating elevated serum glucagon levels.

Glucagonoma arises from alpha-2 cells in the pancreatic islets. Of all glucagonomas, approximately three-fourths are malignant and have usually metastasized to the liver, regional lymph nodes, or adrenal gland. About 25% are benign and confined to the pancreas. Surgical removal of the primary lesion and debulking of any major metastases is indicated if technically feasible. Particularly in unresectable cases, the use of SMS 201-995, the long-acting somatostatin analog, may normalize serum glucagon levels, improve the rash, and result in weight gain (50,51).

The second pancreatic tumor that may result in diabetes is the somatostatinoma. Patients with somatostatinoma typically exhibit diabetes mellitus, diarrhea, and intestinal malabsorption, and dilatation of the gallbladder with gallstones. The syndrome results from secretion of somatostatin by an islet cell tumor of the pancreas, which in most cases is malignant and accompanied by hepatic metastases. The diagnosis is confirmed by measuring increased concentrations of somatostatin in the serum. However, the manifestations may be mild enough so that the somatostatin syndrome is unsuspected until histologic evidence of metastatic islet cell carcinoma is apparent. Surgery is necessary if the disease is localized. More often, chemotherapy with combinations of streptozotocin and doxorubicin is the only treatment possible due to widespread disease (51).

REFERENCES

1. Clements RS Jr, Bell DS. Diagnostic, pathogenetic and therapeutic aspects of diabetic neuropathy. *Spec Top Endocrinol Metabol* 1982;3:1.
2. Niakan E, Haraita Y, Comstock JP. Diabetic autonomic neuropathy. *Metabolism* 1986;35:224.
3. Diani AR, Davis DE, Fix JD, Swartzman J, Gerritsen GC. Morphometric analysis of autonomic neuropathology in the abdominal sympathetic trunk of the ketonuric diabetic Chinese hamster. *Acta Neuropathol* (Berl) 1981;53:293.
4. Lincoln J, Bokar JT, Crowe R, Griffith SG, Haven AJ, Burnstock G. Myenteric plexus in streptozotocin-treated rats. Neurochemical and histochemical evidence for diabetic neuropathy in the gut. *Gastroenterology* 1984;86:654.
5. Schmidt RE, Nelson JS, Johnson EM. Experimental autonomic diabetic neuropathy. *MJ Pathol* 1981;103:210.
6. Belai A, Lincoln J, Millner P, Crowe R, Loesch A, Burnstock G. Enteric nerves in diabetic rats: Increase in vasoactive intestinal polypeptide but not substance p. *Gastroenterology* 1985;89:967.
7. Goyal RK, Spiro HM. Gastrointestinal manifestations of diabetes mellitus. *Med Clin North Am* 1971;55:1031.
8. Yang GR, Arem R, Chan L. Gastrointestinal tract complications of diabetes mellitus. Pathophysiology and management. *Arch Intern Med* 1984;141:1251.
9. Loo DF, Diodos WJ, Soergel KH, Arndorfer RC, Helm JF, Hogan WJ. Multi-peaked eosphageal peristaltic pressure waves in patients with diabetic neuropathy. *Gastroenterology* 1985;88:485.
10. Vela AR, Ballart LA. Esophageal motor manifestations in diabetes mellitus. *Am J Surg* 1970;119:21.
11. Russell CO, Gannan R, Coatsworth J, Neilsen R, Allen F, Hill LD, Pope CE II. Relationship among esophageal dysfunction, diabetic gastroenteropathy, and peripheral neuropathy. *Dig Dis Sci* 1983;28:289.
12. Lake-Bakaar G, Teblick M. Drugs and gut motility. In: Ackermans LMA, Johnson AG, Read NW, eds. *Gastric and gastroduodenal motility.* New York: Prager Publishers, 1984;301.
13. Gillian JS, Kurtz RC. Treatment of Candida esophagitis. *Gastroenterology* 1983;85:971.
14. Brady PG, Richardson K. Gastric bezoar formation secondary to gastroparesis diabeticorum. *Arch Intern Med* 1977;137:1729.

15. Feldman M, Smith HJ, Simon TR. Gastric emptying of solid radioopaque markers: Studies in healthy subjects and diabetic patients. *Gastroenterology* 1984;87:895.
16. Malagelada J-R, Rees WDW, Mazzotta LJ, Go VL. Gastric motor abnormalities in diabetic and postvagotomy gastroparesis: Effect of metoclopramide and bethanecol. *Gastroenterology* 1980;78:286.
17. Camilleri M, Malagelada J-R. Abnormal intestinal motility in diabetics with a gastroparesis syndrome. *Eur J Clin Invest* 1984;14:420.
18. Wooten RL, Meriwether TW. Diabetic gastric atony: A clinical study. *JAMA* 1961;176:1082.
19. Achem-Karam SR, Funikoshi A, Vinik AI, Owyang C. Plasma motilin concentration and interdigestive migrating motor complex in diabetic gastroparesis: Effect of metoclopramide. *Gastroenterology* 1985;88:492.
20. Ricci DA, Saltzman MB, Meyer C, Callachan C, McCallum RW. Effect of metoclopramide in diabetic gastroparesis. *J Clin Gastroenterol* 1985;7:25.
21. Roon AJ, Mason GR. Surgical management of gastroparesis diabeticorum. *Calif Med* 1972;116:58.
22. Karlstrom L, Kelly KA. Roux-Y gastrectomy for chronic gastric atony. *Am J Surg* 1989;157:44.
23. Dotevall G. Gastric secretion of acid in diabetes mellitus during basal conditions and after maximum histamine stimulation. *Acta Med Scand* 1961;170:59.
24. Feldman M, Schiller LR. Disorders of gastrointestinal motility associated with diabetes mellitus. *Ann Int Med* 1983;98:378.
25. McNally EF, Reinhard AE, Schwartz PE. Small bowel motility in diabetics. *Am J Dig Dis* 1969;14:163.
26. Keshavarzian A, Iber FL. Intestinal transit in insulin requiring diabetics. *Am J Gastroenterol* 1986;81:257.
27. Nowak JV, Harrington B, Kalbfleisch JH, Amatruda JM. Evidence for abnormal cholinergic neuromuscular transmission in diabetic rat's small intestine. *Gastroenterology* 1986;91:124.
28. White NH, Waltman SR, Krupin T, Santiago JV. Reversal of neuropathic and gastrointestinal complications related to diabetes mellitus in adolescence with improved metabolic control. *J Pediatr* 1981;99:41.
29. Fedorak RN, Field M, Chang EB. Treatment of diabetic diarrhea with clonidine. *Ann Intern Med* 1985;102:197.
30. Tsai S-T, Vinik AI, Brunner JF. Diabetic diarrhea and somatostatin. *Ann Intern Med* 1986;104:894.
31. Anuras S, Schirazi SS. Colonic pseudo-obstruction. *Am J Gastroenterol* 1984;79:525.
32. Schiller LR, Santa Ana CA, Schmulen C, Hendler RS, Harford WV, Fordtran JS. Pathogenesis of fecal incontinence in diabetes mellitus. *N Engl J Med* 1982;307:1666.
33. Beigelman PM. Severe diabetic ketoacidosis (diabetic coma). *Diabetes* 1971;20:490.
34. Campbell IW, Duncan LJP, Innes JA, MacGuish AC, Munro JF. Abdominal pain and diabetic metabolic decompensation: Clinical significance. *JAMA* 1975;233:166.
35. Eckfeldt JH, Leatherman JW, Levitt MD. High prevalence of hyperamylasemia in patients with acidemia. *Ann Intern Med* 1986;104:362.
36. Vinicor F, Lehrner LM, Karn RC, Merritt AD. Hyperamylasemia in diabetic ketoacidosis: Sources and significance. *Ann Intern Med* 1979;91:200.
37. Leiber MM. The incidence of gallstones and their correlation with other disease. *Ann Surg* 1982;135:394.
38. Strom B, Tamragouri R, Morse M, et al. Oral contraceptives and other risk factors for gallbladder disease. *Clin Pharmacol Ther* 1986;39:335.
39. Ponz de Leon M, Ferenderes R, Carulli N. Bio-lipid composition and bile acid pool size in diabetes. *Dig Dis Sci* 1978;23:710.
40. Stone BG, Gavaler JS, Belle SH, et al. Impairment of gallbladder emptying in diabetes mellitus. *Gastroenterology* 1988;95:170.
41. Turrill FL, McCarron M, Mikkelson WP. Gallstones in diabetes: An ominous association. *Am J Surg* 1961;102:184.
42. Mudth ED. Cholecystitis and diabetes mellitus. *N Engl J Med* 1962;267:642.
43. Walsh DB, Eckhauser FE, Ramsburg SR, et al. Risk associated with diabetes mellitus in patients undergoing gallbladder surgery. *Surgery* 1982;91:254.
44. Tucker LE, Anwar A, Hardin W, et al. Risk factors for cholecystectomy. *South Med J* 1983;76:1113.
45. Pickleman J, Gonzales RP. The improving results of cholecystectomy. *Arch Surg* 1986;121:930.
46. Ransohoff DF, Miller GL, Forsythe SB, Hermann RE. Outcome of acute cholecystitis in patients with diabetes mellitus. *Ann Intern Med* 1987;106:829.
47. Pellegrini CA. Asymptomatic gallstones: Does diabetes mellitus make a difference? *Gastroenterology* 1986;91:245.
48. Hickman MS, Schwesinger WH, Page CP. Acute cholecystitis in the diabetic: A case control study of outcome. *Arch Surg* 1988;123:409.

49. Friedman LS, Roberts MS, Brett AS, Marton KI. Management of asymptomatic gallstones in the diabetic patient: A decision analysis. *Ann Int Med* 1988;109:913.
50. Sackmann M, Delius M, Sauerbruch T. Shockwave lithotripsy of gallbladder stones: The first 175 patients. *N Engl J Med* 1988;318:393.
51. van Heerden JA, ReMine WH, Weiland LH, McIlrath DC, Ilstrup DM. Total pancreatectomy for ductal adenocarcinoma of the pancreas: Mayo Clinic experience. *Am J Surg* 1981;142:308.
52. Altimari AF, Bhoopalam N, Odorsio T, Lange CL, Sandberg L, Prinz RA. Use of a somatostatin analog (SMS 201-995) in the glucagonoma syndrome. *Surgery* 1986;100:989.
53. Bolt RJ, Tesluk H, Esquivel C, Domz CA. Glucagonoma—an underdiagnosed syndrome? *West J Med* 1986;144:746.
54. Kelly TR. Pancreatic somatostatinoma. *Am J Surg* 1983;146:671.

Surgical Management of the Diabetic Patient,
edited by Michael Bergman and Gregorio A. Sicard.
Raven Press, Ltd., New York © 1991.

24

Urologic Complications of Diabetes

Todd J. Garvin

*Division of Urology, University of New Mexico School of Medicine,
Albuquerque, New Mexico 87131*

COMPLICATED RENAL INFECTIONS

Emphysematous Pyelonephritis

Emphysematous pyelonephritis is a rare but life-threatening renal infection characterized by gas formation within the kidney. Over 85% of the reported cases have been in diabetic patients. The clinical presentation is generally one of febrile illness with flank pain and infected urine, initially indistinguishable from uncomplicated pyelonephritis. *Escherichia coli* is most commonly recovered organism by urine culture. The clinical condition of the patient does not improve, however, or may frankly deteriorate, despite appropriate antibiotic therapy.

At this point, radiographic evaluation (by virtually any modality) demonstrates the presence of gas within the kidney (particularly within the renal parenchyma). Gas formation is the result of fermentation of the glucose-rich urine and interstitial fluid of the kidney. A plain abdominal radiograph of the kidney and upper bladder (KUB) generally is the simplest test to confirm this diagnosis (1). If overlying bowel gas obscures the possible intrarenal gas, further investigation with sonography or non-contrast computed tomography (CT) scan must be promptly undertaken; again the demonstration of gas within the kidney is pathognomonic (2). Intravenous contrast is used sparingly in these cases, in order to minimize the possibility of contrast-induced nephropathy (see Chapter 6).

Emphysematous pyelonephritis is of particular concern to urologists, because prompt surgical treatment is necessary once the diagnosis is established. Initial management requires fluid resuscitation, control of diabetes, and broad-spectrum antibiotic coverage. Antibiotic therapy alone, however, has led to mortality rates in excess of 75%. Nephrectomy is definitive therapy, with survival rates over 90%. There have been isolated reports of patient survival following percutaneous drainage in combination with aggressive antibiotic therapy (3); this approach allows needed hemodynamic stabilization until definitive surgical therapy can be rendered.

Xanthogranulomatous Pyelonephritis

Xanthogranulomatous pyelonephritis is another unusual but serious renal infection for which diabetic patients have a predilection. (Approximately one-sixth of reported cases have been in diabetic patients.) Xanthogranulomatous pyelonephritis (XGP) is a chronic infection characterized by infiltration of the renal parenchyma with lipid-laden macrophages ("foam cells"). The clinical presentation can resemble acute pyelonephritis, or may be more insidious, with vague flank pain, recurrent episodes of cystitis, or unexplained fevers or weight loss. Most patients present with flank tenderness or a palpable flank mass. *Proteus mirabilis* has been the causative organism commonly identified in some series, although others have found *E. coli* and other common coliform organisms with equal frequency (4).

The macrophage infiltrate in XGP may lead to tumefactive growth within the kidney, which may develop focally (5) or throughout the kidney. The microscopic appearance of foam cells within the xanthoma closely resembles clear-cell adenocarcinoma of the kidney, and pathologic confusion may result, particularly during frozen section. The XGP mass is demonstrable as a poorly enhancing solid mass within the kidney on intravenous urogram, CT scan, or sonogram. These radiographic findings are highly suggestive of renal malignancy. Frequently an area of poorly functioning renal parenchyma is identified in association with an obstructing calculus (in the extreme case, a staghorn calculus is identified amid a completely nonfunctioning renal unit). Further clouding the preoperative diagnosis of XGP is the tendency for tumefactive XGP growth to extend beyond the renal capsule, at times with apparent extension beyond Gerota's fascia and involvement of adjacent viscera. Xanthogranulomatous pyelonephritis may also be associated with hepatic dysfunction (without demonstrable mass involvement of the liver) and this syndrome (like the paraneoplastic syndrome seen with renal cell carcinoma) should resolve following nephrectomy.

Because the diagnosis of carcinoma usually cannot be excluded before surgical exploration, radical nephrectomy is generally the procedure of choice. In cases where XGP is diagnosed preoperatively, consideration can be given to partial nephrectomy, rather than radical nephrectomy. Surgical removal of all infected tissue remains essential for cure. Because diabetic nephropathy may also develop in these patients, a renal parenchyma-sparing procedure appears preferable (4). This course can only be safely undertaken, however, when preoperative imaging clearly shows the remaining kidney tissue to be normal.

Perinephric Abscess

Diabetic patients are prone to form renal or perinephric abscesses as complications of acute pyelonephritis. This possibility must be borne in mind when a diabetic patient with apparent pyelonephritis fails to respond with clinical improvement and progressive defervescence after 48 hours of appropriate intravenous antibiotic therapy. Careful physical examination is mandatory, as a mass may be palpable over the affected kidney. Radiologic evaluation must assess for ureteral obstruction (resulting in pyonephrosis) or abscess formation. Computed tomography scan is the most accurate modality for this evaluation, although hydronephrosis or loculated fluid collection may also be demonstrated on sonography. The finding of either pyonephrosis or perinephric abscess is an indication for emergent drainage, either via percutaneous aspiration with insertion of a drainage catheter, or via surgical incision. Recovery after drainage and antibiotic therapy should be complete (6).

Renal Papillary Necrosis

Renal papillary necrosis (RPN) develops when there is progressive ischemia in the tissue of the tip of the papilla. Diabetes is the most common underlying angiopathic condition causing papillary necrosis, although RPN may also be seen with sickle-cell anemia, chronic pyelonephritis, or interstitial nephritis due to analgesic (particularly phenacetin) abuse (7). Among diabetic patients with RPN, 80% are women, and 60% have a history of urinary tract infections.

Papillary necrosis is often asymptomatic. Occasionally, patients present with gross hematuria, accompanied by flank pain. Urologic evaluation of the hematuria reveals the characteristic excretory urogram findings of loss of papillary tissue, leading to a "notched" impression of the pyramidal contour that projects into the renal pelvis. A radiolucent mobile filling defect may also be seen, representing the sloughed papillary tissue. Generally no specific therapy is needed. There is concern that repeated episodes of papillary necrosis can occur, which may ultimately cause progressive deterioration of renal function. Occasionally, the sloughed papilla is of sufficient size to occlude the ureteropelvic junction (or ureter) while passing (like a kidney stone) to the bladder. In these cases, urologic surgical intervention may be needed to remove the obstructing tissue (by percutaneous or ureteroscopic extraction), or at least to decompress the kidney until the papillary tissue passes (8).

Fungal Infections

Genitourinary infection with fungus, particularly *Candida albicans* may develop in the diabetic patient, especially during episodes of poorly controlled hyperglycemia, if a foreign body (such as catheter or stent) is left indwelling in the urinary system, or if the patient is receiving broad-spectrum antibacterial therapy. Candiduria is likely to clear when the blood glucose level is brought under control, the foreign body is removed, or the antibiotics are stopped (9). Persistence of candidal infection raises the suspicion that a bezoar of hyphal material ("fungus ball") has formed in the collecting system. Such a fungus ball may be demonstrated as a radiolucent filling defect on excretory or retrograde urography, or as an echogenic mass on sonography. Surgical removal of the fungus ball is necessary to clear the infection: this may be accomplished percutaneously. Ureteric obstruction by the bezoar requires urgent decompression to prevent overwhelming fungal sepsis. Systemic antifungal therapy (amphotericin B) must be given as well, both during the surgical manipulation, and until any renal parenchymal infection has been cleared, with documented absence of fungal growth on follow-up urine cultures (10).

See Chapter 8 for a more detailed discussion of the problem of fungal infections in the diabetic patient.

BLADDER DYSFUNCTION

Neurogenic Bladder

Loss of appreciation of bladder sensation is the neurologic defect classically described with diabetes mellitus (also noted in tabes dorsalis, syringomyelia, and pernicious anemia). (See Chapter 11 for a more detailed discussion of the pathophysiology of diabetic autonomic neuropathy.) The onset of symptoms is usually insidious. Clinical presentation may occur because of urinary tract infection, incontinence, or voiding difficulty. Catheterization may reveal a large residual volume. On cystometry, appreciation of filling is delayed or absent, there are usually no uninhibited detrusor contractions, and the bladder may be of large capacity (11).

The result of this abnormality is that the bladder is capable of normal filling, but there may be failure to empty the bladder. Emptying failure can be the result of either: failure to sense that the bladder is full, with failure to make an effort to void as a result; or progressive loss of contractile ability of the detrusor muscle, as a result of progressive overdistension with ever greater bladder capacity. Incontinence rarely is a presenting complaint, unless the bladder remains chronically full to the point of overflow.

Diagnosis

The urodynamic assessment of a patient with neurogenic bladder begins with the patient completing a bladder chart for 5 days. With such a chart, the patient records the time of voiding and amount voided as precisely as possible for every single void throughout the day. The bladder chart allows cystometry to be performed within appropriate limits for that patient. For instance, if a large residual volume is present on each of several occasions, low pressures measured at low bladder volumes are not going to be clinically relevant—far more important will be the bladder pressures recorded with the bladder nearly full. From the perspective of the upper urinary tract, the pressure changes that exist at the usual residual volume (and greater) are the relevant pressures in determining upper-tract conditions.

In addition to recording voided volumes, the urologist should determine the residual volume after voiding on each of several occasions. This is most often accomplished by simple in-and-out catheterization to drain the bladder, in the doctor's office (or at home, if the patient has been instructed in appropriate self-catheterization technique). Alternatively, in patients who resist catheterization, the bladder volume after voiding can now be estimated fairly reliably by transabdominal sonography, where this technology is available.

Formal urodynamic assessment is based upon fluid fill cystometry. Many urologists prefer to perform this study in conjunction with fluoroscopic imaging of the bladder, in order to monitor the opening of the bladder neck and the sequence of sphincter events with detrusor contraction. Although such analysis is frequently helpful in those with spinal cord injury or myelodysplastic patients, who frequently have elements of sphincter dyssynergia in combination with detrusor abnormalities, the diabetic patient typically does not present such a complex scenario, and nonfluoroscopic cystometry often suffices. Adult patients with normal (or increased) bladder capacities can be studied with moderate or fast filling (100 ml/min), although a slower filling rate is necessary to determine the maximal bladder capacity. The appreciation of bladder sensation is assessed during bladder filling, including note of any sense of temperature change with filling, the first sensation of fullness, and the feeling of urgency. A diabetic patient may report none of these three usual sensations. Bladder filling is stopped at the characteristic bladder capacity indicated by the patient's bladder chart and known postvoid residual volume. The common finding with diabetic bladder dysfunction is for bladder pressure to remain *low* (10 cm of water or less), even with filling to the high volumes characteristically carried in the bladder.

The potential of the lower urinary tract to damage the upper tracts is proportional to the pressure in the bladder (12). A chronically sustained increase in bladder pressure is likely to be particularly harmful. The normal resting pressure in the collecting system is very low (usually < 10 cm of water); with peristalsis, upper tract pressure can rise transiently to approximately 15–20 cm of water. As long as the diabetic bladder maintains pressures below this level (even with large filling volumes), the risk to the upper tracts is small.

Treatment

The achievement of a low intravesical pressure storage and emptying system has been established as the mainstay of neurogenic bladder management. In classic diabetic sensory bladder dysfunction, intravesical pressure should remain low as long as the bladder is not filled beyond a certain critical threshold volume. As long as the patient is able to void spontaneously, the bladder should be able to empty while still filled below this range. Thus, the first therapeutic approach may be instruction of the patient in timed voidings. Based on the recorded voiding pattern in the bladder chart, the patient is instructed in making a conscious effort to void at frequent enough intervals (typically every 4–6 hours) to keep the bladder volume below the level where the pressure starts to rise. The patient needs to follow the clock in making the effort to void, rather than wait for the sense of bladder fullness, which may not be forthcoming until much later. Some patients may need to set an alarm clock to awaken once during the night to void as well, to adhere to the prescribed schedule.

Detrusor contractility is typically *normal* in the diabetic neuropathic bladder, which has strictly sensory impairment. However, bladder contractility may begin to diminish as chronic overdistention leads to progressive fibrosis of the bladder wall. If the patient continues to have significant residual urine volume in the bladder despite spontaneous voiding, assistance in bladder emptying will be necessary. This assistance may take the form of pharmacologic agents, or of instrumentation (catheterization) to insure bladder emptying.

The administration of cholinergic agents occasionally effects improved detrusor contraction. Bethanechol chloride is the cholinergic agonist most commonly used, because it is resistant to acetylcholinesterase and acts selectively on the smooth muscle of the gastrointestinal tract and the urinary bladder (13). Bethanechol appears to be most beneficial in patients with normal control over the striated urinary sphincter (which should be intact in most diabetic patients). Oral doses of at least 50 mg four times daily have been recommended, and responses can vary due to differences in gastrointestinal absorption (14).

Since its introduction by Guttman and Frankel in 1966 (15), intermittent catheterization has become a common method of bladder evacuation in appropriate patients with neurogenic dysfunction. Lapides et al. (16) modified the technique by advocating outpatient clean self-intermittent catheterization. The technique is easily applied and learned in a sterile manner in the institutional setting and with a clean technique at home.

The applicability of long-term intermittent catheterization depends on factors such as patient intelligence, reliability, hand control, educational support, and financial factors. With proper selection, a high compliance rate and low morbidity in the upper tracts will be seen on a long-term basis.

There is seldom any benefit from contemplation of surgical reconstruction of the bladder. Permanent disruption of bladder function, either through indwelling catheter or urinary diversion (ileal conduit) may be considered as a last resort if appropriate intermittent catheterization is unable to prevent progressive deterioration in the upper tracts.

Recurrent Infections

The problem of recurrent bladder infections has been discussed in detail in Chapter 8. In general, bladder infections in the diabetic patient are promulgated by the higher rate of bacteriuria in the diabetic bladder (17,18), and by impaired host defenses at the bladder level, including inappropriate bacterial adherence to the urothelium of the bladder wall, and impaired clearance of bacteria by phagocytosis (19). Diabetic patients are more disposed to ascending infection from the bladder to the upper tract with resulting frank pyelonephritis (20). For this reason, antibiotic treatment is necessary to eradicate infection once it is established in the bladder. However, judicious choice of antibiotic must be made, and the temporal course of treatment must be limited, so as to minimize the risk of fungal overgrowth in the upper tracts that can otherwise be the result (see "Fungal infections" above). In general, surgical intervention is not required during the management of recurrent bladder infections, and so the majority of diabetic patients never come to the urologist's attention.

It should be borne in mind that the patient with persistent relapsing infections, or failure to improve on appropriate antibiotic therapy, even though diabetic, should be evaluated for a possible contributing structural or neurogenic abnormality. To this end, an intravenous pyelogram reveals any structural abnormality (stone, ureteral stricture or diverticulum, bladder diverticulum) likely to cause persistent infection. In the patient who cannot tolerate intravenous contrast, a plain abdominal radiograph excludes the majority of calculi, and a renal sonogram reveals any underlying hydronephrosis or focal obstruction. Determination of the postvoid residual urine volume (by straight bladder catheterization) reveals any significant degree of bladder emptying failure (*vide supra*).

Risk of Bladder Cancer

Over the last two decades, there has been concern over the possible bladder carcinogenicity of artificial sweeteners, and the attendant risk sweetener use confers to diabetic patients. In particular, animal studies showed tumor development in the offspring of rats fed high doses of saccharin, when the saccharin exposure began *in utero* and continued after birth (21). Rats exposed to saccharin doses approximating usual human consumption, however, had no significant bladder tumor risk.

Several epidemiologic studies have failed to substantiate any positive relationship between artificial sweeteners and bladder cancer (22). Bladder cancer mortality rates were not found to be elevated among diabetic patients in the United States and Great Britain. However, one recent Canadian study has shown a small increase in risk of bladder cancer among diabetic patients (relative risk of about 1.6), which was independent of artificial sweetener use (23). Overall, the relative risk contributed by diabetes is certainly an order of magnitude smaller than other potentially avoidable bladder cancer risks, such as occupational exposures (aniline dyes, aromatic amines) or smoking (24). There are no unusual clinical features of bladder cancer in the diabetic patient that require any departure from standard urologic management of this malignancy.

SEXUAL DYSFUNCTION

Impotence

Male erectile insufficiency (impotence) is the diabetic complication most likely to require a urologist's attention. It is estimated that erectile insufficiency develops in between one- and two-thirds of diabetic men during their lifetimes. This means that impotence is a more common complication of diabetes than either retinopathy or nephropathy (25,26). Furthermore, diabetes mellitus is the most common organic causative factor identified in impotent men, accounting for 40% of men presenting for evaluation of sexual dysfunction (27).

In diabetic men, impotence may be the first symptom of previously undiagnosed diabetes (as has been observed in 10–20% of impotent men presenting to some sexual dysfunction clinics) (28). Impotence can also be a secondary symptom after several years of diabetes or a temporary phenomenon associated with poor diabetic control. It should be emphasized that not all patients with diabetes become impotent, and that even if diabetes is present the dysfunction may be totally psychogenic (29,30).

Mechanisms of Normal Erections

The normal process of penile erection requires a coordinated interplay of nervous stimuli and vasoactive responses (31). The initiating stimulus for erection can be tactile stimulation of the penile skin. Other stimuli, such as visual erotic stimulation or erotic fantasy, presumably act at a cerebral/brainstem level. The stimulation then is transmitted to the erectogenic centers of the lumbosacral spinal cord. The induction of erection is largely mediated by sacral parasympathetic fibers that emerge from the pelvic plexus and course along the inferolateral margins of the bladder and prostate bilaterally before sending terminal cavernous branches along the length of the corpora cavernosa.

The neurotransmitters involved in initiating erection have not been definitely identified. Erection may be induced despite blockade of both adrenergic and cholinergic transmission. Neuropeptides (such as vasoactive intestinal polypeptide and substance P) and prostaglandins have been proposed as possible effectors (32). In addition, there is a contributory effect of cholinergic stimulation, which acts upon the penile corporal smooth muscle to induce its relaxation, through the action of an endothelium-derived relaxation factor (which may be nitric oxide) liberated from the endothelial cells that line the vascular spaces of the corpora cavernosa.

The initial hemodynamic event of erection is vasodilatation of the helicine arterioles within the corpora cavernosa. These arterioles are terminal branches of the internal pudendal artery, derived from the hypogastric artery. This vasodilation is accompanied by relaxation of the trabecular smooth muscle within the corpora cavernosa, which allows expansion of the vascular lacunae within the corpora (33). The resulting increase in the intracavernous blood flow elevates the intracavernous pressure, from its resting value of 25–30 mm Hg to the level of diastolic blood pressure, producing visible penile tumescence. With increasing tumescence, the venous drainage of the cavernous spaces becomes occluded. This appears to be the result of passive compression of the subtunical plexus of venules, which course beneath the tunica albuginea linearly for a course of several mm before perforating the tunica albuginea to form visible emissary veins external to the corpora. The emissary veins ultimately drain to the deep and superficial dorsal veins of the penis, and thence to the periprostatic venous plexus and hypogastric veins. Occlusion of the cavernovenous drainage allows further increase of intracavernous pressure to the systolic or suprasystolic level associated with full penile rigidity. With venous occlusion, a full erection is maintained by only a small ongoing arterial inflow (as little as 10 ml/min). Additional compression of the penile crura, by action of the levator ani and bulbocavernosus muscles, helps produce full erection.

In addition, there is probably a requirement for circulating testosterone for normal male sexual function. Testosterone is not required for the neurovascular cascade that produces erection, but appears to be a central nervous system requirement for the initiation of the CNS impulses that lead to erection. The level of testosterone is also generally correlated with the patient's libido. However, there are uncommon cases of men who have been castrated in adult life (traumatically, or for treatment of prostate cancer) who retain normal sexual drive and normal erectile ability.

The process of detumescence is brought about by sympathetic nerve activity, which is electrically measureable within the corpus cavernosum (34), producing release of norepinephrine. Vasoconstriction of the penile arteries, and contraction of the cavernosal smooth muscle to its baseline tonic state, produce decreased penile blood flow, and detumescence proceeds rapidly once the venoocclusive pathway is reopened (35)

Diabetes mellitus may interfere with the normal erection process at any one of several mechanistic levels. The end result of any such interference can be erectile impotence. Recognition and assessment of the various phases of the erection process is essential to the diagnosis and proper treatment of the impotent diabetic man.

Mechanisms of Erectile Disorder in Diabetic Men

Neurologic

The peripheral neuropathy associated with diabetes mellitus contributes to impairment of the reflex activity that produces erections (36–38). This may reflect loss of afferent sensory imput from penile stimulation, due to defective conductance of penile cutaneous nerves (39). Furthermore, changes within the skin itself have been identified (thickening of the skin, with reduced conduction of pressure to deeper dermal structures including sensory corpuscles), that may be a further impediment to transmission of stimulation that normally initiates erection (40).

Penile autonomic neuropathy can also contribute to impaired erectile response (34). Central autonomic neuropathy has been demonstrated in a majority of selected series of impotent patients (41). There is also histologic evidence of abnormality of the autonomic innervation of the penis (42,43).

The general pathophysiology of diabetic neuropathy is discussed in greater detail in Chapter 11.

Vascular

Large-vessel atherosclerosis can produce impaired penile blood flow in the diabetic patient. Studies have shown that one-half of diabetic men have abnormal penile blood pressure demonstrable by Doppler flow study (44,45).

Diabetic men may also have small-vessel occlusive disease, which is not readily detectable by penile-brachial index measurement. In these cases, angiography indicates very sclerotic terminal vessels in the distribution to the cavernous arteries. The results of Doppler duplex flow measurements in the cavernous artery itself have shown restricted vasodilatory response in 60% of diabetic men (33).

Penile Myopathy

Recent investigation of penile smooth-muscle physiology has indicated that the corporal smooth muscle in diabetic men is intrinsically abnormal (46). As a result, the corporal smooth-muscle relaxation, which is associated with the initial hemodynamic phase of erection and which is required for full tumescence, is impaired. This has been demonstrated with both direct electrical stimulation and pharmacologic (cholinergic) stimulation (*in vitro*) of penile smooth-muscle tissue from diabetic men. These end-organ changes preclude normal erection, even in the face of normal arterial perfusion.

Hormonal

Diabetes mellitus may be associated with measurable perturbation of the pituitary-gonadal axis (47). This most often is the result of Leydig cell dysfunction, with diminished production of testosterone in response to luteinizing hormone (LH) stimulation in both diabetic men (48) and experimental animals (49). The usual response to this deterioration is increased pituitary drive, however, in many diabetic men the LH level remains inappropriately depressed, indicating a contribution of hypothalamo-pituitary dysfunction as well. Diabetic patients have also been found to have an above-average incidence of hyperprolactinemia (50). Prolactin-associated impotence is often accompanied by clinically evident gynecomastia, and loss of libido. The testosterone level is usually, but not invariably, depressed by the prolactin elevation.

Psychological

Several studies of diabetic men have shown characteristic changes of depression and loss of libido, which may antedate the onset of impotence (51). The percentage of patients with psychogenic impotence among all impotent diabetic men may be as high as 25–45%, based on nocturnal penile tumescence screening (30).

Evaluation

Initial Clinical Evaluation

The initial evaluation of any impotent man begins with an appropriately focused history and physical examination. During this evaluation, the examiner must inquire about the onset and duration of impotence, and if there is any residual erectile activity whatsoever (including the reflex erection normally accompanying a full urinary bladder on first arising in the morning), if there is any association of erectile difficulty with particular sexual positions, techniques, or partners. Some of these findings (impotence associated with an extramarital affair or with a specific sexual partner) may be clues to psychological, versus physical, etiology of impotence (51).

Other potential comorbidities can also be assessed during the initial history and physical, such as the history of hypertension, myocardial infarction, cerebrovascular accident, peripheral claudication symptoms, and smoking history. These can raise the suspicion of underlying vascular disease that may be associated with vasculogenic impotence (52).

In cases where there is concern that the etiology may be psychological rather than organic, it may be helpful to evaluate spontaneous nocturnal penile tumescence (NPT). Normal men almost invariably have spontaneous erection events during rapid-eye-movement (REM) sleep. These spontaneous erections are preserved in men with psychogenic impotence, but are diminished if organic factors prevent full erection (27,53).

Monitoring of NPT can conveniently be measured in the ambulatory setting with the RigiScan (Dacomed Corp., Minneapolis, MN). The RigiScan continuously measures both tumescence and rigidity at both the base and tip of the penis. Figures 1 and 2 illustrate typical RigiScan records from normal and impotent patients. Some authors have suggested that sleep disturbances (due to anxiety, sleep apnea, periodic leg movements) can interfere with NPT results even if the erectile mechanisms remain intact. Performance of NPT testing in a full sleep laboratory has been their standard recommendation. However, the ambulatory use of RigiScan over several nights provides a cost-effective method for eliminating these interfering influences without the expense of overnight hospitalization (53).

Even more simply, NPT can be demonstrated by breakage of a nonelastic band, such as SnapGauge (Dacomed Corp.), or even a strip of postage stamps, worn around the penis. This method of screening for evidence of spontaneous erectile activity is quite economic. These home units provide no information, however, about the number of erection events, and they may give misleading results because of trauma during normal sleep movements or improper patient application.

Many clinicians believe they are able to identify the patient with psychogenic impotence during the course of the clinical interview, and thus spare these patients protracted evaluation of organic factors when psychological therapy is the indicated form of intervention. In some cases, the value of NPT testing is to provide documentation for medico-legal reasons of the existence and severity of an organic erectile problem prior to launching into surgical or other invasive treatment.

Hormonal

Endocrinologic evaluation is generally accomplished by measurement of serum levels of testosterone and prolactin (54). Impotence has also been reported in men

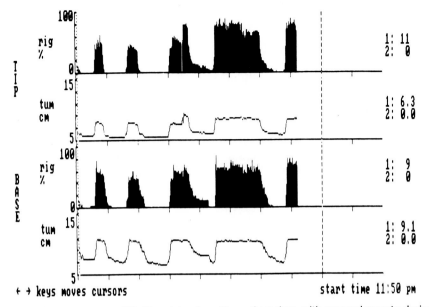

FIG. 1. Penile tumescence (RigiScan) tracing. Normal tracing, with several events during the course of the night, each marked by both tumescence and rigidity at the tip (upper two channels) and base (lower two channels) of the penis. (Courtesy of Dacomed Corp., reproduced with permission.)

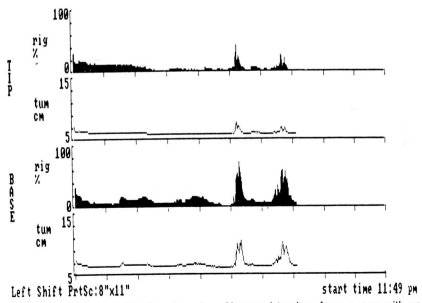

FIG. 2. Penile tumescence (RigiScan) tracing. Abnormal tracing, from a man with vascular disease and impotence. Despite occasional partial tumescence at the base (bottom channel), the erection events are rare and short lived, and the tip of the penis never develops tumescence or rigidity over 20%. (Courtesy of Dacomed Corp., reproduced with permission.)

with clinically silent hypothyroidism. This may only be detectable by detection of an elevated serum thyrotropin (TSH) level, even in the face of thyroid hormone levels within the normal range (55).

Neurologic

Although peripheral sensory neuropathy can be demonstrated by measurement of conduction velocities in the extremities in impotent patients (56), the most meaningful neurologic tests involve assessment of the sensory afferent path from the penis to the level of the sacral spinal cord. The level of tactile sensation can be assessed using a biothesiometer for reproducible and quantifiable production of tactile stimulation. An elevated sensory threshold is detectable with this device, and is believed to correspond to sensory neuropathy (57,58).

The latency of the bulbocavernosus reflex also depends on afferent conduction via the dorsal penile nerve. To measure this latency, electrical stimulation is applied along the penile shaft, activating the dorsal nerve, which carries impulses through the sacral erection center and pudendal nerve to the bulbocavernosus muscle. An electrode in (or over) the bulbocavernosus muscle can record these impulses, allowing determination of the latency time. Normal latency times are 35 msec or lower (59). An abnormality of this latency is detectable in over 60% of the diabetic impotent population (60,61). Although there are conflicting interpretations of these results (62), it is believed by some that this abnormal reflex latency indicates a significant degree of neuropathy contributing to impotence in these men.

Although there is reason to suppose that autonomic neuropathy affects the vasomotor regulation of penile hemodynamics and leads to impotence, there are no readily available clinical tests that assess this function. There is some hope for measuring penile skin temperature changes as a reflection of sympathetic activity in the penis (63,64). Even this dermal vasculature, however, is not the same as the erectile vasculature, so there is some dissociation of the results.

Vascular

Virag (65) is credited with the initial demonstration of the ability of certain vasodilatory substances to produce erections upon injection into either the hypogastric or penile arteries, or into the cavernous spaces of the penis. Stemming from this observation, this technique has been developed for its diagnostic capability. By applying a vasoactive injection into the corpora cavernosa, the cascade of vascular events, involving both relaxation of the cavernous smooth muscles and vasodilatation of the cavernous arteries with increase in penile blood flow, ultimately developing full erection, can be observed. The substances used may be papaverine, papaverine in combination with phentolamine, or prostaglandin E1. The standard dosages are shown in Table 1.

The vasoactive injection technique (31) involves use of a rubber band around the base of the penis, with injection of the chosen agent into the corpus cavernosum, using an insulin syringe with a fine (28–30 gauge) needle. Injection into only one corpus is sufficient, because of extensive transseptal vascular communications between the right and left corpora cavernosa. The site of injection is compressed by direct manual pressure for about 2 minutes; the rubber band is then removed. During

TABLE 1. *Vasoactive agents for intracavernous injection*

Agent	Usual dose
Papaverine HCl	30 mg in 1 ml
Phentolamine	0.2–1 mg in 1 ml (in combination with papaverine)
Prostaglandin E1 (Prostin VR, Upjohn)	20 μg in 0.5 ml

Papaverine:phentolamine combinations are often prepared in batches of 300 mg papaverine:1 (or 2) mg phentolamine in 10–12 ml total volume. Aliquots of as little as 0.15 ml of this combination may be effective.

The usual doses given above induce erection in nearly all normal men, and over 75% of men with mild vascular insufficiency. Some authors routinely begin diagnostic testing with much smaller doses (one-fourth or one-half of the usual dose), in order to assess erectile response without inducing prolonged erection.

Much smaller doses than usual (one-fourth or less) should be used in the initial testing of men with penile denervation (e.g., spinal cord injury), who may be hyperresponsive to vasoactive stimulation.

this time, and for the next 10 minutes, the patient begins to develop penile tumescence. The patient is allowed to view erotic material or to apply manual stimulation to enhance the erection. To avert orthostatic hypotension that can be the result of the initial systemic effect of the vasoactive agent, the patient is kept supine for 10 minutes. He is then observed in the standing position. This change of posture is important in order to get the full compressive value of the pelvic floor musculature upon the cavernous and crural veins draining the penis, making full erection possible. The degree of erection is assessed after 10 and 20 minutes of observation. In addition, the patient may be asked to exercise (e.g., climb a stair) to observe for any diminution of erection with this activity.

Lue (66) has described a "penodynamic" test, based on the application of this vasoactive injection. The schematic results are shown in Table 2. The patient who rapidly attains an erection, but then rapidly experiences detumescence during 20 minutes observation in the office, is likely to be discovered to have venoocclusive insufficiency. Loss of erection with exercise suggests the "external iliac steal syndrome," whereby blood is shunted away from the penis in order to maintain perfusion to the lower extremities. The patient who never achieves tumescence may have either profound venous leak, or significant arterial stenosis, or interference from anxiety or discomfort. The patient who has a normal result may have either detectable sensory neuropathy (*vide supra*), or psychogenic impotence. (Some patients with mild arterial insufficiency are able to respond with a full erection in the face of vasoactive stimulation, indicating at least a degree of arterial reserve.) The opportunity of artificial induction of erection also allows assessment of such characteristics as curvature of the penis with erection (as a result of Peyronie's disease), which may also interfere with normal erectile function (67).

TABLE 2. *Penodynamic test results*

Tumescence	Detumescence	Diagnosis
Fast	Fast	Venogenic
Fast	Slow	Normal
Slow	Slow	Arteriogenic
Slow	Fast	Mixed/penile myopathy

Modified from Lue (66)

Interpretation of an abnormal response to vasoactive injection depends on several factors. The vasoactive injection cannot distinguish reliably between severe arterial and venous insufficiency. The patient may have significant arterial stenosis ("failure to fill"), or excessive escape of blood via penile veins ("failure to store"), and in either case the vasoactive injection may not correct these influences and an inadequate erection results.

There are other caveats to keep in mind. Cigarette smoking causes vascular spasm through the direct action of nicotine. It has been observed that the acute effect of smoking a single cigarette can be to prevent the normal response to papaverine injection. Therefore, a patient who smokes, and who has a negative response to papaverine injection, should have the test repeated, after smoking cessation, in order to obtain a more meaningful result (68). In cases where the patient seems to be significantly anxious or uncomfortable due to the injection itself, the examiner should consider repeating the test on another occasion before concluding that the patient has a significant vascular abnormality. Finally, the patient with an unusually long or capacious phallus may require a larger than standard dose of vasoactive medication to achieve full erection; in such cases repeat testing with a larger dose is recommended. It is generally not necessary to exceed 60 mg papaverine (with up to 1 mg phentolamine) or 40 μg prostaglandin E1 in such cases.

Once an abnormal response to vasoactive injection has been documented, an effort is made to delineate the status of arterial supply to the penis. The standard method that has been used is noninvasive evaluation of penile arterial perfusion using measurement of the resting dorsal penile artery pressure by Doppler stethoscope, or with pulse-volume recording. The penile systolic pressure is then compared to that in the systemic (brachial) circulation and a penile-brachial index (PBI) is calculated as the ratio of these two pressures. A normal value of PBI is generally greater than 0.75. This test in use for many years, is helpful when markedly abnormal (27), but has been subject to criticism, however, because the dorsal penile artery, most often measured in the PBI test, is not the artery involved in the majority of hemodynamic responses leading to erection. Assessment of the cavernous arteries is more germane to assessing erectile status, and these are not routinely accessible for PBI measurement. It is now possible to quantify the bloodflow in the cavernous arteries of the penis, particularly after vasoactive injection, by Doppler flow measurement, or through high-resolution sonography for precise measurement of cavernous arterial diameter (69). The equipment to carry out these measurements is not yet widely available.

Studies have shown that the patient with significantly reduced PBI probably has clinically significant atherosclerosis throughout the circulatory system, and risks a significant vascular event (myocardial infarction, cerebrovascular accident) within the next 2 years, even with no history of anginal symptoms (70). This fact needs to be borne in mind in planning future management of the patient, and treadmill testing or even coronary angiography may need to be considered for his overall well-being.

For the patient with demonstrated arterial insufficiency who may be considered a candidate for revascularization surgery (*vide infra*), arteriography is necessary to delineate the site(s) of stenosis and the status of any distal runoff. Arteriography should be carried out after vasoactive injection to observe the penile arterial supply in a state of maximal blood flow; arteriography in the unstimulated state often falsely suggests poor perfusion or stenosis of the cavernous arteries, when those same arteries are fully capable of normal vasodilatory response after vasoactive stimulation (71).

Patients who have an abnormal response to vasoactive injection and normal arterial parameters are suspected of venoocclusive insufficiency. However, myopathy of penile smooth muscle may produce the same pattern of response. Dynamic cavernosometry and cavernosography have been developed to confirm the status of the venoocclusive mechanism. Many normal men will not demonstrate full action of the venoocclusive mechanism unless full smooth muscle relaxation is produced by vasoactive intracavernous injection (papaverine or prostaglandin E1). Thus, the technique of pharmacologic cavernosometry (72–74) has been developed. In this technique, a standard vasoactive injection is given, as described above. After 15–20 minutes, when maximal response has been achieved (there is generally no erection in these patients), infusion of saline solution into the corpus cavernosum is begun via butterfly cannula, at a rate of 1 ml/sec, and the cavernous pressure is monitored "dynamically" as it changes in response to infusion. The rate of infusion is adjusted so that erection (and pressure over 100 mm Hg) is produced, and then flow is reduced to the minimal level allowing erection to be maintained; this value is termed the pharmacologic erectile maintenance flow (PEMF). Values of PEMF above 30 ml/min are indicative of abnormal venous leak. Once the PEMF is determined, if it is abnormal, infusion of radiographic contrast into the corpus allows fluoroscopic observation of the routes of venous egress from the penis, with the determination of which vein(s) may be responsible for the venoocclusive insufficiency.

Management

Just as the etiologic role of diabetes in the development of impotence may be multifactorial, the management of impotence in the diabetic man may require attention to several different aspects of sexual function. The problem of male sexual dysfunction does not develop in a vacuum. Many couples profit from joint counseling and therapy in helping to cope with one partner's sexual dysfunction, even when there is an identified and treatable physical cause that can be corrected. The devastating psychological consequences of impotence should not be underestimated (75). Although specialists in the field of sexual counseling are found in many communities, very often the task of counseling the couple with sexual dysfunction, leading them to reasonable expectations of what can be achieved with various forms of therapy, and helping them to adapt and accommodate to various changes that can occur with the progression or treatment of sexual dysfunction, falls on the urologist or primary care physician.

General Medical Management

Attention to control of blood glucose levels has been associated with improved sexual satisfaction (if not demonstrable change in erections per se) in a number of impotent diabetic man. In addition, smoking cessation needs to be advocated among men who smoke which may improve sexual performance in one-third of men (76).

Hormonal

Patients with subnormal serum testosterone levels should be offered testosterone replacement. There is no value, however, in supplying excess testosterone to men whose endogenous levels are normal. Testosterone replacement can be given orally or parenterally. Intramuscular injection is generally recommended because of greater reliability of absorption. Long-acting testosterone preparations allow the convenience of injections only every 2–4 weeks. Commonly used doses are 400 mg testosterone enanthate or 400 mg testosterone cypionate every 4 weeks. Testosterone levels should be measured at the trough (just prior to injection) after 2 or 3 months of replacement, in order to verify that the testosterone level is being adequately replaced into the normal range. Serum levels may be more consistently maintained by doses of 200 mg every 2 weeks.

When testosterone levels are low because of primary testicular failure, accompanied by increased levels of pituitary LH, the prospects for improved sexual function after testosterone normalization are good. However, in cases where combined pituitary and testicular failure have developed (resulting in failure of LH to increase despite the testosterone fall), it has been observed that testosterone replacement is less likely to yield patient satisfaction and return of erections (55).

Reasonable care should be taken to exclude prostatic malignancy before beginning testosterone replacement to avoid iatrogenic promotion of an androgen-sensitive tumor. Because liver dysfunction can develop after testosterone administration (oral or intramuscular), testosterone treatment should be avoided in patients with known history of liver disease. In addition, monitoring of liver function tests every 6 months while receiving testosterone is recommended.

Hyperprolactinemia that is not caused by macroscopic pituitary adenoma can be treated with bromocriptine. Usual doses are 2.5–5.0 mg daily; side effects are few. Prolactin levels should decline to normal within 1 month. Although bromocriptine treatment also suppresses prolactin levels in patients with pituitary tumors, surgical removal is preferred to avoid complications from progressive intracranial mass.

Pharmacologic

Several drugs have enjoyed anecdotal reputations for enhancement of sexual performance. One of the few drugs to have proven value in placebo-controlled studies is yohimbine. Yohimbine, an alpha-2-adrenergic antagonist, has demonstrated efficacy in treatment of impotent men, including both organic and psychogenic etiologies (77,78). The action of yohimbine is apparently at a central level, perhaps involving potentiation of sexual excitation, rather than any penile hemodynamic impact (79). Nonetheless, for diabetic men with only mild degrees of neurogenic or vascular impairment, or with a significant component of psychological interference with erectile function, yohimbine may provide a valuable adjunct to sexual counseling or other conservative therapy.

Other agents that have recently been recommended for supportive therapy in the impotent patient include isoxsuprine (a beta-adrenergic agonist) and trazodone (a tricyclic antidepressant with particularly limited anticholinergic side effects) (80). In fact, priapism has been reported with trazodone use in men with normal potency.

External Assistance

Several devices have been designed and marketed over the last decade to provide reversible assistance in inducing erections. These devices generally include a cylinder component into which the flaccid penis is inserted. A vacuum is then created within the cylinder, usually by hand pump action (or by oral suction on a vent tube). The vacuum acts to draw blood into the penis, which becomes progressively engorged in a simulation of the normal penile hemodynamics. Once the penis has become fully engorged, a constricting ring (rubber) is applied over the base of the penis to impede egress of blood from the corpora. At this point, the penis should be sufficiently erect to allow penetration. Once intercourse is completed, the constricting ring is removed (care must be taken not to leave it in place over 30 minutes), and detumescence results.

Success in supplementing erectile performance has been reported with the ErecAid (Osbon Medical Systems, Inc., Augusta, GA) (81), Response (Smith-Collins Pharmaceuticals, Inc., West Chester, PA) and Correctaid (Synergist, Ltd., Houston, TX) (82,83) devices, among others. These reports have included diabetic patients in 25–100% of the patients reported. Advantages of these systems include reversibility, ease of application, minimal toxicity (ocasional mild ecchymosis), and low cost (compared to the expenses of surgery). On the other hand, not all patients are able to reproduce an erection with these external suction devices. Between one-third and two-thirds of men are able to operate the suction devices properly and achieve adequate simulation of erection. There may be impaired response because of severe arterial disease (regardless of the negative pressure applied to the corporal spaces externally), or because of significant venous leak (especially from the cavernosal and crural veins proximal to the point of constriction applied by the external ring).

Although there is some evidence that the external vacuum and constriction may produce a net *reduction* in penile blood flow, there are minimal physical sequelae of their proper use. The external suction assistance devices offer many impotent men an adequate functional erection result, at least temporarily. If nothing else, use of these devices may provide an interim solution that is relatively benign, until the patient is medically and mentally ready for a more invasive or definitive form of therapy.

Penile Injection

Impotent patients who have a satisfactory erection response after trial vasoactive injection (*vide supra*) can be offered such injections (self-administered) for stimulation of the native erection process on a therapeutic basis. Patients most likely to respond well to this treatment are those with neuropathy or psychological factors primarily causing their erectile dysfunction, with normal (or only mildly impaired) vascular responses (see Table 3). As for the vascular diagnostic process, prostaglandin E1 is the preferred vasoactive agent for self-injection. Auto-injection of vasoactive substances by the patient requires slight adjustments, compared with the diagnostic vasoactive injection described previously (84,85). The dose of medication used should be titrated according to the patient's erection response, with the aim of achieving a satisfactorily rigid erection with limited effect so as not to produce pri-

TABLE 3. *Indications and contraindications for vasoactive injection therapy*

Indications
  Neurogenic impotence
  Psychogenic impotence (in conjunction with counseling, sex therapy)
  Mild arterial insufficiency
  Mild venoocclusive insufficiency
Contraindications
  Sickle-cell disease
  Coagulopathy
  Limited manual dexterity
  Severe psychiatric disturbance
  Unwillingness to return for follow-up

apism of several hours' duration. For self-injection, the patient can usually omit use of the rubber band around the base of the penis (manual compression of the injection site provides a similar concentration of the drug within the corpora of the penile shaft during the first few minutes of action). Patients also find injection in the standing (or sitting upright) position more comfortable than the supine position assumed in the doctor's office.

Patients who are being treated with vasoactive auto-injection need to be carefully instructed in the proper self-injection technique, and should perform satisfactory self-injection under the physician's observation in the office before commencing a course of home self-injections. The patient must also be alerted to the possibility of prolonged erection or frank priapism developing after injection. In such cases, the patient needs to know that medical attention must be sought promptly (within the first 4–6 hours of erection), to minimize the risk of permanent corporal fibrosis and impotence.

Patients on a program of self-injection need to return for periodic examinations, both to monitor the quality of their response to injections, to insure that no episodes of prolonged erections have been developing, and to check for development of corporal fibrosis. In patients performing auto-injection of papaverine/phentolamine solutions, palpable corporal nodules developed with increasing frequency the longer self-injections were performed, in up to 20% of men. Animal studies (86) have shown that prostaglandin E1 solution causes significantly less local tissue irritation and consequent fibrosis than papaverine solution, at least in the short run. However, the mechanical act of repeated injection may still be expected to produce risk of fibrosis when repeated over years.

Although both papaverine and prostaglandin E1 have been marketed in the United States for several years, the Federal Food and Drug Administration has not approved either drug for the indication of injection treatment for impotence. In fact, one manufacturer of papaverine (Eli Lilly & Co., Indianapolis, IN) has included a specific statement disclaiming this use of papaverine in the prescribing information insert supplied with the medication. This fact may expose the physician who prescribes these drugs in the setting of impotence treatment to legal repercussions should adverse complications develop in a patient so treated. It is important that the patient be informed at the outset of treatment that this is not an FDA-approved use of the drug, that complications such as corporal fibrosis and priapism may develop, that priapism must be treated as a medical emergency if it does occur, and that the long-term consequences (5 years or longer) of auto-injection therapy are not known. It is most prudent to obtain a signed record of informed consent from the patient, including explicit acknowledgement of these risks, before commencing auto-injection treatment (87).

Vascular Surgery

Several vascular procedures have been devised and advocated over the last decade for treatment of vasculogenic impotence. These fall into the broad categories of venous ligation procedures for patients with venoocclusive insufficiency (88), and arterial revascularization (usually by anastomosis of the inferior epigastric artery into the penile vasculature) (89). These procedures are mentioned in this context primarily to *discourage* consideration of such reconstruction in the diabetic patient. Elaborate vascular reconstruction has been associated with very limited duration of favorable results in even highly selected patients who are otherwise healthy and ideal operative candidates. The tendency of diabetes to produce multiple insults on the erectile mechanism, including relatively intractable damage to the corporal smooth muscle and penile innervation, dooms any revascularization to ultimate failure. Thus, diabetes has been a *contraindication* for consideration of these procedures in nearly all authors' hands.

Penile Prosthesis Surgery

Impotence that fails to respond to other forms of therapy can be managed definitively by surgical insertion of a penile prosthesis. All penile prostheses in current use contain paired cylinders that are inserted in the corpora cavernosa, which act to simulate the erect corpora and provide sufficient rigidity for penetration.

Penile prostheses are generally of two types—inflatable and non-inflatable. The models presently available in each class (and their manufacturers) are itemized in Table 4. The noninflatable (or malleable) prostheses are simpler in design, being

TABLE 4. *Penile prosthesis models*

Model	Manufacturer
Noninflatable	
AMS 600	American Medical Systems, Inc.
Flexirod (Finney)	Medical Engineering Corp.
Jonas (silicone-silver)	C.R. Bard, Inc.
Mentor malleable (Small-Carrion)	Mentor Corp.
Positionable/Noninflatable	
DuraPhase	Dacomed Corp.
OmniPhase (spring-activated)	Dacomed Corp.
Inflatable	
"Three-piece" (separate pump and reservoir)	
AMS 700CX	American Medical Systems, Inc.
Alpha-1	Mentor Corp.
Mentor inflatable	Mentor Corp.
"Two-piece" (combined pump/reservoir, separate from cylinders)	
GFS	Mentor Corp.
GFS Mark II	Mentor Corp.
UniFlate 1000 (Surgitek)	Medical Engineering Corp.
Self-contained (pump/reservoir within cylinder)	
FlexiFlate (Surgitek)	Medical Engineering Corp.
Dynaflex	American Medical Systems, Inc.

composed of solid cylinders (primarily silicone) with a central core of either metal wire (silver or stainless steel) or polymer to provide stiffness. The OmniPhase and DuraPhase prostheses are sometimes termed "positionable"; they contain an arrangement of plastic plates along a spring-loaded cable as their internal structure, to allow greater flexibility along the length of the shaft while retaining rigidity. Noninflatable prostheses do not change in length or girth after insertion–they are always potentially rigid enough for intercourse. (See Figure 3.)

With inflatable prostheses, the corporal cylinders are sealed tubes (of reinforced silicone, polyurethane, or similar polymer), which remain flaccid at rest. These cylinders are attached via connecting tubing to a fluid reservoir, which may be placed either beneath the anterior abdominal wall or within the scrotum (depending on the specific design used and the fluid volume the reservoir must accommodate). (See Figure 4.) Interposed between the reservoir and the corporal cylinders is a pump, palpable in the scrotum, that the patient compresses manually to inflate the cylinders with fluid, which causes erection. Also located with the pump is a release valve to allow fluid to exit from the cylinders and return to the reservoir, for detumescence. The self-contained inflatable prostheses (Dynaflex, Flexi Flate) have no scrotal components, rather the reservoir is contained within the posterior portion of the cylinder and fluid is transferred into an anterior chamber, producing stiffening of the cylinder by compression of the pump which is located in the distal penile shaft.

There are relative merits and drawbacks to each prosthesis design. Advantages of the malleable prosthesis include simplicity and durability of the prosthesis itself, ease of preparation for intercourse, and simplicity of the insertion procedure. The

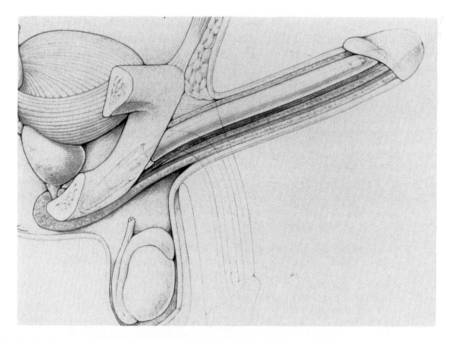

FIG. 3. Penile prosthesis, malleable type. Schematic view of AMS 600 model in position within corpora cavernosa. (Courtesy of American Medical Systems, Inc., Minnetonka, MN. Medical illustration by Michael Schenk, reproduced with permission.)

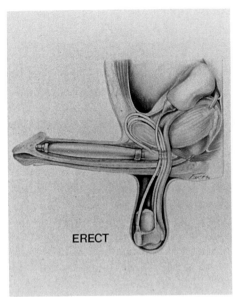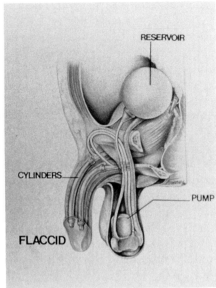

FIG. 4. Penile prosthesis, inflatable ("three-piece") type. Schematic view of AMS 700CX model in position, in both the *flaccid* (deflated) and *erect* (inflated) states. (Courtesy of American Medical Systems, Inc., Minnetonka, MN. Medical illustration by Michael Schenk, reproduced with permission.)

malleable prostheses can have the disadvantage of appearing constantly erect, however, which makes concealment difficult, particularly in gymnasiums and public bathrooms. The major advantage of the inflatable designs is that they simulate more nearly the normal flaccid penis when not inflated, which allows for more comfortable concealment under clothing and offers less restriction to athletics or other physical activities. The manipulation necessary for inflation may not be easily accomplished, however, if the patient has limited manual dexterity; some patients experience additional discomfort from the presence of scrotal hardware. The cost of inflatable prostheses is generally higher (by a thousand dollars or more) than malleable designs. The reliance on proper hydraulic operation for proper inflation and deflation also makes inflatable designs vulnerable to obstruction or mechanical malfunction.

The procedure for insertion of penile prosthesis is similar for both inflatable and noninflatable types. Most surgeons use either an infrapubic or longitudinal penoscrotal midline incision (90). The procedure can be performed under spinal, general, or (in an appropriately compliant and tolerant patient) local anesthesia. Increasingly, surgeons are offering to perform insertion on an outpatient basis if the patient's general medical condition permits, although many patients are hospitalized for 24 to 48 hours. Most men are reasonably comfortable and able to return to work by 7 to 10 days after surgery. Intercourse is delayed until 6 weeks postoperatively to allow reasonably secure healing, particularly of the corporotomy incisions.

Results of penile prosthesis insertion, in terms of satisfactory surgical result, adequate simulation of erection, and patient and partner satisfaction with subsequent intercourse, are generally favorable (good to excellent) in 80–90% of patients, with all models of prosthesis (91,92). Unfavorable results can be attributed to improper sizing of the prosthesis (which may lead to persistent discomfort if either too long or too short), difficulty with concealment of the noninflatable types, or difficulty with hydraulic manipulation of the inflatable types. Mechanical failure of the noninflatable types is extremely rare (although cases of cable fatigue have been noted with the OmniPhase and DuraPhase models). Mechanical failure of the inflatable models is a real concern, primarily due to kinking in connecting tubing, fluid leak from points of tubing connection, or development of fibrous capsule around the fluid reservoir, which can prevent complete deflation of the prosthesis. Mechanical failures requiring revision may develop in 10–20% of inflatable prostheses over 5–10 years of follow-up.

Certain risks of complications are inherent in penile prosthesis insertion, regardless of design. The gravest risk is that of infection. Infection that develops in the penile prosthesis is potentially disastrous, as fulminant sepsis can develop if adequate treatment is delayed. Infection of the prosthesis almost invariably requires removal of the prosthesis, and drainage of the penile corpora. After removal of the prosthesis, the native erectile tissue has been destroyed, so there is no prospect for return of spontaneous erections. A period of healing (usually at least 3 months) is necessary before reinsertion of the prosthesis can be contemplated. At that point, severe corporal fibrosis may have developed which can make redilation of the corpora and reinsertion of the prosthesis impossible.

Prevention of prosthetic infection is of paramount importance. At the time of surgery, this requires scrupulous attention to sterile surgical technique, careful inspection of the scrotal skin and surgical site preoperatively to ensure there are no evident abrasions or potentially infected skin lesions, and refusal to combine penile prosthesis insertion with any other potentially contaminated surgical procedure (such as cystoscopy or urologic instrumentation). Perioperative prophylactic antibiotics are routinely used, including coverage for *Staphylococcus epidermidis*. Some surgeons now perform prosthesis insertion in a sterile filtered-air environment to minimize potential for intraoperative contamination (93). After a penile prosthesis is inserted (just as a prosthetic vascular graft), the patient is advised to take antibiotic prophylaxis (typically employing a cephalosporin, or combination of ampicillin and an aminoglycoside) for any future procedures that may carry a risk of bacteremia, including dental cleaning, cystoscopy, sigmoidoscopy, or gastrointestinal surgery.

Preoperative counseling about the nature and implications of penile prosthesis surgery is critical to the patient's ultimate satisfaction with the result (94). Ideally this counseling will involve both the patient and his partner. The tendency of many patients (and couples) is to view the penile prosthesis as a "quick fix" for full restoration of youthful potency and vigor. It is important that the couple develop an appreciation of the irreversibility of the step to reliance on prosthesis for erection. They must also understand that the prosthesis carries with it a *lifelong* risk of potentially life-threatening infection, which must be matched by a lifelong commitment to necessary self-protection with antibiotic prophylaxis. The patient can expect to feel "different" because of the foreign presence of the prosthesis in the penis, and many men complain of a sense of penile or perineal "heaviness" from the prosthesis, which may take several months to get used to, even when the acute postoperative discomfort has resolved. The partner also will likely notice that the penis with prosthesis feels stiffer and somehow "artificial," compared with past experience. If impotence has caused a suspension in sexual activity for months or years, the couple needs to be especially gentle when first reexploring intercourse, and extra lubrication is often helpful. Penile sensation and ability to reach orgasm should not be affected—positively or negatively—with the prosthesis in place (95).

The chief effect of the prosthesis is to provide rigidity, which can make penetration possible; neither penile length nor girth necessarily matches the remembered dimensions of youth. The length of the penis is certainly *not* augmented. Some urologists provide a written enumeration of these specific expectations for the patient to review (and sign) as part of the documentation of informed consent for surgery. After explicitly reviewing these caveats, the surgeon and the couple can decide on the particular model of prosthesis with which they are most comfortable, and can face the impending surgery with expectations for reasonably reliable and satisfying results.

Retrograde Ejaculation

Retrograde ejaculation is a condition in which the normal ejaculation of semen via the penile urethra is impaired or absent. Normal antegrade ejaculation is the result of the contraction of the bulbourethralis muscles, which forcibly contract upon the prostatic and bulbar urethra while the bladder neck is simultaneously closed. Retrograde ejaculation can be the result of a lack of coordination of these two processes, with the result that seminal fluid is projected into the bladder instead of out the penis. The process of seminal emission and ejaculation is under completely separate neural control from the process of penile erection. Thus, retrograde ejaculation does not signify impotence, and some impotent patients retain normal orgasm and ejaculation. The semen analysis in cases of retrograde ejaculation is marked by a very low ejaculate volume (less than 1 ml). In addition, urine obtained after ejaculation reveals multiple motile spermatozoa.

In diabetic men, retrograde ejaculation is most often caused by autonomic neuropathy. There has been some effort to improve ejaculatory performance by administrating alpha-adrenergic agonists (such as ephedrine sulfate, 60 mg, or phenylpropanolamine, 25–75 mg), given 1 hour before intercourse (96). These drugs tend to increase sympathetic tone and contract the bladder neck. Patients in whom antegrade ejaculation fails to develop may have successful fertilization if the postmasturbatory urine, previously alkalinized by oral bicarbonate, can be obtained and the sperm concentrated by gentle centrifugation of the urine. This specimen then is used for artificial insemination (97). Electrical stimulation of ejaculation has also been reported with some fertilizing success, with similar recovery of sperm from the bladder for processing and insemination (98).

Female Sexual Dysfunction

The phenomenon of female sexual dysfunction has only recently begun to be clinically appreciated (99). This phenomenon is much less amenable to external observation than the male erectile process. Our understanding of the normal physiological processes involved, and their pathological alterations in diabetes, has been correspondingly slow to emerge. It has been possible, however, for several areas of sexual dysfunction to be identified in diabetic women (100).

A difficulty that is also analogous to male impotence is the failure of vasocongestion and muscular relaxation of the vaginal walls, which produces normal congestion and lubrication with sexual excitement. A significant percentage of diabetic women are found to have this difficulty with normal vaginal arousal, which in turn makes coitus significantly uncomfortable, if not impossible. Diabetic women with sensory neuropathy may progress through normal vaginal congestion/lubrication, yet have difficulty responding to labial and clitoral stimulation, and thus have significant obstacles to reaching orgasm. In addition, diabetic women are predisposed to vaginal candidiasis, which can produce discomfort with vaginal manipulation and present a further obstacle to full sexual response. Monilial vaginal infection can at least be objectively diagnosed and treated. Other conditions of female sexual dysfunction are not yet amenable to diagnostic evaluation in the way that impotence is, nor is effective therapy yet available for female vascular insufficiency or neuropathy. It may be hoped, by analogy with the male situation, that efforts at optimized glycemic control may be associated with minimized vascular complications and preservation of normal functioning, but there is as yet no evidence of this effect.

The urologist may not yet have surgical intervention available to assist the diabetic woman with sexual dysfunction, but he may provide a significant service to the couple in an educational and counseling role. It is important for the patient and her partner to recognize that problems with sexual satisfaction in this setting may well have a physical basis. Without this realization, psychological tensions can develop within the relationship, revolving around the partner's "failure to satisfy," with progressive performance anxiety, hostility, and resentment on both sides (100).

REFERENCES

1. Ouellet LM, Brook MP. Emphysematous pyelonephritis: an emergency indication for the plain abdominal radiograph. *Ann Emerg Med* 1988;17:722–724.
2. Pfeffer D, Stein BS. The diagnosis and treatment of emphysematous pyelonephritis. *Infect Urol* 1988;1:97–99.
3. Hudson MA, Weyman PJ, van der Vliet H, Catalona WJ. Emphysematous pyelonephritis: successful management by percutaneous drainage. *J Urol* 1986;136:884–886.
4. Malek RS, Elder JS. Xanthogranulomatous pyelonephritis: a critical analysis of 26 cases and of the literature. *J Urol* 1978;119:589–593.
5. Elder JS, Marshall FF. Focal xanthogranulomatous pyelonephritis in adulthood. *Johns Hopkins Med J* 1980;146:141–147.
6. Lurie DK, Plzak L, Deveney CW. Management of intraabdominal abscesses. *Infect Surg* 1988;(Aug):477–496.
7. Groop L, Laasonen L, Edgren J. Renal papillary necrosis in patients with IDDM. *Diabetes Care* 1989;12:198–202.
8. Dowd JB, Gregoriades C. Surgical management of renal papillary necrosis. In: Kaufmann JJ, ed. *Current urologic therapy,* 2nd ed. Philadelphia: W.B. Saunders, 1986;54–56.
9. Wise GJ, Goldberg P, Kozinn PJ. Genitourinary candidiasis: diagnosis and treatment. *J Urol* 1976;116:778–780.
10. Michigan S. Genitourinary fungal infections. (Review). *J Urol* 1976;116:390–397.
11. Galloway NTM. Classification and diagnosis of neurogenic bladder dysfunction. *Probl Urol* 1989;3:1–22.
12. McGuire EJ, Woodside JR, Borden TA, Weiss RM. Prognostic value of urodynamic testing in myelodysplastic patients. *J Urol* 1981;126:205–209.
13. Herschorn S. The management of neurogenic bladder dysfunction: emphasis on pharmacologic manipulation and intermittent catheterization. *Probl Urol* 1989;3:23–39.
14. Sonda LP, Gershon C, Diokno A, Lapides J. Further observations on the cystometric and uroflowmetric effects of bethanechol chloride on the human bladder. *J Urol* 1979;122:775–777.
15. Guttman L, Frankel H. The value of intermittent catheterization in the early management of paraplegia and tetraplegia. *Paraplegia* 1966;4:63.
16. Lapides J, Diokno AC, Silber SJ, Lowe BS. Clean, intermittent self-catheterization in the treatment of urinary tract disease. *J Urol* 1972;107:458–461.

17. Sawers JS, Todd WA, Kellett HA, et al. Bacteriuria and autonomic nerve function in diabetic women. *Diabetes Care* 1986;9:460–464.
18. Keane EM, Boyko EJ, Reller LB, Hamman RF. Prevalence of asymptomatic bacteriuria in subjects with NIDDM in San Luis Valley of Colorado. *Diabetes Care* 1988;11:708–712.
19. Nielsen KT, Christensen MM, Madsen PO. Risk factors for urinary tract infections. *Infect Urol* 1989;2:67–71.
20. Roberts JA. Pathophysiology of pyelonephritis. *Infect Urol* 1988;1:33–38.
21. U.S. Congress, Office of Technology Assessment. *Cancer testing technology and saccharin.* Washington, DC: U.S. Government Printing Office, 1977.
22. Kessler II. Cancer mortality among diabetics. *J Natl Cancer Inst* 1970;44:673–686.
23. Risch HA, Burch JD, Miller AB, Hill GB, Steele R, Howe GR. Dietary factors and the incidence of cancer of the urinary bladder. *Am J Epidemiol* 1988;127:1179–1191.
24. Morrison AS. Advances in the etiology of urothelial cancer. *Urol Clin North Am* 1984;11:557–566.
25. McCulloch DK, Campbell IW, Wu FC, Prescott RJ, Clarke BF. The prevalence of diabetic impotence. *Diabetologia* 1980;18:279–283.
26. Kaiser FE, Korenman SG. Impotence in diabetic men. *Am J Med* 1988;85(suppl 5A):147–152.
27. Montague DK, James RE, DeWolfe VG, Martin LM. Diagnostic evaluation, classification, and treatment of men with sexual dysfunction. *Urology* 1979;14:545–548.
28. Deutsch S, Sherman L. Previously unrecognized diabetes mellitus in sexually impotent men. *JAMA* 1980;244:2430–2432.
29. Baum N, Neiman M, Lewis R. Evaluation and treatment of organic impotence in the male with diabetes mellitus. *Diabetes Educ* 1988;14:123–129.
30. Melman A, Tiefer L, Pedersen R. Evaluation of first 406 patients in urology department based center for male sexual dysfunction. *Urology* 1988;32:6–10.
31. Lue TF, Tanagho E. Physiology of erection and pharmacological management of impotence. *J Urol* 1987;137:829–836.
32. Saenz de Tejada I, Goldstein I, Krane RJ. Local control of penile erection; nerves, smooth muscle, and endothelium. *Urol Clin North Am* 1988;15:9–15.
33. Fournier GR, Lue TF. Vasculogenic impotence: physiology, diagnosis, and treatment. *Monogr Urol* 1988;9:20–31.
34. Wagner G, Gerstenberg T, Levin RJ. Electrical activity of corpus cavernosum during flaccidity and erection of the human penis: a new diagnostic method? *J Urol* 1989;142:723–725.
35. Bosch R, Berard F, Aboseif S, Lue T, Tanagho E. The phases of detumescence: correlation with hemodynamic events. *J Urol* 1989;141 (part 2:187A).
36. Fowler CJ, Ali Z, Kirby RS, Pryor JP. The value of testing for unmyelinated fibre, sensory neuropathy in diabetic impotence. *Br J Urol* 1988;61:63–67.
37. Parys BT, Evans CM, Parsons KF. Bulbocavernosus reflex latency in the investigation of diabetic impotence. *Br J Urol* 1988;61:59–62.
38. Saenz de Tejada I, Goldstein I. Diabetic penile neuropathy. *Urol Clin North Am* 1988;15:17–22.
39. Levy DM, Karanth SS, Springall DR, Polak JM. Depletion of cutaneous nerves and neuropeptides in diabetes mellitus: an immunocytochemical study. *Diabetologia* 1989;32:427–433.
40. Comer A, Patrick AW, Bell D, et al. Relationship of skin thickness to duration of diabetes, glycemic control, and diabetic complications in male IDDM patients. *Diabetes Care* 1989;12:309–312.
41. Ellenberg M. Impotence in diabetes: the neurologic factor. *Ann Intern Med* 1971;75:213–219.
42. Faerman I, Glocer L, Fox D, Jadzinsky MN, Rapaport M. Impotence and diabetes; histological studies of the autonomic nervous fibers of the corpora cavernosa in impotent diabetic males. *Diabetes* 1974;23:971–976.
43. Lincoln J, Crowe R, Blacklay PF, Pryor JP, Lumley JSP, Burnstock G. Changes in the vipergic, cholinergic and adrenergic innervation of human penile tissue in diabetic and non-diabetic impotent males. *J Urol* 1987;137:1053–1059.
44. Buvat J, Lemaire A, Buvat-Herbaut M, Guieu JD, Bailleul JP, Fossati P. Comparative investigations in 26 impotent and 26 nonimpotent diabetic patients. *J Urol* 1985;133:34–38.
45. Virag R, Bouilly P, Frydman L. Is impotence an arterial disorder? *Lancet* 1985;2:181–184.
46. Saenz de Tejada I, Goldstein I, Azadzoi K, Krane RJ, Cohen RA. Impaired neurogenic and endothelium-mediated relaxation of penile smooth muscle from diabetic men with impotence. *N Engl J Med* 1989;320:1025–1030.
47. Schöffling K, Federlin K, Ditschuneit H, Pfeiffer EF. Disorders of sexual function in male diabetics. *Diabetes* 1963;12:519–527.
48. Murray FT, Wyss HU, Thomas RG, Spevack M, Glaros AG. Gonadal dysfunction in diabetic men with organic impotence. *J Clin Endocrinol Metab* 1987;65:127–135.
49. Anderson JE, Jones D, Penner SB, Thliveris JA. Primary hypoandrogenism in experimental diabetes in the Long-Evans rat. *Diabetes* 1987;36:1104–1110.

50. Mooradian AD, Morley JE, Billington CJ, et al. Hyperprolactinemia in male diabetics. *Postgrad Med J* 1985;61:11–14.
51. Martin LM. Impotence in diabetes: an overview. *Psychosomatics* 1981;22:318–329.
52. Morley JE. Impotence in older men. *Hosp Pract* 1988;(Apr 15):139–158.
53. Kessler WO. Nocturnal penile tumescence. *Urol Clin North Am* 1988;15:81–86.
54. Maatman TJ, Montague DK. Routine endocrine screening in impotence. *Urology* 1986;27:499–502.
55. Baskin HJ. Endocrinologic evaluation of impotence. *South Med J* 1989;82:446–449.
56. Palmer JDK, Fink S, Burger RH. Diabetic secondary impotence: neuropathic factor as measured by peripheral motor nerve conduction. *Urology* 1986;28:197–200.
57. Lin JT, Bradley WE. Penile neuropathy in insulin-dependent diabetes mellitus. *J Urol* 1985;133:213–215.
58. Robinson LQ, Woodcock JP, Stephenson TP. Results of investigation of impotence in patients with overt or probable neuropathy. *Br J Urol* 1987;60:583–587.
59. Kaneko S, Bradley WE. Penile electrodiagnosis. Value of bulbocavernosus reflex latency versus nerve conduction velocity of the dorsal nerve of the penis in diagnosis of diabetic impotence. *J Urol* 1987;137:933–935.
60. Barron SA, Mazliah J, Hoch Z, Bental E. A non-invasive electrophysiological indicator of organic impotence in diabetic men. *Electromyogr Clin Neurophysiol* 1988;39–43.
61. Daniels JS. Abnormal nerve conduction in impotent patients with diabetes mellitus. *Diabetes Care* 1989;12:449–454.
62. Desai KM, Dembny K, Morgan H, Gingell JC, Prothero D. Neurophysiological investigation of diabetic impotence. Are sacral response studies of value? *Br J Urol* 1988;61:68–73.
63. Parkhouse N, LeQuesne PM. Impaired neurogenic vascular response in patients with diabetes and neuropathic foot lesions. *N Engl J Med* 1988;318:1306–1309.
64. Ajjam ZS, Barton S, Corbett M, Owens D, Marks R. Quantitative evaluation of the dermal vasculature of diabetics. *Q J Med* 1985;215:229–239.
65. Virag R, Frydman D, Legman M, Virag H. Intracavernous injection of papaverine as a diagnostic and therapeutic method in erective failure. *Angiology* 1985;35:79–87.
66. Lue TF. A simple office penodynamic test. *J Urol* 1989;141(part 2:288A).
67. Zentgraf M, Baccouche M, Junemann K-P. Diagnosis and therapy of erectile dysfunction using papaverine and phentolamine. *Urol Int* 1988;43:65–75.
68. Glina S, Reichelt AC, Leao PP, Dos Reis JMSM. Impact of cigarette smoking on papaverine-induced erection. *J Urol* 1988;140:523–524.
69. Robinson LQ, Woodcock JP, Stephenson TP. Duplex scanning in suspected vasculogenic impotence: a worthwhile exercise? *Br J Urol* 1989;63:432–436.
70. Morley JE, Korenman SG, Kaiser FE, Mooradian AD, Viosca SP. Relationship of penile brachial pressure index to myocardial infarction and cerebrovascular accidents in older men. *Am J Med* 1988;84:445–448.
71. Bookstein JJ. Penile angiography: the last angiographic frontier. *AJR* 1988;150:47–54.
72. Malhotra CM, Balko A, Wincze JP, Bansal S, Susset JG. Cavernosography in conjunction with artificial erection for evaluation of venous leakage in impotent men. *Radiology* 1986;161:799–802.
73. Bookstein JJ. Cavernosal venocclusive insufficiency in male impotence: evaluation of degree and location. *Radiology* 1987;164:175–178.
74. Puyau FA, Lewis RW, Balkin P, Kaack MB, Hirsch A. Dynamic corpus cavernosography: effect of papaverine injection. *Radiology* 1987;164:179–182.
75. Bernstein G. Counseling the male diabetic patient with erectile dysfunction. *Med Asp Hum Sex* 1989;23(Apr):20–23.
76. Elist J, Jarman WD, Edson M. Evaluating medical treatment of impotence. *Urology* 1984;23:374–375.
77. Reid K, Morales A, Harris C, et al. Double-blind trial of yohimbine in treatment of psychogenic impotence. *Lancet* 1987;2:421–423.
78. Susset JG, Tessier CD, Wincze J, Bansal S, Malhotra C, Schwacha MG. Effect of yohimbine hydrochloride on erectile impotence: a double-blind study. *J Urol* 1989;141:1360–1363.
79. Orvis BR, Breza J, Aboseif SR, Lue TF. The effect of yohimbine on penile erection. *J Urol* 1988;139, (part 2:256A).
80. Nelson RP. Nonoperative management of impotence. *J Urol* 1988;139:2–5.
81. Wiles PG. Successful non-invasive management of erectile impotence in diabetic men. *Br Med J* 1988;296:161–162.
82. Glugla M, Draznin B. Treatment of impotence with vacuum-operated erection assistance device (letter). *Diabetes Care* 1988;11:445–446.
83. Asopa R, Williams G. Use of the "Correctaid" device in the management of impotence. *Br J Urol* 1989;63:546–547.

84. Zorgniotti AW, Lefleur RS. Auto-injection of the corpus cavernosum with a vasoactive drug combination for vasculogenic impotence. *J Urol* 1985;133:39–41.

85. Williams G, Mulcahy MJ, Kiely EA. Impotence: treatment by autoinjection of vasoactive drugs. *Br Med J* 1987;295:595–596.

86. Aboseif SR, Breza J, Bosch RJLH, et al. Local and systemic effects of chronic intracavernous injection of papaverine, prostaglandin E1, and saline in primates. *J Urol* 1989;142:403–408.

87. Baum N. Treatment of impotence; 1. Nonsurgical methods. *Postgrad Med* 1987;81(7):133–136.

88. Lue TF. Penile venous surgery. *Urol Clin North Am* 1989;16:607–611.

89. Goldstein I. Penile revascularization. *Urol Clin North Am* 1987;14:805–813.

90. Kabalin JN, Kessler R. Penile prosthesis surgery. *Monogr Urol* 1989;10:21–32.

91. Beaser RS, Van der Hoek C, Jacobson AM, Flood TM, Desautels RE. Experience with penile prostheses in the treatment of impotence in diabetic men. *JAMA* 1982;248:943–948.

92. Whitehead ED. Diabetes-related impotence and its treatment in the middle-aged and elderly: Part II. *Geriatrics* 1987;42(Aug):77–85.

93. Fishman IJ. Complicated implantations of inflatable penile prostheses. *Urol Clin North Am* 1987;14:217–239.

94. Krauss DJ, Bogin D, Culebras A. The failed penile prosthetic implantation despite technical success. *J Urol* 1983;129:969–971.

95. Mobley DF. When a patient requests a penile prosthesis. *Med Asp Hum Sex* 1987;21(May):30–36.

96. Davis RS, Cockett ATK. Retrograde ejaculation. In: Garcia C-R, Mastroianni MD Jr, Amelar RD, Dubin L, eds. *Current therapy of infertility—3*. Toronto: B.C. Decker, 1988;247–248.

97. Lipshultz LI. Subfertility. In: Kaufman JJ, ed. *Current urologic therapy,* 2nd ed. Philadelphia: W.B. Saunders, 1986;452–457.

98. Hellstrom WJG, Stone AR, Deitch AD, deVere White RW. The clinical application of aspiration deoxyribonucleic acid flow cytometry to neurologically impaired men entering an electroejaculation program. *J Urol* 1989;142:309–312.

99. Hollander P. The need to address sexual dysfunction in diabetes. *Postgrad Med* 1986;79:15–18.

100. Kolodny RC, Masters WH, Johnson VE. Sexual dysfunction in diabetic women. In: *Textbook of sexual medicine*. Boston: Little Brown, 1979;136–142.

Surgical Management of the Diabetic Patient,
edited by Michael Bergman and Gregorio A. Sicard.
Raven Press, Ltd., New York © 1991.

25

Renal Transplantation in the Diabetic Patient

M. Wayne Flye

Division of Surgery, Microbiology, and Immunology, Department of Surgery,
Washington University Medical Center,
St. Louis, Missouri 63110

DEVELOPMENT OF RENAL TRANSPLANTATION

In 1902 Ullmann of Vienna performed the first kidney transplants into the necks of dogs (using magnesium tubes as stents for the vascular connections); the organs functioned for several days (1). The kidneys quickly succumbed to what was later shown to be rejection. Between 1904 and 1910, the French surgeon Alexis Carrel and his American associate Charles Guthrie performed a series of experiments, first at the University of Chicago and subsequently at Rockefeller University, that focused attention on the therapeutic possibilities of renal transplantation (2). While laying the foundation for modern blood vessel surgery, they successfully transplanted kidneys, hearts, and other organs into animals. Carrel noted, however, that after a short period the organ failed to function and that "the physiological disturbance could not be considered as brought about by the surgical factors, but rather because of the influence of the host, that is, the biological factors" (3). His technique for vascular anastomosis is still used today. In addition, he experimented with hypothermic preservation and the immune response. He insisted on strict asepsis, noting that most of his dogs died of infection. By 1914, Carrel wrote:

> the surgical side of the transplantation of organs is now complete because we are able to perform transplantation of organs with perfect ease and excellent results from an anatomical standpoint, but as yet these methods cannot be applied to human surgery for the reason that homoplastic transplantations are almost always unsuccessful from the standpoint of the functioning of the organs. All of our efforts must now be directed toward the biologic methods which will prevent the reaction of the organisms against foreign tissue and allowing the adapting of homoplastic grafts to their hosts (4).

Jaboulay transplanted the kidneys from a pig and a goat to the limbs of humans with chronic renal failure in 1906 and each functioned for one hour. These were the first recorded human transplants, although Ullmann reported in 1914 that he had performed similar transplants in 1902 (5). In 1909, after performing more than 100 kidney transplants in dogs, Ernest Unger transplanted a kidney from a human stillborn baby into a baboon. The kidney never functioned. Similarly, the transplantation of an ape's kidney into a young girl dying of renal failure was not successful. Unger, therefore, concluded that there was a biochemical barrier to transplantation. For the next several decades only sporadic attempts were made at either experimental or clinical transplantation, with minimal success.

In 1946 the Peter Bent Brigham Hospital initiated its major interest in transplantation when Hufnagel, Hume and Landsteiner transplanted a cadaveric kidney into a young woman dying of acute renal failure. Because she was believed to be too sick to move to the operating room, the kidney was anastomosed to her brachial vessels on the ward. It immediately produced urine and the patient improved. Although the graft had to be removed after 48 hours, the patient entered the diuretic phase and did well (6). The first transplant from a living relative was performed in 1953 when a mother donated a kidney to her son, whose solitary kidney was damaged in a road accident. This kidney functioned for nearly one month without immunosuppression before being rejected. Although clinical renal transplantation was introduced at the Peter Bent Brigham Hospital by Hume and associates in 1951 (7), during the next 7 years functioning allografts were achieved in patients with renal failure only when the recipient fortuitously had an identical twin donor (8).

The first kidney transplant between identical twins was performed on December 23, 1954, at the Peter Bent Brigham Hospital; the transplanted kidney functioned well and the patient's condition improved. In contrast to the 13 previous human homotransplants, in which the kidneys were anastomosed to the femoral vessels, the kidney was electively placed in the pelvis and the ureter was directly implanted in the bladder. Previous transplants had used a cutaneous ureterostomy with resulting infection and hydronephrosis. From 1958 through 1962, sporadic efforts at total body irradiation by Murray in Boston and Hamburger in Paris provided little success in patients receiving nonidentical twin kidneys and often led to the death of the recipient from over immunosuppression and resulting infection. The concurrent development of dialysis soon encouraged more extensive trials of transplantation. The major breakthrough in human renal transplantation began with the introduction of azathioprine in 1962 (9). Azathioprine was soon combined with prednisone, and this combination became the foundation for clinical immunosuppressive therapy until the introduction of cyclosporin A (later cyclosporine) in 1980. From 1965 through 1980, a variety of adjunctive procedures were combined with azathioprine and prednisone in an effort to improve graft acceptance and diminish rejection. These measures included the administration of antilymphocyte or antithymocyte globulin, splenectomy, thoracic duct drainage, and the use of radiation therapy to the renal allograft during acute rejection. Although surgical techniques developed and expertise increased in immune modulation (especially the appreciation of the morbidity and mortality of over immunosuppression), there was only modest improvement in allograft survival from these adjunctive techniques.

After Jean Borel appreciated the potency of cyclosporin A in the mid-1970s, clinical trials began in the United States, in the United Kingdom, and in Europe in 1979. It immediately became apparent that this was a powerful immunosuppressive agent. The initial combination of cyclosporin A (cyclosporine) with low-dose prednisone (10), and the subsequent addition of azathioprine for triple drug therapy (11), has provided an exceptionally effective immunosuppressive regimen in terms of both patient and graft survival and fewer infectious complications. Preliminary observations with the new immunosuppressant, FK506, indicate that it is more potent than cyclosporine and has less nephrotoxicity (12).

Before the advent of cyclosporine, one of the most effective methods of immunosuppression was the use of blood transfusions—both donor-specific (i.e., from the renal donor) in patients receiving kidneys from living relatives, and from random donors for cadaveric kidney recipients. The one-year survival results for one haplotype-identical donor allografts from a living relative improved from 65 to nearly 90% (13), whereas the 1-year survival results with random blood transfusions for cadaveric recipients improved approximately 20%. The explanation for the effectiveness of donor-specific blood transfusions remains uncertain but possibly involves formation of antiidiotypic antibodies that may act in tandem with immunosuppressive therapy to modify the immune response and allow long-term graft survival (14).

Transplantation (using living relatives or cadaveric donors) is one of the treatment options for chronic renal failure. Others include hemodialysis (home or in-center), peritoneal dialysis, continuous ambulatory peritoneal dialysis (CAPD), or continuous cyclic peritoneal dialysis (CCPD). When risk factors are controlled, there is little difference in short-term (less than 5 years) patient survival for these different modes of treatment (15); however, there is significant improvement in long-term survival in patients treated by transplantation compared with those treated with dialysis (Fig. 1) (16). In addition, the quality of life and degree of rehabilitation achieved in patients treated with transplantation are clearly superior when compared with those patients maintained on dialysis (17). Seventy-nine percent of all transplant recipients functioned at nearly normal levels, compared with 47 and 59% of those patients treated

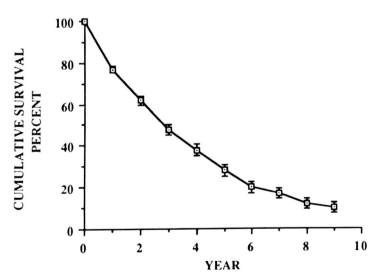

FIG. 1. Cumulative survival curve and 95% confidence intervals for 720 patients with diabetes mellitus started on chronic dialysis between 1966 and 1986. The mean age for these patients was 52 years, and there were 1.5 mean comorbid conditions per patient at the start of dialysis. Approximately 50% of the patients survived 3 years and 10% of the patients were alive 9 years after beginning dialysis. Although not shown, there is no difference in patients with diabetes mellitus types I and II, although the type I patients are younger and have fewer comorbid conditions. This is in part due to the fact that the younger, healthier type I patients more quickly received a renal transplant (From Jacobson SH et al., ref. 27.)

with CAPD or hemodialysis, respectively. The cost of renal transplantation is approximately $36,000 for the first year and, if successful, about $4,000/year thereafter (18). The introduction of cyclosporine has already reduced the length of hospitalization of transplant recipients by about 50%, and it is estimated that total costs will be similarly decreased. This contrasts with the cost of hemodialysis at well over $20,000/year for life. Rehabilitation and the return to work of the transplant recipient not only provides savings in dialysis expenses and welfare payments but also benefits the patients' families. Therefore, there is a medical consensus that kidney transplantation is the treatment of choice for most patients with end-stage renal failure (19). Approximately 8,500 transplants are performed annually in North America.

Treatment of Chronic Renal Failure Due to Diabetes Mellitus

The incidence of end-stage renal failure (ESRD) in North America is approximately 60 individuals/million population (20). In the adult population, transplantation is most often performed for chronic glomerulonephritis, chronic pyelonephritis, or diabetic nephropathy.

Diabetes Mellitus

Chronic renal failure (CRF) develops in approximately one-half of all type I and an undefined but lesser proportion of type II diabetic patients. Diabetic patients constitute about one-fourth of end-stage renal disease patients in the United States, and a lesser but steadily increasing proportion in Europe. In general it has been found that diabetic patients suffer inordinately high morbidity and mortality compared to nondiabetic CRF patients. The costs in human terms are enormous and are reflected in dollar expense as well.

The treatment of ESRD in the United States presently costs over $2.5 billion annually. Because diabetes mellitus represents the primary diagnosis for nearly one-fourth of all patients with ESRD, the care of these patients represents a significant cost. A recent review of 244 patients with diabetes in the Michigan Kidney Registry showed that the average annual charges for ESRD treatment for diabetic patients was $29,671, which were $4,695 higher than charges for nondiabetic patients. The difference for dialysis was $12,437, whereas it was only $4,998 for those treated with transplantation. Of the total difference in charges for diabetic and nondiabetic patients, the majority (84.3%) could be explained by differences in charges for physician services and medical supplies (21). There was only a very small difference in charges for outpatient services.

Diabetic nephropathy develops over approximately a 20-year time scale and is histologically in evidence very early in the disease process (22). Attention to these major areas may optimize survival and rehabilitation, however. Hypertension has long been recognized as a major risk factor for arteriosclerotic complications in both those who are diabetic and those who are not (23). Effective control of hypertension clearly slows the decline of renal function in diabetic nephropathy (24).

Available evidence indicates that the detection of small but abnormal amounts of albumin in the urine enables the prediction of which diabetic patients are at risk for the development of clinical nephropathy both in type I and type II diabetes. The average duration of diabetes before the onset of proteinuria in type I diabetes is 17.3

years, and the time from onset of proteinuria to renal failure is 4.0 years (25). Control of hypertension can often result in reduction of microalbuminuria to normal levels (24).

Regimens of multiple-dose insulin guided by frequent finger-stick blood glucose level determinations have enabled diabetic patients to approach the ideal of 24-hour euglycemia. Maintenance of near-euglycemia can normalize virtually every aspect of abnormal metabolism in these patients. To date, the studies of the influence of glycemic control on the progression of diabetic glomerulosclerosis have produced both positive and negative results (26).

MANAGEMENT OF THE UREMIC DIABETIC

The diabetic patient who reaches the late stages of chronic renal insufficiency is clearly at greater risk for morbidity and death from nonrenal systemic manifestations. In particular, retinopathy with blindness (17%), neuropathy (49%), occlusive coronary artery disease (21%), cardiovascular and peripheral vascular disease (26%) pose major problems (27). Their magnitude is manifested in reports of higher mortality for uremic diabetic patients, whether treated with hemodialysis or renal transplantation, compared with nondiabetic patients.

Only a decade ago it was rare for diabetic patients with ESRD, unlike patients with other causes for renal failure, to be accepted for renal replacement therapy. Recently the attitude toward the treatment of terminal diabetic nephropathy has changed considerably, however. Patients with ESRD from diabetes mellitus can now choose among these successful treatments: hemodialysis, continuous ambulatory peritoneal dialysis (CAPD), or renal transplantation. Diabetic renal failure usually occurs in the age groups favored for acceptance for dialysis, the young and middle-aged. Diabetic patients thus make up a large and growing patient population on dialysis.

Hemodialysis

Although Kolff and Berk demonstrated the technical feasibility of hemodialysis in 1943 using glass or metal tubes for intermittent cannulation of arteries and veins, this method required the ligation of the vessels after each use (27). A major improvement occurred when Quinton and associates (28) utilized rigid polytetrafluoroethylene tubing as the conduit material. Thrombosis and infection continued to occur, however. The problem of an external shunt was largely alleviated in 1966 when Brescia and colleagues (29) developed a side-to-side arteriovenous (AV) fistula by anastomosing the radial artery to the cephalic vein in the wrist, resulting in high blood flow in the superficial venous system of the forearm, which could be repeatedly punctured. Although this is considered the best method of creating venous access, there are patients who have an inadequate radial artery or cephalic vein. Inadequate vessels are a greater problem for the diabetic patient than for other ESRD groups. Consequently, a subcutaneous autogenous loop of saphenous vein or bovine heterograft was placed between the brachial artery and a vein in the forearm (30). Currently, an artificial graft material, polytetrafluoroethylene (PTFE), has become more widely used when a primary AV fistula cannot be created (31). This process requires ingenuity, because the interposed grafts usually fail after a period of time and must be revised, or a new access site must be created. The initial perferred sites are in the forearm, followed by upper arm access. The lower extremities are only used as a last resort.

Peritoneal Dialysis

An increasingly used mode of dialysis is via exchange across the peritoneal membrane. Although this method was successful as early as 1960, problems of fluid leakage and infection limited its usefulness. Introduction of a rigid catheter with a collar sewn to the subcutaneous tissue prevented leakage. Current catheters have polyester cuffs that prevent leakage and decrease infection when incorporated into the surrounding tissue. Peritoneal dialysis has now come to be widely used in both the acute and chronic setting. Short-term peritoneal dialysis is used for acute renal failure until recovery is complete or while a venous access site is maturing. CAPD is indicated for patients who desire home dialysis (although home hemodialysis is also possible); for patients with no available vascular access sites; for patients with repeated venous access site infections; for patients with an unstable cardiovascular system; for patients with bleeding problems, for example, peptic ulcer; for Jehovah's witnesses; for patients greater than 65 years of age; and for small children. This mode of dialysis is often more acceptable to patients than hemodialysis, which restricts activity more (32). After one year, 85% of catheters will still be functioning; this rate decreases to 50% at the end of 2 years. As new catheters are developed, their longevity rates may improve. In patients awaiting transplantation, the transplant operation must not coincide with a bout of peritonitis or infection at the catheter site.

Dialysis in the Diabetic

The early results of hemodialysis of diabetic patients were poor, but recently have improved dramatically. At the Hennepin County Medical Center, Minneapolis, Minnesota, between 1966 and 1986 there were no differences in survival for diabetic patients on hemodialysis or peritoneal dialysis. Thirty percent survived 5 years, and 10 percent survived 9 years on dialysis (Fig. 1). There was also no difference in survival between type I and type II diabetes mellitus in spite of the fact that type I patients were younger than type II patients (41 versus 64 years) and had fewer complications at the beginning of dialysis (1.2 versus 1.8 comorbid conditions). An explanation for the lack of survival difference for the type I and II patients is that young, healthy diabetic patients with fewer complications were selected for renal transplantation, thus skewing the type I patient toward poorer results (27). Particularly poor survival figures were noted in type I patients older than 60 years. These older patients now make up approximately one-half of all diabetic patients accepted for dialysis, and have a mortality rate three times that of younger patients. The results of dialysis are improving even though these patients have an increasing number of comorbid conditions thought to mitigate against successful long-term outcome. Even though the number of comorbid conditions has increased from 0.8 to 1.1 per patient from 1966 to 1986, the 5-year survival for patients <61 years has improved from 10 to 45% (Fig. 2). If these factors are controlled, much of the difference in survival between transplantation and dialysis disappears.

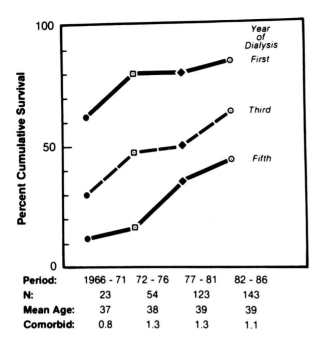

Period:

	1966 - 71	72 - 76	77 - 81	82 - 86
N:	23	54	123	143
Mean Age:	37	38	39	39
Comorbid:	0.8	1.3	1.3	1.1

FIG. 2. Improvement in cumulative survival rates occurring in young (<61 years) patients with type I diabetes mellitus started on chronic dialysis at different time periods. It is obvious that there has been a remarkable improvement with an increase in 1-year survival rates from 60 to 85% (From Jacobson SL et al., ref. 27.)

The most common cause of death in dialyzed diabetic patients is cardiovascular disease, causing 51% of deaths. On the other hand, most of the patients without preexisting vascular disease at the beginning of dialysis die of infections, 14% of total deaths. One-fourth die because of the decision to terminate dialysis: It is 4–10 times more common for diabetic patients than nondiabetic patients <60 years of age to die because dialysis is discontinued (33).

THE TRANSPLANTATION PROCEDURE

Selection and Preparation of the Renal Recipient

With improving results and the increasing safety of transplantation, there has been a gradual relaxation in the stringent recipient selection criteria, so now the majority of patients presenting with renal failure are considered suitable transplantation candidates (34).

The only absolute contraindications are active infection or malignant disease that cannot be adequately controlled; however, in the presence of severe malnutrition, incapacitating systemic disease, or severe cardiovascular disease, especially in the diabetic patient, transplantation must be approached with great care. There are also relative contraindications in patients in whom there exists a high probability of recurring disease in the newly transplanted kidney. These diseases include rapidly progressive glomerulonephritis with a high titer of antiglomerular basement membrane antibodies, oxalosis, sickle-cell disease, or an immunologic disease in the "active phase," for example lupus erythematosus or Wegener's granulomatosis.

Graft loss from recurrent diabetic nephropathy is a relatively rare occurrence with only two renal grafts being lost at 12.5 and 13.5 years post-transplant in 265 uremic type I diabetic recipients transplanted at the University of Minnesota from 1966 to 1978 (35). The incidence of diabetic nephropathy may increase with time, however, because serial renal allograft biopsies taken post-transplant have shown characteristic light and election microscopic diabetic changes. The rate of recurrence is highly variable, however, and did not correlate with the duration of prior diabetes, the donor source, age of the recipient or donor, degree of HLA disparity, or dose of immunosuppressive medications.

Pretransplantation Evaluation

Clinical assessment of the potential recipient may be performed on an outpatient or inpatient basis (36). The original renal disease must be clearly defined, and symptoms of cardiovascular disease, urinary tract infection, bladder dysfunction, or other systemic disease must be elicited. The major risk factors that have an impact on the recipient with or without transplantation include age and the presence of diabetes mellitus, arteriosclerotic cardiovascular disease, malignant disease, or chronic pulmonary disease. A careful physical examination should document coexisting cardiovascular, gastrointestinal or genitourinary disease, assess pulmonary reserve, define potential sources of infection, including dental caries, and assess the gynecologic risks for females. The laboratory evaluation should include routine hematologic assays to document leukopenia or thrombocytopenia, liver function tests to identify patients in whom the metabolism of cyclosporine may be abnormal, a hepatitis and HIV-III profile, viral titers, and throat and urine cultures.

A voiding cystourethrogram (VCUG) is performed in all patients to evaluate the urinary tract for evidence of outflow obstruction or vesicoureteral reflux. A normal VCUG demonstrates a functioning bladder with no abnormalities of the bladder wall, no ureteral reflux, an unobstructed urethra, and no residual urine volume after voiding. Full cystometric evaluation should be performed in patients with evidence of bladder dysfunction. This is especially important for the diabetic patient because bladder dystonia is a frequent problem. A contracted bladder can be expanded by hydrodilatation, and such a bladder generally enlarges satisfactorily following transplantation. Lower urinary tract obstruction (e.g., prostatic hypertrophy) should be corrected before transplantation. In a small proportion of patients with irreversible structural or neurogenic dysfunction, an ileal conduit should be fashioned prior to transplantation (20). In the occasional patient, the dysfunction of bladder may be managed by frequent catheterization after transplantation.

Bilateral nephrectomy is now performed infrequently and only for specific indications such as persistent upper urinary tract infection, uncontrollable renin dependent hypertension, polycystic kidneys with significant pain, persistent infection, bleeding or excessive kidney size, gross vesicoureteric reflux predisposing to infection, and Goodpasture's syndrome. Only rarely are there indications for native nephrotomy in the potential diabetic recipient. In many patients, this selective policy avoids the consequent severe fluid restriction, anemia with its increased risk of sensitization by repeated transfusion, hyperkalemia, and vitamin D deficiency. In the anephric state there is a direct relationship between the patient's plasma volume and blood pressure. When required, nephrectomy via a bilateral flank approach offers more rapid patient recovery and decreased operative morbidity than does a trans-peritoneal approach.

Patients with a history of gastroesophageal disease should undergo upper gastro-intestinal endoscopy to define the site and activity of an ulcer and to biopsy any gastric ulceration to exclude malignancy. Pretransplantation parietal cell vagotomy in patients with significant ulcer disease, along with appropriate medical therapy, has almost completely eliminated upper gastrointestinal bleeding as a complication of steroid use. Diabetic gastroparesis can become a significant problem in the im-mediate post-transplantation period. In patients with symptomatic cholelithiasis and probably in those with asymptomatic stones seen with ultrasonography, cholecys-tectomy should be performed before the transplantation procedure to eliminate the risk of cholecystitis and possible sepsis after transplantation. Patients with colonic disease, especially those with previous episodes of diverticulitis, should be evaluated with barium enema and colonoscopy, and, if appropriate, should be treated with surgical resection prior to transplantation. Patients with adequately treated primary tumors may be considered for transplantation after a tumor-free interval of 2 years, but metastatic disease or the continued presence of a primary tumor is an absolute contraindication to transplantation.

Because ESRD is associated with a high incidence of coronary artery disease (CAD), particularly in diabetic patients, screening for CAD is an important aspect of pretransplant evaluation. Even in those patients selected for transplantation, car-diovascular disease is the major source of postoperative mortality. Unfortunately, clinical assessment is unreliable with both false-positives and false-negatives (silent ischemia). Routine exercise tests have limited application because patients with ESRD frequently are unable to complete a maximal test due to anemia, debility, peripheral vascular disease, or peripheral neuropathy.

There are now several studies that examine the prognostic influence on survival of coronary artery stenosis diagnosed by angiogram. Fifty-seven of 170 patients (33%) reported had >50% stenosis of at least one coronary artery on coronary an-giogram (37). Because there is a high reported incidence of irreversible acute exac-erbation of severe chronic diabetic renal failure occurring after intravascular dye, it has been considered unethical to use the coronary angiogram to select patients one would not wish to have undergo dialysis. Although coronary artery bypass surgery may reduce the risk associated with transplantation, greater morbidity and mortality in the first 3 months after bypass are seen in these patients. These results, therefore, limit the usefulness of this procedure.

Patients may also be evaluated noninvasively by echocardiography, exercise ra-diotopic angiography, and stress thallium 201 scans (38). The dipyridamole single photon emission computed tomography (SPECT) thallium imaging has 67–95% sen-sitivity in detecting CAD in patients without renal disease (39). When used in a se-lected high-risk group of patients with ESRD, dipyridamole SPECT thallium imaging had poor sensitivity when compared with follow-up coronary angiography and clin-ical follow-up of 19 patients (42%) with an obstructon of >50% of at least one cor-onary artery. Fourteen had a positive thallium scan, but seven of these were false-positives (sensitivity 37%, specificity 73%) (40). Five of the six patients who died of cardiac causes over a mean follow-up period of 25 months had normal thallium im-aging but all had significant coronary disease at cardiac catheterization.

The predominant mechanism of action of dipyridamole is coronary vasodilation, which produces regional hyperemia in proportion to flow reserve of each coronary vessel. There are reasons to suspect that the most common course of a false-negative dipyridamole SPECT thallium imaging would be a reduced coronary hyperemic response. Because adenosine, which mediates the vasodilator effects of dipyridamole, is increased in patients with ESRD (41) this may produce a reduced vascular responsiveness to dipyridamole and the high false-negative rate. Therefore, dipyridamole SPECT thallium imaging is not a reliable nonevasive technique for screening for CAD in patients with ESRD (40).

Immunologic Assessment

The recipient's ABO blood group should be determined and complete human leukocyte antigen (HLA) typing should be performed for the A, B, C and DR loci. Compatibility of ABO has traditionally been assumed to be obligatory in renal transplantation because, even within families, the crossing of this major histocompatibility barrier produces such poor results. Sutherland and coworkers (42) further emphasized this requirement, demonstrating graft survival to be inferior even in ABO compatible but nonidentical donor-recipient combinations.

The degree of antibody sensitization is measured by detection of cytotoxic antibodies in the recipient's serum against a panel of T and B lymphocytes. The more highly sensitized a patient is, the longer the waiting time generally is to obtain a crossmatch-negative cadaveric donor. Prior to transplantation of either a cadaveric kidney or one from a living relative, a final T cell (and in some transplantation centers B cell) crossmatch is performed to identify preformed antibodies that are specific to that donor. This final negative crossmatch has largely eliminated immediate (hyperacute) rejection.

In those individuals with a living donor who is crossmatch negative, ABO-compatible, and HLA-identical, an elective operation can be performed with a 95% chance for long-term graft survival with less immunosuppression and the chance for fewer complications. In recipients whose donors are one- and two-haplotype mismatched living relatives, an 85% 2-year allograft survival rate can be obtained with donor-specific transfusions under the protection of azathioprine (43), or with cyclosporine without the need for transfusions (44). With donor-specific transfusions, however, sensitization or post-transfusion hepatitis can occur, whereas with cyclosporine no recipients are eliminated by sensitization, but they are subjected to the risk of cyclosporine toxicity. There is a difference in the incidence of sensitization to donor-specific transfusions among patients even with the protection of azathioprine. In one-haplotype combinations, recipients with a panel reactive antibody (PRA) level of less than 10% have a sensitization rate of 6%, whereas in patients with a PRA of more than 10%, a 56% incidence of donor-specific transfusion sensitization occurs (45). The antibodies appear within 2 weeks of the transfusion, they possess anti-T cell properties, and they are generally of broad specificity and persistent duration consistent with amplification of a previous antigenic exposure. This latter group should especially be considered for treatment with cyclosporine rather than with donor-specific transfusions.

In cadaveric donor recipients, non-donor-specific blood transfusions also improved graft survival, prior to the use of cyclosporine (46). Because a similar beneficial effect occurs in patients receiving cyclosporine, many centers have stopped the policy of deliberate transfusion with five or more units prior to transplantation.

Because transfusion of a single unit of blood may induce broadly reactive antibodies directed at public antigenic determinants on the HLA molecule, it seems appropriate that many cadaveric donor recipients come to transplantation without having received transfusions because cyclosporine use is already more important in the immunosuppressive regimen for cadaveric organs than for organs from living relatives.

In potential recipients of both cadaveric organs and organs from living relatives, existing antibody sensitization remains the major obstacle to transplantation, an effect that has not yet been overcome by current therapy. Approximately 20% of the more than 20,000 patients currently awaiting kidney transplantation in Europe and North America are so highly sensitized that the provision of a satisfactory graft is improbable or impossible. Although natural antibodies may occur, broadly reactive sensitization is normally caused by pregnancy, prior transplantation, or blood transfusion.

Although livers and hearts may in certain instances be transplanted across a positive T cell crossmatch, the immunologic consequences appear to be different for the kidney, and this barrier is rarely breached. Autoreactive IgM anti-T or anti-B cell antibodies do not appear to be deleterious, however, and may be removed by absorption or treatment with dithiothreitol (DTT) (47). Accumulating evidence suggests that a history of a positive donor-specific T cell crossmatch is not predictive of outcome in a first or subsequent graft if the current crossmatch result is negative (48), even when stratified for length of prior graft survival, which itself represents a significant risk factor. Positive crossmatches with noncurrent sera apparently can also be ignored in living donor transplants. This approach reduces the waiting time for a transplant and permits transplantation in increasing numbers of sensitized patients.

Refinements in sensitivity and specificity may further increase the discriminative value of the crossmatch. Anti-HLA class I antibodies of the IgG class inhibitable by a monoclonal antibody PA2.6 appear particularly damaging (47). T cell immunofluorescence flow cytometry (49) or antihuman globulin-enhanced microcytotoxicity assay (50), as well as assays involving Cr-51 release, antibody dependent cellular cytotoxicity (ADCC), and enzyme-linked immunosorbent assay labeling, can detect antibodies below the threshold of sensitivity of the standard complement dependent cytotoxicity (CDC) technique. Each of these methods, however, tends to increase the relative number of false-positives reactions (i.e., decreased diagnostic specificity), resulting in increased donor exclusion.

Immunosuppressive therapy may also influence the predictive value of crossmatch testing. Kerman and coworkers (51) reported that the association between 1-year graft loss and a positive Cr-51 release crossmatch was significantly reduced in patients receiving cyclosporine (14) in contrast to those receiving azathioprine (17). This and other studies suggest that newer immunosuppressive agents and protocols may reduce the risk of graft loss from rejections that are associated with low levels of presensitization. Nevertheless, graft loss from hyperacute or accelerated rejection can occur when the standard crossmatch is negative but the antiglobulin crossmatch is positive (52).

The target cell specificity is also important. Although positive crossmatches against T cells are detrimental, those associated with autoreactive antibodies are not. The risks of reversible and irreversible rejection reactions associated with antibodies against donor B cells, monocytes, or endothelial cells remain uncertain. These uncertainties are compounded by other factors, such as immunoglobulin class, temperature sensitivity, target antigen, and clinical factors, such as cyclosporine use and mode of sensitization. Current evidence suggests that of the various "non-T-cell" reactive anti-donor leukocyte antibodies that are often identified, those that are IgG, warm reactive, and recognize donor HLA-DR have the greatest risk for rejection (53).

Because of these recent findings (i.e., that the natural loss of anti-donor lymphocytotoxic antibodies may allow for renal transplantation and that better immunosuppressive therapy may reduce the risk of graft loss from rejection reactions associated with low levels of anti-donor antibodies), the active removal of anti-donor antibodies by plasma exchange has received attention as a possible means of avoiding donor exclusion, especially following donor-specific transfusions. However, the removal of preformed antibody has proved particularly difficult. In many subjects, the elimination of transfusions or conversion to peritoneal dialysis allows the gradual disappearance of antibody, and titers decline over the subsequent 12–24 months. The use of cyclophosphamide combined with plasma exchange three times weekly has been reported to reduce specific anti-HLA antibody eight- to 60-fold in small numbers of patients, with a 5–60% reduction in panel reactivity (54), although this has not been widely employed. Fauchald and colleagues (55) did report that T lymphocyte crossmatches became negative after plasma exchange or pheresis in four of five patients and that no hyperacute rejection was seen following transplantation from the specific donors.

Although the beneficial role of matching for antigens of the HLA-A and -B series (class I antigens) is well established in the selection of donors who are living relatives, the value of HLA-A and -B matching to the survival of cadaveric renal grafts remains controversial. It is generally agreed that matching for the HLA-C locus has little or no importance. Matching for HLA-DR antigens (class II antigens) appears to have more influence on the outcome of transplantation than does HLA-A and -B matching, which is not a surprising finding because animal experiments indicate that class II antigen identity is more important to allograft survival than is class I antigen identity (56). Before the advent of cyclosporine, zero or one DR mismatches had significantly better one-year graft survival than did mismatches for both DR antigens. The early results with cyclosporine administration suggests, however, that this drug is capable of overriding many effects of mismatching for primary grafts (57). There are data to suggest, however, a 15–25% increase in renal graft survival in the highly sensitized individual, independent of the immunosuppressive therapy employed, when there is compatibility at both class I and class II loci (52). The provision of a well-matched, crossmatch negative graft for such individuals is difficult, necessitating a donor pool calculated at between 5×10^2 and 2×10^5, depending on the degree of sensitization, the phenotype, and the match.

Kidney Donor Selection

Living Donor

The use of living donors for kidney transplantation in general is justified because

1. The increase in graft survival exceeds that obtained with cadaveric donor transplantation by 10–15% at 1 year and increases with continued follow-up
2. There exists the ability to arrange transplantation at an optimum time with a lessened chance of acute tubular necrosis (ATN) and early rejection

3. There is a chronic inability of cadaveric organ donation to fulfill the increasing demand for organ transplantation.

Despite these compelling reasons and the resulting psychologic benefit in many cases, the use of a living donor is acceptable only if there is no significant morbidity or mortality (58). This has been supported by a mortality risk of less than 0.05% and a 5-year life expectancy that is comparable with the normal population. An important concern raised in the rat model was that continued hyperfiltration in the remnant kidney might jeopardize long-term renal function. However, follow-up studies over 10–15 years in large numbers of renal donors have provided no evidence of such functional deterioration (59).

In the patients treated at the University of Minnesota, the actual graft functional survival rate at 10 years of 62% for diabetic recipients of HLA-identical grafts was significantly higher than the 28 and 22% 10-year rates for HLA-mismatched living related and cadaver donor grafts, respectively (Fig. 3B). These graft survival rates are lower than those for nondiabetic uremic recipients of 80%, 54%, and 39% for HLA-identical sibling, HLA-mismatched, and cadaver donors, respectively (35), (Fig. 3C). When the graft has functioned for more than 10 years there continues to be poorer survival for the diabetic recipient than for the nondiabetic (Fig. 4A graft survival for the diabetic versus nondiabetic at 15 years of 37 versus 75%, respectively). In this late period, immunologic events appear to be equivalent, with no difference between HLA identical, HLA mismatched and cadaveric for diabetic or nondiabetic recipients (Fig. 4B and 4C).

The living donor is generally between 18 and 65 years of age, in good physical health, and without structural or functional renal disease. Unsuspected hypertension, subclinical diabetes, or significant cardiopulmonary disease must be eliminated. It is especially important that family members being evaluated for donation to a diabetic recipient be carefully tested for incipient diabetes by a glucose tolerance test. A normal creatinine level clearance and intravenous pyelogram assures normal renal function, and renal arteriography demonstrates the renal vasculature preoperatively (60). It is especially important that potential volunteers be protected from family pressures to donate against their will, especially in the case of minors.

Nephrectomy

In the nephrectomy procedure, a flank incision is generally used with or without removal of the tip of the twelfth rib. The preoperative arteriogram shows the number, size, and origin of the renal arteries, aiding in the choice of the right or left kidney. Ideally, the left kidney, with a single renal artery, is preferable because the left renal vein is longer. The external and internal oblique muscles are divided, and the transversus muscle is split. The retroperitoneal space is entered directly over the kidney by incising Gerota's fascia, and the greater curvature of the kidney and the upper pole are dissected free and the hilar renal artery and vein are exposed. Ligation of the adrenal and gonadal veins is required on the left side. The renal artery, which is then identified slightly cephalad and posterior to the renal vein, is dissected to its aortic origin. Care is taken to prevent excessive traction on the renal artery, which may cause spasm and decreased renal perfusion. This may be prevented or reversed by periarterial application of 20% lidocaine or papaverine. Great care should be taken not to skeletonize the ureter, which should be mobilized with its

A.

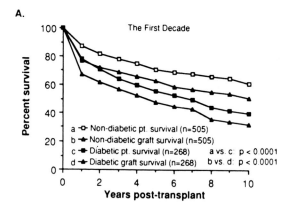

B.

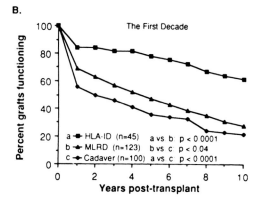

C.

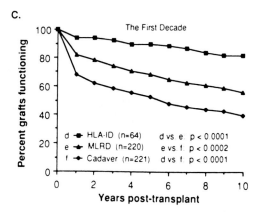

FIG. 3. Actual 10-year patient and graft functional survival rate curves for adult recipients of primary renal allografts between 1966 and 1978 at the University of Minnesota. Patient and graft survival for 265 diabetic and 505 nondiabetic recipients. (A). Graft survival according to donor source for diabetic (B) and nondiabetic (C) recipients (From Najarian JS et al., ref. 35.)

blood supply and a generous amount of periureteral fat. After dissection over the iliac bifurcation, the ureter is ligated and divided close to the bladder. If the donor is well hydrated and renal vasospasm has been minimal, urine should be seen issuing from the proximal end of the divided ureter. Mannitol (12.5 g) or furosemide (5–10 mg) is useful in promoting a brisk diuresis.

Attention is given to coordination with the simultaneously conducted recipient operation. When the recipient iliac vessels and bladder have been prepared, the do-

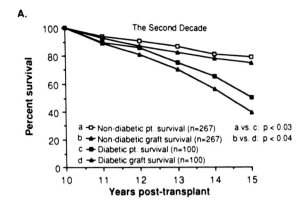

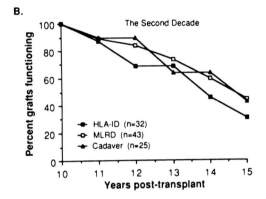

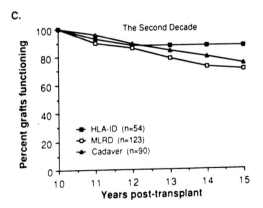

FIG. 4. Actuarial patient and graft functional survival rate for 100 diabetic and 267 nondiabetic recipients who have already survived for 10 years post-transplantation (A) according to the donor source for diabetic (B) and nondiabetic (C) recipients (From Najarian JS et al., ref. 35.)

nor renal artery and then the vein are clamped and divided. Blood is flushed from the kidney and is core cooled with several hundred millimeters of a 4°C (39.2°F) heparinized Euro-Collins solution. The kidney is also immersed in a basin filled with the cold electrolyte solution and is transported to the recipient operating room. After the donor vessels are oversewn, the incision is closed without drainage. The remaining kidney is monitored for urine output, and a chest radiograph is taken in the recovery room to detect any pneumothorax.

Cadaveric Donor Nephrectomy

In patients for whom there is no living donor, a cadaveric kidney is used. Although in the United States there are an estimated 20,000 brain-dead patients/year who would be good donors, only 2,500 actually donate their organs for transplantation (61). Public education about the need for and acceptability of organ donation is needed. Cadaveric donation requires the declaration of brain death and surgical recovery, preferably by the "en bloc" technique. Increasingly, this is part of a multiple organ recovery effort coordinated with several surgical teams (62,63). Ideally, the donor should be less than 35 years of age; however, with the current shortage of donors, 60 to 65 years is the accepted upper age limit for cadaveric renal donor consideration. Generally, the creatinine clearance level declines annually after the age of 50 years so that the creatinine clearance level of a normal 60-year-old has decreased by 35% (64). The potential donor must have good renal function, as evidenced by normal serum blood urea nitrogen (BUN) and creatinine levels (a terminal increase in creatinine levels to 3 mg/dl is acceptable), and must be free of diabetes, significant hypertension, sepsis, drug abuse, acquired immune deficiency syndrome (AIDS), and malignant disease (except primary central nervous system tumors and low-grade skin cancers).

An en bloc technique for bilateral nephrectomy is preferred for the following reasons: warm ischemia time is decreased, renal arterial spasm is decreased, the kidneys may be initially washed out through the aorta, the chances of renal artery intimal disruption are decreased, the technical problems associated with recognition and management of multiple renal arteries are minimized, and there is greater flexibility in the use of the kidneys. The kidneys may be recovered via a median sternotomy and suprasternal notch to symphysis pubis midline incision or a bilateral subcostal incision plus a midline xiphoid to pubis incision. The abdomen is thoroughly explored for unsuspected disease. The mesocolon is freed from the cecum to the diaphragm and medially to the midline. The entire bowel is freed, wrapped in a towel, and rotated to the upper left out of the abdomen. The ureters are freed with adventitia along their entire length. The kidneys are mobilized without dissection near the hilum. The ureters are severed deep in the pelvis and urine production is noted. Systemic heparin (10,000 units for an adult) is given, the distal aorta is ligated proximal to the bifurcation, and the aortic perfusion cannula is ligated in place proximally. When the other organs in a multiple organ recovery are ready, the vena cava is ligated distally and a cannula is inserted proximally to allow controlled decompression of blood and fluid during perfusion. A proximal aortic clamp is applied (at the aortic arch for cardiac recovery, above the celiac axis artery for liver recovery, and above the renal arteries for kidney recovery alone) and retrograde perfusion through the aortic cannula with cold (0° to 4°C) solution is immediately begun *in situ*. (Ligation and division of the superior mesenteric artery allows easier access for clamping the aorta when kidneys alone are to be recovered.) Ventilation by anesthesia may now be stopped. The kidneys are removed en bloc and placed in a basin of cold solution on another sterile table. The kidneys are flushed until they are completely blanched, usually with a solution such as Collins' solution. Under cold protection, extraneous tissue is removed and the kidneys are separated with an aortic cuff for each kidney. Each kidney is placed in double sterile plastic bags, is surrounded with flush solution, and is then placed into a plastic jar packed in ice.

The time of proximal aortic clamping and any warm ischemia time must be recorded. Warm ischemia is the time from aortic cross-clamping until the kidneys have been flushed with iced solution and any time during the transplant operation before the renal vessels are reperfused. This time should be kept to a minimum because injury occurs much more rapidly in this situation than under cold protection.

Unlike recipient selection with a living donor, with cadaveric donors, recipient selection usually occurs after renal recovery, and the organ must be preserved for a number of hours. This is usually accomplished by core cooling with an intracellular composition solution, such as Collins' solution, and hypothermic storage or pulsatile machine perfusion (65). Excellent clinical response has resulted from cold storage up to 24 hours. Although some have advocated storage at 4°C for up to 48 hours, a high incidence of ATN results with less than optimal renal function (66). Continuous hypothermic machine perfusion provides more effective preservation beyond 24 hours (67).

Recipient Surgery

Dialysis is generally performed in the 12–36 hours before transplantation to control volume, blood pressure, potassium, and acidosis. The patient's dry weight is the minimum weight that has been achieved with dialysis. The patient's estimated dry weight compared with the present weight helps estimate fluid status before surgery.

General anesthesia is preferred by most transplant surgeons, although spinal anesthesia is also satisfactory. Good relaxation is necessary during the vascular and ureteral anastomoses. Immediately prior to surgery, 100–200 ml of an antibiotic solution are instilled via a clamped Foley catheter to distend the bladder and facilitate its identification and dissection.

Using the extraperitoneal approach, the donor kidney is placed in either the right or left lower quadrant (through an oblique incision just above the inguinal ligament). Although the dissection is generally contralateral to the side of the donor kidney to facilitate renal vein to iliac vein approximation, a more important consideration is to avoid sites of previous transplantation or other operations (e.g., appendectomy, herniorrhaphy, or bladder or ureteral operation) or of peritoneal dialysis catheters. The smallest possible dissection is done to accomplish adequate exposure of the planned anastomotic sites. Lymphatics that are divided in exposing the iliac vessels are ligated to prevent prolonged lymph drainage or lymphocele formation that might subsequently obstruct the ureter. Exposure of the bladder is facilitated by dividing the inferior epigastric vessels and, in female patients, the round ligament. Division of the spermatic cord is to be avoided, because testicular ischemia and atrophy are often the result. Care should be exercised in retraction of the lower surgical margin because a disabling femoral neuropathy may result from nerve compression.

The usual vascular anastomoses are as follows: the end of the donor renal artery to the recipient's divided internal iliac (hypogastric) artery and the end of the donor renal vein to the side of the external iliac vein. However, if there is significant disease of the internal iliac artery or if the contralateral internal iliac artery has been ligated during a previous transplantation operation (especially in male patients because bilateral internal artery ligation can result in impotence), an end-to-side anastomosis of the renal artery to the external iliac artery should be used. Some surgeons favor the external iliac anastomosis because less dissection is required and stenosis may be less likely, especially if a Carrel patch of donor aorta, including the renal artery orifice, is used. This is especially applicable if there are multiple renal arteries arising from the Carrel patch. If several arteries are present that have not been preserved on the aortic patch, they may be anastomosed to form a common orifice, or the smaller arteries can be anastomosed to the side of the larger renal artery. This part of the operation can be performed deliberately under magnification during hypothermic protection by immersion in a basin of cold saline. Even a small accessory artery should be preserved because occlusion of the end arteries will cause renal infarcts. It should be remembered that interruption of venous blood supply can be as lethal as interruption of the arterial blood supply; however, the small accessory vein may be ligated because venous collateral circulation is almost always adequate.

The hemodynamic and pharmacologic status of the patient must be optimized before the release of vascular clamps. Upon release of the clamps, the kidney should turn from gray to pink. Dopamine may be administered if the kidney appears mottled after adequate fluid administration (68). The blood pressure should be monitored every minute for several minutes following release of the clamps. Even if cardiac filling pressures are adequate initially [central venous pressure (CVP) >5 cm H_2O], they may fall within a few hours after renal transplantation as the kidney begins to function. The patient may require 2–4 liters of fluid to restore adequate circulating volume. This fall appears to be out of proportion to the urine output, suggesting a decrease in vascular resistance as occurs following bilateral nephrectomy (69). Urine output should be replaced milliliter for milliliter with one-half normal saline in the immediate revascularization period. If large volumes of urine are the result, hyponatremia and hypokalemia can develop. In this case, less than the urine output should be cautiously replaced to allow the kidney to begin to regulate output.

Although the blood supply of the ureter has multiple origins with three anastomoses within the ureteral adventitia, the transplanted ureter receives a blood supply only from the renal vessel branches that occur in the hilar and upper periureteral fat. Small aberrant vessels can be easily overlooked when there is no circulation, which sometimes occurs in cadaveric donor nephrectomy. A divided accessory artery to the lower pole of the kidney is especially important because it may contribute the blood supply to a segment of the collecting system or ureter and its ligation may lead to necrosis and urinary fistula. Therefore, a lower pole branch should always be implanted. Because the ureteric blood supply lies in the adventitia, the ureter must be meticulously removed with adequate surrounding tissue. This is best done by sharp dissection of the ureter in the cadaveric donor or in the living donor. Blunt dissection by the surgeon's finger, although rapid, should never be done. In addition, the ureter must be long enough to prevent tension at the ureterovesical anastomosis after implantation, as tension is the second most common cause of urinary fistula after transplantation. Prevention of these complications is directly related to strict adherence to technical details in organ procurement, management of multiple arteries, renal preservation, and renal implantation. Rejection is a possible, but probably infrequent, mechanism in the development of ureteral leaks.

The most common method for reconstruction of ureteral drainage is by modified Politano-Leadbetter technique of ureteroneocystostomy. The ureteroneocystostomy is performed in men by placing the ureter posterior to the spermatic cord and creating a submucosal tunnel through the right or left posterior lateral bladder wall (through an anterior midline cystotomy incision). It is important that the extravesicular ureter is not twisted or under any tension when the kidney is properly positioned. Likewise, it is important to minimize the length of the donor ureter to decrease the risk of ischemic necrosis. After a ureteral mucosal-to-bladder mucosal anastomosis, a ureteral stent may be placed to differentiate urine output from the transplanted kidney from that of the native kidneys. The anterior cystostomy is closed in three layers. A ureteroneocystostomy prevents reflux of urine by its submucosal tunnel, and it is possible even if the native ureters are absent or diseased. The risks of this technique include the possible exposure of the wound to the contents of a contaminated bladder, ureteral tip necrosis or stenosis, and postoperative hematuria and bladder clots. Although ureteric duplication is relatively uncommon, a kidney with a double ureter can be used successfully if it is dissected en bloc with its common adventitial sheath and periureteral fat, so that the ureteral blood supply is protected. The ureters may be implanted separately or brought through a generous submucosal tunnel side by side.

Extravesicular ureteroneocystostomy, pyeloureterostomy, or ureteroureterostomy can also be used for ureteral reconstruction. The extravesicular ureteroneocystostomy does not necessitate opening the bladder, and hematuria is reduced but reflux is probably more common. Anastomosis of the donor ureter or pelvis to the recipient ureter is an alternative approach that is particularly valuable if the bladder is known to have bacterial contamination or has been entered on several occasions for transplant ureteroneocystostomy or for previous urologic surgery (70). The advantages of this technique include the assurance of an adequate blood supply to both the proximal donor and the distal recipient ureters, the absence of reflux, the avoidance of opening the bladder, less risk of postoperative hematuria, and the lack of a need for indwelling catheters. There is, however, a much greater risk of urinary fistula developing, which frequently requires a transplantation nephrectomy.

More patients now receiving renal transplants have ileal loops. A "loopogram" should be obtained during the initial evaluation and if gross ureteral reflux is present, a decision should be made as to the advisability of pretransplantation nephrectomy. The ileal loop can be anchored into the lower abdominal quadrant so that a retroperitoneal approach can be used for transplantation, and easy access to the loop is assured. The ureter can then be anastomosed to the ileum with interrupted full thickness absorbable sutures (71).

The Period Following Transplantation

Unless the transplanted kidney has suffered ischemic injury, diuresis usually begins within minutes after revascularization. Unlike the kidney from a living donor, the cadaveric kidney frequently has a period of ATN that results from suboptimal donor factors or from prolonged preservation. Diuresis (often of 100 to 1,000 ml/hour) may be the result of osmotic load secondary to uremia or high glucose concentrations in the intravenous fluids; total blood, fluid, and electrolyte overload from chronic uremia; and proximal tubular damage from allograft ischemia. In the early postoperative period, adequate fluid replacement is given to match urine volume and, if necessary, diuretics are given to ensure a continuing diuresis. Inadequate replacement of fluid may lead to oliguria and impaired renal function, which may interfere with the ability to diagnose early rejection, urinary obstruction, or vascular occlusion. Conversely, if transplant function is minimal, volume overreplacement may result in congestive heart failure. Hyperkalemia is particularly apt to occur in this setting and prompt dialysis or administration of the ion exchange resin sodium polystyrene sulfonate (Kayexalate), 25 to 50 g orally or by enema, with careful monitoring of plasma potassium levels, is necessary. Fluids should be replaced with 0.45% (one-half normal) saline with or without isotonic glucose, according to blood glucose levels. Rarely is potassium replacement required. After 12–24 hours, fluid replacement normally may be allowed to lag behind the urine output until the urine volume returns to normal levels. For the diabetic recipient it is especially important to monitor blood glucose levels because levels exceeding the renal threshold can increase the urine osmotic load with a resulting excessive diuresis and possible hypovolemic. The freshly transplanted kidney temporarily loses its ability to regulate urine volume.

The Foley catheter is usually left in the bladder from 3 to 5 days. By using the retroperitoneal approach, intestinal ileus is usually minimal and the patient can begin oral intake after full recovery from anesthesia. By the first postoperative day, the patient should be encouraged to ambulate. Perioperative antibiotics are used for 24–48 hours to decrease the incidence of wound infections. Trimethoprim-sulfamethoxazole is given chronically for prophylaxis against urinary tract infections and may provide protection against *Pneumocystis carinii* (72). Renal toxicity from trimethoprim-sulfamethoxazole is possible, however, especially in patients receiving cyclosporine. Antacids or H_2 blockers, or both, are given in the immediate period after transplantation or during the treatment of rejection to protect against ulcer formation, and nystatin is given as prophylaxis against monilial infections. Hypertension, which is especially common in cyclosporine-treated patients, should be managed conventionally with drugs such as hydralazine, hydrochlorothiazide, or α-methyldopa. The antihypertensive agent chosen must be evaluated for its so-called compatibility with the diabetic state.

After renal transplantation, the patient could have a completely uneventful course, in which case renal function returns to normal within 3–5 days with a kidney from a living relative or within 7–15 days with a cadaveric kidney. The most important management aspect after transplantation is the awareness of complications that can impair or alter renal function. Causes for impaired renal function include acute and hyperacute rejection; ATN; cyclosporine nephrotoxicity; arterial, venous, or ureteral complications; pseudorejection due to laboratory error; and the sudden onset of diabetes. Several weeks to months after transplantation, ureteral stenosis or development of a lymphocele can cause renal dysfunction due to obstruction. The routine use of radionuclide scans and the duplex Doppler scan generally allows the appropriate diagnosis to be made (73). When there is still doubt, a percutaneous needle biopsy with or without ultrasound guidance is usually diagnostic.

The radionuclide scan is not invasive and may be obtained often to evaluate both renal perfusion and excretory function. Unfortunately, it is relatively nonspecific and is most useful when serial studies are compared for changes. In addition to the usefulness of the real-time image of the ultrasonic component, duplex Doppler studies allow precise definition of the vessels and assessment of vascular flow characteristics. In acute rejection, the diastolic flow is decreased, probably reflecting an increased vascular impedance in the allograft microcirculation and a pulsatility index can be calculated. The sensitivity for acute rejection with Doppler studies is greater for vascular rejection and lower when rejection is limited to the interstitium (74).

Immunosuppression

The current methods of immunosuppression are undergoing substantial change (75). From 1965 to 1983, the standard immunosuppressive regimen included azathioprine and prednisone. Azathioprine was usually started at a dosage of 3–5 mg/kg/day and gradually reduced to maintain the recipient's white blood cell count at greater than 4,000 cells/mm^3. Corticosteroids (prednisone) were essential in the management of patients (76). Prednisone started initially in the range of 2 to 5 mg/kg/day, was reduced rapidly to a total dose of 30 mg/day by 1–2 months after transplantation, and was then decreased gradually to 10–15 mg/day at 1 year. In some circumstances, especially in an effort to stimulate pediatric growth, conversion to alternate-day prednisone dosage (usually twice the daily dose) was employed in stable patients after 1 year to diminish the side effects of steroids. If rejection ensued, high doses of steroids (0.5–1 g of methylprednisolone intravenously or 100–300 mg of prednisone orally) were given for 3–5 days and were then tapered rapidly to maintenance levels as the rejection subsided. When corticosteroids are used in higher doses immediately after transplantation or for the treatment of rejection, blood glucose levels may increase dramatically in the diabetic recipient. The resulting increased insulin requirements should be regulated by close blood glucose monitoring.

Antilymphocyte or antithymocyte heterologous antiserum (ALS or ATG) prepared by repeated inoculation of human lymphocytes into animals (e.g., rabbits and horses) initially was found to be of marginal benefit when used prophylactically (as an adjunct to azathioprine and prednisone) in the early 1970s (77,78). Subsequently, however, ALG was found to be very effective in reversing rejection crises, even in patients who had failed to respond to high-dose steroid therapy (79). This observation was at variance with experimental results in rodents, but after confirmation in a multicenter randomized study, ALG treatment of rejection was adopted by many transplantation centers.

The documented effectiveness of ALG in antirejection treatments was the stimulus for the exploration of the developing technology of monoclonal antibody production for the same purpose. The highly specific mouse antihuman antibodies were shown to remove virtually all circulating T lymphocytes within minutes without affecting other blood elements, as often occurred with polyclonal ALG (80). OKT$_3$ pan-T cell monoclonal antibodies have been very effective in aborting rejection crises, but require other immunosuppression to prevent rejection recurrence and can be rendered ineffective by the rapid development of antibodies against the mouse protein. The future application of this monoclonal specificity against T helper and other lymphocyte subsets is theoretically quite attractive but must still be explored.

A subsequent randomized clinical trial of OKT$_3$ monoclonal antibody confirmed that rejection was reversed in 94% of cases, with a 1-year cadaveric renal allograft survival of 62% compared with 45% in patients treated for rejection with corticosteroids (81). During the administration of OKT$_3$ antibody (5 mg/day by the intravenous route for 7–14 days), other immunosuppressive therapy is reduced by one-half to avoid excessive immunosuppression. The long-term implications of the therapeutic use of monoclonal antibodies pertain not only to treating graft rejection but also to their potential use in eliminating activated cell clones and attempting to achieve specific unresponsiveness.

The fungal derivative cyclosporin A was noted by Borel (82) in 1974 to have im-

munosuppressive qualities. Cyclosporine operates selectively to block gene tran-
scription for IL-2, IFN-γ and related lymphokines in the responding lymphocyte.
Cyclosporine may also decrease graft immunogenicity by reducing major histocom-
patiblity complex (MHC) class II antigen expression (83). Failure to display inhibition of IL-2 or IFN-γ generation during the first three months after the transplantation procedure correlates closely with early graft rejection and facilitates its
differentiation from nephrotoxicity (84).

Initially when used alone, cyclosporine A was found to be quite toxic and was
associated with infections, tumors, and renal failure (85). The subsequent combination of smaller doses with prednisone dramatically improved renal and liver allograft
success (up to 90% initial success with cadaveric kidneys (86). More recently, cyclosporine has been combined with both azathioprine and prednisone in "triple-drug
therapy" (11). The early experience of administering cyclosporine at 15–17 mg/kg/
day appears to have been excessive (87). Excellent results have been obtained for
cadaveric kidney recipients with 5–10 mg/kg/day of cyclosporine combined with azathioprine or ATG globulin and prednisone (88–90).

Initial low-dose cyclosporine therapy has been particularly helpful during the early
period after transplantation in avoiding nephrotoxic effects that may produce acute
renal dysfunction and the need for prolonged dialysis. Steroids are still used for antirejection therapy, even with "triple-drug therapy"; however, the total dose of steroids tends to be considerably less than that for azathioprine-prednisone-treated patients, primarily because rejection episodes occur less frequently. In fact, elevation
of serum creatinine levels in patients treated with cyclosporine is most frequently
due to nephrotoxicity and not to rejection. This nephrotoxicity appears to be synergistic with renal damage from other causes, such as ischemia. For this reason, at
some centers cyclosporine is not begun until diuresis begins after transplantation.
Monitoring blood or serum cyclosporine levels does not always reliably correlate
with immunosuppression or nephrotoxicity, but it may be useful in evaluating toxic
or subtherapeutic levels caused by malabsorption, the patient's failure to take the
medicine, or activation of the P-450 cytochrome enzyme system by drugs such as
phenobarbital and phenytoin. Therefore, in the absence of other factors suggesting
rejection, cyclosporine may be empirically lowered for several days. A renal biopsy
may be needed if the creatinine level does not improve, and in instances of prolonged
hypercreatinemia, it may be necessary to discontinue the cyclosporine. Patients on
cyclosporine tend to have a persistently higher creatinine level than that of azathioprine patients treated with azathioprine (1.7–2.3 mg/dl versus 1.4 mg/dl). There is
uncertainty about the long-term importance of cyclosporine nephrotoxicity and the
possible development of irreversible interstitial fibrosis (90). Therefore, some authors advocate substitution of azathioprine for cyclosporine in all patients who have
stable graft function after a few months. Most authors agree that the 10–20% improvement in cadaveric graft survival with cyclosporine versus azathioprine justifies
the early risks of cyclosporine nephrotoxicity.

The introduction of cyclosporine has also improved patient survival, presumably
because of a decreased incidence and severity of infections. Although the inductive
phase of the immune response and the synthesis of lymphokines by T lymphocytes
are inhibited, other aspects of the immune response that are important in warding
off bacterial and viral infections are not depressed to the same extent by cyclosporine as by conventional immunosuppression (91). Older patients, recipients of extrarenal transplants, and high immune responders especially benefit from cyclosporine.

These effects of this drug explain in part the present policy of more liberal application of renal transplantation. Although there are new problems associated with the use of cyclosporine, its introduction has been a major advance in the quest for more specific and effective immunosuppression.

Results of Renal Transplantation

The treatment of ESRD has improved markedly in the past 30 years. Before transplantation, renal failure was uniformly fatal, but with the advent of cyclosporine a 1–2-year renal graft survival of 77–95% is now possible for both cadaveric donor grafts and grafts from living relatives. The considerably better results with transplants from living relatives versus cadaveric donor grafts continues to justify the use of the former, especially for two haplotype-identical sibling donors, in whom graft survivals of 95–100% are reported. Unfortunately, most patients with ESRD do not have suitable available living donors and must depend upon a cadaveric donor. The number of transplants from living relatives has remained relatively constant, and the increasing numbers have primarily reflected increased cadaveric transplants.

The mortality associated with transplantation from a living donor is only about half as great as that from a cadaveric donor (92). The improvement in patient survival (which occurred prior to the use of cyclosporine) was probably mainly attributable to a striking decrease in severe infections because of a general policy to diminish the intensity of immunosuppression, especially when rejection seemed inevitable (93). Cyclosporine further improved graft and patient survival by decreasing the incidence of rejection and associated infection that often accompanies the treatment of rejection. One-year patient survival rates of 95–98% can now be achieved (94). Because the mortality rate for the first year of dialysis is 10% even if the transplant fails, early nephrectomy and return to dialysis does not increase patient mortality.

The cause of the ESRD accounts for some of the differences in transplantation outcome. Collective studies by Terasaki (95) at UCLA confirm what others have also shown, that diabetic patients have lower survival, which in turn affects graft survival (Fig. 5). There was a relatively greater difference in functional and graft survival rates for diabetic patients than for nondiabetic patients. As in dialysis, however, the results of renal transplantation on diabetic patients have improved markedly during the last decade. Sixty-five percent of diabetic patients survive 5 years compared with 83% for patients with glomerulonephritis. When patient deaths are excluded, however, graft survival does not vary between diabetic patients and nondiabetic patients (95), (Fig. 6). Three-year patient survival rates for recipients of HLA-identical kidneys was 100% compared with 80% for recipients of cadaver kidneys (27).

The results of second and third renal transplants are markedly influenced by the reason for failure of the first graft. If the first transplant was rejected for immunological reasons, second-graft survival is significantly less, whereas technical loss has a minimal impact on the second graft. Terasaki (95) reports that immunologic failure produces a 20% difference at 1 year and a 17% difference at 2 years. Early loss of the first transplant from acute rejection decreases the chances for survival of the second transplant, whereas slow, chronic rejection of the first graft does not have the same adverse effect. Cytotoxic antibodies do not influence second-graft survival if the pretransplantation crossmatch is negative.

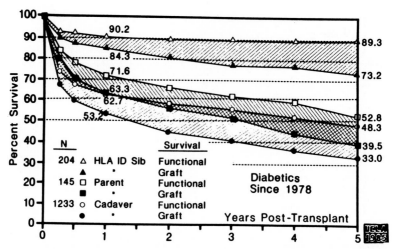

FIG. 5. Graft survival rates are influenced by patient survival because, conventionally, patient death is counted as graft loss. The upper line in each of the categories represents the functional survival rate at which death was counted as lost to follow-up. Because death played a greater role in graft loss for diabetic than nondiabetic patients, there was a relatively larger difference in functional and graft survival rates in diabetic patients who have undergone transplant operation since 1978. In addition, the role of death was almost the same for related donor transplants as for cadaver donors, which contrasts with the lesser effect of death for living donors in nondiabetic patients. The functional survival rate was high for diabetics, indicating that the immunologic rejection process in diabetic patients was no different than for patients with other underlying diseases, and that the lower graft survival rate was attributed to deaths. The difference in functional survival rates at 5 years was 16% for HLA-identical sibling donors, 13% for parental donors, and 15% for cadaver donors (From Terasaki PI, et al., ref. 95.)

In most series, the graft survival rate for black recipients is about 10% lower, even when the organs are from living relatives and black-to-black recipients (95). This is important because blacks are at higher risk for renal failure from diabetic nephropathy than are whites. The best results that have been reported are for white-to-white transplantation. Socioeconomic factors are not believed to play a role, as patient survival is the same regardless of race. The poor results for blacks may reflect poorer HLA matching, since more than 98% of the HLA-A, and -B loci polymorphisms have been identified for whites, but far fewer have been identified for blacks.

Complications after Renal Transplantation

Visual acuity has always been well preserved following renal transplantation of diabetic patients. Although blindness develops in five percent of the eyes of diabetic patients during the first year after transplantation, stable eyesight was achieved in 54% of patients who underwent transplant during 3.5 years of follow-up (27).

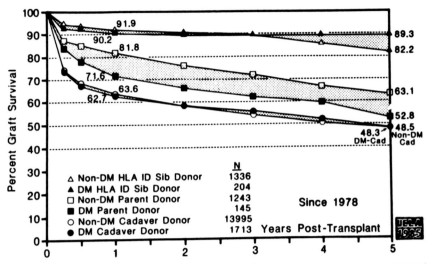

FIG. 6. Comparison of functional survival rates in diabetic versus nondiabetic patients in first transplants since 1978. If deaths were excluded, the graft function was the same for HLA-identical sibling donor and cadaver donor transplants into diabetic and nondiabetic patients. The parental donor transplants had a much lower functional survival rate for diabetic patients due to the higher death rate for diabetic recipients (From Terasaki PI et al., ref. 95.)

Amputations are still a major complication because approximately 15% of diabetic patients who have undergone transplant surgery have an amputation within 3 years (27). Bentley et al. (96) found that in a group of 26 diabetic renal allograft recipients, 31% had had an amputation of the lower extremity by 10 years post transplant. Fifty-four percent of diabetic patients who survived more than 10 years were able to return to employment or homemaking duties immediately after transplantation, but only 23% remained fully rehabilitated after 10 years. Retinopathy and peripheral vascular disease were the main causes of increasing disability.

Combination Renal-Pancreas Transplantation

Pancreas transplantation is the only therapy for diabetes mellitus that is capable of restoring a normal state of carbohydrate metabolism resulting in normalization of glycosylated hemoglobin levels. There is significant evidence that a successful pancreas transplant is capable of ameliorating the secondary complications of diabetes, in particular those of neuropathy and gastroenteropathy. The presence of a functioning pancreas transplant has been shown to prevent the occurrence of diabetic nephropathy in the renal graft, and also to reverse changes of diabetic nephropathy in the native kidneys of patients who have received only pancreas transplants prior to the development of ESRD (97). Retinopathy continues to be the most refractory complication (98). Encouraging results have been noted, however, in successful

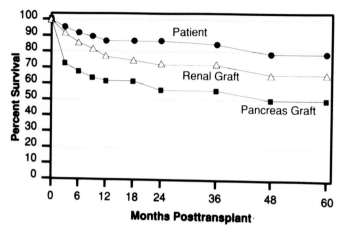

FIG. 7. Patient, renal and pancreas survival after simultaneous renal-pancreas transplantation at the University of Iowa from March 1984 to March 1989 in 51 patients (From Wright FH, et al. In: Terasaki PI, ed. *Clinical transplants 1988.* Los Angeles: UCLA Tissue Typing Laboratory, 1988;73–77.).

long-term pancreas recipients, and recent data suggest that glycosylated hemoglobin correlates strongly with the incidence and progression of diabetic retinopathy (99).

There is increasing interest in the simultaneous transplantation of both the kidney and pancreas from the same donor for diabetic patients with ESRD. The results for this combination of transplanted organs are continually improving. At the University of Iowa, the 12-month patient survival of 87% was similar for both kidney alone and simultaneous kidney-pancreas transplants (Fig. 7). The renal graft survival of 75% also approached the survival of kidney transplanted alone, and the pancreas graft survival was 62%. Survival figures have improved with the use of a more aggressive cardiac evaluation, including coronary angiography if indicated, and a decreased incidence of early pancreatic graft thrombosis. The University of Iowa's 12-month patient survival for 27 pancreas recipients from July 1986 to October 1988, increased to 96% with this approach.

CONCLUSION

The treatment of ESRD now has a better 5-year prognosis than do most malignancies. Although dialysis can be used for maintaining patients awaiting transplantation or as primary treatment for those patients unsuitable for transplantation because of age or other serious illness, the primary aim should be successful transplantation. Although the results of treatment for diabetic patients with ESRD are not as good as for nondiabetic patients, the results have improved markedly and diabetic patients should be treated as are other patients with ESRD. Particular attention should be given to the treatment of the systemic complications of diabetes mellitus. With improving results, simultaneous kidney-pancreas transplants should also be considered for selected diabetic patients. Because many victims of ESRD are relatively young, successful transplantation can be quite gratifying.

REFERENCES

1. Ullmann E. Experimentelle nierentransplantation. *Wien Klin Wochenschr* 1902;15:281.
2. Carrel A. La technique operatoire des anastomoses vasculaires et la transplantation des visceres. *Lyon Med* 1902;99:859.
3. Carrel A. Remote results of the replantation of the kidney and of the spleen. *J Exp Med* 1910;12:146.
4. Moseley J. Alexis Carrel, the man unknown. Journey of an idea. *JAMA* 1980;244:1119.
5. Graybar GB, Tarpey M. Kidney transplantation. In: Gelman S, ed. *Anesthesia and organ transplantation*. Philadelphia: W.B. Saunders, 1987;61.
6. Moore FD. Give and take: the development of tissue transplantation. Philadelphia: W.B. Saunders 1964;14.
7. Hume DM, Merrill JP, Miller BF, et al. Experiences with renal homotransplantation in the human: Report of nine cases. *J Clin Invest* 1953;24:227.
8. Murray JE, Harrison JH. Successful management of fifty patients with kidney transplants including eighteen pairs of twins. *Am J Surg* 1963;105:205.
9. Murray JE, Merrill JP, Harrison JH, et al. Prolonged survival of human-kidney homografts by immunosuppressive drug therapy. *N Engl J Med* 1963;268:1315.
10. Starzl TE, Weil R, Iwatsuki S, et al. The use of cyclosporine A and predinsone in cadaver kidney transplantation. *Surg Gynecol Obstet* 1980;151:17.
11. Canafax DM, Sutherland DER, Simmons RL, et al. Combination immunosuppression. Three drugs (azathioprine, cyclosporine, prednisone) for mismatched related and four drugs (+ALG) for cadaver renal allograft recipients. *Transplant Proc* 1985;17:2671.
12. McCarthy J, Fung J, Jain A, et al. The effects of FK506 on renal function after liver transplantation. *Transplant Proc* 1990;22:17.
13. Salvatierra O, Vincenti F, Amend W, et al. Deliberate donor-specific blood transfusions prior to living related renal transplantation: a new approach. *Ann Surg* 1980;192:543.
14. Kahan BD. Donor specific transfusions—a balanced view. *Prog Transplant* 1985;1:115.
15. Hellerstedt WL, Johnson WJ, Ascher NL, et al. Survival rates of 2728 patients with end stage renal disease. *Mayo Clin Proc* 1984;59:776.
16. Vollmer WM, Wahl PW, Blagg CR. Survival with dialysis and transplantation in patients with end stage renal disease. *N Engl J Med* 1983;308:1553.
17. Evans RW, Manninen DL, Garrison LP, et al. The quality of life of patients with end stage renal disease. *N Engl J Med* 1985;312:553.
18. Blagg CR. Dialysis or transplantation? *JAMA* 1983;250:1072.
19. Hanto DW, Simmons RL. Renal transplantation: clinical considerations. *Radiol Clin North Am* 1987;25:239.
20. Canadian Renal Failure Registry. 1984 report. Montreal: The Kidney Foundation of Canada, 1985.
21. Smith DG, Harlan LC, Hawthorne VM. The charges for ESRD treatment of diabetics. *Clin Epid* 1989;42:111–118.
22. Castills S, Tejani A, Nicostin A, et al. Diabetic nephropathy: Early renal changes in adolescent insulin dependent diabetics. *Diabetic Nephrology* 1984;3:15–18.
23. Manis T, Friedman EA. Current thinking on the management of the uremic diabetic. *Semin Nephrol* 1986;6:183–185.
24. Parving HH, Adersen AR, Smidth NM, et al. Diabetic nephropathy and arterial hypertension. The effects of antihypertensive treatment. *Diabetes* 1983;32(Suppl. 2):32.
25. Kussman MJ, Goldstein HH, Gleason RE. The clinical course of diabetic nephropathy. *JAMA* 1976;236:1861.
26. Friedman EA. Race and diabetic nephropathy. *Trans Proc* 1987;2:77–81.
27. Jacobson SH, Fryd D, Sutherland DER, Kjellstrand CM. Treatment of the diabetic patient with end-stage renal failure. *Diabete Metab Rev* 1988;4:191–200.
28. Quinton WE, Dillard DH, Scribner BH. Cannulation of blood vessels for prolonged hemodialysis. *Trans Am Soc Artif Intern Org* 1960;6:104.
29. Brescia MJ, Cimino JE, Appel K, et al. Chronic hemodialysis using venipuncture and a surgically created arterio-venous fistula. *N Engl J Med* 1966;275:1089.
30. Hertzer NR. Circulatory access for hemodialysis. In: Rutherford RB, ed. *Vascular surgery*. Philadelphia: W.B. Saunders, 1984.
31. Tellis VA, Kohlberg WI, Bhat DJ. Expanded polytetrafluoroethylene graft fistula for chronic hemodialysis. *Ann Surg* 1979;189:101.
32. Olcott C, Feldman CA, Coplon NS, et al. Continuous ambulatory peritoneal dialysis: Technique of catheter insertion and management of associated surgical complications. *Am J Surg* 1983;146:98.
33. Neu S, Kjellstrand CM. Stopping long-term dialysis. *N Engl J Med* 1986;314:14–20.

34. Keown PA, Stiller ER. Kidney transplantation. *Surg Clin North Am* 1986;66:517.
35. Najarian JS, Kaufman DB, Fryd DS, McHugh L, et al. Survival into the second decade following kidney transplantation in type I diabetic patients. *Transplant Proc* 1989;21:2012–2015.
36. Steinmuller DR. Evaluation and selection of candidates for renal transplantation. *Urol Clin North Am* 1983;10:217.
37. Philipson JD, Carpenter BJ, Itzkoff J, et al. Evaluation of cardiovascular risk for renal transplantation in diabetic patients. *Am J Med* 1986;81:630–634.
38. Gattiker H, Lerch R, Ratib O, et al. Two dimensional exercise echocardiography. Comparison with ECG, myocardial scan with thallium 201 and coronaography. *Schweiz Med Wochenschr* 1987;117:1028.
39. Leppo J, Boucher CA, Okada RD, et al. Serial thallium 201 myocardial imaging after dipyridamole infusion: diagnostic utility in detecting coronary stenosis and relationship to regional wall motion. *Circulation* 1982;66:649.
40. Marwick TH, Steinmuller DR, Underwood DA, Hobbs RE, et al. Ineffectiveness of dipyridamole spect thallium imaging as a screening technique for coronary artery disease in patients with end-stage renal failure. *Transplantation* 1990;49:100–103.
41. Melissinos K, Delidou A, Grammenou S, et al. Study of the activity of lymphocyte adenosine deaminase in chronic renal failure. *Clin Chim Acta* 1983;135:9.
42. Sutherland DER, Fryd DS, Ascher NL, et al. Detrimental effect of ABO mismatching in renal transplantation. *Transplant Proc* 1987;19:711.
43. Anderson CB, Tyler JD, Sicard GA, et al. Renal allograft recipient pretreatment with immunosuppression and donor specific blood. *Transplant Proc* 1985;17:1047.
44. Kahan BD, Van Buren CT, Flechner SM, et al. Clinical and experimental studies with cyclosporine in renal transplantation. *Surgery* 1985;97:125.
45. Colombe BW, Lou CD, Salvatierra O Jr, et al. Two patterns of sensitization demonstrated by recipients of donor specific transfusion. *Transplantation* 1987;44:509.
46. Werner-Favre C, Jeannet M, Harder F, et al. Blood transfusion, cytotoxic antibodies and kidney graft survival. *Transplantation* 1979;28:343.
47. Chapman JR, Taylor CJ, Ting A, et al. The positive cross-match: Antibody class and specificity correlate with graft outcome. *Transplant Proc* 1987;19:725.
48. Cardella CJ, Falk JA, Nicolson MJ, et al. Successful transplantation in patients with T cell reactivity to donor. *Lancet* 1982;2:1240.
49. Thistlewaite JR, Buckingham M, Stuart JK, et al. T cell immunofluorescence flow cytometry: cross match results in cadaver donor renal transplantation. *Transplant Proc* 1987;19:722.
50. Fuller TC, Cosimi AB, Russell PS. Use of an antiglobulin-ATG reagent for detection of low levels of alloantibody—improvement of allograft survival in presensitized patients. *Lancet* 1973; 1:573.
51. Kerman RH, Flechner SM, Van Buren CT, et al. Successful transplantation of cyclosporine-treated allograft recipients with sero-logically positive historical, but negative preoperative donor cross matches. *Transplantation* 1985;40:615.
52. Suranyi MG, Hall BM, Duggin GG, et al. T cell presensitization in renal transplantation. *Transplant Proc* 1987;19:896.
53. Sanfilippo F. Cross match testing in renal transplantation. Literature scan: *Transplantation* 1986;2.
54. Taube DH, Williams DG, Cameron JS, et al. Renal transplantation after removal and prevention of resynthesis of HLA antibodies. *Lancet* 1984;I:824.
55. Fauchald P, Leivestad T, Bratlie A, et al. Plasma exchange and immunosuppressive therapy before renal transplantation in highly sensitized patients. *Transplant Proc* 1987;19:727.
56. Pescovitz MD, Thistlethwaite JR Jr, Sharp T, et al. Class II histocompatibility complex-matched renal allografts in swine: Summary of current results and continuing studies. *Transplant Proc* 1985;17:686.
57. Kahan BD, Van Buren CT, Flechner SM, et al. Cyclosporine immunosuppression mitigates immunologic risk factors in renal transplantation. *Transplant Proc* 1983;15:2469.
58. Velosa JA, Anderson CF, Torres VE, et al. Long-term renal status of kidney donors: Calculated small risk of kidney donation. *Transplant Proc* 1985;17:100.
59. Weiland D, Sutherland DER, Chavers B, et al. Information on 628 living related kidney donors at a single institution with long term follow up in 472 cases. *Transplant Proc* 1984;16:5.
60. Harrison LH, Flye MW, Seigler HF. Incidence of anatomical variants in renal vasculature in the presence of normal renal function. *Ann Surg* 1978;188:83.
61. Kolata G. Organ shortage clouds new transplant era. *Science* 1983;221:32.
62. Rosenthal JT, Shaw BW Jr, Hardesty RL, et al. Principles of multiple organ procurement from cadaveric donors. *Ann Surg* 1983;198:617.
63. Starzl TE, Hakala TR, Shaw BW, et al. A flexible procedure for multiple cadaveric organ procurement. *Surg Gynecol Obstet* 1984;158:223.

64. Rowe JW, Andres R, Tobin JD, et al. The effects of age on creatinine clearance in man: A cross-sectional and longitudinal study. *J Gerontol* 1976;31:155.
65. Barry JM. Procurement and preservation of cadaver kidneys. *Urol Clin North Am* 1983;10:205.
66. Barry JM, Fischer S, Lieberman C, et al. Successful human kidney preservation by intracellular electrolyte flush followed by cold storage for more than 48 hours. *J Urol* 1983;129:473.
67. Grundman R, Strumper R, Eichmann J. The immediate function of the kidney after 24 to 72 hour preservation. *Transplantation* 1977;23:437.
68. Grodin W, Scantlebury V, Warmington N. Dopaminergic stimulation of renal blood flow and renal function after transplantation. *Anesthesiology* 1984;61:A129.
69. Williams GM. Clinical course following renal transplantation. In: Morris PJ ed. *Kidney transplantation*. New York: Grune and Stratton, 1984;335.
70. Jaffers GJ, Cosimi AB, Delmonico FL, et al. Experience with pyeloureterostomy in renal transplanation. *Ann Surg* 1982;196:588.
71. Glass NR, Uehling D, Sollinger H, et al. Renal transplantation using ileal conduit in five cases. *J Urol* 1985;133:666.
72. Cuvelier R, Pirson Y, Alexander GPJ, et al. Late urinary tract infection after transplantation: Prevalence, predisposition and morbidity. *Nephron* 1985;40:76.
73. Flye MW, Rigsby CM, Desire G, et al. Diagnosis of renal allograft rejection by radionuclide scintigraphy, pulsed Doppler scanning, Indium 111 labeled platelet scintigraphy and renal biopsy. *Transplant Proc* 1986;18:705.
74. Rigsby CM, Taylor KJW, Weltin G, et al. Renal allografts in acute rejection: Evaluation using duplex sonography. *Radiology* 1986;158:375.
75. Morris PJ. Immunosuppression in renal transplantation. *Transplant Proc* 1985;17:1153.
76. Dupont E, Wybran J, Toussaint C. Glucocorticosteroids and organ transplantation. *Transplantation* 1984;37:331.
77. Birtch AG, Carpenter CB, Tilney NL, et al. Controlled clinical trial of antilymphocyte globulin in human renal allografts. *Transplant Proc* 1971;3:762.
78. Turcotte JG, Feduska NJ, Haines RF, et al. A clinical trial of antithymocyte globulin in renal transplant recipients. *Arch Surg* 1973;106:484.
79. Hardy MA, Nowygrad R, Elberg A, et al. Use of ATG in treatment of steroid resistant rejection. *Transplantation* 1980;29:162.
80. Cosimi AB, Robert BC, Burton RC, et al. Use of monoclonal antibodies to T cell subsets for immunologic monitoring and treatment in recipients of renal allografts. *N Engl J Med* 1981;305:308.
81. Ortho Multicenter Transplant Study Group: A randomized clinical trial of OKT3 monoclonal antibody for acute rejection of cadaveric renal transplants. *N Engl J Med* 1985;313:337.
82. Borel JF, Feurer C, Gubler HU, et al. Biological effects of cyclosporin A: a new antilymphocyte agent. *Agents Actions* 1976;6:468.
83. Milton AD, Spencer SC, Fabre JW. Absence of class II major histocompatibility complex antigen induction in cyclosporine A-treated recipients of heart and kidney allografts in the rat. *Transplant Proc* 1987;19:192.
84. Kahan BD, Pellis NR, Leinikki, et al. Pharmacodynamic assays of the immunosuppressive action of cyclosporine therapy in transplant recipients. *Transplant Proc* 1987;19:1695.
85. Calne RY, Rolles K, White DJ, et al. Cyclosporin A initially as the immunosuppressant in 34 recipients of cadaveric organs. 32 kidneys, 2 pancreas and 2 livers. *Lancet* 1979;2:1033.
86. Rosenthal JT, Hakala TR, Iwatsuki S, et al. Cadaveric renal transplantation under cyclosporine-steroid therapy. *Surg Gynecol Obstet* 1983;157:309.
87. Merian RM, While DJG, Thirv S, et al. Cyclosporine: five years' experience in cadaveric renal transplantation. *N Engl J Med* 1984;310:148.
88. Calne RY, White DJG. The use of cyclosporin A in clinical organ grafting. *Ann Surg* 1982;196:330.
89. Canadian Multicentre Transplant Study Group. A randomized clinical trial of cyclosporine in cadaveric renal transplantation. *N Engl J Med* 1983;309:809.
90. Klinmalm G, Sundelin B, Bohman SO, et al. Interstitial fibrosis in renal allografts after 12 to 46 months of cyclosporin treatments: beneficial effects of low doses in early post-transplantation period. *Lancet* 1984;2:954.
91. Cohen DJ, Rolf L, Rubin MF, et al. Cyclosporine: A new immunosuppressive agent for organ transplantation. *Ann Intern Med* 1984;101:667.
92. Krakauer H, Grauman JS, McMullan MR, et al. The recent U.S. experience in the treatment of end-stage renal disease by dialysis and transplantation. *N Engl J Med* 1983;308:1558.
93. McDonald JC, Vaughn W, Filo RS, et al. Cadaver donor renal transplantation by centers of the South-Eastern Organ Procurement Foundation. *Ann Surg* 1984;200:536.
94. Tilney NL, Milford EL, Araujo JL, et al. Experience with cyclosporine and steroids in clinical renal transplantation. *Ann Surg* 1984;200:605.

95. Terasaki PI, Toyotome A, Mickey MR, et al. Patient, graft and functional survival rates: An overview. In: Teraski PI ed. *Clinical kidney transplants 1985*. Los Angeles, UCLA Tissue Typing Lab, 1985;1.

96. Bentley FR, Sutherland DER, Mauer SM, et al. The status of diabetic renal allograft recipients who survive for ten or more years after transplantation. *Transplant Proc* 1985;17:1573–1578.

97. Bilous RW, Mauer SM, Sutherland DER, Steffes MW. Glomerular structure and function following successful pancreas transplantation for insulin independent diabetes mellitus. *Diabetes* 1987;36:43A.

98. Ramsay RC, Goetz FC, Sutherland DER, et al. Progression of diabetic retinopathy after pancreas transplantation for insulin-dependent diabetes mellitus. *N Engl J Med* 1988;318:208.

99. Klein R, Klein BEK, Moss SE, et al. Glycosylated hemoglobin predicts the incidence and progression of diabetic retinopathy. *JAMA* 1988;260:2864.

100. Cowie CC, Port FK, Wolfe RA, et al. Disparities in incidence of diabetic end-stage renal disease according to race and type of diabetes. *N Engl J Med* 1989;321:1074–1079.

101. Beckseth RO, Kjellstrand CM. Radiologic contrast-induced nephropathy. *Med Clin North Am* 1984;68:351–370.

102. Sutherland DER, Fryd DS, Payne WD, Ascher N, et al. Kidney transplantation in diabetic patients. *Transplant Proc* 1987;2:90–94.

103. Eskstrand A, Gronhagen-Riska C, Groop L, Kuhlback B, et al. Outcome of patients with diabetic nephropathy after kidney transplantation. *Acta Med Scand* 1987;222:251–260.

104. Solders G, Wilczek H, Gunnarsson R, Tyden G, et al. Effects of combined pancreatic and renal transplantation on diabetic neuropathy: A two-year follow-up study. *Lancet* 1987;1232–1235.

105. Passlick J, Grabensee B. CAPD and transplantation in diabetics. *Clin Neph* 1988;30:(Suppl. 1)518–523.

106. Zander E, Schulz B, Jutzi E, et al. Frequency and therapy of end-stage renal disease due to diabetic nephropathy in the German Democratic Republic. *J Diab Compl* 1989;3:120–123.

107. Grenfell A, Bewick M, Parsons V, et al. Non-insulin-dependent diabetes and renal replacement therapy. *Diab Med* 1988;5:172–176.

108. Brunner FP. End-stage renal failure due to diabetic nephropathy: Data from the EDTA registry. *Diab Neph EDTA* 1988;127–135.

109. Miller DG, Levine SE, D'Elia JA, Bistrian BR. Nutritional status of diabetic and nondiabetic patients after renal transplantation. *Am J Clin Nutr* 1986;44:66–69.

110. Brunner FP, Brynger H, Callah S, et al. Renal replacement therapy in patients with diabetic nephropathy, 1980–1985. *Nephr Dial Trans* 1988;3:585–595.

Surgical Management of the Diabetic Patient,
edited by Michael Bergman and Gregorio A. Sicard.
Raven Press, Ltd., New York © 1991.

26

Pancreas and Islet Transplantation for the Treatment of Type I Diabetes Mellitus

Christopher S. McCullough and David W. Scharp

Division of General Surgery, Section of Organ Transplantation, The Islet Transplant Center, Washington University School of Medicine, St. Louis, Missouri 63110

The discovery of insulin in 1922 by Banting and Best had a profound effect on medicine and the prognosis for diabetic patients (1). There was a dramatic improvement in life expectancy due to the ability to control acute metabolic crises. At the Joslin Clinic in the preinsulin era the median survival for juvenile onset diabetes from the time of diagnosis of disease was 20 months (2). At the same institution from 1939–1959, the 10-year survival rate for a similar group of patients was greater than 95%. With increased longevity came the clinical appearance of the chronic complications of diabetes (e.g., retinopathy, nephropathy, neuropathy, and accelerated atherosclerosis), which previously were unknown because of the brief survival following onset of the disease. Specific treatments directed at these complications have been developed (e.g., laser therapy of diabetic retinopathy, renal transplantation, and reconstructive vascular surgery); however, prevention of these complications has been much more difficult to achieve. Though early mortality from ketoacidosis is now comparatively rare, the median survival for type I diabetes is still approximately 25 years less than for the population as a whole (2).

The exact relationship between the hyperglycemia and insulin deficiency of type I diabetes and the pathophysiology of the morbid complications of the disease remains uncertain. In animal models there is ample evidence to link hyperglycemia and insulin deficiency with retinopathy, nephropathy, and vascular disease (3–5). Unfortunately, no animal model exactly mimics human diabetes, and extrapolation of animal studies to human clinical disease must be done carefully. Both retrospective and prospective clinical studies tend to confirm the hypothesis that the onset and the severity of the morbid complications of type I diabetes mellitus are closely linked to the degree of metabolic control (6–13). Potential problems have been identified with both retrospective and prospective studies; however, the bulk of evidence strongly suggests that the complications of type I diabetes may be ameliorated or even prevented by physiologic glucose level control.

Attaining physiologic control of the underlying metabolic derangements of type I diabetes has been a difficult goal to achieve. The native pancreas secretes insulin continuously in response to blood glucose levels and other secretagogues, and maintains blood glucose levels within an exquisitely narrow range. Intermittent insulin injections, even multiple times per day, do not provide the same degree of continuous tight control of the normal pancreas. Continuous insulin delivery systems based on algorithms can provide tighter control of blood glucose levels than with exogenous injections and are often more convenient for the compliant and motivated patient. Currently, such systems lack a direct feedback loop from the blood glucose level and consequently do not provide physiologic control. In addition, such systems carry the real risk of inducing severe hypoglycemia (14). There is active research into durable sensors that will provide accurate feedback for a truly closed system; however, such sensors are not yet clinically practical (15). Currently, pancreas and islet transplantation are the only insulin replacement therapies which can offer the potential for physiologic glucose control.

The essential objective of transplantation for the patient with diabetes is to achieve insulin independence after transplantation of insulin-producing tissue providing sufficient metabolic control to prevent or at least stabilize diabetic complications. This means that the transplants must be done early in the course of the disease, which makes this kind of transplantation prophylactic. The use of immunosuppression as we know it today would, therefore, not be acceptable because of its risks. In addition, the fact that type 1, insulin-dependent diabetes mellitus (IDDM) is an autoimmune disease implies that the potential for autoimmune recurrence in the grafted islet tissue must also be considered. Thus, the challenge for both pancreas and islet transplantation is to achieve the objective of preventing complications while avoiding the use of standard immunosuppression and minimizing the potential of autoimmune recurrence. These goals need to be met in order for transplantation to become a practical alternative to insulin therapy.

PANCREAS TRANSPLANTATION

Pancreas transplantation is performed in patients with type I diabetes mellitus with the dual objectives of obtaining a normoglycemic state without the need for exogenous insulin and having a beneficial effect on the morbid complications of diabetes. Since 1978, the number of pancreas transplants performed per year has been steadily increasing. To date, over 2,000 pancreas transplants have been performed (16). Currently, the results of both graft function and patient survival are approaching those of renal transplantation (17).

Though experimental work on pancreas transplantation began in the last century (18), it was not until 1966 that the first pancreas transplant in a human was performed at the University of Minnesota (19). The graft functioned immediately and the patient was normoglycemic without the need for insulin administration. With the immunosuppressive medications available at that time, graft loss from rejection was high. Results were also adversely affected by a high incidence of technical problems such as thrombosis, leakage of exocrine secretions, sepsis, and suboptimal graft preservation. As a consequence, pancreas transplantation was performed infrequently at a few dedicated centers throughout the world. By the time cyclosporine was introduced in 1978, many of the technical problems had been satisfactorily resolved. Since 1978 there has been a steady increase in the number of pancreas transplants performed each year (16). Currently, over 2,000 pancreas transplants have been performed worldwide.

The vast majority of pancreases used for transplantation are obtained from cadaver donors. Living, related pancreas donation was pioneered at the University of

Minnesota (20) and this institution continues to have the most experience with this procedure (21,22). Most other centers, uncomfortable with the potential for short-term and long-term morbidity in the living donor, have elected to use brain-dead cadaver donors as the sole source of organs for pancreas transplantation.

Nearly any cadaver donor from whom other solid organs are being obtained can be a pancreas donor. Many cadaver organ donors are hyperglycemic as a consequence of CNS trauma, administration of large doses of exogenous steroids, dextrose in intravenous fluids, and the glycolytic action of exogenous catecholamines. Hyperglycemia, under these circumstances, is not a contraindication to pancreas donation if the donor has no prior history of diabetes. Likewise, hyperamylasemia per se is not a contraindication to pancreas donation. Maxillofacial trauma can cause hyperamylasemia by injury to the parotid glands. Blunt or penetrating CNS trauma can be associated with hyperamylasemia without evidence of injury to any other organ system (23). Direct pancreatic trauma or gross pathology identified in the pancreas at the time of procurement preclude the use of the gland for whole-organ transplantation. Such a gland might still be used for obtaining islets for transplantation, however.

In the past, the shared blood supply of the pancreas and the liver created controversy as to whether both organs could be safely obtained from the same donor and function optimally in the respective recipients. It is now clear that simultaneous procurement of both the liver and a whole pancreas graft can be achieved safely in nearly all circumstances (24,25). It may be necessary to reconstruct the arterial supply and/or extend the portal vein of the pancreas with the donor iliac artery or vein (26). In the rare circumstance where the anatomy absolutely precludes the simultaneous procurement of a whole pancreas graft and the liver, the liver is given priority as the life-saving organ. In these circumstances, the pancreas may be used as a segmental graft (distal pancreas) or obtained in its entirety for islet transplantation after the liver has been removed.

Currently, the University of Wisconsin solution (ViaSpan, manufactured by Du Pont) is favored as the preservation vehicle of choice (27,28). Use of this cold storage solution has allowed successful storage of the pancreas for up to 24 hours. This important achievement may allow for organ sharing based on optimal human leukocyte antigen (HLA) matching.

Various technical approaches to pancreas transplantation have been taken at different centers. These differences lie mainly in the management of pancreas exocrine secretions, using all or a segment of the pancreas for transplantation, and in the route of venous drainage—either systematically or by venous drainage directed into the portal system.

When the pancreas is transplanted, it maintains essentially all of its usual functions involving both endocrine and exocrine systems. The management of the exocrine component has been a difficult problem in the historic development of pancreas transplantation. Currently, three methods are used: drainage of the exocrine secretions into the small bowel, drainage into the urinary bladder, or obliteration of exocrine function by injection of the pancreatic duct with a polymer at the time of transplantation. Enteric drainage should be regarded as the most physiologic approach; however, the incidence of sepsis is increased with this procedure and the exocrine secretions of the pancreas cannot be monitored. Consequently, biopsy of the graft requires either a percutaneous or an open technique. Bladder drainage, although not physiologic, is associated with fewer complications and allows the direct monitoring of pancreatic exocrine function (17). The ability to monitor exocrine function through the quantification of urinary amylase is the current mainstay of monitoring for pancreas graft rejection. In addition, biopsy of the pancreas can be performed with relative safety using a transcystoscopic technique (29). Polymer injection of the pancreatic duct offers the advantage of eliminating the problems associated with the acute leakage and the chronic loss of pancreatic exocrine secretions. This technique precludes the ability to monitor exocrine function, however, and has been associated with a progressive fibrosis of the exocrine portion of the gland and potentially impaired endocrine function (30). Despite the purported advantages or disadvantages of a single technique of exocrine management, the International Pancreas Transplant Registry, directed by Dr. David E.R. Sutherland at the University of Minnesota, shows that in a comparison of technically successful grafts between 1983 and 1988 there was no significant difference in 1-year patient (84–86%) or functional graft survival (63–66%) between techniques (16).

Either the entire pancreas or a segment consisting of the body and tail of the pancreas can be used for pancreas transplantation. Although transplantation of the entire pancreas would provide endocrine reserve that has the potential to enable a graft to retain function after a rejection episode, both techiques provide sufficeint islet mass to produce normoglycemia and insulin independence. Again, the International Registry data indicate no difference in functional graft survival up to 4 years (16). It is now possible to safely obtain both the whole pancreas graft and the liver for transplantation from the same cadaver donor; many centers in this country favor using the whole pancreas graft. Use of the whole pancreas allows inclusion of a segment of duodenum to be included with the transplant. This facilitates the anastomosis to either the urinary bladder or to the small bowel for the management of exocrine secretions.

Providing venous drainage from the pancreas graft into the portal system is more physiologic than the use of systemic venous drainage; this technique has only been used at a small number of centers (31–34). By far the more common and technically easier technique is to anastomose the venous outflow of the pancreas to the iliac veins or to the inferior vena cava (35), resulting in systemic insulin delivery. This may be viewed as analogous to insulin injection therapy where the hormone is delivered directly into the systemic circulation. The arterial anastomosis is determined by the choice of venous drainage. As the most common arrangement of venous drainage is into the cava or iliac veins, the most convenient approach for arterial anastomosis is therefore well into the common or external iliac artery.

The immunosuppression protocols used for pancreas transplantation are generally similar to those for kidney transplantation. As a consequence, patients who receive a combined pancreas and kidney transplantation from the same donor [approximately two-thirds of grafts reported to the International Registry between 1984 and 1988 (16)] should incur no additional immunosuppressive morbidity over and above what would have been required for their kidney transplant alone. Each transplantation center has its own protocol for the management of immunosuppression and therefore no standard approach has been formulated. Similarly, no single center has accumulated a large enough series to study specific protocols in a randomized, prospective fashion. Much has been extrapolated from the kidney transplant experience. General trends can be seen in the International Registry data as analyzed by Sutherland and Moudry-Munns (16). Combination therapy including cyclosporine, prednisone, and azathioprine is associated with superior graft survival when compared with regimens that do not include either cyclosporine or azathioprine. The elimination of glucocorticoids may be desirable from the standpoint of glucose homeostasis (36), but this is not done routinely. Elimination of steroids from the immunosuppression regimen has been associated with an increased risk for rejection episodes in kidney transplant recipients (37,38). Induction quadruple therapy with the addition of either a polyclonal antilymphocyte globulin or monoclonal antibody (OKT-3), as is frequently used in renal transplantation, has not been associated with an improvement in pancreas graft survival in those cases that have been reported to the International Registry (16).

Among solid organ transplants, the pancreas is unique in that an entire organ is transplanted for the therapeutic effect provided by a small portion (approximately 2%) of the cells contained therein. It is perhaps paradoxical that at the same time it is the nonendocrine portion of the native pancreas that expresses the vast majority of HLA antigens that are responsible for organ rejection. The native pancreas has a measurable level of expression of class I and II transplantation (HLA) antigens (39). These are predominantly seen within the vascular endothelium, ducts, and the exocrine portion of the pancreas. Normally the Islets of Langerhans have a very low level of HLA expression (40). Normal endocrine cells within the pancreas do not express HLA Class II (DR) antigens, which is limited to the microvascular endothelium and dendritic cells interspersed between the endocrine cells of the islets (39,41). Following this discordant distribution of HLA antigens, it appears that on both histologic and clinical grounds cellular rejection of the pancreas graft is initiated in the nonendocrine portion (42,43). Extensive work by Sibley, based on the experience at the University of Minnesota, has shown that the mononuclear cell infiltrate associated with acute pancreas graft rejection is predominantly seen in the vasculature and the ductal and acinar epithelium (39,44). The Islets of Langerhans generally show minimal or no involvement. Similarly, in bladder drained pancreas grafts a significant fall in the urinary amylase secretion rate often heralds an acute rejection episode, while the blood glucose level remains under good control (45).

There is good evidence to support that matching of HLA antigens between donor and recipient has a beneficial effect on the outcome of cadaver donor kidney transplants (46,47). This is particularly true for matching at the DR loci. Evidence is now accumulating that supports the conclusion that matching for the HLA-DR loci has a positive effect on the functional graft survival of pancreas transplants as well. Data extracted from the International Registry demonstrate that matching for HLA-A and -B loci had little if any effect on graft survival. Conversely, matching for DR antigens significantly improved the 1-year functional graft survival rate from 61 to 84% for technically successful cases (16). These findings have been supported by similar results in single centers with extensive experience. So et al. (48) from the University of Minnesota found that for all technically successful cases the functional graft survival was 69% when there was matching for one or two DR loci versus 50% when there was no DR match between donor and recipient.

Rejection is the primary cause of loss of graft function in technically successful pancreas transplants (49). Monitoring techniques for acute rejection in the pancreas graft are not as sensitive and specific as would be desired. Observations from multiple centers have shown that the return of hyperglycemia is probably a late finding and is associated with significant injury to the graft (50). Such patients have a poor prognosis for recovery of adequate graft function even if treatment successfully reverses the rejection. As acute rejection cannot, at this time, be prevented safely in all cases, methods need to be developed to detect rejection at an early stage; successful treatment would therefore leave the patient euglycemic and independent of exogenous insulin. In those patients who receive a simultaneous pancreas and kidney transplant from the same donor, an acute rejection episode frequently involves both transplanted organs. Elevation of the serum creatinine level is a sensitive marker for acute rejection in the transplanted kidney. Confirmation of renal allograft rejection can be easily accomplished by percutaneous renal allograft biopsy with minimal morbidity for the patient. Demonstration of rejection in the transplanted kidney does not prove the presence of rejection in the simultaneously transplanted pancreas, and isolated rejection of one or the other of these grafts has been reported; however, treatment of the documented renal allograft rejection simultaneously treats rejection in the pancreas graft. Perhaps as a consequence, patients who are recipients of a simultaneous pancreas and kidney transplant have a significantly better functional pancreas graft survival than patients who receive a pancreas transplant after having had a kidney transplant, or nonuremic diabetics who receive a pancreas transplant only (16).

In the early experience with pancreas transplantation, technical complications were not infrequent and the result was often graft loss, patient morbidity and mortality. Refinements in the techniques of exocrine management have significantly reduced the incidence of leakage with abscess formation or pancreaticocutaneous fistula. If leakage does occur, prompt surgical management may salvage a functioning graft (51). If there is gross infection, however, graft removal may be the most prudent course of action.

Graft thrombosis has historically been a major cause of pancreatic graft failure (52,53), which has been attributed to unfavorable hemodynamics within the pancreatic graft (54). The pancreas is a relatively low-flow organ and therefore stagnation with thrombosis has been thought to be more likely. Aggressive anticoagulation has been used to reduce the incidence of thrombosis (55). Although aggressive anticoagulation may reduce the incidence of graft thrombosis, the risk of serious bleeding complications is significantly increased. Current reports suggest that the incidence of graft thrombosis occurs less frequently than in the past. Careful construction and alignment of the vascular anastomoses, particularly the venous anastomosis, improved organ preservation, and modest anticoagulation with antiplatelet agents and low-dose heparin probably accounts for the significant decrease in the incidence of graft thrombosis that was once a common cause of early graft failure.

On a long-term basis, several complications can be the result of the use of a whole pancreaticoduodenal graft with bladder drainage. These include metabolic acidosis from loss of bicarbonate in the urine (56), hyponatremia (57), and symptomatic urinary tract inflammation (53,56). Mild cases of these metabolic complications often are successfully managed medically with oral replacement of bicarbonate or sodium. Severe cases have been successfully treated by surgical conversion from bladder drainage to enteric drainage (58).

Graft pancreatitis may occur either early or late following pancreas transplantation. Some degree of hyperamylasemia immediately following transplantation is expected and probably reflects preservation effect of the graft. In these circumstances the rise in amylase is usually modest and begins to return towards normal levels within 3–6 days. Marked pancreatitis shortly following transplantation may reflect inadequate preservation or excessively long cold or warm ischemic periods. If severe, this may necessitate graft removal. Pancreatitis or hyperamylasemia can also occur late following transplantation. Infrequently, this may represent a rejection episode (59) although more often the cause is not definitely identified and may be attributable to reflux in bladder-drained grafts. Treatment should include bladder decompression with a Foley catheter. Recurrent episodes of pancreatitis could require conversion to enteric drainage (60).

Since the first pancreas transplant in 1966, there has been a steady improvement in both patient and functional graft survival. Currently, for the International Pancreas Transplant Registry, the 1-year actuarial patient survival rate is reported as 88%, and the functional graft survival rate is 55% (16). These data represent a compilation from all reporting centers. Some individual centers have reported patient survival rates greater than 90% and graft survival rates greater than 80% at 1 year (17). The improvement in patient and graft survival is due to a combination of many factors, including technical improvements, better organ preservation, improved immunosuppression, and increased ability to monitor and detect rejection.

Following successful pancreas transplantation, diabetic patients become insulin independent and generally have a normal fasting blood glucose level. The response to either oral glucose tolerance tests or to intravenous glucose tolerance tests, however, are frequently moderately abnormal (54,61). This may be due, in part, to metabolic effects of the steroids and cyclosporine used for immunosuppression (62). When the 24-hour metabolic profiles of diabetic recipients of a pancreas transplant are compared with those of nondiabetic recipients of a kidney allograft on similar immunosuppression, they are found to be very similar (63,64). Hemoglobin A1C levels generally are significantly reduced and return to normal levels in many patients (65). Patients who have their pancreatic graft drained into the systemic venous circulation manifest resting and stimulated hyperinsulinemia (64,65). Unlike serum insulin levels, serum glucagon levels remain in the normal range (64), reflecting an appropriate physiologic response to normal or near-normal blood glucose levels.

Although the immediate results of pancreas transplantation on metabolism are fairly well established, the data concerning the long-term effect of successful pancreas transplantation on the morbid complications of diabetes are only recently becoming available. In general, it appears that establishing insulin independence and normoglycemia has a beneficial effect on these complications (as described in the following paragraphs). It is clear, however, that in many patients with long-standing disease, much of the pathology is irreversible and the best that can be expected is stabilization.

When a diabetic patient receives a normal kidney, recurrence of the diabetic nephropathy, based on histologic examination, is an almost universal occurrence (66,67). Conversely, it has been reported that a diabetic kidney transplanted into a nondiabetic recipient shows reversal of the characteristic histologic changes of diabetic nephropathy (68). Pancreatic transplantation has been shown to protect the simultaneously or previously transplanted kidney from recurrent diabetic nephropathy (69,70). It is not known whether successful pancreas transplantation, performed early in the course of the disease, will prevent or reverse pathologic changes in the native kidney.

Although the data concerning prevention or stabilization of diabetic changes in the transplanted kidney are clear and consistent among various groups, the results with regard to diabetic retinopathy are less straightforward. Studies comparing diabetic patients who received a pancreas alone (71) or a pancreas and a kidney (72) to similar diabetic cohorts who lost their pancreatic graft showed no significant difference between the two groups as far as stabilization or progression of retinopathy. Similar findings of the lack of significant change in retinopathy have been reported by other investigators (73–75). When small numbers of patients with early retinopathy (69,72) or nonuremic recipients of a pancreas alone (76) are examined, however, there is a trend towards stabilization of retinal changes. Longer follow-up may demonstrate an advantage with pancreas transplantation in this group of patients with established retinopathy. The absence of convincing improvement or even prevention of progression of established retinopathy should not be surprising. In an experimental dog model, failure to correct experimental hyperglycemia within 2 months after onset is associated with the development of diabetic retinopathy (77). The nonenzymatic glycosylation of tissue proteins caused by hyperglycemia may lead to progressive cross-linkage of structural proteins despite reinstitution of normoglycemia (78). These changes, in turn, may lead to progressive retinal deterioration (79). These findings suggest that successful pancreas transplantation at an earlier phase of the disease may be more successful in preserving visual acuity.

The effects of pancreatic transplantation on established diabetic neuropathy are also not definitive. Kennedy et al. (80), working at the University of Minnesota, showed definite continuous improvement in neurophysiologic parameters over 42 months. A control group of nontransplanted diabetic patients showed progressive deterioration using the same neurophysiologic parameters. In contrast to neurophysiologic parameters, clinical evaluation of this same group of patients showed no significant changes over the period of study. The Minnesota study did find that motor-nerve function parameters were more apt to improve than sensory-nerve parameters. They also noted that patients with minimal abnormalities improved the most (80). Other investigators, however, have found no significant improvement in diabetic neuropathy with successful pancreas transplantation or have attributed any improvement to elimination of uremia in patients who received both a pancreas and a kidney (81). Evaluation of established diabetic autonomic neuropathy by several groups has failed to demonstrate any improvement following pancreas transplantation (80–82).

Although there is an appreciation that diabetes is associated with accelerated atherosclerosis, little is known about the impact of pancreas transplantation on the course of this disease process in diabetic patients. Pancreas transplantation in long-standing diabetic patients has not been shown to prolong survival. Indeed, the most frequent cause of death in patients with established, functioning pancreas allografts is cardiovascular.

In summary, pancreas transplantation, if technically successful and not abrogated by rejection, is the only current insulin replacement therapy that can consistently establish a near-normoglycemic state with insulin independence. Most pancreas transplants have been performed in patients with advanced diabetes and established secondary complications. As a consequence, the impact on the secondary complications has not been dramatic. The available evidence, however, strongly suggests that successful pancreas transplantation at an earlier stage of the disease, before establishment of irreversible pathologic changes, prevents many of the morbid complications of diabetes. More effective and safer immunosuppression must be developed before this mode of therapy can be offered to diabetic patients in the earliest phases of their disease.

ISLET TRANSPLANTATION

Whereas technical and immunosuppressive developments have resulted in clinical improvements having an impact on pancreas transplantation throughout the 1980s, islet transplantation has been relying on animal studies to prove feasibility because the main barrier to clinical application has been the inability to isolate sufficient numbers of islets to achieve insulin independence (83). The first patient to achieve insulin independence following islet transplantation was reported in the literature in 1990 (84). This was accomplished through developments in the islet isolation processing and the use of islets from two cadaver donated pancreata. This result has been accomplished a second time with current islet function for over 4 months with normalized glucose tolerance testing. Thus, during the 1990s the development of islet transplantation should advance through the use of clinical trials in diabetic patients to determine its feasibility in comparison to pancreas transplantation in patients with type I diabetes.

The ability to isolate islets from the pancreas began in 1967 in the guinea pig pancreas using a mixture of enzymes found in collagenase preparations produced by bacteria (85). Lacy (86) demonstrated that distension of the pancreatic duct increased the yield of isolated islets, apparently by breaking the islet-acinar interface. The first demonstrations of the feasibility of islet transplantation were by Ballinger and Lacy (86) and Barker's group (87) in 1972 in a diabetic rodent model. The direct injection of islets into the portal vein led to a more efficient model of islet transplantation (88), which has been the basis for a large number of animal islet transplant studies. This topic summarizing the development of the animal research has been recently reviewed (83,89–92). The basic information from these studies confirms that islet transplantation can provide long-term metabolic control without the need for insulin therapy in the rodent and canine models of diabetes. In addition, transplantation of islet tissue before diabetic complications develop in rodents can prevent the complications of the disease. Thus, the first two prerequisites for long-term success in diabetic patients have been demonstrated by animal research. The latest achievement of insulin independence in diabetic patients demonstrates that this objective has also been met in man.

The major impediment to practical application of transplanting insulin-producing islet tissue in diabetic patients early in the course of their disease is the need to prevent rejection of the transplanted islet tissue. Whole pancreas transplantation relies on classic immunosuppression, which is now fairly successful. Yet, the use of these drugs is not practical for the younger diabetic patient requiring a prophylactic transplant to prevent the complications due to the toxicity of the immunosuppressants. The use of purified islet tissue has the potential to be a major advantage over pancreas transplantation in this regard. There are two technical approaches available for islet transplantation because they are small, cellular organs that can be manipulated *in vitro* prior to transplantation. The two approaches are immunoalteration, in which the purified islets are treated *in vitro* to eliminate donor immune cells; and immunoisolation, in which the islets are protected by various membranes at the time of transplantation (93). Snell (94) in 1957, suggested that the barrier to transplantation was not cellular antigens per se from the transplanted organs, but the donor immune cells that were included in the transplanted organ. These passenger immune cells are the antigen-presenting cells that come into contact with the recipient T lymphocytes, converting them to the killer cells specific for the grafted tissue. Although this idea was not developed for many years, the establishment of islet transplantation provided an opportunity to test this concept.

Preliminary rodent results of immunoaltered islets confirmed this concept (93,95,96). In other words, purified islets could be treated *in vitro* to remove the donor antigen presenting cells which could then be successfully transplanted without long-term immunosuppression as either allografts or xenografts. There have now been several *in vitro* methods of treating the islets, which include 7 days of 24°C culture, high oxygen exposure, the use of several types of antibodies directed against the antigen-presenting immune cells, ultraviolet light, and other types of processing that selectively rid the islets of these cells. In addition, transient treatment of the recipient has also been successful, such as the use of antilymphocyte sera or immunosuppressants combined with the *in vitro* treatments. Thus, the concept of immunoalteration of islets has been proven in rodents. Effective clinical trials in patients are presently required to determine if the human immune system will react in a similar fashion.

The second advantage of using purified islets is the ability to encapsulate them in various types of devices to permit their function while preventing the recipients immune system from attacking the grafts (93). The feasibility of this approach in the short-term has been documented, but long-term graft acceptance has been prevented to date due to biocompatibility problems with the membranes used in these devices. The body so far has walled off these devices by fibrosis, which stops diffusion, leading to death of the islets. New biomaterials are being tested to find those not susceptible to this process. Another approach to immunoisolation is to place a biochemical membrane around the islets directly or the production of microcapsules of alginate and polylysine (97). This approach is promising, however, details regarding the long-term success and the ability to encapsulate and transplant large numbers of islets by this method must still be determined.

Thus, in terms of islet transplantation, the era of the 1990s should be one of continuing clinical trials to prove the feasibility of transplanting with a combination of various immunosuppressants to determine the optimal regimen for the patient who needs immunosuppression for a kidney transplant. This time should also be one of determining the practical feasibility of immunoalteration and immunoisolation approaches in large animal models and clinical trials in diabetic patients. In terms of pancreas transplantation, the 1990s should be a time of documenting the practical aspects of this technique and comparing them with those of islet transplantation. Success in these studies should determine whether the concept of transplanting insulin-producing tissue can be a practical alternative therapy for the diabetic patient that can prevent the complications and avoid the current risks of immunosuppression.

REFERENCES

1. Banting FG, Best CH. The internal secretion of the pancreas. *J Lab Clin Med* 1922;7:251.
2. Krolewski AS, Warram JH, Christlieb AR. Onset, course, complications, and prognosis of diabetes mellitus. In: Marble A, Krall LP, Bradley RF, Christlieb AR, Soeldner JS, eds. *Joslin's diabetes mellitus*, 12th ed. Philadelphia: Lea & Febiger, 1985;251–277.
3. Engerman R, Bloodworth JMB Jr, Nelson S. Relationship of microvascular disease in diabetes to metabolic control. *Diabetes* 1977;26:760.
4. Bloodworth JMB Jr, Engerman RL. Diabetic microangiopathy in the experimentally diabetic dog and its prevention by careful control with insulin. *Diabetes* 1973;22(Suppl. 1):290.

5. Howard CF Jr. Aortic atherosclerosis in normal and spontaneously diabetic *Macaca nigra*. *Atherosclerosis* 1979;33:479.
6. Job D, Eschwege E, Guyot-Argenton C, et al. Effect of multiple daily insulin injections on the course of diabetic retinopathy. *Diabetes* 1976;25:463.
7. Eschwege E, Job D, Guyot-Argenton C, et al. Delayed progression of diabetic retinopathy by divided insulin administration: a further follow-up. *Diabetologia* 1979;16:13.
8. Miki E, Kuzuya T, Ide T, Nakao K. Frequency, degree, and progression with time of proteinuria in diabetic patients. *Lancet* 1972;1:922.
9. Takazakura E, Nakamoto Y, Hayakawa H, et al. Onset and progression of diabetic glomerulosclerosis. A prospective study based on serial renal biopsies. *Diabetes* 1975;24:1.
10. Pirart J. Diabetes mellitus and its degenerative complications: a prospective study of 4,400 patients observed between 1947 and 1973. (Part 1). *Diabetes Care* 1978;1:168.
11. Pirart J. Diabetes mellitus and its degenerative complications: a prospective study of 4,400 patients observed between 1947 and 1973. (Part 2). *Diabetes Care* 1978;1:252.
12. Tchobroutsky G. Relationship of diabetic control to development of microvascular complications. *Diabetologia* 1978;15:143.
13. Hanssen KF, Dahl-Jorgensen K, Lauritzen T, Feldt-Rasmussen B, Brinchmann-Hansen O, Deckert T. Diabetic control and microvascular complication: the near-normoglycaemic experience. *Diabetologia* 1986;29:677.
14. Ungar RH. Meticulous control of diabetes: benefits, risks and precautions. *Diabetes* 1982;31:479.
15. Pfeiffer EF. On the way to the automated (blood) glucose regulation in diabetes: the dark past, the grey present and the rosy future. *Diabetologia* 1987;30:51.
16. Sutherland DER, Moudry-Munns KC. International pancreas transplant registry report. In: Terakai PI, ed. *Clinical transplants 1988*. Los Angeles: UCLA Tissue Typing Laboratory, 1988; 53–64.
17. Sollinger HW, Stratta RJ, D'Alessandro AM, Kalayoglu M, Pirsch JD, Belzer FO. Experience with simultaneous pancreas-kidney transplantation. *Ann Surg* 1988;208:475.
18. Hedon E. Sur la consummationdusucre ches le chien apres l'extirpadon de pancreas. *Arch Phys Norm Path* 1893;5:154.
19. Kelly WD, Lillehei RC, Merkel FK, et al. Allotransplantation of the pancreas and duodenum along with the kidney in diabetic nephropathy. *Surgery* 1967;61:827.
20. Sutherland DER, Goetz FC, Najarian JS. Living related donor segmental pancreatectomy for transplantation. *Transplant Proc* 1980;12(Suppl. 2):19.
21. Bolinder J, Gunnarsson R, Tyden G, Brattstrom C, Ostman J, Groth CG. Metabolic effects of living related pancreatic graft donation. *Transplant Proc* 1988;20:475.
22. Kendall DM, Sutherland DER, Najarian JS, Goetz FC, Robertson RP. Effects of hemipancreatectomy on insulin secretion and glucose tolerance in healthy humans. *N Engl J Med* 1990;322:898.
23. Hesse UJ, Najarian JS, Sutherland DER. Amylase activity and pancreas transplants. *Lancet* 1985;2:726.
24. Dunn DL, Schlumpf RB, Gruessner RWG, et al. Maximal use of liver and pancreas from cadaveric organ donors. *Transplant Proc* 1990;22:423.
25. Spees EK, Orlowski JP, Temple DR, Kam I, Karrer IF. Efficacy of simultaneous cadaveric pancreas and liver recovery. *Transplant Proc* 1990;22:427.
26. Ngheim DD, Schulak JA, Corry RJ. Duodenopancreatectomy for transplantation. *Arch Surg* 1987;122:1201.
27. Barr D, Munn SR, Carpenter HA, Perkins JD. A prospective comparison of two preservation solutions in human pancreaticoduodenal transplantation. *Transplant Proc* 1990;22:529.
28. D'Alessandro AM, Sollinger HW, Hoffman RM, et al. Experience with Belzer UW cold storage solution in simultaneous pancreas-kidney transplantation. *Transplant Proc* 1990;22:532.
29. Perkins JD, Engen DE, Munn SR, Barr D, Marsh CL, Carpenter HA. The value of cystoscopically-directed biopsy in human pancreaticoduodenal transplantation. *Clin Transplantation* 1989;3:306.
30. Heptner W, Neubauer HP, Schleyerbach R. Glucose tolerance and insulin secretion in rabbits and dogs after ligation of the pancreatic duct. *Diabetologia* 1974;10:193.
31. Calne RY. Paratopic segmental pancreas grafting: a technique with portal venous drainage. *Lancet* 1984;1:595.
32. Sutherland DER, Goetz FC, Abouna GM, et al. Use of recipient meseneric vessels for revascularization of segmental pancreas transplants. *Transplant Proc* 1987;19:2300.
33. Gil-Vernet JM, Fernandez-Cruz L, Andreu J, Figuerola D, Caralps A. Clinical experience with pancreaticopyelostomy for exocrine pancreatic drainage and portal venous drainage in pancreas transplantation. *Transplant Proc* 1985;17:342.
34. Tyden G, Wilczek H, Lundgren G, et al. Experience with 21 intraperitoneal segmental pancreatic transplants with enteric or gastric exocrine diversion in humans. *Transplant Proc* 1985; 17:331.

35. Sutherland DER, Ascher NL, Najarian JS. Pancreas Transplantation. In: Simmons RL, Finch ME, Ascher NL, Najarian JS, eds. *Manual of vascular access, organ donation, and transplantation.* New York: Springer-Verlag, 1984;237–254.
36. Cantarovich D, Dantal J, Murat A, Soulillou JP. Normal glucose metabolism and insulin secretion on CyA-treated nondiabetic renal allograft patients not receiving steroids. *Transplant Proc* 1990;22:643.
37. Christinelli L, Brunori G, Setti G, et al. Withdrawal of methylprednisolone at the sixth month in renal transplant recipients treated with cyclosporine. *Transplant Proc* 1989;19:2021.
38. Brown MW, Forwell MA. Rejection reaction after stopping prednisolone in kidney-transplant recipients taking cyclosporine. *N Engl J Med* 1986;314:183.
39. Sibley RK, Sutherland DER. Pancreas transplantation: an immunohistologic and histopathologic examination of 100 grafts. *Am J Path* 1987;128:151.
40. Daar AS, Fuggle SV, Fabre JW, Ting A, Morris PJ. The detailed distribution of HLA-A, B, C antigens in normal human organs. *Transplantation* 1984;38:287.
41. Daar AS, Fuggle SV, Fabre JW, Ting A, Morris PJ. The detailed distribution of MHC class II antigens in normal human organs. *Transplantation* 1984;38:293.
42. Severyn JA, Olson L, Miller J, et al. Studies on the survival of simultaneous canine renal and segmental pancreatic allografts. *Transplantation* 1982;33:606.
43. Groth CG, Lundgren G, Arner P, et al. Rejection of isolated pancreatic allografts in patients with diabetes. *Surg Gynecol Obstet* 1976;143:933.
44. Sutherland DER, Casanova D, Sibley RK. Role of pancreas graft biopsies in the diagnosis and treatment of rejection after pancreas transplantation. *Transplant Proc* 1987;19:2329.
45. Perkins JD, Munn SR, Marsh CL, Barr D, Engen DE, Carpenter HA. Safety and efficacy of cystoscopically directed biopsy in pancreas transplantation. *Transplant Proc* 1990;22:665.
46. Cho YW, Terasaki PI. UCLA registry: long-term survival. In: Terasaki PI, ed. *Clinical transplants 1988.* Los Angeles: UCLA Tissue Typing Laboratory, 1988;277.
47. Cicciarelli J, Corcoran S. An update on HLA matching, including HLA "epitope" matching: a new approach. In: Terasaki PI, ed. *Clinical transplants 1988.* Los Angeles: UCLA Tissue Typing Laboratory, 1988;329.
48. So SKS, Minford EJ, Moudry-Munns KC, Gillingham K, Sutherland DER. DR matching improves cadaveric pancreas transplant results. *Transplant Proc* 1990;22:687.
49. Tyden G. Pancreatic graft rejection. In: Groth CG, ed. *Pancreatic transplantation,* Philadelphia: W. B. Saunders, 1988;249–267.
50. Dubernard JM, Traeger J, Touraine JL, Malik MC, Martin X, Devonec M. Patterns of renal and pancreatic rejection in double-grafted patients. *Transplant Proc* 1981;13:305.
51. Gruessner RWG, Dunn DL, Tzardis PJ, Nakhleh RI, Najarian JS, Sutherland DER. Complications occurring after whole organ duodenopancreatic transplantation: relation to the allograft duodenal segment. *Transplant Proc* 1990;22:578.
52. Dubernard JM, Traeger J, Martin X, Faure JL, Devonec M. Pancreatic transplantation in man: surgical technique and complications. *Transplant Proc* 1980;12:40.
53. Sutherland DER, Goetz FC, Najarian JS. One hundred pancreas transplants at a single institution. *Ann Surg* 1984;200:414.
54. Groth CG. Surgical complications following pancreatic transplantation. In: Groth CG, ed. *Pancreatic transplantation,* Philadelphia: W.B. Saunders, 1988;219–238.
55. Tollemar J, Tyden G, Brattstrom C, Groth CG. Anticoagulation therapy for prevention of pancreatic graft thrombosis—benefits and risks. *Transplant Proc* 1988;20:479.
56. Munda R, Tom WW, First MR, Alexander JW. Pancreatic allograft exocrine urinary tract diversion: pathophysiology. *Transplantation* 1987;43:95.
57. Raab HAA, Niles JL, Cosimi AB, Tolkoff-Rubin NE. Severe hyponatremia associated with combined pancreatic and renal transplantation. *Transplantation* 1989;48:157.
58. Burke GW, Gruessner R, Dunn DL, Sutherland DER. Conversion of whole pancreaticoduodenal transplants from bladder to enteric drainage for metabolic acidosis or dysuria. *Transplant Proc* 1990;22:651.
59. Stratta RJ, Sollinger HW, Groshek M, et al. Differential diagnosis of hyperamylasemia in pancreas allograft recipients. *Transplant Proc* 1990;22:675.
60. Boudreaux JP, Nealon WH, Carson RC, Fish JC. Pancreatitis necessitating urinary undiversion in a bladder-drained pancreas transplant. *Transplant Proc* 1990;22:641.
61. Pozza G, Traeger J, Dubernard JM, et al. Endocrine responses of type 1 (insulin dependent) diabetic patients following successful pancreas transplantation. *Diabetologia* 1983;24:244.
62. Yale JF, Roy RD, Grose M, Seemayer TA, Murphy GF, Marliss EB. Effects of cyclosporin on glucose tolerance in the rat. *Diabetes* 1985;34:1309.
63. Sutherland DER, Najarian JS, Greenberg BZ. Hormonal and metabolic effects of a pancreatic endocrine graft. Vascularized segmental transplantation in insulin-dependent diabetic patients. *Ann Int Med* 1981;95:537.
64. Pozza G, Bosi E, Secchi A, et al. Metabolic control of type 1 diabetes after pancreas transplantation. *Br Med J* 1985;291:510.

65. Landgraf R, Landgraf-Leurs MMC, Burg D. Long-term follow-up of segmental pancreas transplantation on type I diabetes. *Transplant Proc* 1986;18:1118.
66. Mauer SM, Barbosa J, Vernier RL, et al. Development of vascular diabetic lesions in kidneys transplanted into patients with diabetes mellitus. *N Engl J Med* 1976;295:916.
67. Mauer SM, Goetz FC, McHugh LE, et al. Long-term study of normal kidneys transplanted into patients with type I diabetes. *Diabetes* 1989;38:516.
68. Abouna GM, Al-Adnani MS, Kremer GD, Kumar SA, Daddah SK, Kusma G. Reversal of diabetic nephropathy in human cadaveric kidneys after transplantation into non-diabetic recipients. *Lancet* 1983;2:1274.
69. Bohman SO, Wilczek H, Tyden G, Jaremko G, Lundgren G, Groth CG. Recurrent diabetic nephropathy in renal transplants placed in diabetic patients and the protective effect of simultaneous pancreatic transplantation. *Transplant Proc* 1987;19:2290.
70. Bilous RW, Mauer SM, Sutherland DER, Najarian JS, Goetz FC, Steffes MW. The effects of pancreas transplantation on glomerular structure of renal allografts in patients with insulin-dependent diabetes. *N Engl J Med* 1989;321:80.
71. Ramsay RC, Goetz FC, Sutherland DER. Progression of diabetic retinopathy after pancreas transplantation for insulin dependent diabetes mellitus. *N Engl J Med* 1988;318:208.
72. Konigsrainer A, Miller K, Kieselbach G, et al. Course of diabetic retinopathy after pancreas transplantation. *Transplant Proc* 1990;22:689.
73. Munda R, First MR, Kranias G, Pedersen S, Alexander JW. Long-term effects of successful pancreas-allograft transplantation. *Diabetes* 1989;38(Suppl. 1):263.
74. Ulbig M, Kampik A, Landgraf R, Land W. The influence of combined pancreatic and renal transplantation on advanced diabetic retinopathy. *Transplant Proc* 1987;19:3554.
75. Bandello F, Vigano C, Secchi A, et al. Diabetic retinopathy in patients submitted to successful pancreas-kidney allografts. *Diabetes* 1989;38(Supplement 1):265.
76. Sutherland DER, Kendall DM, Moudry KC, et al. Pancreas transplantation in nonuremic, type I diabetic recipients. *Surgery* 1988;104:453.
77. Engerman RL, Kern TS. Experimental galactosemia produces diabetic-like retinopathy. *Diabetes* 1984;33:97.
78. Monnier VM, Kohn RR, Cerami A. Accelerated age-related browning of collagen in diabetes mellitus. *Proc Natl Acad Sci* 1984;81:583.
79. Merimee TJ. Diabetic retinopathy: a synthesis of perspectives. *N Engl J Med* 1990;322:978.
80. Kennedy WR, Navarro X, Goetz FC, Sutherland DER, Najarian JS. Effects of pancreatic transplantation on diabetic neuropathy. *N Engl J Med* 1990;322:1031.
81. Solders G, Wilczek H, Persson A, Wilczek H, Tyden G, Groth CG. Effects of combined pancreatic and renal transplantation on diabetic neuropathy: a two-year follow-up study. *Lancet* 1987;2:1232.
82. Schaffenhaus K, Heidbreder E, Land W, et al. Diabetic autonomic neuropathy after simultaneous transplantation: progressively across the Rubicon? *Transplant Proc* 1986;18:1136.
83. Scharp DW, Lacy PE. Islet transplantation: a review of the objectives, the concepts, the problems, the progress and, the future. In: Sutherland DER, Dubernard JM, eds. *Transplantation of the pancreas*. The Netherlands: Martinus Nijhoff Publishers, 1989;455–478.
84. Scharp DW, Lacy PE, Santiago JV, et al. Insulin independence after islet transplantation into Type I diabetic patient. *Diabetes* 1990;39:515–518.
85. Moskalewski S. Isolation and culture of the islets of Langerhans of the guinea pig. *Gen Comp Endocrinol* 1965;5:342–353.
86. Ballinger WF, Lacy PE. Transplantation of intact pancreatic islets in rats. *Surgery* 1972;72:175–186.
87. Reckard CR, Ziegler MM, Barker CF. Physiological and immunological consequences of transplanting isolated pancreatic islets. *Surgery* 1973;74:91–99.
88. Kemp CB, Knight MJ, Scharp DW, Ballinger WF, Lacy PE. Effects of transplantation site on the results of pancreatic islet isografts in diabetic rats. *Diabetologia* 1973;9:489–491.
89. Sutherland DER. Pancreas and islet transplantation. I. Experimental studies. *Diabetologia* 1981;20:161–185.
90. Gray DWR, Morris PJ. Developments in isolated pancreatic islet transplantation. *Transplantation* 1987;43:321–331.
91. Scharp DW. Isolation and transplantation of islet tissue. *World J Surg* 1984;8:143–151.
92. Lacy PE, Scharp DW. Islet transplantation in treating diabetes. *Ann Rev Med* 1986;37:33–40.
93. Scharp DW, Mason NS, Sparks RE. Islet immunoisolation: the use of hybrid artificial organs to prevent islet tissue rejection. *World J Surg* 1984;8:221–229.
94. Lafferty KJ, Prowse SJ. Theory and practice of immuno-regulation by tissue treatment prior to transplantation. *World J Surg* 1984;8:187–197.
95. Lacy PE. Experimental immunoalteration. *World J Surg* 1984;8:198–203.
96. Bach FH, Morrow CE, Sutherland DER. Immunogenetic considerations in islet transplantation. The role of Ia antigen in graft rejection. *World J Surg* 1984;8:204–206.
97. Fan MY, Lum ZP, Fu XW, Levesque L, Tai IT, Sun AM. Reversal of diabetes in BB rats by transplantation of encapsulated pancreatic islets. *Diabetes* 1990;39(4):519–522.

Surgical Management of the Diabetic Patient,
edited by Michael Bergman and Gregorio A. Sicard.
Raven Press, Ltd., New York © 1991.

27

Diabetes and Pregnancy

Donald R. Coustan

*Department of Obstetrics and Gynecology, Brown University Program in Medicine,
and Department of Obstetrics and Maternal-Fetal Medicine, Women & Infants'
Hospital of Rhode Island, Providence, Rhode Island 02905*

Pregnancy exerts dramatic effects upon glucose metabolism in both normal woman and those with diabetes. Furthermore, the presence of maternal diabetes has an adverse impact upon the outcome of pregnancy. This chapter briefly describes these phenomena, and then considers approaches to management of the "surgical" situations that arise during diabetic pregnancy: tocolysis, labor and delivery, and cesarean section.

THE EFFECTS OF PREGNANCY ON DIABETES MELLITUS

Pregnancy is accompanied by dramatic changes in glucose metabolism. In normal pregnant women there is an "accelerated starvation" during periods of fasting, with a fall in circulating glucose levels and a more rapid increase in ketone acid concentrations (1). Relative resistance to the effects of insulin occurs, presumably in an attempt to make glucose, the primary fuel for fetal growth and energy, more available to the developing conceptus. Although the precise pathophysiologic mechanism for this insulin resistance has not been elucidated, a number of hormones that are present in increased amounts during pregnancy have been associated with insulin resistance. These include human placental lactogen (hPL) or human chorionic somatomammotropin (hCS), estrogens, progesterone, and corticosteroids. The normal pregnant woman is capable of compensating for these changes with a marked increase in insulin production and release, so that normal values for glucose tolerance during pregnancy are somewhat lower than in the nonpregnant state (2).

When a woman with diabetes becomes pregnant, the above physiologic changes can have a severe impact on her diabetic control. Insulin requirements increase markedly, and it is not unusual for the insulin dose to be doubled or more by the third trimester (3). Diabetic ketoacidosis may occur at lower circulating glucose levels because of the insulin resistance that is present (4). Caloric requirements increase because of the needs of the growing conceptus. Because of the need for improved metabolic control during pregnancy (see below), hypoglycemia may be more of a problem than is usually the case in nonpregnant individuals, particularly during early pregnancy. Fortunately, the tendency toward marked fluctuations in glucose levels seen in some patients with diabetes, generally known as "brittleness," tends to be ameliorated, particularly during the latter half of pregnancy (5). Thus, pregnancy can be viewed as a period of increasing insulin requirements, increasing tendency toward diabetic ketoacidosis, an early increase in the tendency toward hypoglycemia, with a later increase in stability of control despite the need for more insulin.

THE EFFECTS OF DIABETES ON PREGNANCY

Before the discovery of insulin in the early 1920s diabetic pregnancy was associated with an almost 50% maternal mortality rate and a similarly high perinatal mortality rate (6). The availability of insulin was followed by an almost immediate decrease in maternal death rates, such that at present the effects of diabetes and the effects of pregnancy are best thought of as additive, the maternal mortality rate being approximately the sum of the maternal mortality rate for the general population plus the mortality rate associated with having diabetes for a given 9-month period of time. Exceptions exist, such as the woman who has suffered a previous myocardial infarction and thus has a markedly increased mortality risk associated with pregnancy (7). The perinatal mortality rate (i.e., fetal deaths after 20 weeks' gestation plus neonatal deaths during the first 29 days of life) took a much longer time to fall, but that level is now near the background rate in most large perinatal centers (8).

A number of technologic advances have contributed to the lowering of perinatal mortality rates. These include blood transfusions, improved anesthetic and surgical techniques, and antibiotic therapy, which have made cesarean section a safer mode of delivery in situations where this is necessary. In addition, the advent of neonatal intensive care units in the 1960s, which enabled prematurely delivered infants to survive with greater regularity, improved the survival rate for infants of diabetic mothers (IDMs). Other techniques, such as fetal heart-rate monitoring to evaluate respiratory status *in utero,* amniocentesis to determine fetal lung maturity, and ultrasound to determine fetal age, anatomy and growth, have allowed a more accurate determination of the optimal delivery date. However, it is my view that the most significant improvement in the prevention of perinatal death and morbidity has been the advocacy of improved maternal metabolic control to normalize the milieu in which the fetus develops.

First delineated by Jorgen Pedersen, (9) the "Pedersen Hypothesis" states that fetal hyperinsulinemia is the underlying cause of the various adverse outcomes encountered by IDMs. This fetal hyperinsulinemia is caused by fetal hyperglycemia, which is caused by maternal hyperglycemia, because maternal glucose is freely taken up by the fetus. Because maternal insulin does not cross the placenta to any appreciable extent, Pedersen assumed that it was the high glucose level that was responsible for the problems. This concept was later expanded to include other metabolic fuels that can act as secretogogues for the fetal pancreas, and is now called the "modified Pedersen hypothesis" (10). Empiric support for the Pedersen hypothesis came from studies describing a correlation between third-trimester mean maternal glucose levels and perinatal mortality rates among diabetic pregnancies (11,12), and from the demonstration that metabolic profiles in normal pregnant women during the third trimester exhibit mean plasma or serum glucose levels between approximately 70–110 mg/dl (13–15).

In addition to higher perinatal mortality rates, maternal hyperglycemia-fetal hyperinsulinemia has been associated with neonatal morbidities (16) such as macrosomia, hypoglycemia, plethora, and respiratory distress syndrome, and possibly childhood obesity (17–20) in IDMs. Therefore, current therapy of diabetes in pregnancy is designed to normalize maternal circulating glucose levels. This has been made practical by the advent of self glucose monitoring, which is now standard in the care of diabetic pregnancy.

TOCOLYSIS

Controversy exists as to whether preterm labor occurs more frequently among pregnant diabetic individuals (21,22). Even if the rate is similar to that in the general population, approximately 5% of diabetic pregnancies will be complicated by this problem. In addition, abdominal surgery during the second and third trimesters of pregnancy may be followed by preterm labor, and thus tocolysis may become necessary during the immediate postoperative period. It is not clear whether the labor is due to the surgery or to the underlying condition for which surgery was necessary. This clinical problem is of particular importance because the most commonly used pharmacologic agents for treatment of preterm labor (tocolytic agents) are beta adrenergic agonists such as ritodrine and terbutaline. This class of drugs can cause severe hyperglycemia and ketoacidosis in pregnant women with diabetes (23,24). Although these agents also cause augmented insulin release, (25) this effect is less important in type I diabetic patients with islet cell atrophy, and may also be insufficient to prevent hyperglycemia in type II diabetic patients who retain pancreatic function but are quite insulin resistant.

Should it be necessary to prescribe tocolytic therapy for a pregnant woman with diabetes, intravenous magnesium sulfate is an appropriate choice (26). It is not a beta adrenergic agonist, and does not cause hyperglycemia. The usual starting dose is 4–6 g given iv over 20–30 minutes, followed by maintenance at a continuous infusion rate of 2–4 g/hr (27). Although there have not been adequately controlled trials, most clinicians aim for serum magnesium levels of 5–8 mg/dl. Potential side effects of magnesium sulfate tocolysis include pulmonary edema, and, more frequently lethargy, muscle weakness, chest pain, and a generalized warm feeling. Overdosage or impaired renal function with resultant decreased excretion of magnesium can cause respiratory depression (generally at levels of 13 mg/dl) and even respiratory arrest (at serum concentrations around 14.5 mg/dl) (27). Thus, careful attention must be paid to serum levels and other clinical indicators, such as the loss of deep tendon reflexes, which may occur at levels of 9–13 mg/dl. Once parenteral tocolysis has been accomplished, oral tocolysis may be desirable for the long term. Although oral terbutaline or ritodrine are commonly used in nondiabetic individuals, many investigators are now using oral magnesium (gluconate or oxide) in an attempt to avoid the hyperglycemia accompanying the use of the former agents. Although efficacy has not yet been proven, the usual recommended dose of magnesium gluconate is 1 g (two 500 mg tablets) every 4 hours (28). Serum levels achieved with this route of administration are considerably lower than with the intravenous approach.

When situations arise that necessitate the use of beta adrenergic agonist tocolysis, great care must be exercised to maintain glucose homeostasis in the pregnant woman with diabetes. Whether ritodrine or terbutaline is utilized, circulating glucose levels should be monitored every 1–2 hours during the infusion. Particularly in the type I diabetic patient, we initiate a constant insulin infusion at approximately 5 units/hr at the same time we start the beta adrenergic agonist. The use of higher insulin infusion rates has been found necessary when beta adrenergic tocolysis is combined with the use of corticosteroids to induce lung maturity in diabetic pregnancies (29). On the other hand, the use of insulin infusion rates of 1 unit/hr when starting tocolysis has been associated with unacceptably high glucose levels during the early hours of therapy (30). The ritodrine or terbutaline is usually infused in a glucose-containing, salt-free solution, in order to avoid pulmonary edema, which has been reported to be highly associated with saline infusion (31,32). Although one study has shown that the use of glucose-containing infusates is associated with a greater elevation in plasma glucose levels (33), as might be expected, this problem can be anticipated with insulin infusions; pulmonary edema is much more difficult to reverse. One must be ready to infuse additional glucose in case the need for insulin has been overestimated, but this has rarely been necessary in our experience. The hyperglycemia observed with these agents is often transient, so that it is necessary to monitor circulating glucose levels frequently and decrease the insulin infusion rate once the glucose normalizes. Other problems encountered with beta adrenergic agonists include hypokalemia, maternal and fetal tachycardia, tremulousness, and, rarely, myocardial ischemia and/or pulmonary edema (34). Maternal anemia, twin gestation, and possibly the concomitant use of glucocorticoids may be other predisposing factors. It is prudent to obtain an electrocardiogram prior to initiating beta adrenergic tocolysis. The hypokalemia rarely requires intervention, because it is the result of potassium being driven to the intracellular compartment, presumably as a result of glucose and insulin release.

Maintenance with oral beta adrenergic agonists may be used, but deterioration of diabetic control has been noted, as well as the appearance of gestational diabetes in individuals known to have had normal glucose metabolism earlier in pregnancy (35,36). Thus, great care must be exercised with these agents.

MANAGEMENT OF DIABETES DURING LABOR

The infant of a diabetic mother is prone to neonatal hypoglycemia in direct proportion to the maternal (and cord blood) glucose level at delivery (37,38). Thus, one of the prime considerations in the metabolic management of diabetes during labor is to maintain relatively normal circulating glucose levels in the mother. A number of studies have shown that fewer than half of women with insulin-treated diabetes require any extra insulin during early labor, despite receiving a continuous glucose infusion (39,40). It is as if labor is a form of exercise that can substitute for insulin. On the other hand, a proportion of women with diabetes do require insulin throughout labor, and most require insulin during the late first stage and throughout the second stage of labor in order to avoid marked hyperglycemia. It is thus necessary to monitor circulating glucose levels frequently, every 1–2 hours in our center, to assess the need for insulin. The bedside use of a glucose reflectance meter serves this purpose quite efficiently. Insulin, when necessary, is administered as a continuous iv infusion via an infusion pump or other accurate infusion device; subcutaneous (sc) insulin has too long a delay in absorption and too prolonged an action to be used during the metabolically dynamic period of labor.

Now that preterm delivery is not automatic, many women with diabetes begin labor spontaneously, at a variable length of time after the last subcutaneous insulin injection. We generally insert an iv line on admission, and administer dextrose 5% in 0.5 normal saline at a constant rate of 125 ml/hr. If the glucose level exceeds 120 mg/dl we begin administering insulin. This can be accomplished with a separate infusion of insulin in normal saline, using a second pump, so that the glucose infusion rate can be kept constant while the insulin infusion rate is varied. An alternative approach used in our center is to add the insulin to the already infusing dextrose in 0.5 normal saline, starting at a concentration of 1 unit/dl of infusate. The infusion rate is always kept at 125 ml/hr, so that the glucose infusion is constant. Thus, a theoretical 1.25 units of insulin is infused each hour. If the glucose level does not stabilize after 2–3 hours at this rate, the concentration of insulin in the infusate can be doubled, so that at an infusion rate of 125 ml/hr, 2.5 units of insulin per hour will be given. If the glucose concentration falls to below 80 mg/dl we usually halve the insulin concentration. The major advantage of this system over the use of two independent infusions is the need for fewer infusion pumps and infusion sets. The most important thing to keep in mind is that the endpoint is the circulating glucose level in the mother, not some arbitrary insulin dose. When the mother arrives in labor during the time of absorption of her last subcutaneous insulin dose, it is important to watch for rapid changes in glucose levels as the injected insulin reaches its peak and then disappears. Remember that the mother will not be consuming her usual meals during labor, so that the insulin injected will have effects that are less predictable.

It is not uncommon for women with diabetes to undergo planned induction of labor at term when the fetal lungs are known to be mature and the cervix is "ripe" (i.e., favorable for induction) (41). Such an induction is relatively easier to manage from the metabolic standpoint than is spontaneous labor. When an induction is planned, it is scheduled to begin in the early morning. The patient takes her usual insulin injection(s) the night before, and eats her usual meals and snacks. No food is consumed after midnight, and insulin is not administered in the morning on the day of induction. An iv line is established, and 5% dextrose in 0.5 normal saline is infused at 125 ml/hr, as described above. Glucose levels are measured every 1–2 hours, and insulin is added to the infusate if levels above 120 mg/dl are detected, as described above. As injected sc insulin is not available, planned inductions appear to progress more easily than spontaneous labor. However, it is still common for glucose levels to increase markedly during the second stage of labor, and close attention must be paid at this time lest severe maternal hyperglycemia cause severe neonatal hypoglycemia.

Current obstetric practices include the liberal use of anesthesia and analgesia for labor and delivery. Conduction anesthesia, particularly continuous lumbar epidural analgesia, is commonly used, and should not be withheld merely because the mother has diabetes. Some common sense precautions are necessary, however. When conduction anesthesia/analgesia is administered, it is common for a "pharmacologic sympathectomy" to occur, with decreased vasomotor tone, decreased venous return, and hypotension. In order to prevent these complications, most anesthesiologists administer a liter or more of crystalloid before initiating anesthesia, so as to "fill up the tank," preventing hypovolemia. If that fluid contains glucose, its rapid infusion may be associated with fetal and neonatal acidosis (42,43), so only glucose-free solutions should be used for this purpose.

MANAGEMENT OF DIABETES DURING CESAREAN SECTION

The approach to management during planned cesarean section is similar to that for induction of labor. The patient eats her usual meals and takes her usual insulin dose the evening before surgery. She eats nothing after midnight, and the surgery is planned for the early morning. An iv line is established, but only normal saline or Ringer's lactate solutions are administered, because the baby will be delivered before any appreciable changes from the usual maternal fasting glucose level has occurred. Glucose levels are measured to ensure that the mother's usual normal fasting glucose level has been attained, and the cesarean section is then performed. Should a particularly high or low glucose level be detected, the surgery should be deferred for however long it takes to reestablish a relatively normal level, provided that there is no other urgent indication for delivery.

Once the baby has been delivered, a glucose infusion is established and insulin is added, if necessary, to maintain reasonable circulating glucose levels. It should be remembered that the patient is no longer pregnant, and so the very tight control that had been necessary for the protection of the fetus can now be relaxed. Glucose values between 80 and 150–200 mg/dl are perfectly acceptable for such patients.

POSTPARTUM MANAGEMENT

Insulin requirements are usually minimal in the post-cesarean section patient who has not begun to eat. Hypoglycemia may occur, particularly in a patient who had a large dose of intermediate acting insulin given sc prior to delivery. The diabetic woman who has delivered vaginally will be less likely to demonstrate severe insulin sensitivity, probably because she is eating normally during the immediate postpartum period. Once a diet is introduced, we usually give approximately half of the patients's *prepregnancy* insulin dose, working our way up gradually until she is in reasonably good control.

One of the most important aspects of care, and one that is often neglected, is the support such patients need for the reestablishment of reasonable diabetic control at a time when the demands of new parenthood may seem overwhelming. In our Diabetes in Pregnancy Program, we have noticed that many of our patients have difficulty disengaging from the intensive care and attention they receive during pregnancy. It is often helpful to invite mother and baby back for a visit 2–3 weeks postpartum so as to ease the transition to nonpregnant care. Plans must be solidified for diabetes care, and habits of frequent self-monitoring and close attention to personal health, which have been learned during pregnancy, should be encouraged for the nonpregnant state as well.

SUMMARY

The management of surgical problems in pregnancy complicated by diabetes should be guided by the need to maintain relatively normal glucose levels, and by the principle that glucose crosses the placenta freely while insulin does not. Pregnancy is associated with a state of relative insulin resistance. Once the pregnancy has been successfully concluded, the diabetes can be managed as in the nonpregnant state, except that increased insulin sensitivity tends to occur for the few days following delivery.

REFERENCES

1. Felig P, Lynch V. Starvation in human pregnancy: hypoglycemia, hypoinsulinemia, and hyperketonemia. *Science* 1970;170:990–992.
2. National Diabetes Data Group. Classification and diagnosis of diabetes mellitus and other categories of glucose intolerance. *Diabetes* 1979;28:1039–1057.
3. Rudolf MCJ, Coustan DR, Sherwin RS, et al. Efficacy of the insulin pump in the home treatment of pregnant diabetics. *Diabetes* 1981;30:891–895.
4. Coustan DR. Diabetic ketoacidosis. In: Berkowitz RL, ed. *Critical care of the obstetric patient.* New York: Churchill Livingstone, 1983;411–429.
5. Lev-Ran A, Goldman JA. Brittle diabetes in pregnancy. *Diabetes* 1977;26:926–930.
6. Williams JW. The clinical significance of glycosuria in pregnant women. *Am J Med Sci* 1909;137:1.
7. Hare JW. Diabetic neuropathy and coronary heart disease. In: Reece EA, Coustan DR, eds. *Diabetes mellitus in pregnancy: principles and practice.* New York: Churchill Livingstone, 1988;515–522.
8. Gabbe SG. Diabetes mellitus in pregnancy: have all the problems been solved? *Am J Med* 1981;70:613–618.
9. Pedersen JL. *The pregnant diabetic and her newborn.* Baltimore: Williams and Wilkins, 1967;128–129.
10. Freinkel N. Of pregnancy and progeny. *Diabetes* 1980;29:1023–1035.
11. Harley JMG, Montgomery DAD. Management of pregnancy complicated by diabetes. *Br Med J* 1965;1:14–18.
12. Karlsson K, Kjellmer I. The outcome of diabetic pregnancies in relation to the mother's blood sugar level. *Am J Obstet Gynecol* 1972;112:213–220.
13. Gillmer MDG, Beard RW, Brooke FM, Oakley NW. Carbohydrate metabolism in pregnancy. Part I—Diurnal plasma glucose profile in normal and diabetic women. *Br Med J* 1975;3:399–404.
14. Lewis SB, Wallin JD, Kuzuya H, et al. Circadian variation of serum glucose, C-peptide immunoreactivity and free insulin in normal and insulin-treated diabetic pregnant subjects. *Diabetologia* 1976;12:343–350.
15. Cousins L, Rigg L, Hollingsworth D, Brink G, Aurand J, Yen SSC. The 24-hour excursion and diurnal rhythm of glucose, insulin and C-peptide in normal pregnancy. *Am J Obstet Gynecol* 1980;136:483–488.
16. Coustan DR. Hyperglycemia-hyperinsulinemia: effect on the infant of the diabetic mother. In: Jovanovic L, Peterson CM, Fuhrmann K, eds. *Diabetes and pregnancy: teratology, toxicity and treatment.* New York: Praeger, 1986;131–156.
17. Vohr BR, Lipsitt LP, Oh W. Somatic growth of children of diabetic mothers with reference to birth size. *J Pediatr* 1980;97:196–199.
18. Pettit DJ, Knowler WC, Bennett PH, Aleck KA, Baird HR. Obesity in offspring of diabetic Pima Indian women despite normal birth weight. *Diabetes Care* 1987;10:76–80.
19. Oh W, Gelardi NL, Cha C-J. Maternal hyperglycemia in pregnant rats: its effect on growth and carbohydrate metabolism in the offspring. *Metabolism* 1988;37:1146–1151.
20. Green OC, Winter RJ, Depp R, et al. Fuel-mediated teratogenesis: prospective correlations between authropometric development in childhood and antepartum maternal metabolism. *Clin Res* 1987;35:657A.
21. Cousins L. Obstetric complications. In: Reece EA, Coustan DR, eds. *Diabetes mellitus in pregnancy: principles and practice.* New York: Churchill Livingstone, 1988;455–468.
22. Mimouni F, Miodovnik M, Siddiqi TA, Berk MA, Wittekind C, Tsang R. High spontaneous premature labor rate in insulin-dependent diabetic pregnant women: an association with poor glycemic control and urogenital infection. *Obstet Gynecol* 1988;72:175–180.
23. Schilthuis MS, Aarnoudse JG. Fetal death associated with severe ritodrine induced ketoacidosis. *Lancet* 1980;1:1145.
24. Mordes D, Kreutner K, Metzger W, Colwell JA. Dangers of intravenous ritodrine in diabetic patients. *JAMA* 1982;248:973–975.
25. Lipshitz J, Vinik AI. The effects of hexporenaline, a β2-sympathomimetic drug, on maternal glucose, insulin, glucagon, and free fatty acid levels. *Am J Obstet Gynecol* 1978;130:761–764.
26. Hill WC, Katz M, Kitzmiller JL, Burr RE. Tocolysis for the insulin-dependent diabetic woman. *Am J Obstet Gynecol* 1984;148:1148–1150.
27. Creasy R. Preterm labor. In: Eden RD, Boehm FH, eds. *Assessment and care of the fetus: physiological, clinical, and medicolegal principles.* Norwalk, CT: Appleton and Lange, 1990;622–625.

28. Martin RW, Gaddy DK, Martin JN Jr, Lucas JA, Wiser WL, Morrison JC. Tocolysis with oral magnesium. *Am J Obstet Gynecol* 1987;156:433–434.
29. Barnett AH, Stubbs SM, Mander AM. Management of preterm labour in diabetic pregnancy. *Diabetologia* 1980;18:365–368.
30. Miodovnik M, Peros N, Holroyde JC, Siddiqi TA. Treatment of premature labor in insulin-dependent diabetic women. *Obstet Gynecol* 1985;65:621–627.
31. Philipsen T, Eriksen PS, Lynggard F. Pulmonary edema following ritodrine-saline infusion in premature labor. *Obstet Gynecol* 1981;58:304–308.
32. Ferguson JE III, Hensleigh PA, Kredenster D. Adjunctive use of magnesium sulfate with ritodrine for preterm labor tocolysis. *Am J Obstet Gynecol* 1984;148:166–171.
33. Perkins RP, Varela-Gittings F, Dunn TS, Argubright KF, Skipper BJ. The influence of intravenous solution content on ritodrine-induced metabolic changes. *Obstet Gynecol* 1987;70:892–895.
34. Benedetti TJ. Maternal complications of parenteral β-sympathomimetic therapy for premature labor. *Am J Obstet Gynecol* 1983;145:1–6.
35. Main EK, Main DM, Gabbe SG. Chronic oral terbutaline tocolytic therapy is associated with maternal glucose intolerance. *Am J Obstet Gynecol* 1987;157:644–647.
36. Angel JL, O'Brien WF, Knuppel RA, Morales WJ, Sims CJ. Carbohydrate intolerance in patients receiving oral tocolytics. *Am J Obstet Gynecol* 1988;159:762–766.
37. Light IJ, Keenan WJ, Sutherland JM. Maternal intravenous glucose administration as a cause of hypoglycemia in the infant of the diabetic mother. *Am J Obstet Gynecol* 1972;113:345–350.
38. Andersen O, Hertel J, Schmolker L, Kuhl C. Influence of the maternal plasma glucose concentration at delivery on the risk of hypoglycaemia in infants of insulin-dependent diabetic mothers. *Acta Paediatr Scand* 1985;74:268–273.
39. Golde SH, Good-Anderson B, Montoro M, Artal R. Insulin requirements during labor: a reappraisal. *Am J Obstet Gynecol* 1982;144:556–559.
40. Jovanovic L, Peterson CM. Insulin and glucose requirements during the first stage of labor in insulin-dependent diabetic women. *Am J Med* 1983;75:607–612.
41. Coustan DR. Delivery: timing, mode and management. In: Reece EA, Coustan DR, eds. *Diabetes mellitus in pregnancy: principles and practice.* New York: Churchill Livingstone, 1988;525–536.
42. Lawrence GF, Brown VA, Parsons RJ, Cooke ID. Feto-maternal consequences of high-dose glucose infusion during labour. *Br J Obstet Gynaecol* 1982;89:27–32.
43. Kenepp NB, Shelley WC, Gabbe SG, Kumar S, Stanley CA, Gutsche BB. Fetal and neonatal hazards of maternal hydration with 5% dextrose before cesarean section. *Lancet* 1982;1:1150–1152.

Surgical Management of the Diabetic Patient,
edited by Michael Bergman and Gregorio A. Sicard.
Raven Press, Ltd., New York © 1991.

28

Surgery for Obesity in the Diabetic Patient

Norman B. Ackerman

*Department of Surgery, New York Medical College, Metropolitan Hospital Center,
New York, New York 10029*

The association of obesity and diabetes mellitus has been recognized for many years. The incidence of diabetes increases with age and with the degree of obesity. In the study reported by Rimm and associates (1), prevalence of diabetes ranged from 0.7% incidence in women aged 20–29 years who were 10% over ideal weight, to 8.1% in woman 50–59 years who were at least 85% overweight.

Obesity is extremely common in the United States and in much of the Western world. It has been estimated that 25–45% of adult Americans over the age of 30 years are more than 20% overweight (2). The term "morbid obesity" has been used to define those individuals who are massively overweight and either already have or will likely develop medical problems related to their obesity. Patients in this category are at least 100 lbs overweight. The incidence of morbid obesity in the United States is not known precisely, but has been thought to range between 400,000 and 9 million people. The estimate of 7 million Americans has been frequently quoted recently. Women are four times more likely to be morbidly obese than men.

Abnormalities of glucose metabolism and clincially significant diabetes mellitus are among the most common medical problems associated with morbid obesity. In Drenick's study (3), 54% of his grossly obese male patients had "either frank or chemical diabetes." He estimated that it took at least 20–25 years of gross obesity for diabetes to develop in 50% of this morbidly obese population. O'Leary (4) reported that more than 70% of morbidly obese patients had diabetes or abnormal glucose tolerance tests. Clinically significant diabetes requiring medical therapy has been estimated to be 4.5–5 times more prevalent in the morbidly obese population than in the general population (1,5). Approximately 7 or 8% of morbidly obese patients in several series had clincial diabetes. In our experience, 8% of our morbidly obese patients required insulin or oral medication for diabetes.

The potential consequences of diabetes in this morbidly obese population are grave, particularly in patients who have lost and then regained substantial weight. The development of severe ketoacidosis has been described in these patients (3). Drenick (6) reported that diabetes as a cause of death was three times more common in the morbidly obese patients in his series than in the general population. In addition, he noted that the "presence of diabetes contributed to the excess mortality as a cofactor in the genesis of cardiovascular deaths and possibly in the mechanisms leading to thromboembolic and infectious diseases" (3). By "excess mortality," he referred to his series of 200 morbidly obese men of whom, at an average following period of 7.6 years, 50 had died as consequence of a variety of medical problems. Other authors have confirmed the potential seriousness of diabetes in the morbidly obese patient.

SURGICAL APPROACHES FOR MORBID OBESITY

In view of the medical problems, including diabetes, associated with morbid obesity, it is clear that an effective regimen for inducing weight loss is a necessity. Virtually all morbidly obese patients give a long history of attempts to lose weight by dietary control. Group therapy programs such as Weight Watchers or TOPS have had only very modest success in this group. Experiences with behavior modification techniques have generally been disappointing, and total weight loss may average as little as 10–15 lbs. "Crash" and fad diets have been disappointing and often dangerous. Total fasting under a physician's care for up to 3 months has produced weight loss from 30–90 lbs. Regaining weight after stopping these diets, however, is extremely common. It has been estimated that the success rate of significant weight loss maintained for at least 2 years is less than 5% in the morbidly obese population, and possibly closer to 1–2%. Other nonoperative means of causing weight loss in these patients have also been unsuccessful. There are currently no anorectic drugs available that are both safe and effective for long periods. Although exercise is beneficial in many respects, weight loss from exercise alone is relatively inconsequential. Other procedures such as hypnosis and acupuncture have little value. Most recently, the gastric balloon technique has been discontinued because of the dangers of gastric rupture, perforation, or bleeding.

At this time, the only successful methods of producing significant weight loss in the morbidly obese individual are operative procedures. There have been two basic techniques that have been used extensively in clinical experience. Weight loss in the older procedure, the intestinal or jejunoileal bypass, occurs mostly as a result of decreased absorption of ingested calories; in the newer procedure, gastric bypass, weight loss is the result of significant decreases in oral caloric intake.

CRITERIA FOR SURGERY

Most surgeons who perform these operations have developed a rigid set of criteria that must be satisfied before considering the use of surgery. The criteria generally include the following:

1. Patients must be morbidly obese, at least 100 lbs over ideal weight.
2. There must be a definite history of attempts to lose weight by dietary control. The patient and surgeon must be firmly convinced that the dietary approach has been given an adequate trial.
3. Obesity due to correctable endocrine problems must be ruled out. Assessment of thyroid and adrenal function is of particular importance.
4. Patients should represent a reasonable operative risk.
5. The presence of obesity-related conditions, such as diabetes, hypertension, Pick-

wickian syndrome, and degenerative arthritis are positive factors that intensify the need for surgery.

6. Patients must be reliable enough to follow directions, take medications when pre-scribed, and keep follow-up appointments.

7. Age limits have been extended, and in our experience range from teenage to 65 years.

INTESTINAL BYPASS

These procedures were first developed in the late 1950s, although the first report of a large series was that of Payne and DeWind in 1969 (7). In these operations, approximately 90% of the small intestine was bypassed, with absorption of calories and nutrients occurring only in the remaining 10%. The two major variations of this procedure were an end-to-side operation (end of jejunum anastomosed to side of terminal ileum) and an end-to-end operation (end of jejunum to end of ileum). The actual lengths of jejunum and ileum varied in different series, but ranged from 5–16 inches of jejunum and 2–14 inches of ileum, with the length of functioning intestine totaling 18–20 inches.

After intestinal bypass, most patients experienced a major loss of weight. Average weight loss, in the experience reported by most surgeons, varied between 33–40% of preoperative weight. There was a wide range of weight loss, from 10–65% with an average of 38% in our experience. Ninety-seven percent of our patients lost at least 20% of their preoperative weight, and 92% had at least a 25% weight loss. Weight loss appeared to depend on a decreased intake of food in addition to malabsorption of carbohydrates, fats, and proteins. Almost two-thirds of the patients noted a de-crease in appetite. Although some observers believed that this was an attempt by patients to prevent diarrhea, there was some evidence that there may be a physio-logical explanation for the change in eating habits. Experimental studies in rats dem-onstrated a decreased caloric intake after intestinal bypass. Malabsorption played a major role in producing weight loss because caloric reduction alone did not account for the total loss of weight occurring in intestinal bypass patients. In our experience, patients consumed 2½–4 times more calories per day after intestinal bypass than after gastric bypass, but had a slightly greater weight loss (8).

Although the weight loss after intestinal bypass was very satisfactory, the opera-tion has come into relative disfavor because of the numerous early and late compli-cations. Diarrhea developed in all patients after surgery. Diarrhea was due to in-creased intestinal transit time, decreased absorption of fluids, and increased concentration of bile salts and fatty acids reaching the colon. As a consequence of diarrhea and malabsorption, problems such as electrolyte deficiencies (particularly potassium, magnesium, and calcium), vitamin deficiencies (fat-soluble vitamins), and anal problems (hemorrhoids, anal fissure, papillitis, inflammation, and pain) were common. Other major complications included hepatic failure (probably due to protein malnutrition), calcium oxalate kidney stones, and arthralgias. Some of these complications began suddenly, often several years after the bypass operation. Many patients, at least 25%, have undergone surgery again, with takedown of the intestinal bypass and conversion to a gastric bypass or gastroplasty. At this time, these latter operations are the procedures of choice for morbid obesity.

GASTRIC BYPASS AND GASTROPLASTY

In the late 1960s Mason developed an operative procedure for weight loss that drastically restricted caloric intake by reducing the size of the stomach (9). Through the years the original procedure has gone through a great number of modifications and variations, although the original concept of a small gastric reservoir has remained. In the hands of various surgeons, the reservoir has ranged in size from about 15 ml capacity to about 50 ml. It is of equal importance to make the outlet of this reservoir narrow and restrictive so that the distention after eating will persist for many hours. As a result of this distention, appetite is curbed for a prolonged period after eating, and patients are able to limit food intake, comfortably, to two or three small meals per day. The size of this gastric outlet stoma varies from about 5–12 mm.

The two basic procedures have been the gastric bypass and the gastroplasty (Fig. 1). In the former operation, the reservoir is created by transecting and suturing the stomach, or more commonly, partitioning the stomach with stainless steel staples, and performing a narrow gastrojejunostomy, using either a loop of jejunem or Roux-en-Y. In these operations, the distal stomach, duodenum, and a foot of proximal jejunum are bypassed. In the latter procedure, the gastroplasty, food goes directly from the proximal gastric reservoir through a narrow stoma into the distal stomach, without bypassing any of the digestive tract. The most popular gastroplasty is the vertical-banded gastroplasty, also developed by Mason (10).

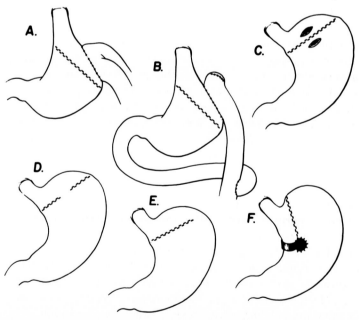

FIG. 1. Variations of gastric bypass and gastroplasty procedures. (A) Gastric bypass with loop gastrojejunostomy. This technique is preferred by author. (B) Gastric bypass with Roux-en-Y gastrojejunostomy. (C) Gastrogastrostomy. (D) Gastroplasty with gap in mid-portion of staple line. (E) Gastroplasty with gap in greater curvature. (F) Vertical banded gastroplasty. (From Ackerman NB: Gastric and intestinal bypass procedures. In: Fromm D, ed. *Gastrointestinal surgery,* New York: Churchill Livingstone, 1985;475–518).

Weight loss after these operations has been approximately the same as the intestinal bypass, with the average varying from about 25–40% of preoperative weight. The range of weight loss is wide. In our experience with gastric bypass, weight loss varied from 10–61%, with an average of 35%. Ninety-three percent of patients lost at least 20% of their preoperative weight, and 90% lost at least 25%. These figures may be improving because of more effective stapling devices. Weight loss appeared to be related solely to the restricted caloric intake of these patients. In our patients, average preoperative caloric intake of 6–7,000 cal/day decreased to 740 cal/day at 3 months postoperatively and 1,280 cal/day at 6 months (8). Similarly, carbohydrates decreased from 699 g/day to 73 and 129 at 3 and 6 months, proteins from 206 g/day to 35 and 55, and fats from 251 g/day to 36 and 61. However, because gastric bypass patients seem to lose about 10% more of their preoperative weight than patients who have undergone vertical-banded gastroplasty (36% versus 26%) (11), other factors may be involved, possibly with some caloric malabsorption.

The gastric bypass and gastroplasty operations are currently the procedures of choice for morbid obesity. Probably more than 25,000 of these operations are performed annually in the United States. Perioperative complications such as splenic injury, gastric perforations, and intraabdominal abscesses are uncommon in most surgeons' experience. Later problems including obstruction, ulceration, and iron deficiency are also uncommon, and in contrast to intestinal bypasses, late metabolic problems do not occur. The major side effect of these procedures is vomiting, which occurs soon after surgery in virtually all patients. Vomiting can be caused by several mechanisms, such as eating more than the capacity of the gastric reservoir, eating certain foods that are not tolerated in the early postoperative state, (especially red meat, and greasy, spicy foods), late stenosis of the outlet stoma, and emotional problems in the postoperative patient. With appropriate therapy and time these problems resolve and vomiting stops. In a small number of patients late failures resulting in some regain of weight may occur as a consequence of staple line breakdown, stomal dilatation or reservoir enlargement. A second operation to correct the problem may be necessary. Fortunately, the most common of these problems, staple line breakdown, appears to be virtually eliminated in our experience since the development of the four-row stapler (U.S. Surgical TA90B).

EFFECTS OF INTESTINAL BYPASS ON DIABETES

After intestinal bypass, a very rapid improvement in diabetes was uniformly experienced. Even as early as 10 days after operation marked improvements were seen in oral glucose tolerance tests in morbidly obese patients (12). Patients with preperative elevated fasting plasma glucose levels often showed significant improvements by the time they were discharged from the hospital 8 or 9 days after operation.

We have studied a group of 24 patients with elevated preoperative fasting plasma glucose levels (13). The mean value in this group of patients was 184 mg/dl. After intestinal bypass, patients were maintained on intravenous fluids for 3–4 days, and then were advanced from a liquid to a full, regular diet over the remaining time in the hospital. Discharge generally occurred 9 or 10 days after operation. In 17 patients, plasma glucose levels decreased or administered hypoglycemic therapy was discontinued, or both, before discharge from the hospital (Fig. 2). The other seven patients had either no change or too few tests to demonstrate a trend.

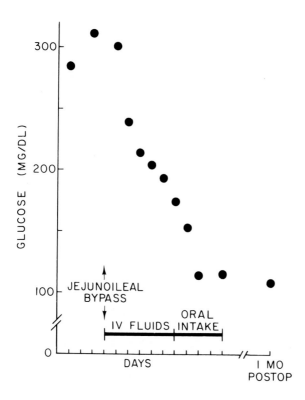

FIG. 2. Fasting plasma glucose levels of 43-year-old woman weighing 372 pounds showed a marked improvement immediately after intestinal bypass. (From Ackerman NB. Observations on the improvements in carbohydrate metabolism in diabetic and other morbidly obese patients after jejunoileal bypass. By permission of *Surgery, Gynecology and Obstetrics* 1981;152:581–586).

    Later follow-up of these 24 patients revealed that 12 had normal fasting plasma glucose levels by 1 month after surgery. Most of the others responded similarly over the next few months. The mean fasting plasma glucose level 1 month after operation was 126 mg/dl. Eventually all but two patients became normoglycemic, and fasting plasma glucose levels in these two patients were almost normal. Of interest is the fact that the fasting plasma glucose level became normal at a time when mean weight loss was only 13% of original preoperative weight. These patients were still very obese. At an average late follow-up time of 19 months the mean fasting plasma glucose level was 101 mg/dl. None of the patients requires hypoglycemic therapy or restricted diets.

    Eight of our patients were studied with oral glucose tolerance tests at varying intervals from 1–12 months after intestinal bypass. In all of these patients, including those who were clinically diabetic, a normal, but flattened glucose tolerance curve was seen at the time of the first postoperative test, as early as 1 month (Fig. 3). There appeared to be little change in time, although some investigators eventually noted a more rounded curve (12). The mean sum of fasting, 1-hour, 2-hour, and 3-hour plasma glucose levels was 821 before operation and 385 at the time of the first postoperative test. This latter figure is within the normal range, and the difference is significant. Similarly, in the experience of Bendezu and assoicates (14), the sum of fasting, 1/2-hour, 1-hour and 2-hour plasma glucose levels decreased from 596 preoperatively to 385 postoperatively.

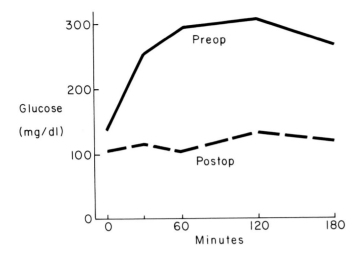

FIG. 3. Oral glucose tolerance test before and 1 month after intestinal bypass in 37-year-old woman with diabetes who weighed 337 pounds before surgery. (From Ackerman NB. Observations on the improvements in carbohydrate metabolism in diabetic and other morbidly obese patients after jejunoileal bypass. By permission of *Surgery, Gynecology and Obstetrics* 1981;152:581–586).

In our studies, serum immunoreactive insulin levels were measured in seven patients during the preoperative oral glucose tolerance test (13). Fasting levels were elevated in all patients and became markedly elevated during the 3 hours of the study (Fig. 4). Postoperatively, as early as 1 month after operation, serum insulin levels were markedly decreased in fasting and postglucose periods. Insulin levels eventually became normal in our experience and in that of others (14–16).

In contrast to the rapid improvement in the oral glucose tolerance test after intestinal bypass, intravenous glucose tolerance tests showed little change at 3 months after operation in our experience. In the experience of Ahmad and associates (16), intravenous glucose tolerance tests generally improved by 5–10 months although results were not uniform. Further improvements were seen at 10–15 months. The differences noted in oral and intravenous glucose testing suggest the possible role of decreased oral carbohydrate absorption in the intestinal bypass patient.

We have followed 12 morbidly obese patients who were clinically diabetic (13). Six required daily insulin injections, and six were receiving oral hypoglycemic agents. In the patients taking insulin, mean fasting plasma glucose levels averaged 233 mg/dl, and mean preoperative weight was 271 lbs. Immediately after intestinal bypass, insulin was no longer required by five patients and they were discharged from the hospital without medication. The other patient discontinued insulin injections within a month. Normal fasting plasma glucose levels occurred at an average postoperative time of 2 months when mean weight loss was 11%. At 17 months after operation, the mean plasma glucose level was 103 mg/dl.

Of the six patients taking oral hypoglycemic agents, preoperative fasting plasma glucose levels averaged 166 mg/dl and weight was 289 lbs. Immediately after operation all six had marked improvement in plasma glucose levels and all have discontinued their therapy. At 17 months after intestinal bypass the mean fasting plasma glucose level was 96 mg/dl. Our experience with morbidly obese diabetic patients undergoing intestinal bypass is matched by all other investigators studying similar patients.

The mechanisms responsible for the rapid and long-lasting improvements in diabetes after intestinal bypass are not fully understood. There are probably several

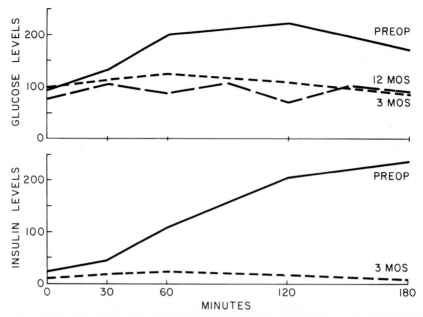

FIG. 4. Plasma glucose and insulin levels during oral glucose tolerance test before and 3–12 months after intestinal bypass in 34-year-old man who weighed 299 pounds before surgery. (From Ackerman NB. Observations on the improvements in carbohydrate metabolism in diabetic and other morbidly obese patients after jejunoileal bypass. By permission of *Surgery, Gynecology and Obstetrics* 1981;152:581–586).

important factors involved. It is unlikely that weight loss per se was responsible for the earliest improvements in these patients. Fasting plasma glucose levels often fell to normal by the time the patient was discharged from the hospital, and weight loss at that time was relatively negligible. On the other hand, at a time several months after operation when weight loss had been significant, this factor probably contributed to the overall amelioration of the diabetes.

Dietary changes undoubtedly were responsible for some of the improvements noted. Many patients spontaneously modified their diet after intestinal bypass. There was often a decrease in carbohydrate ingestion, and many patients reported a loss in their desire for excessive sweets. Total caloric intake decreased, in some patients as much as 50%. The effects of decreased carbohydrate intake on diabetes has been known for many years and has been a major therapeutic approach to the disease. In addition to this, decreased absorption of carbohydrates, fats, and proteins are known to occur after intestinal bypass. The presence of a flattened postoperative oral glucose curve suggests glucose malabsorption. The combination of decreased oral intake and decreased absorption of carbohydrates and protein probably accounted for most of the improvements after intestinal bypass, and these mechanisms are probably specific for this type of operation. These changes may also be responsible, at least initially, for improvement in insulin sensitivity seen in these patients. The role of certain intestinal polypeptides [such as glucose-dependent insulinotropic polypeptide(GIP)] and their postoperative changes have been studied, and may also play a role in the improvements in diabetes after intestinal bypass.

EFFECTS OF GASTRIC BYPASS ON DIABETES

Major improvements in carbohydrate metabolism and diabetes also occur after gastric bypass, although some of the mechanisms involved may be different from those with intestinal bypass. Improvements documented after gastric bypass are often more gradual, particularly in clinically treated diabetic patients.

We have studied 13 patients who were found to have abnormal fasting plasma glucose levels and/or abnormal oral glucose tolerance curves (17). These patients were not clinically diabetic. The mean fasting plasma glucose level was 147 mg/dl. After undergoing gastric bypass, the patients improved. At an average time of 2 months after surgery, with a range of 1 to 5 3/4 months, all fasting plasma glucose tests were normal. At 2 months after operation, mean weight loss was 18% of original weight. Other investigators have reported similar experiences.

Many of our patients had abnormal oral glucose tolerance tests before surgery. It is difficult to perform oral glucose tolerance tests after gastric bypass because patients often are unable to swallow and retain the sweetened glucose solution. However, when successfully performed, an improved parabolic glucose tolerance curve is generally seen (Fig. 5). This is in contrast to the flattened curves noted after intestinal bypass. Comparisons of the oral glucose tolerance tests before and after gastric bypass in 12 morbidly obese patients were made by Sirinek and associates

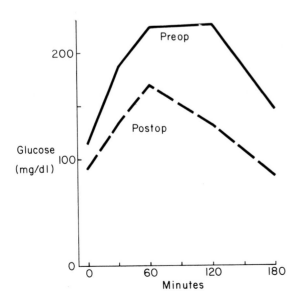

FIG. 5. Oral glucose tolerance test before and after gastric bypass in 51-year-old woman who weighed 337 pounds before surgery. (From Ackerman NB. Gastric and intestinal bypass procedures. In: Fromm D, ed. *Gastrointestinal surgery,* New York: Churchill Livingston, 1985; 475–518).

(18). At 3–4 months after surgery, improvements in the oral glucose tolerance tests were observed by these investigators.

Fasting serum insulin levels were elevated in all our patients where such studies were performed as well as by other investigators (18–20). When studied 3–4 months after gastric bypass fasting serum insulin levels and serum insulin measurements obtained during oral glucose tolerance tests significantly decreased as compared to preoperative testing (18). Similar decreases in serum insulin levels have been observed during intravenous glucose tolerance tests, as reported by Hale and coworkers (19). These improvements were seen 3 months after surgery, and further decreases were noted at 12 months postoperatively. In all these studies, considerable weight loss, in the range of 21–25%, had occurred at the period of postoperative testing. Weight loss resulted in a marked improvement in sensitivity to insulin. Glucose disappearance during intravenous glucose tolerance testing improved in patients studied 5–11 months after gastric bypass, but levels did not become normal in any patient (22). We have had similar experiences in our patients.

A group of 27 clinically diabetic and morbidly obese patients has been studied by us before and after gastric bypass. Fifteen of these patients required daily insulin injections, from 20–260 units of neutral protamine Hagedorn (NPH) insulin per day. Their fasting plasma glucose level averaged 281 mg/dl and mean weight was 294 lbs. Twelve of the 15 patients (80%) have been able to discontinue insulin completely at an average postoperative time of 2 months (3 weeks to 4 3/4 months). This is a more gradual improvement as compared with the intestinal bypass patients. Weight loss in the gastric bypass patients at the time when insulin was completely discontinued averaged 17% of original weight (9–28%). The three patients who still need insulin have all greatly decreased their dose (260 units to 50 units; 60 units to 5 units; 48 units to 15 units) and are more stable. Other investigators have had similar experiences; for example, Herbst and associates (21) reported that 14 of 21 insulin-dependent diabetic patients were able to discontinue insulin by 6 weeks after operation, and the other seven patients decreased insulin doses by 72%.

Twelve of our patients were maintained before surgery on oral hypoglycemic agents for control of diabetes. Their fasting plasma glucose level averaged 229 mg/dl and mean weight has 300 lbs. At an average postoperative time of 3 months (ranging from immediately after surgery to 9 3/4 months), 10 of the 12 patients (83%) were able to discontinue all medications. Average weight loss was 18% (12–27%) of original weight. One of the patients who continues to need medication was able to reduce her dosage, but she is still considerably obese. The other patient was able to discontinue her drugs at 9 3/4 months after surgery, but in spite of some additional weight loss she was again started on a low dose of oral hypoglycemic pills. The other 10 patients continue to remain without the need for medication.

There are probably multiple reasons for improvement in diabetes after gastic bypass, and study of this issue continues. In contrast to the effects of intestinal bypass, decreased absorption of carbohydrates is probably not a factor, although Pories and coworkers (20) have suggested that the bypass of the antrum and duodenum may play a role. The greatly reduced food intake, which includes reduction of carbohydrates, fats, and proteins, undoubtedly is a major factor (8). The early postoperative improvements in diabetes are probably related to this. As weight loss continues, it certainly plays an increasing role in maintaining the early clinical improvement in diabetes. Associated with these changes, greater insulin sensitivity plays its role.

There may be other factors involved in the complete picture. Sirinek and associates (18) have reported that serum GIP was markedly increased in obese diabetics before surgery, and became significantly decreased after gastric bypass. This may be related to the postsurgical bypass of the duodenum and proximal jejunum, which are the sites of highest concentration of GIP. The known relationship between GIP and release of insulin suggests that this may be an important factor in the improvement in diabetes in these gastric bypass patients.

EFFECTS OF CONVERSION OF JEJUNOILEAL BYPASS TO GASTRIC BYPASS ON DIABETES

Although many patients who have had intestinal bypass surgery continue to enjoy good results from the operation, many others, perhaps 25–50% of these patients, have needed additional surgery and reversal of their bypass. Reasons for reversal include the development of major metabolic and physical complaints described earlier, and, less commonly, unsatisfactory weight loss or substantial regain of weight. Simple takedown of the intestinal bypass has not been satisfactory because of the tendency to regain all of the lost weight. Instead, the procedure of choice has been to combine takedown of the intestinal bypass and conversion to a gastric bypass at one operation.

We have had several diabetic patients who became normoglycemic after intestinal bypasses, but ultimately needed conversion to gastric bypass (22). All of these patients have remained normoglycemic after conversion to gastric bypass, even if there has been some regain of weight after the second operation (Fig. 6).

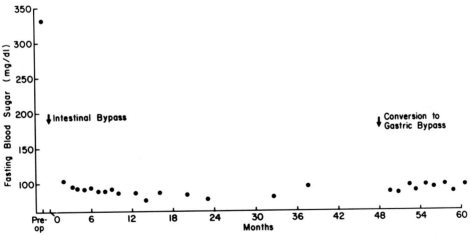

FIG. 6. Diabetic patient with normal fasting plasma glucose levels remained normal after conversion to gastric bypass, even after some increase in weight. (From Ackerman NB. Metabolic consequences from conversion of jejunoileal bypass to gastric bypass. By permission of *Annals of Surgery* 1982;196:553–559).

CONCLUSION

Morbidly obese patients who have abnormalities in carbohydrate metabolism, including clinical evidence of diabetes, respond well to the various operations performed to promote major weight loss. Although the mechanisms responsible for improving diabetes may be somewhat different in the intestinal and gastric bypass procedures, the end results are similar. After either of these operations, virtually all diabetic patients note improvement in their disease, and most become normoglycemic without the need for medication.

At this time, the gastric bypass operations are the procedures of choice because of the substantial weight loss occurring with relatively few complications. Because of the beneficial effect on diabetes, the presence of this condition in a morbidly obese individual should be a positive factor in recommending the performance of a gastric bypass.

REFERENCES

1. Rimm AA, Werner LH, Van Yserloo B, Bernstein RA. Relationship of obesity and disease in 73,532 weight-conscious women. *Public Health Rep* 1975;90:44–51.
2. Bray GA, Davidson MB, Drenick EJ. Obesity: a serious symptom. *Ann Intern Med* 1972;77:779–795.
3. Drenick EJ. Definition of health consequences of morbid obesity. *Surg Clin North Am* 1979;59:963–976.
4. O'Leary JP. Overview: jejunoileal bypass in the treatment of morbid obesity. *Am J Clin Nutr* 1980;33:389–394.
5. Bray GA, Barr RE, Benfield JR, Castelnuovo-Tedesco P, Drenick EJ, Passaro E. Intestinal bypass operation as a treatment for obesity. *Ann Intern Med* 1976;85:97–109.
6. Drenick EJ, Bale GS, Seltzer F, Johnson DG. Excessive mortality and causes of death in morbidly obese men. *J Am Med Assoc* 1980;243:443–445.
7. Payne JH, DeWind LT. Surgical treatment of obesity. *Am J Surg* 1969;118:141–147.
8. Rogus J, Blumenthal SA. Variations in dietary intake after bypass surgery for obesity. *J Am Diet Assoc* 1981;79:437–441.
9. Mason EE, Ito C. Gastric bypass. *Ann Surg* 1969;170:329–339.
10. Mason EE. Vertical banded gastroplasty for obesity. *Arch Surg* 1982;117:701–706.
11. Pories WJ, Flickinger EG, Meelheim HD, et al. The effectiveness of gastric bypass (GB) over gastric partitioning in morbid obesity (MO). *Ann Surg* 1982;196:389–399.
12. Baden H. Bypass operations in the treatment of obesity. *Ann Chir Gynaecol* 1974;63:365–370.
13. Ackerman NB. Observations on the improvements in carbohydrate metabolism in diabetic and other morbidly obese patients after jejunoileal bypass. *Surg Gynecol Obstet* 1981;152:581–586.
14. Bendezu R, Wieland RG, Green SG, Hallberg MC, Marsters RW. Certain metabolic consequences of jejunoileal bypass. *Am J Clin Nutr* 1976;29:366–370.
15. Nolan S, Danowski TS, Clara DW, et al. Prospective study of jejunoileal bypass in obesity. *Obesity Bariatric Med* 1975;4:156.
16. Ahmad V, Danowski TS, Nolan S, et al. Remission of diabetes mellitus after weight reduction by jejunoileal bypass. *Diabetic Care* 1978;1:158–165.
17. Ackerman NB. Improvement of metabolic problems after gastric bypass for morbid obesity. *J Obesity Weight Regulation* 1984;3:184–189.
18. Sirinek KR, O'Dorisio TM, Hill D, McFee AS. Hyperinsulinism, glucose-dependent insulinotropic polypeptide, and the enteroinsular axis in morbidly obese patients before and after gastric bypass. *Surgery* 1986;100:781–787.
19. Hale PJ, Singh BM, Crase J, Baddeley RM, Nattrass M. Following weight loss in massively obese patients correction of the insulin resistance of fat metabolism is delayed relative to the improvement in carbohydrate metabolism. *Metabolism* 1988;37:411–417.
20. Pories WJ, Caro JF, Flickinger EG, Meelheim HD, Swanson MS. The control of diabetes mellitus (NIDDM) in the morbidly obese with the Greenville Gastric Bypass. *Ann Surg* 1987;206:316–323.
21. Herbst CA, Hughes TA, Gwynne JT, Buckwalter JA. Gastric bariatric operation in insulin-treated adults. *Surgery* 1984;95:209–214.
22. Ackerman NB. Metabolic consequences from conversion of jejunoileal bypass to gastric bypass. *Ann Surg* 1982;196:553–559.

Surgical Management of the Diabetic Patient,
edited by Michael Bergman and Gregorio A. Sicard.
Raven Press, Ltd., New York © 1991.

29

Surgery in the Patient with Diabetic Eye Disease

Aaron Kassoff

Department of Ophthalmology, Albany Medical College, Albany, New York 12208

Numerous studies have concluded that diabetic retinopathy is the leading cause of new blindness in individuals aged 20–74. Approximately 10% of all new cases of blindness, and 20% of those occurring in persons between the ages of 45–74 are due to diabetic retinopathy (1). The duration of diabetes appears to be the strongest risk factor for predicting the presence of diabetic retinopathy (2–4). In patients with insulin-dependent diabetes, where duration may be estimated accurately, diabetic retinopathy is rarely observed during the first 5 years after diagnosis. In individuals who have had diabetes for approximately 10 years, some evidence of retinopathy is found in up to 50% of eyes and within 15–20 years, some 75–95% of patients will reveal clinical evidence of diabetic retinal change. After 20 years duration, some 20–40% of patients will have progressed to proliferative disease. There is some suggestion that in the juvenile diabetic patient the predictive value of duration relates only to those years following puberty.

A second identifying risk factor relates to the age of the patient. In the insulin dependent diabetic patient, when matched for duration, the older the patient was at the time of diagnosis, the more frequent the presence of retinopathy (5). In the older patient, however, it seems that the prevalence of retinopathy decreases with increasing age at diagnosis (4). Although retinopathy occurs in both sexes and all races, there is a higher prevalence of blindness from diabetic retinopathy in black women than in all other groups (1).

The diagnosis of diabetic retinopathy is most often made by visualization of the ocular fundus. Often this examination is done by the nonophthalmologist through undilated pupils. The accuracy of diagnosis, however, can be enhanced significantly by employing dilation. Dilation can be accomplished by using Phenylephrine 2 1/2%, instilled in the eye following a brief screening evaluation of the anterior chamber depth utilizing a pen light to evaluate for an anatomic narrow angle. In this case, light introduced temporally and parallel to the iris plane does not project across to the nasal iris as it does in the eye of normal depth. If drops are instilled prior to the general physical examination, the pupils are usually adequately dilated for examination by the time this is completed. Techniques such as fundus photography and fluorescein angiography can be utilized by the ophthalmologist for purposes of assisting in the diagnosis and follow-up care of the patient. At the least, however, an annual examination of the dilated eye of the diabetic patient is essential in all individuals with insulin dependent diabetes and those with noninsulin dependent diabetes of over 5 years duration (6).

There is a high correlation between the severity of retinopathy and mortality. Survival of the blind diabetic individual is significantly decreased, with an average survival 3.5–5.8 years (7). The coexistence of severe renal disease, systemic hypertension, and arteriosclerotic heart disease account for the majority of deaths. The association of diabetic retinopathy and nephropathy is well established, as is retinopathy and systemic hypertension. It is not clear as to whether hypertension plays a part in the development or acceleration of retinopathy.

The possible relationship between pregnancy and diabetic retinopathy has been a source of concern for some time (8). Significant progression of retinopathy has been observed during pregnancy in many instances, but it is not clear whether or not there is a causal relationship. What seems to be agreed upon, however, is that if a woman enters pregnancy with little or no retinopathy, there is minimal likelihood of significant progression. With moderate degrees of retinopathy, the risk of progression increases and when proliferative disease is present at the time of the onset of pregnancy, there is a significantly high risk for progression of proliferation to vision-threatening disease. It should be noted here that photocoagulation therapy seems to be as effective for the pregnant as well as for the nonpregnant woman.

CLASSIFICATION

Diabetic retinopathy has been divided, with great practical value, into two broad stages (9). The two—background diabetic retinopathy and proliferative diabetic retinopathy—share many of the same characteristic changes. Proliferative retinopathy, by definition, however, includes the presence of neovascular or fibrous tissue growth, whereas background retinopathy shows no such change. In preproliferative diabetic retinopathy, an advanced degree of background change has been recognized in recent years. No actual proliferation is present in such eyes, but recognition of progression to this level is of true clinical importance in order that closer observation be initiated.

Background Diabetic Retinopathy

The earliest sign of diabetic retinopathy is the presence of microaneurysms, seen as small red dots in the retina. Their appearance may change with time as they become occluded or obliterated. Small round "dot" hemorrhages and larger "blot" hemorrhages occur in deeper retinal layers. The smaller ones are often indistinguishable from true microaneurysms on clinical examination and are often evanescent. Not uncommonly, hard exudates are also seen. These are small lipid deposits that have precipitated from leaking damaged blood vessels. They vary in size from small flecks to larger accumulations and may, at times, arrange themselves in a circular pattern surrounding specific leaking areas, which can be defined by fluorescein angiography. They may be located anywhere in the posterior fundus, but have greatest threat for potential visual loss when they are noted in the area of the macula, the area of the retina responsible for sharp central visual acuity. (Fig. 1.)

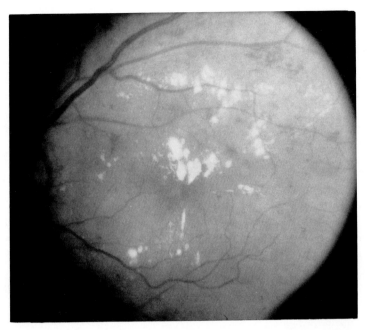

FIG. 1. Background diabetic retinopathy. Microaneurysms, dot and blot hemorrhages, hard exudates.

Preproliferative Diabetic Retinopathy

At this level, in addition to dot and blot hemorrhages and hard exudates, several other features are found. Microinfarctions of the nerve fiber layer of the retina, seen as soft exudates, are fluffy, often feathery patches of whitish appearance in the posterior fundus. Intraretinal microvascular abnormalities (IRMA) may be seen as fine, telangiectatic networks within the retina. Venous caliber abnormalities, appearing as beading may also be identified (Fig. 2). This group of lesions, particularly in combination, suggests a more advanced degree of retinopathy. Although progression to true proliferation is not inevitable in such eyes, the likelihood of neovascular change developing is substantially increased and more frequent observation is warranted.

Proliferative Diabetic Retinopathy

In this stage of the disease, neovascularization with or without fibrous tissue proliferation may be seen on the surface of the retina or extending forward into the vitreous cavity. These new vessels can be seen as neovascularization of the optic disc (NVD) appearing as fine strings, networks, or tufts (Fig. 3). Often in company with whitish-yellow fibrous tissue, these vessels can extend along the vascular ar-

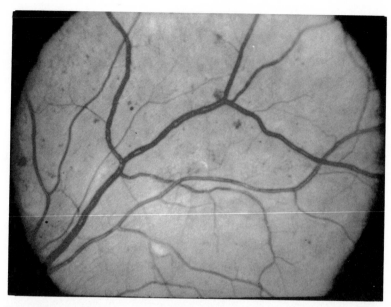

FIG. 2. Preproliferative diabetic retinopathy—venous caliber abnormalities (beading), intra-retinal microvascular abnormalities, soft exudates.

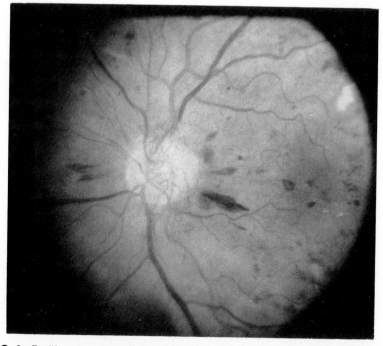

FIG. 3. Proliferative diabetic retinopathy—new vessels at the optic disk (NVD).

cades temporal to the optic nerve. In general, the presence of NVD constitutes a more significant threat to vision than does neovascularization elsewhere (NVE). These latter may also appear as small, petaled, flower-like structures or may seem more stringy (Fig. 4).

The basic cause for the development of neovascularization is thought to be retinal ischemia. Recent evidence has suggested that endothelial cell proliferation resulting in neovascularization is stimulated by angiogenic factors released by hypoxic retina (10).

Once neovascularization has developed, the likelihood of visual loss secondary to vitreous hemorrhage increases significantly. It therefore becomes critical that eyes with or at risk of developing new vessels be identified promptly and before symptoms occur so that proper therapeutic interventions may be offered.

Macular Edema

Macular edema defined as thickening of the retina at or close to the center of the macula, is most accurately diagnosed by the ophthalmologist using stereoscopic techniques. This is the most frequent cause of significant visual loss in the patient with diabetic retinopathy (11). The nonophthalmologist may recognize a loss of the normal foveolar light reflex and a general loss of clarity of structures in the area. The most important clue to the presence of macular edema, however, is the presence of hard exudates in the region. Although such exudates do not inevitably accompany

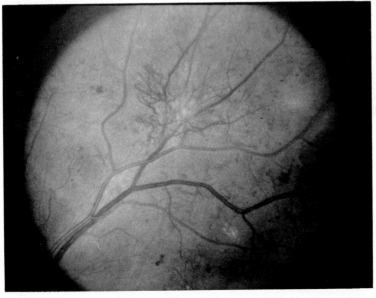

FIG. 4. Proliferative diabetic retinopathy—new vessels elsewhere (NVE).

retinal thickening, or vice versa, their presence suggests leakage from incompetent vessels and the possibility of edema threatening the center of vision. Macular edema may accompany the changes seen in either background, preproliferative, or proliferative retinopahty.

NONOCULAR SURGERY IN THE PATIENT WITH DIABETIC EYE DISEASE

General Considerations

In order to assess the possibilities of ocular complications consequent to nonocular surgery in the diabetic patient, it is critical that the surgeon be aware of the presence of retinopathy. This can be most accurately done by examination of the retina through dilated pupils. In general, concern is warranted only in those individuals with evidence of proliferative change or macular edema. In eyes with no retinopathy or showing only background or preproliferative change, most surgical procedures can be approached without true concern for ocular complications.

Proliferative Diabetic Retinopathy

Several studies have pointed out that the onset of vitreous hemorrhage from neovascularization has most often been noted upon awakening or while at physical rest (12). In addition, such hemorrhage can accompany strenuous exercise or a Valsalva Maneuver. Increased intravascular pressure may be induced by a head-down position, coughing, or postoperative vomiting, and may predispose the general surgical patient to intraocular bleeding from preexisting neovascularization (13). Recognition of proliferative disease and institution of measures to reduce the likelihood of bleeding seem to be reasonable precautions. Such possibilities may lead the obstetrician to consider a caesarean section as an alternative to active labor in the pregnant woman with proliferative diabetic retinopathy.

The postoperative recuperative period is often one of relative immobility and restricted ability to travel. These factors can impose a prolonged delay in initiating laser photocoagulation for proliferative disease. When elective surgery is contemplated, it is an advantage for laser treatment to precede the surgery in an effort to prevent hemorrhage.

Recent studies have indicated that the use of aspirin in the patient with proliferative diabetic retinopathy does not increase the risk of vitreous hemorrhage and there is therefore no contraindication to its postoperative use, when indicated (14). The use of heparin or coumadin, however, appears to increase the likelihood of bleeding from neovascularization. When possible, operative procedures, such as cardiac surgery, which necessitate the use of these agents, should be delayed until laser photocoagulation has been completed.

Vitreous Hemorrhage

The presence of vitreous hemorrhage should be noted before surgery. Many patients with such hemorrhage are advised to maintain a head-up position in order to facilitate settling of the blood to the inferior portion of the glove. In such cases it is wise to maintain this attitude during the surgery, if at all possible.

Blood Glucose and Blood Pressure Control

There is some speculation that sudden hypertensive episodes independent of or related to periods of hypoglycemia may be a factor in the acute onset of vitreous hemorrhage. Careful monitoring of these parameters is of particular importance in patients with proliferative diabetic retinopathy. It has also been recognized that, on occasion, deterioration of glucose control, often associated with hypertension, can lead to the onset of macular edema. At times when regulation is reestablished, remission of macular thickening occurs.

OCULAR SURGERY IN THE PATIENT WITH DIABETIC EYE DISEASE

Before the development of photocoagulation techniques for use in retinal disease, surgical treatment for severe diabetic retinopathy was restricted to pituitary ablation (15). Some ameliorative effect was demonstrated utilizing this technique, but because the systemic consequences of pituitary ablation were so severe, the technique generated limited support from both the medical community and eligible patients. At present, particularly with the increasing availability of laser photocoagulation, it is rarely, if ever, used.

Since the late 1960s and early 1970s, photocoagulation has been performed with increasing frequency and success in patients with diabetic retinopathy. The earliest treatments were performed using Xenon-arc photocoagulators, but such procedures gradually evolved and are now almost exclusively performed using laser photocoagulators, taking advantage of their inherent flexibility, ease of use, and precision. All photocoagulation techniques utilized for the treatment of diabetic retinal disease take advantage of the ability of pigmented tissue to absorb light and convert it to heat, producing a measured degree of tissue coagulation. The instrument most frequently used at present is the argon laser photocoagulator, which produces light of a green or blue-green color. Red krypton laser light is utilized to some advantage in special situations and, more recently, laser photocoagulation has been performed with laser-produced light of other colors. The procedures are routinely performed on an outpatient basis, and while generally comfortable with just topical anesthesia, at times a retrobulbar injection of a local agent is found to be helpful.

Most laser instruments have been adapted so that treatment can be applied using a standard slit lamp arrangement, viewing the ocular fundus through a contact lens. A variety of such lenses that vary in magnification and field of view is available. Most treatment sessions can be accomplished within 20–30 minutes, which patients and physicians generally tolerate without undue stress.

Proliferative Diabetic Retinopathy

Some controversy regarding the benefits of laser photocoagulation in the treatment of diabetic retinopathy led to the creation of a large-scale, multi-centered, randomized clinical trial, the Diabetic Retinopathy Study (DRS), the results of which were first presented in 1976 (16). It was clearly demonstrated that the use of photocoagulation in a so-called pan-retinal technique could reduce the incidence of severe visual loss by 50% over a 5-year period in high-risk eyes. The DRS identified eyes with such high risks as those with the presence of vitreous or preretinal hemorrhage with neovascularization at the optic nerve or elsewhere in the posterior pole, or eyes in which new vessels cover at least one-third of the optic nerve, even without evidence of hemorrhage. Untreated, the risk of severe visual loss is 25–40% over 2 years. Prompt photocoagulation, even in the presence of excellent vision, reduces the rate of severe visual loss by approximately 50%.

During panretinal photocoagulation (PRP), 1,200 to 1,500 or more separate, moderately heavy laser photocoagulation burns are focused in a tight pattern in the midperipheral and peripheral retina, avoiding the central area around the macula (Fig. 5). The technique also usually includes focal, direct photocoagulation of neovascular networks flat on the retinal surface. Although the mechanism by which beneficial effect achieved is not fully understood, it is likely that ischemic areas of retina are destroyed, reducing the stimulus for new vessel growth or changing the necessary conditions for maintenance of those vessels already present.

If, within 4–6 weeks, no regression of vessels has occurred, additional photocoagulation may be necessary, either by adding more peripheral spots or placing new photocoagulation burns between treatment scars (17). When the presence of vitreous blood prevents the use of argon laser photocoagulation, use of the krypton laser may allow penetration of the opacity so that photocoagulation may be performed without waiting for the vitreous haze to clear.

Dividing the full treatment into several treatment sessions does not compromise the efficacy of treatment, but has the advantage of allowing the patient a more comfortable experience and reducing the likelihood of inducing macular edema. Often

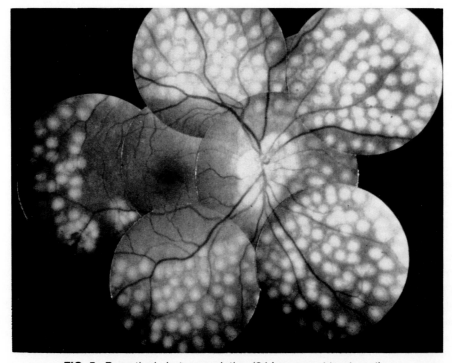

FIG. 5. Panretinal photocoagulation (24 hours post treatment).

associated with macular edema, (18) PRP has been noted to induce a loss of visual acuity of small degree in some eyes. PRP is twice as likely to produce such loss in eyes with preexisting macular edema then in eyes without. The effect of PRP in reducing the incidence and extent of vitreous hemorrhage from proliferative vessels in high risk eyes, however, outweighs the dangers attributable to induced macular edema.

Fortunately, although it has been noted that panretinal photocoagulation produces a variety of complications on rare occasions, the procedure is recognized as generally safe. Corneal abrasions may occur secondary to manipulation of the contact lens used for treatment, and are related to a fragile epithelial surface often seen in diabetic patients. Only rarely are burns of the ocular lens produced, particularly when cataracts of a brown color are present. Permanent pupillary dilatation can occur in a treated eye and accomodative power may be diminished. In some eyes, panretinal photocoagulation may induce an exudative change in the choroidal layer with swelling of the ciliary body and an acute glaucoma. Usually this is self-limited and resolves without significant sequellae.

Probably the most important potential complication involves constriction of the visual field (19). Although many patients note no visual effects, a significant number report difficulties related to visual field abnormalities, such as insecurity while using stairs. This induced loss is superimposed upon visual field loss already present resulting from retinal ischemia or vascular occlusion. At times, photocoagulation burns can induce hemorrhage from a focally treated blood vessel or may occlude a vessel supplying the macular region, with consequent visual loss.

In eyes in which panretinal photocoagulation is not possible due to vitreous hemorrhage or previous extensive photocoagulation, peripheral cryotherapy of the retina can be performed. Utilizing this technique, retinal neovascularization may regress and vitreous hemorrhage resorb.

Diabetic Macular Edema

Although vision loss from vitreous hemorrhage secondary to neovascularization of the retina may be most devastating, the most frequent cause of legal blindness in the diabetic population is macular edema. The Early Treatment Diabetic Retinopathy Study (ETDRS), another large-scale multi-centered clinical trial, has recently been completed (20). In this trial, the effect of focal photocoagulation was evaluated and compared with the natural history of macular edema. In a group of clearly defined eyes with "clinically significant macular edema," a beneficial treatment effect was recognized, with a decrease of approximately 50% in the rate of moderate visual loss from baseline at all levels of initial vision.

Fluorescein angiography is helpful in defining the location and extent of leakage from microaneurysms and incompetent retinal blood vessels. Focal photocoagulation is directed to discrete leaks and a small grid pattern to areas of diffuse leakage or capillary nonperfusion.

Complications have not been recognized with sufficient frequency or severity to warrant withholding such treatment in eyes at risk. However, the potential of an inadvertent foveal burn while treating close to center and the occasional production of a paracentral scotoma suggest that treatment in eyes with excellent vision be carefully considered.

Vitrectomy

Since the early 1970s, significant advances have been made in the instrumentation and techniques of vitrectomy. Although still a procedure with potential serious complications, it has afforded the opportunity for good vision to many patients whose eyes have not responded to photocoagulation or in whom such treatment was not possible due to complicating features such as vitreous hemorrhage and/or tractional retinal detachment. Ultrasound evaluation of an eye that cannot be visualized satisfactorily has proven to be an invaluable aid in determining the potential value of vitrectomy surgery.

Vitrectomy is most commonly done for eyes that have longstanding vitreous hemorrhage. Due to the fact that many eyes with such hemorrhage clear spontaneously, it is often advisable to delay surgery for up to 1 year to avoid a possibly unnecessary procedure. The most definitive clinical trial evaluating the use of vitrectomy for diabetic vitreous hemorrhage revealed no significant advantage to a vitrectomy prior to this time (21). The one exception to this finding was in patients with type I diabetes whose vision was significantly more improved with early vitrectomy than by waiting for 1 year. Although vitrectomy provides early visual recovery in successful cases, approximately 20% of eyes undergoing such surgery suffer a loss of vision.

Vitrectomy has also, at times, been utilized for treatment of tractional retinal detachment. When fibrous tissue on the surface of the retinal extending into or across the vitreous cavity contracts, the retina may detach at points of adhesion. Many such detachments do not progress and it is therefore usually recommended that a vitrectomy not be done unless there is treatened or actual macular detachment. When retinal holes complicate tractional retinal detachment, a vitrectomy is often combined with standard retinal detachment surgery.

The surgical techniques used in vitrectomy surgery have undergone constant modification and improvement. Current systems utilize mechanized microsurgical instrumentation that combines suction and cutting modalities with the simultaneous infusion of saline solution to maintain the volume of the eye. Intraocular light sources, diathermy, and laser are now available and have added to the safety and efficacy of the surgery. This surgery may be used to sever fibrous bands releasing traction at attachment points on the retina (or to peel) membranes from the surface of the retina releasing traction in this plane.

The variety and rate of complications from vitrectomy surgery are not inconsequential. Corneal erosion, edema, and opacification can occur. Lens opacities may be induced, which may or may not resolve spontaneously. In as many as one-quarter of surgically treated eyes, a retinal tear can be created during surgery, which requires treatment during the procedure. When this occurs, success of the surgery is significantly diminished.

Another significant and vision threatening complication of vitrectomy is neovascularization of the iris with development of subsequent neovascular glaucoma. Eyes with preexisting iris neovascularization, extensive retinal vascular proliferation, especially untreated, and retinal detachment, are more likely to develop progressive postoperative iris neovascularization. Iris neovascularization and neovascular glaucoma are significantly more common if removal of the lens is done during a vitrectomy to deal with opacities of the lens, which can develop intraoperatively (22). Improvements in irrigating solutions used during the surgery have substantially reduced the incidence of such opacities. When significant cataract exists, it is often recommended that removal be done prior to a vitrectomy. Using an extracapsular technique whereby the posterior lens capsule is not removed, it is possible to avoid the increased incidence of iris neovascularization seen subsequent to extraction of the entire lens.

As mentioned, complications of vitrectomy may be substantial. Postoperative vitreous hemorrhage, which often spontaneously resolves, may, however, require subsequent surgery and a so-called "wash-out" of the blood. Retinal detachment can occur as a result of tears. As in any surgery, intraocular infection can occur, which is often devastating to the eye.

Cataract in the Diabetic Patient

The risk for developing cataracts in diabetic patients is substantially greater than in nondiabetic patients, particularly in patients over 50 years of age (23). This risk increases further with poor control of blood glucose levels and with increasing duration of the disease. The risks of cataract extraction are related to the presence and degree of retinopathy that exists at the time of surgery. In the eye with no diabetic retinal changes, the decision as to when to perform cataract surgery is made based on the same criteria appropriate for the nondiabetic patient. A similar approach is reasonable for the eye with only mild background retinopathy.

An important consideration specific to the patient with diabetic retinopathy is the possible need to perform photocoagulation in an eye in which significant cataract formation compromises such treatment. It is therefore reasonable that panretinal photocoagulation for proliferative diabetic retinopathy, or focal treatment for diabetic macular edema, might be advised earlier than usual in the presence of a rapidly developing cataract. Should either of these manifestations of diabetic retinopathy be stabilized, future cataract surgery can be done more safely. In addition, as long as adequate visualization of the fundus is possible, cataract extraction can be delayed in spite of compromised vision, particularly if the vision in the fellow eye is adequate to serve the visual needs of the patient.

In an eye recognized as having significant retinopathy but in which adequate visualization cannot be achieved due to cataract, it is appropriate to remove the cataract so that the retinopathy can be appropriately treated even though the patient may not be visually handicapped. In an eye with proliferative change of the retina and a cataract that precludes adequate photocoagulation, peripheral cryotherapy can be used in an effort to induce regression prior to cataract extraction.

In view of recent advances in cataract surgery, there has been some debate with regard to the type of surgery to be performed in the individual with diabetes. The first issue of importance relates to the increased incidence of iris neovascularization following cataract extraction. It appears that the incidence of this most serious postoperative complication is substantially reduced by utilization of an extracapsular technique rather than an intracapsular one (24). It is speculated that the presence of an intact lens capsule and anterior vitreous face acts as a barrier to protect against the migration of a vasoproliferative factor from the retina into the anterior segment of the eye stimulating new iris vessel growth.

Another issue of importance is the question of placing an intraocular lens into the eye following extracapsular extraction. The results of several studies have indicated that in most patients the use of such a lens induces no significant complications.

Certain considerations, however, militate against universal use. Although photoco-agulation can usually be done adequately through an intraocular lens, deposits on the lens surface, opacification of the posterior lens capsule, and possible inadequate dilation of the pupil may compromise the ability to perform the procedure in an optimal fashion. In some instances, therefore, it may be advisable to withhold place-ment of an intraocular lens, notwithstanding the recognized advantages of improved vision, convenience, and visual rehabilitation.

Patients with diabetic retinopathy face several potential complications in the period during and just after uneventful cataract surgery. Development or progression of macular hard exudates has been described following surgery (25). Also, following cataract surgery patients with proliferative diabetic retinopathy are exposed to an increased risk of vitreous hemorrhage. When cataract surgery is itself complicated by rupture of the posterior lens capsule or when loss of vitreous occurs during sur-gery, there is an increase in the likelihood of subsequent hemorrhage or macular edema. The increased risk of cataract surgery in the patient with diabetic retinopathy should be clearly conveyed to the patient prior to the procedure.

Glaucoma

Individuals with diabetes have, on average, higher intraocular pressures than peo-ple without diabetes, and the incidence of chronic open angle glaucoma is increased in the presence of diabetes as well (26). At equal intraocular pressures, optic nerve damage from glaucoma in the eye of a person with diabetes appears to be more severe than in the eye of a nondiabetic individual. At the same time, it is the clinical impression of many that elevated intraocular pressure conveys a protective effect with regard to the development of proliferative diabetic retinopathy. In fact, prolif-eration is rarely, if ever, recognized in a patient with established open angle glaucoma.

Therapy of chronic open angle glaucoma in the patient with diabetes is often suc-cessful, utilizing the variety of pharmacologic agents that are now available. When these measures are unsuccessful, laser photocoagulation to the trabecular meshwork in the filtration angle (Argon Laser Trabeculoplasty) may bring about control of in-traocular pressure. This may be desirable as an alternative to immediate filtering surgery because the danger of complications associated with the latter, such as in-duced cataract formation, potential hypotony of the eye, and endophthalmitis may be avoided.

When these measures fail, filtration surgery aimed at creating a communication between the anterior chamber and subconjunctival space is usually performed. Fol-lowing such surgery there is a significantly increased likelihood of cataract formation in such eyes.

Diabetes is a leading cause of neovascularization of the iris (rubeosis iridis) and is most often seen in the presence of proliferative diabetic retinopathy (27). In this condition, neovascular growth may first appear as small wisps of vessels at the pu-pillary margin or in the angle of outflow. This latter change may progress to result in an obliteration of the angle with a consequent elevation of intraocular pressure. Although many patients with neovascularization of the iris show no change over long periods of time, such eyes may progress rapidly, producing an acute, painful attack of neovascular glaucoma that is notoriously most difficult to manage.

Regression of rubeosis iridis may be induced by panretinal photocoagulation. This is most effective when done in eyes with significant new vessels of the iris before extensive damage to the angle structures, when attendant pressure elevation occurs. Other procedures such as cryoablation of the ciliary body may be utilized to reduce aqueous production to yield pressure control. Because good vision is not often seen following this procedure, newer surgical techniques have been attempted in an effort to allow pressure control without tissue destruction. The surgical insertion of a seton into the anterior chamber may allow pressure control while maintaining useful vision.

General Considerations

The majority of ocular surgery is presently done on an outpatient basis utilizing local anesthesia. This practice has the advantage of returning the patient to familiar surroundings and usual diabetic management, and has not resulted in increased complications. When approving the diabetic patient for ocular surgery, the relatively minor impact of such a procedure on general medical status should be appreciated. Often the patient is given a reduced dose of insulin preoperatively, intravenous dextrose and water during surgery, and prior to discharge, insulin as indicated. These considerations are dealt with in detail in another chapter.

REFERENCES

1. Kahn HA, Hiller R. Blindness caused by diabetic retinopathy. *Am J Ophthalmol* 1974;78:58–67.
2. Klein R, Klein BE, Syrjala SE, et al. Wisconsin epidemiologic study of diabetic retinopathy. In: Freidman EA, L'Esperance FA, eds. *Diabetic renal-retinal syndrome*. New York: Grune and Stratton, 1981;21–38.
3. Klein R, Klein BEK, Moss SE, et al. The Wisconsin epidemiologic study of diabetic retinopathy. II. Prevalence and risk of diabetic retinopathy when age at diagnosis is less than 30 years. *Arch Ophthalmol* 1984;102:520–526.
4. Klein R, Klein BEK, Moss SE, et al. The Wisconsin epidemiologic study of diabetic retinopathy. III. Prevalence and risk of diabetic retinopathy when age at diagnosis is 30 or more years. *Arch Ophthalmol* 1984;102:527–532.
5. Frank RN, Hoffman WH, Podgor MJ, et al. Retinopathy in juvenile-onset type I diabetes of short duration. *Diabetes* 1982;31;874–882.
6. American Diabetes Association, Committee on Professional Practice. Eye care guidelines for patients with diabetes mellitus. *Diabetes Care* 1988;11:745–746.
7. Caird FL. Epidemiology of diabetic retinopathy. In: Lynn Jr, Snyder WB, Vaisera, eds. *Diabetic retinopathy*. New York: Grune and Stratton, 1974;43.
8. Dibble CM, Kochenour NK, Worley RJ, et al. Effect of pregnancy on diabetic retinopathy. *Obstet Gynecol* 1982;59:699–704.
9. Benson WE, Brown GC, Tasman W. *Diabetes and its ocular complications*. Philadelphia: WB Saunders, 1988.
10. Patz A. Retinal neovascularization: early contributions of Professor Michaelson and recent observations. *Br J Ophthalmol* 1984;68:42–46.
11. Patz A, Schatz H, Berkow JW, et al. Macular edema—an overlooked complication of diabetic retinopathy. *Trans Am Acad Ophthalmol Otolar* 1973;77:34–42.
12. Tasman W. Diabetic vitreous hemorrhage and its relationship to hypoglycemia. *Mod Prob Ophthalmol* 1979;20:413–414.
13. Kassoff A, Catalano RA, Mehu M. Vitreous hemorrhage and the valsalva maneuver in proliferative diabetic retinopathy. *Retina* 1988;8:174–176.
14. *Clinical Alert to Ophthalmologists:* Scientific Reporting Section of the National Eye Institute, National Institutes of Health. October 1989.
15. Bradley RF, Rees SR. Surgical pituitary ablation for diabetic retinopathy. In: Goldberg MF, Fine SL eds. *Symposium on the treatment of diabetic retinopathy*. PHS Pub. No. 1890, U.S. Department of Health, Education, and Welfare, 1969;171–191.

16. Diabetic Retinopathy Study Research Group. Preliminary report on effects of photocoagulation therapy. *Am J Ophthalmol* 1976;81:383–396.
17. Vine AK. The efficacy of additional argon laser photocoagulation for persistent, severe proliferative diabetic retinopathy. *Ophthalmology* 1985;92:1532–1537.
18. Meyers SM. Macular edema after scatter laser photocoagulation for proliferative diabetic retinopathy. *Am J Ophthalmol* 1980;90:210–216.
19. Diabetic Retinopathy Study Research Group. Photocoagulation treatment of proliferative diabetic retinopathy. Report number 8. *Ophthalmology* 1981;88:583–600.
20. The Early Treatment Diabetic Retinopathy Study Research Group. Photocoagulation for diabetic macular edema. Early treatment diabetic retinopathy study report number 1. *Arch Ophthalmol* 1985;103:1796–1806.
21. The Diabetic Retinopathy Vitrectomy Study Research Group. Early vitrectomy for severe vitreous hemorrhage in diabetic retinopathy. *Arch Ophthalmol* 1985;103:1644–1652.
22. Blankenship G, Cortez R, Machemer R. The lens and pars plana vitrectomy for diabetic retinopathy complications. *Arch Ophthalmol* 1979;97:1263–1267.
23. Klein BEK, Klein R, Moss RE. Prevalence of cataracts in a population-based study of persons with diabetes mellitus. *Ophthalmology* 1985;92:1191–1196.
24. Poliner LS, Christianson DJ, Escoffery RF, et al. Neovascular glaucoma after intracapsular and extracapsular cataract extraction in diabetic patients. *Am J Ophthalmol* 1985;100:637–643.
25. Jaffe GJ, Burton TC. Progression of non-proliferative diabetic retinopathy following cataract extraction. *Arch Ophthalmol* 1988;106:745–749.
26. Becker B. Diabetes mellitus and primary open-angle glaucoma. *Am J Ophthalmol* 1971;71:1–13.
27. Brown GC, Magargal LE, Schachat A, et al. Neovascular glaucoma, etiologic considerations. *Ophthalmology* 1984;91:315–319.

Subject Index